Mental Health in Nursing

Theory and practice for clinical settings

5th edition

Mental Health in Nursing

Theory and practice for clinical settings

5th edition

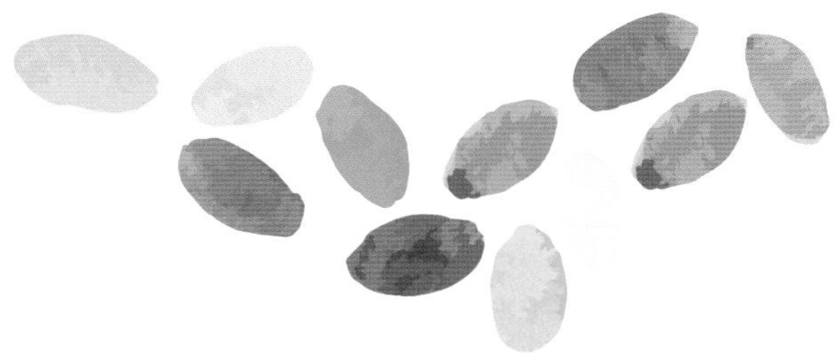

KIM FOSTER, RN, DipAppSc, BN, MA, PhD, CF, FACMHN
Professor of Mental Health Nursing
Australian Catholic University and NorthWestern Mental Health
Australia

PETA MARKS, RN, CMHN, BN, MPH, MCFT, FACMHN
National Project Manager
InsideOut Institute, The University of Sydney and Australian Health Consulting
Australia

ANTHONY J O'BRIEN, BN, MPhil(Hons), PhD, FNZCMHN, ONZOM
Associate Professor, Mental Health Nursing
University of Waikato
New Zealand

TOBY RAEBURN, RN, MN(Hons), PhD, FACMHN, Churchill Fellow
Senior Lecturer and Nurse Practitioner in Mental Health
School of Nursing and Midwifery, Western Sydney University
Australia

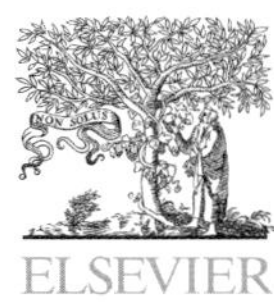

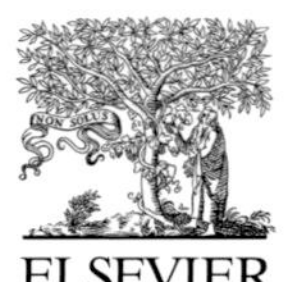

Elsevier Australia. ACN 001 002 357
(a division of Reed International Books Australia Pty Ltd)
Tower 1, 475 Victoria Avenue, Chatswood, NSW 2067

ISBN: 978-0-7295-4339-2

National Library of Australia Cataloguing-in-Publication Data

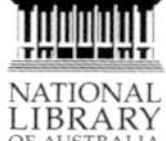

A catalogue record for this book is available from the National Library of Australia

Senior Content Strategist: Libby Houston
Content Project Manager: Shruti Raj
Edited by Matt Davies
Proofread by Melissa Faulkner
Permissions editing and photo research by Sathya Narayanan
Cover and internal design by Georgette Hall
Index by Innodata Indexing
Typeset by New Best-set Typesetters Ltd
Printed in China by 1010 Printing International Limited

Lat digit in the print number: 9 8 7 6 5 4 3 2 1

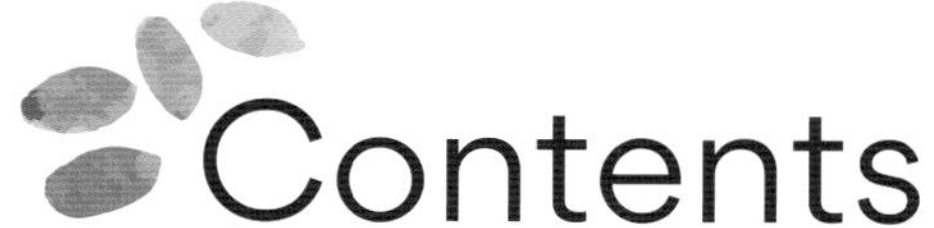

Contents

Foreword
Fay Jackson viii
About the authors xi
Contributors xii
Reviewers xiv
Introduction
Kim Foster, Peta Marks, Anthony J O'Brien and Toby Raeburn 1

Part 1 Positoning Practice 3

Chapter 1 Why mental health matters
Anthony J O'Brien, Toby Raeburn, Peta Marks and Kim Foster 5
Introduction 6
Epidemiology of mental distress and illness 6
Mental health care 10
Cultural safety and mental health care 12
Mental health legislation 13
Mental health and the scope of nursing practice 14
Nursing and mental health 14
Chapter summary 15

Chapter 2 Nursing and mental health in context
Kim Foster, Peta Marks, Anthony J O'Brien and Toby Raeburn 19
Introduction 20
Social ecological approach to mental health nursing practice 20
Effective mental health nursing practice 28
Chapter summary 33
Acknowledgement 33

Chapter 3 The spectrum of mental health and illness
Toby Raeburn, Peta Marks and Kim Foster 37
Introduction 38
Mental health 38
Mental illness 42
Chapter summary 47

Chapter 4 Safety in care, safety at work
Scott Brunero and Scott Lamont 50
Introduction 51
Understanding the context of safety in care and safety at work 51
Models of care 53
Preparedness for creating safety in care and safety at work 54
Principles for engaging consumers in safe care 56
Safety in care during aggression 57
Deliberate self-harm and suicide 58
Manipulation 63
Understanding safety risks in care and at work 63
The legal context 65
Chapter summary 67

Chapter 5 Working with families in mental health
Kim Foster, Sophie Isobel and Kim Usher 71
Introduction 72
Defining 'family' 72
Why work with families? Introducing a strengths-based approach 72
Potential challenges for families when a person has mental illness 73
Addressing challenges and building strengths – family resilience 76
Family and relational recovery 77
Working with families: family-focused practices 79
Chapter summary 84

Chapter 6 Professional self-care
Julie Sharrock 86
Introduction 87
Therapeutic use of self 87
Professional challenges 88
Holistic self-care 91
Lifelong learning and professional development 94
Maintaining a satisfying career 97
Chapter summary 101
Acknowledgement 102

Part 2 Knowledge for Practice 107

Chapter 7 Mental health assessment
Anthony J O'Brien and Mandy Allman 109
Introduction 110
Assessment 110
Methods of mental health nursing assessment 112
Comprehensive assessment process 118
Mental state assessment 123
Clinical formulation 125
Diagnosis 125
Triage 126
Risk assessment 126
Assessing strengths 127

Classification in psychiatry 127
Chapter summary 128

Chapter 8 Legal and ethical issues
Anthony J O'Brien and Scott Trueman 132
Introduction 133
Ethics and professional practice 133
Law and mental health 141
Duty of care and decision-making capacity 151
Chapter summary 152

Chapter 9 Anxiety
Anna Elders 156
Introduction 157
Aetiology of stress, fear and anxiety 157
Anxiety disorders 158
Epidemiology of anxiety disorders 159
Comorbidity 160
Assessment and diagnosis 161
Anxiety disorders 162
Trauma- and stressor-related disorders 167
Treatment and nursing interventions 169
Psychopharmacology 173
Chapter summary 173

Chapter 10 Mood disorders
Greg Clark and Sophie Temmhoff 177
Introduction 178
Types of mood disorders 178
Prevalence of mood disorders 179
Factors contributing to mood disorders 180
The experience of mood disorders 180
Signs and symptoms of mood disorders 180
Physical health and mood disorders 181
Assessment areas 181
Interventions 185
The role of nursing 187
Chapter summary 189

Chapter 11 Substance use and co-occurring mental health disorders
Megan McKechnie 191
Introduction 192
Types of substance use disorders 192
Behavioural addictions 193
Substance use and misuse among specific populations 195
Pharmacology of psychoactive drugs 196
Contributing factors 200
The experience of a substance use disorder 200
Physical health and substance use disorders 209
Assessment areas 209
Interventions 214
Detoxification 215
Relapse prevention 216
Other healing approaches 216
Co-occurring substance use disorders 217
Chapter summary 220

Chapter 12 Psychosis and schizophrenia
Toby Raeburn and Matthew Ball 226
Introduction 227
Prevalence and social determinants 227
The powerful role of language and labels 228
Signs and symptoms 229
Types of psychosis and schizophrenia-related phenomena 230
Alternative approaches to psychosis and schizophrenia-related phenomena 231
Theories of causation/aetiology 234
Nursing interventions 234
Final word regarding stigma 243
Chapter summary 243

Chapter 13 Eating disorders
Peta Marks and Bridget Mulvey 246
Introduction 247
Types of eating disorders 247
Incidence and prevalence 249
Contributing factors 251
Signs and symptoms 254
Assessment 257
Interventions 260
A final word on the nurse's role 268
Chapter summary 268

Chapter 14 Personality disorders
Toby Raeburn and Marika Van Ooyen 273
Introduction 274
What is personality? 274
Types of personality disorder 274
Prevalence 275
Contributing factors 278
The experience of personality disorders 278
Assessment areas 280
Interventions 281
Crisis intervention 281
Chapter summary 285

Chapter 15 Mental disorders of childhood and adolescence
Lucie Ramjan and Greg Clark 288
Introduction 289
Diagnosis in child and adolescent mental healthcare 289
Incidence 289
Developmental issues 291
Mental illness in context 292
Assessment 292
Services available to children and young people 293
The nursing role 294
Engaging with children and adolescents 295
Family work 305
Confidentiality 306
Psychoeducation 307
Legal issues 307
Chapter summary 308

Chapter 16 Mental disorders of older age
Melissa Robinson-Reilly and Peta Marks 311
Introduction 312
Demography of ageing 312
Screening and assessment of older people 313
Biopsychosocial factors and life-stage transition 313
Chronic disease and mental health 314
Screening and observation 315
Mental health disorders in older age 316
Substance use and misuse 322
Schizophrenia 322
Suicide 323
Nursing management of older people 324
Polypharmacy for older age and medication safety 325
Chapter summary 326

Chapter 17 Autism and intellectual disability
Andrew Cashin 331
Introduction 332
Types of disorder 332
Prevalence 336
The experience of inclusion and exclusion 337
Signs and symptoms 337
Physical health and ASD and intellectual disability 340
Key points related to assessment 341
Interventions 342
Deinstitutionalisation 343
Chapter summary 343

Chapter 18 Physical health
Andrew Watkins 345
Introduction 346
Physical health neglect in the mental health system 346
Metabolic syndrome 347
Diabetes 348
Cardiovascular disease 350
Respiratory diseases 355
Oral health 356
Sleep 357
Sexual health 357
When psychiatric symptoms are not a mental illness 359
Chapter summary 359

Chapter 19 Psychopharmacology
Kim Usher and Simeon Evans 365
Introduction 366
Important pharmacological principles 366
Important psychotropic medications 367
Special issues with psychotropic medications 378
Pro re nata antipsychotic medication administration 379
Adherence and concordance with medications 380
Depot or long-acting intramuscular injectable antipsychotics 384
Psychotropic medication use in special populations 384
Chapter summary 387

Part 3 Contexts of Practice 391

Chapter 20 Mental health in every setting
Peta Marks 393
Introduction 394
Chapter summary 398

Chapter 21 Primary care and community
Elizabeth Halcomb, Christopher Patterson and Ros Rolleston 399
Introduction 400
Presentations to primary and community care settings 400
Chapter summary 406

Chapter 22 Emergency care
Justin Chia and Timothy Wand 409
Introduction 410
Approaches to mental health presentations in the emergency setting 410
Chapter summary 414

Chapter 23 Generalist inpatient settings
Catherine Daniel and Cynthia Delgado 416
Introduction 417
Ill-health experiences 417
Chapter summary 423

Chapter 24 Older age care
Melissa Robinson-Reilly and Sharon Rydon 425
Introduction 426
Chapter summary 432

Chapter 25 Perinatal and infant mental health
Julie Ferguson 434
Introduction 435
Chapter summary 442

Chapter 26 Forensic mental health nursing
Tessa Maguire and Brian McKenna 444
Introduction 445
Attitudes 448
Mental health nursing actions and interventions 448
Chapter summary 451

Chapter 27 Mental health settings
Fiona Whitecross 454
Introduction 455
Mental health care settings 455
Chapter summary 462

Glossary 464
Index 475

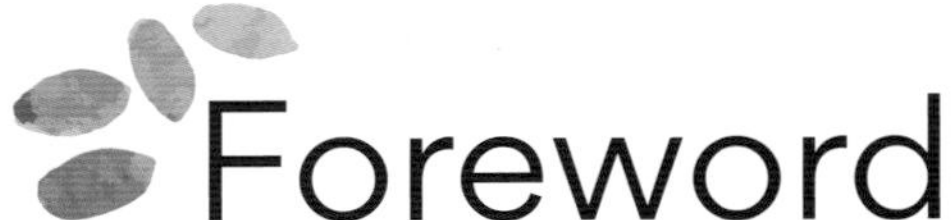

Foreword

Mental Health Nursing: Theory and practice for clinical settings, 5th edition is a text with welcome differences because it draws upon the narratives of people with lived experience of mental health issues who have been under the care and treatment of nurses. It also, bravely, brings into the open lived experience narratives of nurses who themselves have experienced trauma and mental health issues. Because of this, and because of the focus placed on recovery and the humane treatment of people who have experienced trauma and psychological distress, it is an honour to write the foreword for this text. In doing so, I hope to enthuse students and nurses to consider the important role they play in the lives of each person they treat, care for, support and work with. Whether the care is offered in primary, community, inpatient or other clinical settings, the impact nurses have on people with lived experience can have lasting, positive (or detrimental) effects on their life, sense of self, recovery and subsequent outcomes.

This edition focuses on nursing practices embedded in the *Code of ethics for nurses*, the healing power of dedicated nurses and the recognition that every person has a unique and innate value. The authors and editors recognise that great nurses contribute to people's healing and recovery and to living socially and emotionally satisfying lives, contributing to their family, workplace and community.

My career in mental health has had wide dimensions. I have been a lived experience volunteer, peer worker, manager of peer workers and a director of a large public mental health service. I founded Vision in Mind, a national systemic advocacy, consultancy and training body. I was the inaugural Deputy Commissioner with the NSW Mental Health Commission and an executive member of a large specialist community-managed organisation. For years I have written policies, issues papers, strategic plans, guidelines and protocols and have always undertaken these utilising co-design practices. I am also a person with lived experience of trauma and subsequent mental health issues. Through all these experiences I have had the personal and professional honour of working with great mental health nurses who work from a strong human rights base and use strengths-based language, and who practise empathy and holistic care with each person. Nurses working in this way regard people with mental health issues as individuals, not as a diagnosis or problematic behaviours, and do not pathologise the human experience.

High-quality mental health services and nurses work in respectful, multidisciplinary teams including all clinical staff and peer workers. The individual needs of each person in their care are central to everything good nurses do and they respect the lived experience mantra of 'Nothing about me, without me'. The power dynamic is recognised and smoothed out, providing a respectful, holistic and therapeutic alliance with the people they care for and, where appropriate, with their family.

I have also had the unfortunate and traumatising experience of working with nurses who do not practise holistic, therapeutic and empathic care. They use the nurse's station as just one tool in the unequal power dynamic they enjoy and use seclusion and restraint far more often than is needed; they see this as a win, rather than a failure of care. When I was working in the public system, I could look at the roster and know if there was going to be instances of seclusion and restraint by the particular staff who were rostered. I implore student nurses and practising nurses to work together to ensure these attitudes and outcomes do not prevail in their services. Please work within the spirit of this text and create holistic healing instead of further trauma for all people and staff involved.

Indigenous healing circles and the Open Dialogue model of care are practices that work in holistic ways utilising the community, family, kin and whānau and multidisciplinary teams working together to provide healing supports for individuals, families and communities. I would encourage all services to engage with these practices. I would also encourage nurses to become familiar with the different cultural beliefs around mental health issues and connection to country and community, spirituality and body language. Recognising all aspects of a person's needs and making allowances for these demonstrates respect and care and builds a stronger therapeutic alliance between patients/consumers/people with lived experience, their families and communities.

Until recently, the interconnection between mental and physical health was generally ignored. Doctors and nurses could often be dismissive of consumers' concerns about their physical health and attribute symptoms to 'paranoia', 'being all in their mind', 'hypochondria' or 'just attention seeking'. Discrimination has led to the physical health needs of people with mental health conditions being seen as less important than their mental health, than other people's physical health and than the community's comfort about 'the behaviour' of the person.

Also, the negative impact of mental distress and pharmaceutical treatment on people's health was underestimated and downplayed. Clinicians often point to a person's choices such as diet, lack of exercise, drugs, cigarettes and alcohol use as being the cause of people's physical health issues. However, ethical clinical treatment is transparent about the unwanted effects of prescribed psychiatric medications on people's short- and long-term health. Ethical clinical treatment is also transparent about the risks electroconvulsive therapy (ECT) may have on people's memory and physical health.

To achieve holistic care, preserving memory and the physical health of people with mental health issues must also be seen as a priority in all services including acute, stepped, community and primary healthcare settings. Ethical practices ensure people know what their treatment involves and the possible unwanted side effects of medication, which often includes obesity, metabolic syndrome and a major gap in life expectancy.

Physical illness untreated or inadequately treated increases the burden of disease on the community and on individuals and diminishes speed, likelihood of recovery and the gap in life expectancy.

The relationship between personal and family trauma, social dynamics and environmental impacts on mental and physical health are being increasingly understood. This text outlines a social and ecological approach that integrates the various influences on mental health from biological through to environmental and social. Valuable nurses recognise that the causes of mental health issues include external factors and rarely lie solely within the individual. Childhood and adult abuse, harsh environments, the impact of global warming (fire, floods, drought, earthquakes and destruction of nature), neglect and intergenerational trauma including the destruction of family and communities through war, stolen lands, stolen children, sexual abuse and poverty all contrive to undermine people's lives and wellbeing. Epidemiological studies show that mental health and addiction issues affect up to 50% of people in their lifetime. It would seem obvious by this figure that mental health issues can no longer be seen as crazy, disordered or abnormal, but rather on the spectrum of normal responses to trauma, abuse, neglect and harsh living conditions.

As this text points out, the World Health Organization recommends that mental health care should be based in primary care. While this trend is increasing in Australia and New Zealand, a large percentage of clinical and acute treatment takes place in psychiatric wards.

Throughout my career I have worked in and attended mental health settings across Australia, New Zealand and internationally amid diverse cultures with varying degrees of wealth and poverty. Some services have been exciting, empathic environments exuding hope and healing, even when resources were scarce and the facilities poor. Sadly, my excitement has often been overwhelmed with shame, anger and painful questioning as to why all clinical and community mental health services are not holistic, therapeutic, trauma-informed and person-centred/person-led environments.

I have consulted multiple stakeholders about the reasons for the variations in service quality and outcomes. While mental health certainly needs more funding and resources, contrary to popular narratives I believe the variants do not relate to resources and finances; rather, they are based in individual nurse and clinician attitudes and the collective culture of the services. This can be evidenced by comparisons between services within the same states of Australia. State public services are working under the same funding models and the same policies and protocols yet vary dramatically in culture and outcomes.

Interactions between nurses, clinical staff and people they care for are either empathic, hopeful and respectful cultures engaged in respectful multidisciplinary teams producing outcomes desired by the people accessing the service and staff, or that of a culture that has inequitable power dynamics in which nurses and clinicians primarily pathologise the human experience and see people as the diagnosis, disorder or 'problem behaviour'. The latter culture produces detrimental outcomes including higher instances of seclusion, restraint and suicide and people feeling further marginalised and traumatised by the so-called 'trauma-informed treatment and care' they receive. Such detrimental cultures are also often characterised by workplace bullying, increased staff trauma and burnout. This text speaks to the importance of respect, care and wellbeing for *all* stakeholders.

As previously mentioned, *Mental Health Nursing: Theory and practice for clinical settings* takes the brave and wonderful step of including not only the voices of people accessing services with lived experience but also nurses' stories of their own lived experience. This deserves to be applauded. While the practices of nursing and mental health peer work are very different, nurses with lived experience have a positive impact on service culture and outcomes. Nurses and clinical staff with lived experience are valued and celebrated in this text, as they should be in all workplaces.

The stigma and discrimination shown against people with mental health issues has, in the past, driven nurses to hide their lived experience. This, coupled with workplace bullying and incidents of seclusion, restraint and enforced treatment, leads to trauma for both people being 'treated' and staff, and burnout among good nurses. Cultures such as these intimidate good staff and breed fear in people who need to access mental health services. People often turn to alcohol and drugs to self-medicate and to self-harm or suicide rather than return to a service where they feel unsafe, traumatised and humiliated.

Australia and New Zealand are signatories to the United Nations' declarations and conventions on human and disability rights. Nurses who focus on human rights and the innate value and needs of each person build healing, trusting relationships and workplaces for all stakeholders. Coercion, bullying, seclusion and restraint are non-existent or rare in services focused on respectful interactions. Nurses working in this culture see incidents of seclusion and restraint as failures of the service, rather than the fault of the person in distress.

While this text points out that current laws allow for seclusion and restraint in New Zealand and Australia, it also speaks to the need for these practices to be used as a last resort. However, lived experience advocates declare restrictive practices as abuses against human rights. I hope you will permit me to challenge all nurses to work as if seclusion and restraint were illegal and to consider alternative protocols to meet individual needs such as the support of peer workers. Peer workers use mutual experiences to connect with people and are a calming and hope-filled influence that can lead to a positive shift in the power dynamic between the multidisciplinary team and the people they care for.

The editors of this edition of *Mental Health Nursing: Theory and practice for clinical settings* have engaged chapter authors who focus on the particular aspects of ethical nursing practice. They have used vignettes written from different perspectives and consulted people with lived experience, peer workers, family/carers, clinicians and academics. The use of 'Critical thinking challenges' engages nurses in reflective thinking, learning and practice.

This text draws on lived experience, professional experience and tools to produce a learning experience based in ethical practices and the therapeutic alliances built between caring, respectful nurses and the people they treat and care for, their families and communities.

I commend this text to students and practising nurses at all stages of their careers. I thank the editors and authors for valuing lived experience and producing such a strong human rights–based, recovery-focused mental health guide to good nursing. Working in the ethical way this text demonstrates will, I hope, lead to improved outcomes, increased rates of recovery and healing, decreased rates of suicide and enforced treatment and the cessation of seclusion and restraint.

May nurses' careers be filled with a sense of pride, coupled with respect and humility as they witness how their practices and interactions with people contribute to the positive reframing of lived experience, enriched sense of self, healing and recovery and the ability to lead contributing, meaningful, respected lives.

Fay Jackson, Dip. Ed., BCVA, LEA, EBE
Founder of Vision In Mind
Lived Experience Advocate
Inaugural Deputy Commissioner, NSW
Mental Health Commission
NSW, Australia

About the authors

Kim Foster is a registered nurse with specialist mental health nursing qualifications. She is currently Professor of Mental Health Nursing and leads the Mental Health Nursing Research Unit at the Royal Melbourne Hospital, a joint research partnership between Australian Catholic University and NorthWestern Mental Health. Kim has extensive experience as a mental health nurse academic and educator, having developed and taught mental health curricula at the undergraduate and postgraduate levels across several Australian universities and in Fiji. She has consulted to AusAID and the World Health Organization and has an international reputation as a mental health researcher, with more than 120 publications. Her key research interests include: the resilience and wellbeing of the health workforce; the resilience of individuals and families with challenging health conditions; and the experiences and needs of families where a person has mental illness.

Peta Marks is a credentialled mental health nurse and family therapist working in private practice who specialises in working with people who have eating disorders and their families. Peta has extensive experience undertaking mental health project management at the national level and as a mental health writer and subject matter expert for online learning platforms. She is currently working as the national projects manager for the University of Sydney's InsideOut Institute for Eating Disorder Research and is the lead writer for Mental Health Professionals Online Development (MHPOD).

Anthony J O'Brien graduated as a registered nurse in Dunedin in 1977 and as a psychiatric nurse in Auckland in 1982. Anthony is currently employed at the University of Waikato as an Associate Professor in mental health nursing and as a nurse specialist in liaison psychiatry with the Auckland District Health Board. Anthony's PhD research investigated variation in the use of mental health legislation, including the roles of social deprivation, ethnicity, clinical decision making and service provision. Anthony's research interests are in social issues related to mental health, police and mental health, and advance directives. In 2020 Anthony was made an Officer of the New Zealand Order of Merit in recognition of services to mental health nursing.

Toby Raeburn is a senior lecturer, nurse practitioner and social historian in mental health at Western Sydney University. His interest in research and writing emerged over the two decades he spent working among the homeless and other vulnerable groups in Sydney. Toby has a growing body of publications on topics including mental health history, homelessness and recovery-oriented practice. He is particularly passionate about the empowering potential of history. Toby believes learning and reflecting on history can improve nurses' awareness and ability to cope with the present and can also inform development of vision and purpose for the future.

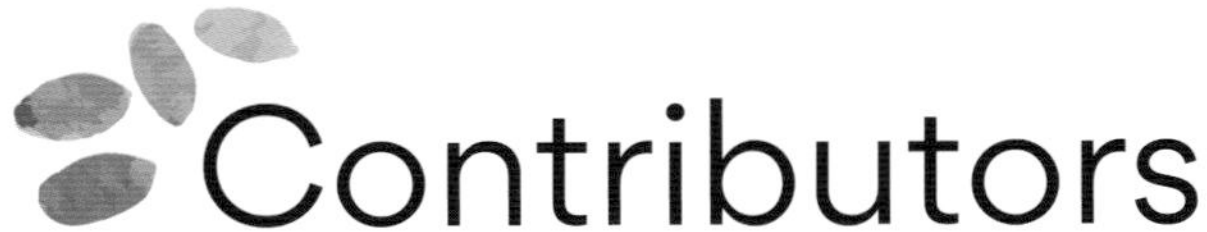

Contributors

Mandy Allman, MNurs, NP
Mental Health & Addictions (across the life span)
New Zealand Nurses Organisation
New Zealand

Matthew Ball, AdvDipCouns (UK) HEDipNurs (UK), MN(NP)
Director and Nurse Practitioner
Humane Clinic
Australia

Scott Brunero, RN, DipAppSc, BHSc, MA(NP), PhD
Casual Academic, Western Sydney University and Southern Cross University
Clinical Nurse Consultant, Prince of Wales Hospital
Australia

Andrew Cashin, RN, NP, DipAppSc, GCPTT, GCHPol, BHSc, MN, PhD, FACMHN, FACN, FACNP
Professor of Autism and Intellectual Disability, Southern Cross University
Honorary Professor, The University of Sydney
Australia

Justin Chia, BScPsych, BN, MNurs(MH)
Transitional Nurse Practitioner (Community Mental Health), Sydney Local Health District
Honorary Lecturer, The University of Sydney
Australia

Greg Clark, RN, NP, BHSc(MHN), MN(AdvPrac), MN(NP), PhD, FACMHN
Academic Course Adviser, Postgraduate Mental Health
Western Sydney University
Australia

Catherine Daniel, RPN, BPsychNurs, PGDip(MH), MN, PhD
Senior Lecturer, Nursing, The Melbourne of School of Health Sciences
The University of Melbourne
Australia

Cynthia Delgado, RN, DipHSc, MN(MH-NP), MACMHN, MACN
Clinical Nurse Consultant, Mental Health
Health Education and Training Institute (HETI)
Australia

Anna Elders, RN, BN, PGCertCAMH, PGDipCBT, MN
Clinical Lead, Nurse Practitioner, Cognitive Behaviour Therapist
Just a Thought (The Wise Group)
New Zealand

Simeon Evans, RMHN, DipHMH, PGCertCBT, PGDipHSc, MN(Hons), FACMHN
Nurse Practitioner
Hunter New England Mental Health
Australia

Julie Ferguson, RN, NP, CMHN, GDipHSM, MN(APMH), MN(NP), FACMHN
Lecturer, Nursing, School of Nursing, Midwifery and Indigenous Health
Charles Sturt University, Bathurst Campus
Australia

Elizabeth Halcomb, RN, BN(Hons), GCICNurs, GCHE, PhD, FACN
Professor of Primary Health Care Nursing
University of Wollongong
Australia

Sophie Isobel, RN, BN, CAMH, GCCAFH, ResMeth
Lecturer, Mental Health Nursing
The University of Sydney
Australia

Scott Lamont, RMN, RN, MN(Hons), PhD
Clinical Nurse Consultant and Casual Academic
Prince of Wales Hospital and Southern Cross University
Australia

Tessa Maguire, RN, BN, PGDipFBS, PGDipFMHN, MMHSc, PhD
Senior Lecturer, Forensic Mental Health Nursing
Centre for Forensic Behavioural Science
Swinburne University of Technology & Forensicare
Australia

Megan McKechnie, NP, DipMH&Addict, BN, MSc, MA
Alfred Mental and Addiction Health
Australia

Brian McKenna, RN, BMHSc(Hons), PhD, FNZCMHN
Professor, Forensic Mental Health
Auckland University of Technology and the Auckland Regional Forensic Psychiatry Services
New Zealand
Adjunct Professor, Centre for Forensic Behavioural Science
Swinburne University of Technology
Australia

Bridget Mulvey, RN, MHN, CNC, BHSc(Nursing), MMH(C&A)
Clinical Nurse Consultant and Coordinator, NSW Eating Disorders Outreach Service
The Insideout Institute for Eating Disorders
The University of Sydney
Australia

Christopher Patterson, RN, BN(Hons), MN(MH)
Lecturer
University of Wollongong
Australia

Lucie Ramjan, RN, BN(Hons), PhD, MACN
Associate Professor
Western Sydney University
Australia

Melissa Robinson-Reilly, RN, DipAppSc, BN, GCOnc, MN(PallCare), MN(NP), PhD, MACN, ACNP
Program Convenor, School of Nursing and Midwifery
University of Newcastle
Australia

Ros Rolleston, BHSc, GCMHN, MN, MACN
Primary Health Nurse Educator and Facilitator
Nowra
Australia

Sharon Rydon, RCompN, BN, MPhil(Nursing)
Clinical Learning and Development Manager
Summerset Group
New Zealand

Julie Sharrock, RN, CertCritCare, CertPsychNurs, AdvDip(GestaltTher), MHSc(PsychNurs), PhD Candidate, FACMHN, MACN, MACSA
Mental Health Nurse Consultant
Private Practice
Australia

Sophie Temmhoff, AdvDipVA
Art mentor, disability support worker and advocate
Western Sydney
Australia

Scott Trueman, RN, MHN, LLB, BCom(Acc), GDLP, GDipMH, MMHN, MPhil, PhD, FACMHN
Adjunct Associate Professor
Queensland Health
Australia

Kim Usher, AM, RN, DipAppSc, BA, MNSt, PhD, FACMHN, FACN
Professor of Nursing
University of New England
Australia

Marika Van Ooyen, RN, BN(IAH), GCN(MH), MEd
Clinical Nurse Consultant
headspace Early Intervention Team – Sydney Local Health District and headspace Camperdown
Australia

Timothy Wand, RN, NP, MN(Hons), PhD
Associate Professor and Nurse Practitioner
The University of Sydney and Sydney Local Health District
Australia

Andrew Watkins, NP, BN, MN
Nurse Practitioner
Thomson Institute, University of Sunshine Coast
Australia

Fiona Whitecross, RN, DipAppSci, BN, MA, FACMHN
Operations Manager, Inpatient Psychiatric Services
Alfred Health
Australia

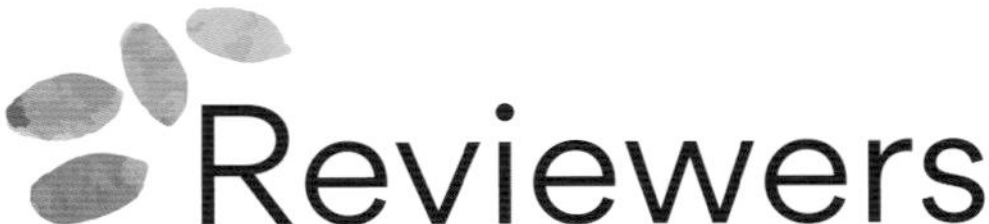

Reviewers

Katheryn Butters, RN, MPhil
Lecturer, School of Nursing
Massey University
New Zealand

Philip Ferris-Day, RN, BSc(Hons), PGCertEdu, PGCertCouns, MMH(Comm)
Lecturer, College of Health
Massey University
New Zealand

Jarrad Hickmott, BAAncHist/Archaeol
Peer Support Worker, Mental Health ICU, Prince of Wales Hospital, Randwick, NSW
Youth Advisor to the board of 'headspace' – The National Youth Mental Health Foundation
Australia

Diana Jefferies, RN, BA(Hons), PhD
Senior Lecturer and Aboriginal and Torres Strait Islander Liaison
School of Nursing and Midwifery, Western Sydney University
Australia

Elijah Marangu, RN, GCHE, MPH, PhD
Lecturer, School of Nursing and Midwifery
Deakin University
Australia

Karen-Lee O'Brien, RN
Mental Health Clinician; Teacher, CERT IV TAE; Associate Lecturer
CQUniversity
Australia

Alana Wilson, GDipMHNurs, GCDiabEd, MNPsych
Lecturer, Mental Health
Holmesglen Institute
Australia

Introduction

Kim Foster, Peta Marks, Anthony J O'Brien and Toby Raeburn

We are very pleased to introduce the fifth edition of this text. This edition signals a new direction, reflected in a name change – *Mental Health in Nursing: Theory and practice for clinical settings*. This change recognises that mental health, in addition to being an area of specialist practice, is part of holistic nursing practice in every setting. In this edition we welcome three new editors who have joined Anthony O'Brien from New Zealand on the editorial team. Kim Foster is a professor from Australian Catholic University and NorthWestern Mental Health and has been a longstanding contributor to the text. She brings extensive experience as a book and chapter author and mental health nurse researcher. Peta Marks is a credentialled mental health nurse and family therapist working in private practice and for the InsideOut Institute for Eating Disorder Research as the national projects manager. Peta has significant experience undertaking mental health project management and content development for online learning platforms. Toby Raeburn is a senior lecturer and nurse practitioner from Western Sydney University who is particularly interested in the history of mental health care and recovery-oriented care. We also gratefully acknowledge the contribution of former editors Katie Evans and Debra Nizette to the fourth and previous editions of the text.

The editorial team has been thankful to partner with Jarrad Hickmott, who contributed as a lived experience consultant. With a growing reputation as a consumer advocate, Jarrad is a peer support worker at Prince of Wales Hospital in Sydney and a youth advisor to the national board of 'headspace', Australia's national youth mental health foundation. Jarrad reviewed numerous chapters and authored several lived experience commentaries throughout. The story of Jarrad's recovery journey is available in both written and video materials associated with the text. We are also sincerely thankful to the many other people with lived experience who were involved as co-authors and contributors in chapters throughout.

This fifth edition builds on the successful foundations of the previous editions. In response to the developing landscape of modern mental health care and the evolving role of nurses in mental health and other service contexts, we have taken a wider perspective on nursing in mental health. As noted, the change of title is an acknowledgement of the fact that all nurses interact with people who have mental health needs in all service contexts. With wide-ranging nursing contexts in mind, we have introduced brand new chapters in Part 3 of this edition, authored by nursing experts from a range of primary health, generalist health and specialist mental health services. We hope the scenarios in Part 3 provide students and nurses who work in diverse contexts with knowledge and confidence by providing information focused on the practical application of mental health nursing skills.

Nurses require historical knowledge in order to be informed members of the profession and to formulate views and opinions grounded in evidence. Another change in this edition is the use of historical anecdotes throughout Parts 1 and 2. The goal is that by providing a range of historical anecdotes students and nurses will become aware that their understanding of what is happening in the present day has parallels and precedents with previous historical periods. It is our hope that as readers interact with the text, awareness will grow that knowledge about mental health is open to different readings and interpretations. Reflecting on history in this way can lead to more enlightened critique and understandings.

Use of varied language is another important way this textbook reflects contemporary practice. In mental health, nurses need to be aware of how language can influence their practice and relationships with people who experience mental ill health. Many different terms can be used to describe a person with lived experience of mental illness, including consumer, patient, client, service user and person with (or experiencing) a mental illness. You will hear all these terms (and more) in clinical practice, depending on the setting and people's preferences, and you will read them all in this text too. In this text, chapter authors use a range of terms to refer to people with lived experience, in acknowledgement that there is no universally accepted term. Most importantly, our language needs to be person-centred rather than illness-focused. For example, we might describe someone as 'a person with a lived experience of psychosis', reminding us that this is a person experiencing an illness or set of symptoms, rather than 'a schizophrenic', which is an objectifying label and implies that the disorder is the dominating feature of the individual. Our approach to language also reflects the view that although a person may experience mental distress or mental illness, they may not necessarily identify as a consumer of mental health services. In every clinical context mental health is part of nursing but may not be the primary reason the person seeks health care.

In this edition the text has been restructured into three sections. Specialist mental health nursing knowledge and skills remain a key focus, particularly in Parts 1 and 2.

Part 1 *Positioning Practice* introduces the context for nursing in mental health, describes the importance of mental health, introduces the social ecological approach to mental health in nursing that frames the text, and explores the mental health nursing knowledge, skills and attitudes needed to provide effective mental health care for individuals and their family or carers. A new chapter also addresses the need for nurses to engage in professional self-care, as this is an essential but often neglected aspect of the nursing role.

Part 2 *Knowledge for Practice* is a core feature of the text, examining specific mental health conditions that people experience, providing a comprehensive description of major mental health problems, their assessment, nursing management and relevant treatment approaches. This section specifically addresses the specialist practice of mental health nursing. It will be of particular interest to nursing students on mental health clinical placements as part of their undergraduate education, and to nurses in their first years of specialist clinical practice in mental health.

Part 3 *Contexts of Practice* is a new section of the text, with chapters demonstrating how mental health nursing knowledge and skills can be integrated into the nursing role and applied across a range of clinical settings – both generalist and mental health settings. This does not mean that mental health knowledge and skills are *only* applicable in these settings – we have included these settings because they are common clinical settings and areas where nurses frequently practice. The chapters in Part 3 have been written by clinical experts and are different in their tone and in how they have been written from other sections of the text.

Existing features of the text have been retained across chapters, including lists of useful websites, nurses' and consumers' stories, key points, key terms and learning outcomes, and critical thinking exercises and exercises for class engagement. In the Part 2 chapters, references to diagnostic classification systems of mental illness have been largely removed, in recognition that diagnosis is imprecise, contested and does not capture individuals' subjective experiences. Nurses focus on people's experiences and their responses to adversity, stress and distress, rather than to diagnoses and symptoms. Of course, diagnostic systems remain a core component of mental health services, and for that reason the Part 2 chapters, as in previous editions, include the language of diagnosis.

Including new chapters means that decisions needed to be made about the length of chapters and the relevance of previous material. In particular, there was a need to consider areas of duplication and where word length could be reduced without loss of core information. Chapters in this edition have been made more concise throughout to enhance readability and usefulness. References have been updated over the whole text, drawing on the most contemporary research and scholarship while retaining core references that situate this fifth edition within the scholarly history of mental health and nursing.

We warmly thank all the chapter authors, people with lived experience, family/carers, clinicians and academics who contributed to this edition, as well as the reviewers who have provided helpful and constructive feedback. We hope the text continues to be widely used because of its contemporary focus and integration of theory and practice.

PART 1

Positoning Practice

CHAPTER 1

Why mental health matters

Anthony J O'Brien, Toby Raeburn, Peta Marks and Kim Foster

KEY POINTS

- There is no health without mental health.
- Mental distress and mental illness are relatively common in Australia and New Zealand, and rates vary between different population groups.
- Nurses care for people who have mental health needs in every practice setting.
- Nurses do not need to be a specialist mental health nurse to respond to mental health needs.

KEY TERMS

- Cultural safety
- Mental distress
- Mental health
- Mental health care
- Mental health legislation
- Mental illness
- Physical health
- Prevalence of mental illness
- Scope of practice
- Suicide

LEARNING OUTCOMES

The material in this chapter will assist you to:

- understand the importance of mental health in every clinical practice setting
- understand the prevalence of mental distress and illness
- identify how physical health problems can affect mental health
- discuss how mental health is seen in New Zealand and Australia's indigenous cultures
- describe the provision of mental health care.

Introduction

Mental health matters. When individuals can live socially and emotionally satisfying lives, families, communities and whole nations benefit. The term 'mental health' refers to a range of experiences that affect the health and functioning of individuals, families, communities, societies and nations. These experiences include everything from happiness and wellness through to mild distress, anxiety and long-term mental illness. The term 'mental health' is often used as a synonym for 'mental illness' but the term properly refers to a state of wellbeing, not illness. It is important to keep this distinction in mind as you read this chapter. Effects of mental ill health can extend to economic impacts through healthcare costs and loss of economic productivity. Such impacts are not just from mental illness, although mental illness does have considerable impact on employment, productivity and quality of life, but also from distress and impaired function. In Chapter 2 we outline a social ecological approach that integrates the various influences on mental health, from biological through to social. Health planners are increasingly recognising that mental health problems can also lead to physical illness, poor recovery after physical illness and impaired social functioning. Successive epidemiological studies have shown that mental health problems are relatively common, with high proportions of the population experiencing a mental health problem at some point in their lives.

Nurses care for people who may be experiencing mental ill health in every clinical setting and in the work of many social agencies such as schools, police services, social welfare services and correctional services. For this reason, mental health is increasingly regarded as an issue for all health professionals and social agencies. For nurses therefore, skills in mental health form an essential part of their clinical skill set. This chapter begins with an overview of the prevalence of mental distress and illness internationally and in Australia and New Zealand. The chapter then outlines some of the central mental health issues including the range of nursing responses available for people with mental health problems and the place of mental health in the nursing scope of practice. Reading this chapter should help you understand why mental health matters in nursing.

Epidemiology of mental distress and illness

To understand the impact of mental health problems it is important to consider their epidemiology, or distribution in the population. Distribution is measured by prevalence and incidence. Prevalence is a measure of the rate of mental illness over a given time period – for example, at a single point in time (point prevalence) or over a year (12-month prevalence). Incidence is the measure of new cases of a disorder – for example, the number of new cases in a year. Both the Australian and New Zealand governments have conducted extensive research into the prevalence of mental health problems. For both countries the most recent national epidemiological evidence on mental illness is now more than a decade old, although recent research has provided more up-to-date evidence of prevalence. The following sections review reports on the prevalence of mental distress and illness internationally and in Australia and New Zealand.

Prevalence of mental distress

Mental distress is an unpleasant mental or emotional state that can impact on enjoyment of life and on personal and social functioning. The experience of distress is a common part of life, although if severe or prolonged it can impact on health and is a risk factor for mental illness. Mental distress can be measured using standardised scales, the most common of which is the Kessler Psychological Distress Scale (K10). Using the K10, the 2015–16 New Zealand Household Survey found that 4–8% of the population experienced high levels of distress, with younger people, Māori and Pacific people and women reporting higher levels (Ministry of Health 2016). In a similar national survey Australians reported higher levels of distress, with 13% of the Australian adult population reporting very high levels (Australian Bureau of Statistics 2018).

Rates of mental distress have been reported to be high in countries as diverse as Norway, the United States and France and even higher in developing countries such as Bangladesh (Islam 2019) and in conflict zones (Jayasuriya et al. 2016; Summers et al. 2019). Distress is also common in people with physical illness – for example, people with diabetes (McCarthy et al. 2019), cancer (Gilbertson-White et al. 2017), cardiac disease (McPhillips et al. 2019) or renal disease (Damery et al. 2019) – and for people experiencing adverse events such as trauma (de Munter et al. 2020), victimisation (Thomas et al. 2016), fire (Maybery et al. 2019) or natural disaster (Inoue & Yamaoka 2017). Despite being a common experience, attempts to reduce levels of mental distress in the community are not always successful. Western countries including Australia and New Zealand have made substantial increases in mental health care provision in recent decades; however, there has been little change in population rates of distress (Tomitaka et al. 2019).

Prevalence of mental illness

According to the World Health Organization (WHO) 'mental, neurological and substance use disorders make up 10% of the global burden of disease and 30% of non-fatal disease burden' (WHO 2019), with one in five children and adolescents experiencing a mental disorder. WHO also reports that depression alone affects 264 million people worldwide and is one of the leading causes of disability (WHO 2018). Depression is also associated with higher rates of unemployment, incarceration and homelessness (Grech & Raeburn 2019).

In developed nations, total government spending on mental health is substantial. In Australia, the quantifiable costs of mental ill health and suicide in 2018–19 were estimated to be from $43 to $51 billion and include health care, education, housing and justice, with health care alone estimated at $18 billion (Productivity Commission 2019). The main societal costs related to mental illness are lost productivity, caused by high unemployment and under-employment of people with mental illness, along with impacts on quality of life and other non-quantifiable costs such as the cost of stigma. In addition, there are social participation impacts as well as the pain and suffering of family and friends who have lost a loved one to suicide.

Australia's 2019 Productivity Commission Inquiry into Mental Health identifies that the cost of lost productivity due to lower employment, absenteeism and presenteeism (working while unwell) ranges from $10 to $18 billion. Informal care costs to family and friends has been valued at $15 billion per annum. There is an approximately $130 billion cost associated with diminished health and reduced life expectancy for people with mental ill health. On an individual level, for example, the annual costs for a person who experiences psychosis in Australia have been evaluated as comprising $40,941 in lost productivity, $21,714 in health sector costs and $14,642 in other costs. Overall this amounts to four times the cost in annual health expenditure for an average Australian adult (Neil et al. 2014).

In New Zealand there are similar costs associated with mental illness. A recent inquiry into mental health and addiction (Ministry of Health 2018) received submissions on the personal, social and economic impacts of mental illness. The Ministry of Health (2017) estimates the annual cost of the burden of serious mental illness, including addiction, in New Zealand at $12 billion or 5% of gross domestic product. In addition to this economic impact there is an estimated $1.5 billion annual cost across government agencies associated with the nearly 60,000 health and disability benefit recipients whose primary barrier to work is mental illness is $1.5 billion. Poor mental health has other indirect costs – for example, the cost of housing for those who cannot work because of mental health problems. This cost is estimated at $1.2 billion over the lifetime of New Zealand's 6,700 social housing tenants receiving benefits and whose primary barrier to work is mental health is $1.2 billion (Ministry of Health 2018).

Historical anecdote 1.1: Early descriptions

Experiences of mental ill health have been described since the beginning of human history in ancient documents such as Egyptian papyri, the Indian Ramayana and the Old Testament of the Bible. The longest lasting historical theory regarding mental ill health was developed by ancient Greek philosophers Pythagoras (570–495 BCE) and Hippocrates (460–377 BCE), who proposed that the human body contains four 'humors': blood, phlegm, yellow bile and black bile. Black bile and phlegm were thought to cause mental ill health, which was believed to be more common in spring and beginning of winter when the humors were 'active'. Humoral theory dominated medical treatment for more than 2,000 years, informing the administration of several painful remedies such as blisters to the head, castor oil, solution of lilac emetic and bloodletting. Each of these 'treatments' were designed to purge the body of the 'black bile and phlegm' thought to be causing mental ill health. Today, we still see the relic of humoral theory in our modern terms 'choleric' and 'sanguine' used to describe different personality types.

Read more about it: *Davison K 2006 Historical aspects of mood disorders. Psychiatry 5(4): 115–8.*

Australian national survey of mental health

The Australian Bureau of Statistics (ABS) conducted a national survey of mental health and wellbeing in 1997 and 2007, which collected information on lifetime and 12-month prevalence of selected mental health problems among people aged 18–65 years. The following information was obtained from the survey report (ABS 2008).

Almost half of all Australians who were surveyed reported a mental health problem at some point in their life, and one in five (20%) experienced a mental health problem within the preceding 12 months. Analysis of survey results showed that anxiety disorders (14%) were the most commonly experienced type of mental health problem in Australia, with the most frequently reported anxiety disorder being post-traumatic stress disorder (6%) followed by social phobia (5%). Affective disorders were reported by 6% of respondents, with the most common affective disorder being depression (4%). Substance use disorders affected 5% of respondents, the most common being harmful use of alcohol, reported by 3% of respondents.

The survey also highlighted significant connections between mental and physical conditions; 11.7% of respondents had both a mental and physical health problem, and 8.5% reported two or more mental disorders. In line with prevalence of discreet mental health problems, the most common comorbidity was anxiety disorder and a physical condition (6%). Comorbidity compounds the impact of individual disorders, resulting in higher rates of relapse, greater impairment, higher use of health services and higher risk of suicidal behaviour.

The survey also showed the gendered distribution of mental disorder in Australia. Women (22%) were more likely to experience mental disorders than men (18%). Compared with men, women reported higher rates of anxiety disorder than men (18% vs 11%) and higher rates of affective disorders (7% vs 5%). Men had more than twice the rate of substance use disorders (7%) compared with women (3%). Rates also varied across age groups, with younger people more likely to have a mental illness than older people. Just over a quarter (26%) of people aged 16–24 reported a mental disorder compared with 6% of those aged 75–85. Substance use disorders were more common among younger people (13%) than in other age groups, while anxiety disorders were more common in people aged 35–44, with a reported rated of 18%. Family and housing status were other factors associated with rates of mental disorder. One-third (34%) of people living in one-parent families reported a mental health problem compared with 19% of those living in couple families. More than half of those who had ever been homeless had a mental health problem, almost three times the rate of those who had never been homeless. Mental health problems were more common in unemployed people (29%) and in people who had ever been incarcerated (41%).

Rates of psychotic disorder were examined in the 2010 Survey of High Impact Psychosis, Australia's second national psychosis survey (Morgan et al. 2012). That survey reported a 12-month prevalence of psychotic disorder of 4.5 in 1,000. Of those diagnosed with a psychotic disorder the most common diagnosis was schizophrenia spectrum disorder (63%). While the overall rate might seem relatively low, especially compared with the rates of depression and anxiety, the impact of psychotic disorder can be profound. Morgan et al. reported that 49.5% of those with a psychotic disorder had attempted suicide over their lifetime, 63.2% experienced significant social impairment and 78.5% were unemployed. The relationship between mental and physical illness is marked, with 54.8% of this sample having metabolic syndrome and therefore at significant risk of developing type 2 diabetes and cardiovascular disease.

Te Rau Hinengaro: the New Zealand mental health survey

Te Rau Hinengaro,[1] the New Zealand Mental Health Survey (Oakley Browne et al. 2006) aimed to describe the mental health state of the entire New Zealand population. Like its Australian counterpart, the survey did not collect data on psychotic disorders. Specific objectives of Te Rau Hinengaro were to describe:

- the one-month, 12-month and lifetime prevalence rates of major mental disorders among those aged 16 or older living in private households, overall and by sociodemographic correlates
- patterns of and barriers to health service use for people with a mental disorder
- the level of disability associated with a mental disorder.

The survey reported a 44.6% lifetime prevalence of mental disorder, with a 12-month prevalence of 20.7%. The latter figure is very close to the 20% 12-month prevalence reported in Australia. In addition to overall prevalence, the survey presented specific findings on age, gender, ethnicity and socioeconomic status.

Mental disorders are more common in young people in New Zealand, with younger people reporting a higher prevalence of disorder in the past 12 months and more likely to report having ever had a disorder. In terms of gender, females reported higher prevalence of anxiety disorder, major depression and eating disorders than males, whereas males reported substantially higher prevalence for substance use disorders than females. Social disadvantage is also associated with mental disorders, with higher rates for people who are disadvantaged in terms of educational qualification, household income or social deprivation. Comorbidity of mental disorders is common, with 37.0% of those experiencing 12-month mental disorders having two or more disorders. Mood disorders and anxiety disorders are most likely to co-occur. The survey also noted that rates of mental and physical comorbidity are high and cause compounding disability, but these rates of comorbidity are not reported in Te Rau Hinengaro.

The prevalence of disorder in any period is higher for Māori and Pacific people than for the 'Other' composite ethnic group. For disorder in the past 12 months the prevalence rates are 29.5% for Māori, 24.4% for Pacific people and 19.3% for 'Other', which indicates that Māori and Pacific people have a greater burden due to mental health problems. Much of this burden appears to be due to the youthfulness of the Māori and Pacific populations and their relative socioeconomic disadvantage.

Suicidality was also reported in Te Rau Hinengaro. Of the New Zealand population, 15.7% reported ever having thought seriously about suicide. In total, 5.5% had ever made a suicide plan and 4.5% had ever made an attempt. These rates are comparable with those of several other developed countries. In the 12 months preceding the survey, 3.2% experienced suicidal ideation, 1.0% made a suicide plan and 0.4% made a suicide attempt. Higher rates of suicidality were reported for women, younger people and for people experiencing social deprivation. Individuals with a mental disorder had elevated risks of suicidal behaviour, with 11.8% of people with any mental disorder reporting suicidal ideation, 4.1% making a suicide plan and 1.6% making a suicide attempt. It is important to remember, however, that many of the individuals reporting suicidal thoughts, plans and even attempts will not have sought professional support. Others will have attended a primary care service for a physical health problem but will not have reported their suicidal thoughts.

[1] The term 'Te Rau Hingengaro' means 'the many minds'.

Critical thinking challenge 1.1

Epidemiological studies show that mental illness and addiction problems are relatively common in our communities, with up to 50% of people experiencing a mental illness (including addiction) in their lifetime. And yet the belief persists that mental illness is uncommon and experienced by only a small minority of people. Why does the belief persist that only a small minority of people experience mental illness? What effect does this belief have on nurses and other primary care clinicians who regularly see many patients with mental health and addiction problems?

Physical and mental health

In 1954 Dr Brock Chisholm, the first Director-General of WHO, stated that 'without mental health there can be no true physical health' (Kolappa et al. 2013). Conversely, it has been argued that 'there is no true mental health without (physical) health' (Kolappa et al. 2013).

Health is defined in the WHO constitution as:

> A state of complete, physical, mental and social wellbeing and not merely the absence of disease or infirmity.
>
> (WHO 2014, p. 1)

As can be seen from the above quote, people are holistic beings with both physical and mental health needs. However, generalist and mental health services are often separated, which has led to an artificial divide between physical and mental health care. This means that the mental health needs of patients in generalist health settings can be overlooked. Similarly, the physical health of people with mental illness in mental health settings may not be prioritised.

People with mental illness have higher rates of physical illness than the general population and do not always receive adequate screening, assessment and treatment for their physical health (Te Pou o Te Whakaaro Nui 2014a; 2017). In addition, people with mental illness have high rates of chronic physical illness, which contributes to higher morbidity and mortality rates. It is therefore important in every practice setting that nurses respond to both the physical health and mental health needs of people with mental illness. Both Australia and New Zealand have strategies to address the health disparities experienced by people with mental illness. The *Equally Well* consensus statements (Mental Health Commission of NSW 2016; Te Pou o Te Whakaaro Nui 2014b) express the commitment of multiple organisations to improving the physical health of people with mental illness. These statements reflect the view that mental health is 'everybody's business', including the whole health sector as well as social agencies, employers, housing providers and police. The physical health of people with mental illness is discussed in detail in Chapter 18.

Nowhere is the relationship between mind and body more evident than in the area of chronic conditions. People with mental illness experience chronic disease at greater rates than the general community in areas including but not limited to respiratory disease, cardiovascular disease, diabetes, chronic pain and cancer. People with mental illness experience a reduction in life expectancy of up to 25 years (Firth et al. 2019), with a meta-analysis of research reporting that up to 14.3% of deaths worldwide, approximately 8 million deaths each year, are attributable to mental disorders (Walker et al. 2015). People with the more enduring forms of psychotic illness struggle to have even their most basic physical health needs met and experience very poor access to regular physical review by a general practitioner and health promotion services (e.g. smoking cessation programs and cancer screening). This lack of appropriate health care contributes significantly to increased risk of chronic disease and premature death.

The relationship between physical and mental health is also important in understanding causes and treatment of physical illness. For example, depressive illness can precede a physical disease. It has been linked to diseases such cardiovascular disease, stroke, colorectal cancer, epilepsy, chronic obstructive pulmonary disease and type 2 diabetes (Olver & Hopwood 2013). In addition, people with any chronic physical disease tend to feel more mental distress than do healthy people (Nasif 2015). Poor physical health brings an increased risk of depression (Caneo et al. 2016), as do the social and relationship problems that are common among chronically ill patients (Gürhan et al. 2019). Understanding the relationship between physical and mental health is crucial for nurses in order to develop strategies to reduce the incidence of co-existing conditions and support those already living with mental illnesses and chronic physical conditions. Everyday behaviours with the potential to positively or negatively affect physical and mental health include sleep, diet, alcohol/drug use and physical exercise (White et al. 2014).

Assisting patients to manage their physical health and mental health is a role for all nurses. Simple ways we can observe a person's physical health status include taking note of their body shape, skin, central adiposity, weight, height, body mass index, blood pressure, heart rate, cholesterol, blood sugar levels, abdominal circumference and fitness level. See Chapter 18 for further nursing strategies.

Critical thinking challenge 1.2

Metabolic syndrome is a cluster of risk factors that predicts development of type 2 diabetes and cardiovascular disease. Rates of metabolic syndrome are high in people taking antipsychotic medication, yet nurses in mental health and primary care settings do not always provide routine screening for metabolic syndrome. Consider your own area of practice or your current clinical placement. Are mental health consumers in that area screened for metabolic syndrome? Do nurses consider this to be part of their practice? If consumers are screened, what interventions are used to reduce the risk of metabolic syndrome?

Self-harm and suicide

In addition to mental disorders, self-harm and suicidality are behaviours that nurses commonly encounter in settings such as primary care and emergency departments, as well as mental health services. Rates of suicide have increased in recent years in both Australia (Harrison & Henley 2014) and New Zealand (Ministry of Health 2019), and for every person who completes suicide there are many more who self-harm (Chan et al. 2016). Self-harm can vary from cutting to relieve distress, to overdoses of prescribed or over-the-counter medication and potentially lethal attempts at suicide. Depression is a common mental disorder and is associated with self-harm and suicidal thoughts.

In general hospital settings patients may sometimes express a sense of hopelessness when faced with ill health, pain, lost function or an adverse prognosis. Such patients may then entertain passive suicidal thoughts – ideas that they would be better off dead or a wish that they would die from their illness. Passive suicidal thoughts are relatively common and may respond to the listening skills and validation of an empathic nurse (Mortier et al. 2018). If passive suicidal thoughts worsen and develop into active suicide plans, the nurse may need to consider referral to a mental health specialist.

Although suicide is statistically rare, it leaves emotional ripple effects on the lives of hundreds of thousands of friends and relatives of people who complete suicide each year. Research suggests many people who complete suicide had recent contact with a health professional (Rhodes 2013), indicating that those considering suicide are not always receiving the psychological support they seek. Certain population groups are at higher risk of suicide. These groups currently include men and young people. In fact, suicide is the leading cause of death in adolescents and young adults in Australia (Australian Institute of Health and Welfare 2019); men over the age of 85 have the highest suicide rate of all age groups (Burns 2016). Other groups that have been identified as being at higher risk of suicide include people from rural and remote communities and Aboriginal and Torres Strait Islander people (Wilson et al. 2018).

Mental health care

Australian mental health service delivery is guided by a national mental health strategy that comprises a national policy and a national plan (the *Fifth National Mental Health and Suicide Prevention Plan* was published in 2017), as well as a statement of rights and responsibilities (Commonwealth of Australia 2012). Each of the states and territories develops and reforms services in accordance with this national strategy. In New Zealand, the Ministry of Health provides national direction for mental health services. In both countries the aim is to provide mental health care to people in the least restrictive environment. In keeping with this, mental health care is provided in a wide range of clinical settings from generalist health settings and primary care, through to specialist mental health services, with the preferred setting for service delivery being in the community wherever possible.

WHO recommends that mental health care should be based in primary care. This is because general practice is usually the first point of contact for people seeking assistance for all health problems – including mental health problems – and a significant number of people with severe mental illness and high care needs receive their mental health care from a general practitioner working in a primary care setting and/or a psychiatrist working in private practice. In addition, the high prevalence of comorbid illnesses and the side effects of psychotropic medications make the need for a strong and well-established links with general practice important. A systematic review by Perkins et al. (2017) identified that generalist healthcare providers in Australia, including nurses, undertake recognition and identification of illness, assessment and care planning, patient education, pharmacotherapy, psychological therapies (and other therapies), ongoing management, physical care and referral for people with mental health problems.

The 'stepped care' model of mental health care is an evidence-based, staged system that includes a hierarchy of interventions that are matched to a person's needs – ranging from least to most intensive (Australian Government Department of Health 2019; Te Pou o Te Whakaaro 2012). Box 1.1 provides some descriptors around the intervention hierarchy in the stepped care model.

In a stepped care arrangement, it's not necessary to start at level 1. The care that people need depends on the severity of their problems, the impact of their experiences on their functioning and how any problems identified may have responded to initial (first-line) interventions. For example, for some people interventions such as relaxation training, sleep hygiene and moderating use of alcohol may be effective in reducing mild anxiety, while others might need specialist assessment, psychological therapy or pharmacological treatment. In addition to improving access to mental health care, as well as detection, early intervention and outcome for consumers, stepped care aims to improve the efficiency and effectiveness mental health service delivery.

Within mental health services, there are many settings in which a nurse may practise (see Chapter 27). The most common of these include inpatient services in general hospitals, crisis teams, community mental health teams and recovery-focused services. Specialist mental health services are delivered in mental health settings by health professionals with specialist mental health qualifications and training, including mental health nurses, psychiatrists, psychologists and mental health–trained social workers and occupational therapists.

Increasingly, people with a lived experience of mental illness are undertaking peer worker roles across primary care, community and inpatient settings (Crane et al. 2016). The essence of these various roles is to provide support based on mutual respect, shared responsibility and mutual agreement about what support is needed (Cleary et al.

Box 1.1 Stepped care model of mental health care in primary health

Level 1: Self-management – for people with no or mild mental illness, designed to prevent the development of illness (or prevent illness from progressing) and focused on helping individuals to manage symptoms themselves. This might include pamphlets about mental health and wellbeing, workbooks about a specific problem or online self-help programs.

Level 2: Low-intensity services – for people with mild to moderate mental illness and might include guided self-help or brief psychological interventions designed to last for a few short sessions.

Level 3: Moderate-intensity services are for people with mild to moderate mental illness but provide more structured, frequent and intensive interventions.

Level 4: High-intensity services are for people with more severe mental illness that is persistent or episodic, but that doesn't carry a high level of risk, complexity or disability. This includes high-intensity services and intensive interventions that might include multidisciplinary support.

Level 5: Acute and specialist community mental health services are for people with severe and persistent needs and those with complex multiagency needs or conditions that include high levels of risk, disability or complexity. These services include intensive team-based specialist assessment and intervention provided by mental health professionals across disciplines.

2018). Similarly, community-managed organisations (also known as non-government organisations or 'NGOs') are increasingly playing a key role in providing support to people with a lived experience of mental illness – through direct service delivery (Balagopal & Kapanee 2019). They complement existing mental health services and strengthen community supports and partnerships. The main types of support provided include: accommodation support and outreach; employment and education; leisure and recreation; family and carer support; self-help and peer-support; helpline and counselling services; and promotion, information and advocacy. While it is critical for nurses to work in an integrated way with community-managed organisations, it is important to remember that NGOs do not provide whole-of-life services, but rather stepping stones for those people who choose to use them. The aim is for people to develop naturally occurring supports within the community or to use other created supports that are accessed by all members of the community.

NURSE'S STORY 1.1

Anna

I undertook my nursing training at a regional base hospital in the mid-1970s. At that time, we lived in nurses' quarters. We had a month-long placement at the local psychiatric hospital and the psychiatric nurse trainees had a placement with us. I had not considered psychiatric (as it was called then) nursing at the time. During my third and final year of training I had a relationship breakup. It was very traumatic for me, mostly because it was so sudden. My then boyfriend was particularly nasty and made some very unkind comments about my appearance. I became quite depressed.

Living in nurses' quarters might lead you to think that everyone would have noticed me getting more and more unhappy, but shared living with hundreds of student nurses also provided quite a lot of anonymity. I went about my shifts and stayed in my room most of the time. I didn't confide in my parents. My mother had suffered from depression and hypochondriasis for many years and I didn't want to burden her or my dad. I didn't want to be like her. I pretended nothing was wrong.

Over the next few months I joined a gym and started going more and more often. I also started dieting, purging and using diuretics. I lost a lot of weight. The depression lifted (I didn't have any formal treatment), but I was getting very thin. I loved it and was proud of my body. By this time, we were also gearing up for the statewide final exams. I was able to handle the stress by working out. My weight was 45 kg and I had a BMI of 17. This was now considered a problem, but not for me.

After a few months one of the gym instructors asked me out and I agreed. That was the turning point. He said that I was looking unwell and he preferred it when I was fit but at a healthy weight. I was very fearful of becoming fat. He encouraged me to change to a 'lifters' high-protein diet and worked with me and encouraged me. I steadily gained weight but not fat. The relationship didn't last, but we have remained good friends ever since.

I moved interstate after my graduate year and tried to get a job at a general hospital in a large regional town, without success. I then considered psychiatric nursing. Although I wasn't previously interested, my personal journey created a curiosity and a greater understanding of the issues that people with mental health problems face and the courtesy stigma that is attached to people who are associated with people with a mental health problem. I am pleased I made the decision. I have never looked back.

Critical thinking challenge 1.3

Nurses meet people with mental health and addiction problems in every clinical setting. For some people, their mental health needs can be met within a general health setting, such as primary care or in a medical ward of a general hospital. Others need referral to a specialist mental health service. How would you assess the mental health needs of a patient in a general health setting? When would you consider referral for a specialist mental health assessment?

Cultural considerations

Australia and New Zealand are culturally diverse countries originally peopled by indigenous populations. Following colonisation and migrant settlement over two centuries, both countries now embrace multiple cultures, although the dominant culture in both countries reflects a Western worldview and values. This dominant worldview has been found to be inadequate in the face of the cultural diversity of both countries.

The indigenous peoples of Australia and New Zealand experience high rates of mental disorder that reflects the history and modern legacy of colonisation (Tapsell et al. 2018; Trueman 2013). 'Mental illness' is a Western construct, however, and so for many indigenous people represents Western ideas of the individual and the relationship between the individual and society. These ideas may be profoundly different from those of people from non-Western cultures. Indigenous Australians and New Zealand Māori have views of health and illness that are informed by their wider cultural beliefs and that support practices unique to those cultures. The way people express mental distress and illness will reflect their cultural beliefs. In New Zealand, for example, the phenomenon of *whakamaa* (shame, self-abasement, shyness, excessive modesty and withdrawal describe some aspects of this concept) is unique to the Māori culture (Tauranga & Moore 2018). For Australian Aboriginal people, individuals who spend long periods of time away from their country (place of birth/Dreaming) can be vulnerable to episodes of unwellness due to their weakened spiritual link with country and community (Vicary & Westerman 2004). Symptoms of a cultural syndrome known as 'longing for country' commonly includes feelings of weakness, nausea and general 'sickness' and somatic complaints, identity confusion and disorientation, which if cultural background is not considered may be misinterpreted by clinicians reliant on Western interpretations as forms of clinical depression or anxiety. Not being able to go home and settle these feelings can lead Aboriginal Australians to further health deterioration. The importance of country might partially explain the profound effect prison has on many Aboriginal people and the high rate of deaths in custody among Australian Aboriginals compared with Westerners (Vicary & Westerman 2004). Connection with land is central to many indigenous people and is often related to issues of mental health.

The increasing ethnic and cultural diversity of Western societies means that diverse individuals attend Western health services with presentations influenced by cultural beliefs and practices different from those of clinicians trained in Western models. Nurses respond to this diversity by developing an understanding of the diversity of cultures in their own societies and by developing cross-cultural communication skills (O'Brien et al. 2017). Services also attempt to provide clinicians from the cultural group of the service user and, in some cases, develop specialty services based on a culturally specific model of treatment. Collaborations between traditional and Western practitioners in mental health care have been further described by NiaNia et al. (2017).

Critical thinking challenge 1.4

Consider the cultural influences on your own identity. What insights does your cultural experience give you into the experience of people from cultures other than your own? In what ways does your cultural background limit your understanding of the cultures of others? What skills and strategies can you use to ensure barriers to cross-cultural communication are effectively addressed?

Cultural safety and mental health care

Nursing is about people of all cultures. Consumers and nurses have diverse cultural backgrounds, and while this diversity makes for rich and rewarding experiences it also brings the possibility of misinterpretations and misunderstandings. Experiences of distress and emotional conflict are embedded in cultural beliefs and traditions, so it is important that every nursing encounter is regarded as one that occurs with the cultural contexts of the nurse and consumer. The populations of Australia and New Zealand are characterised by increasing cultural diversity, and it is important that this diversity is acknowledged by nurses. Australian professional standards for mental health nurses recognise the need for nurses to work with consumers from all cultures (Australian College of Mental Health Nurses 2010), and New Zealand standards require nurses to provide care that is culturally safe (Te Ao Maramatanga 2012). The term 'cultural safety' (kawa whakaruruhau) was developed by New Zealand nurse Irihapeti Ramsden and can be considered the effective nursing of a person/family from another culture by a nurse who has undertaken a process of reflection on their own cultural identity and recognises the impact of their own cultural identity on their nursing practice.[2] The concept of cultural safety has been widely adopted across many countries and health settings (Kurtz et al. 2018) and has been suggested as a model for Australian healthcare standards (Laverty et al. 2017). More recently there has been increasing recognition that individuals carry multiple cultural and other identities (Kang & Bodenhausen 2015), making cultural safety a more complex construct but also one that is more sensitive to the realities of nurses' and consumers' multiple cultural beliefs, values and practices. For this reason, the Nursing Council of New Zealand's definition of 'culture' extends to 'age or generation; gender; sexual orientation; occupation and socioeconomic status; ethnic origin or migrant experience; religious or spiritual belief; and disability' (Nursing Council of New Zealand 2011, p. 5). As can be seen from that definition, culture is seen as construct that applies to many possible identities. A key to cultural safety is the nurse's own self-awareness and sensitivity to the impact of their cultural identity on the care they provide to others. As we have discussed above, the mental health experience of indigenous Australians and New Zealanders is shaped by the historical and contemporary experience of colonisation. Awareness of this history and how it continues within contemporary society is a critical aspect of cultural safety if nurses are to avoid reinforcing the colonial relationship within their nursing practice. This historicising approach provides a foundation for culturally safe practice with all the diverse cultures of Australia and New Zealand. Cultural safety does not require that nurses 'understand' the cultures of all consumers and communities. Such an approach is naïve and risks the nurse assuming cultural expertise they do not have.

[2]Adapted from a definition provided by the Nursing Council of New Zealand (2011).

CASE STUDY 1.1
Zahra

Zahra is a 30-year-old Somalian woman who police found wandering on a busy road. They were unable to engage her in conversation and were also unclear as to whether she was under the influence of alcohol or drugs. They took her to a mental health facility where mental health clinicians were asked to assess her.

The mental health team approached Zahra and introduced themselves. At that moment Zahra became more aware of her surroundings and became agitated. She kept repeating that she was not a prisoner and not to hurt her. Her English was limited but her meaning was clear to all. The mental health team attempted to calm her and requested that the police remain in the area but be unseen. This had a short-term calming effect.

Using an interpreter, the mental health team undertook their assessment and mental state examination. It became evident that Zahra was using multiple substances including cannabis and alcohol. She stated that she was using these substances more and more because they helped her forget the past.

Zahra had experienced terrible hardship including rape, being separated from her family and living in a detention centre for 3 years. As a result, she developed post-traumatic stress disorder.

Many refugees have experienced and witnessed appalling conditions, often perpetrated by people in authority. In Zahra's case staff could not have predicted her response. However, when working with refugees, nurses must be mindful of the possibility of traumatic stress and the associated sequelae, including substance use.

Historical anecdote 1.2: Ancient treatments

Communities as early as 5000 BCE associated mental ill health with mythological and spiritual beliefs such as demonic possession, sorcery and curses. Archaeologists have found the remains of prehistoric human skulls that had holes chipped into them using stone instruments (a treatment known as trephining) in the belief that by opening the skull an evil spirit, thought to be inhabiting a person's head and causing mental ill health, might be released and the individual would be cured. Some who underwent such procedures appear to have survived and lived for many years afterwards as trephined skulls of early humans show signs of healing. Pressure on the brain may have also been incidentally relieved.

Read more about it: *Prioreschi P 1991 Possible reasons for neolithic skull trephining. Anecdotes in Biology and Medicine 34(2): 296–303*

Mental health legislation

Mental health is unique within the healthcare environment in providing legislation that can compel people to accept treatment and, in some cases, to remain in hospital. Treatment without consent under mental health legislation is known as 'compulsory treatment' or 'civil commitment'. Informed consent is normally considered fundamental to providing care in every clinical setting, and treatment without consent is considered unethical. The usual rationale for providing compulsory treatment under mental health legislation is given in terms of risk to the person with mental illness or to another person. It is not enough for risk to be present; the risk must be due to mental illness. Examples include impaired judgement due to mania that might lead people to take actions that are very unsafe, suicidal thoughts together with intentions to act due to depression, or thoughts of harming others in response to voices telling the person to act in a harmful way. These high-risk situations are exceptional and require clinicians to act within the definitions of mental disorder contained in legislation. The purpose of compulsory treatment is to protect the person or others from potential harm. In addition to compulsory treatment in hospital, mental health legislation can also compel patients to accept treatment in community settings under a community treatment order. Although mental health legislation limits some rights of consumers it also provides protections through the right to consult a lawyer and to appeal to a court for a review of legal status. Several Australian states have amended their mental health legislation in recent years to give greater effect to human rights through processes such as supported decision making and advance directives. Mental health legislation is further explored in Chapter 8.

Mental health and the scope of nursing practice

In Australia and New Zealand nursing is regulated by statutory bodies that determine the responsibilities and obligations of nurses. One of the main mechanisms of statutory bodies is through statements of the scope of nursing practice (Lubbe & Roets 2014). Another mechanism is through statements of competencies, which are descriptions of the skills every nurse is expected to demonstrate. Nurses are legally and professionally responsible for working within their nursing scope of practice and for meeting all competencies of their regulatory bodies. There is no regulated scope of practice for mental health nursing in either Australia or New Zealand. Instead the scope is stated in broad terms and applies in every clinical setting.

The Nursing and Midwifery Board of Australia (www.nursingmidwiferyboard.gov.au) cites the following International Council of Nurses scope of practice statement:

> Nursing encompasses autonomous and collaborative care of individuals of all ages, families, groups and communities, sick or well and in all settings.

The Nursing Council of New Zealand also identifies a broad scope of practice for nurses (available at www.nursingcouncil.org.nz):

> Registered nurses utilise nursing knowledge and complex nursing judgment to assess health needs and provide care, and to advise and support people to manage their health [...]. This occurs in a range of settings in partnership with individuals, families, whānau and communities.

Statements of the scope of nursing practice make it clear that mental health care is every nurse's business. Together with the competencies for practice, they encompass the whole range of health care, meaning that nurses are expected to appropriately respond to the full range of needs of all patients. When we understand how common mental health issues are in the community, and how commonly people experience both mental and physical health problems, it is clear that there is a professional obligation for nurses to respond to the whole person, including their physical and mental health needs. The nursing scope of practice clearly reflects that obligation.

Nursing and mental health

As a nurse you will meet people with mental health issues in every area of clinical practice, from primary care through to specialist settings such as intensive care and surgery, and in prisons, schools, workplaces and aged care services. Mental health is both a specialised field of nursing practice and a fundamental part of every nurse's scope of practice. Yet you do not need to be a mental health specialist to respond to people's mental health needs. Fundamental mental health knowledge and skills can be used by all nurses, regardless of setting (O'Brien 2014).

Caring for people's mental health is a vital part of nursing. Patients in every clinical setting have mental health needs that may or may not contribute to their reasons for accessing health services. For many people nurses work with, mental health care is about helping a person maintain a sense of social and emotional wellbeing and seeking to optimise their mental health, which they normally experience as being positive. For others, mental health care may involve some short-term assistance to overcome mild experiences of mental health challenges such as anxiety or low mood. Nurses also commonly care for people who have long-term experience of mental illness such as schizophrenia or bipolar disorder that requires support of varying levels of intensity over many years. It is important for nurses to consider the whole of each person's health needs. Just as a patient with a long-term mental illness might present to their general practitioner with asthma or high blood pressure, a patient with a chronic physical illness such as diabetes might experience episodes of low mood or anxiety.

Responding to a person's mental health needs requires a variety of nursing skills including listening, exploring emotional issues and troubling thoughts, showing empathy, offering encouragement and building on strengths. See Chapter 2 for a discussion of holistic mental health nursing practice and therapeutic mental health nursing skills. Such actions can be incorporated into regular nursing care; they do not have to wait until other needs have been attended to. A nurse who practises holistically will be aware of the needs of each person at the time, will be open to discussing emotional and physical health issues and be comfortable in responding in an informed and helpful way. This may involve seeking guidance from other professionals or making a referral to a specialist service. Such referral or advice seeking is an integral part of the nurse's practice and an acknowledgement of the scope of nursing practice. Mental health is part of the core business of every nurse, whether by the direct care the nurse provides or by referral to a specialist service.

CONSUMER'S STORY 1.1

Maria

I had a difficult childhood and found myself on the streets at the age of 13 doing what I had to do to survive. I married young to a violent man and had four children. I didn't start using drugs until I was in my mid-40s when I was told that speed (methamphetamine) wasn't addictive! Before too long I was injecting and had a $300 a day habit. I even injected it into my neck when I couldn't find a vein in my arm. I was always chasing the dragon (trying to get that incredible feeling of elation experienced at the first taste). I was a junkie, and nothing mattered more than getting my next hit. Not even my kids. Eventually I realised I had a problem, so I walked down to my local GP and asked for some help. I was told they didn't work with people like me. I was stunned but I walked further along the street to another GP and was standing at the reception desk asking if someone would see me when one of the doctors, who just happened to be standing near the desk, invited me into his office right there and then. He referred me to the mental health nurse working at the practice and I saw both of them for the next several years. She (the mental health nurse) would see me at home even when I didn't want to see her! There were times when I wouldn't see her because I'd started using again and I was too ashamed to look her in the eye. But she kept coming back. After 10 years of addiction I've now been clean for more than 2 years. I now have a 'normal' life. I work two jobs but, more importantly, I have a pretty good relationship with my kids and a fantastic relationship with my three gorgeous grandkids. And now I've been cigarette-free for almost 11 months.

Chapter summary

Mental health matters because mental health problems are prevalent in our society, have significant personal, social and economic impacts, present in every clinical setting, and form part of the nursing scope of practice. Mental health is part of health. Mental health problems impact on the course and severity of physical health problems and are associated with worse health outcomes. Mental health consumers experience high rates of physical health disorders, are less likely to have physical health issues attended to and die younger than those in the general population. People with physical illnesses experience worse mental health than those without illness, and mental health problems adversely affect treatment, recovery and quality of life. Nurses have opportunities to use mental health skills to improve consumers' mental and physical health.

Responding to the mental health needs of patients is a professional obligation of nurses. Nurses do not need to be specialists to respond to patients' mental health needs. Fundamental mental health nursing skills such as listening, validating and responding empathically will help meet the mental health needs of patients in all clinical settings. Nurses can also learn and develop skills in specific therapeutic modalities. In some cases, nurses will feel they need to ask for further advice about a patient's needs or to refer the patient to a mental health specialist. Every nurse is not a *specialist* mental health nurse, just as every nurse is not a specialist in diabetes care, coronary care or primary care. But just as mental health is part of health, mental health is part of every nurse's scope of practice.

EXERCISES FOR CLASS ENGAGEMENT

After reading this chapter discuss the following scenarios in small groups.

SCENARIO 1

Mental health is part of the scope of practice of every nurse. However, the mental health needs of consumers in general health settings (such as medical and surgical wards and primary care) are frequently overlooked. Discuss the possible barriers to nurses in general settings responding to consumers' mental health needs. Make a list of the six most important barriers. Consider individual, system and policy-level barriers.

SCENARIO 2

Taking the list made in discussing scenario 1 above, identify strategies that would help nurses in addressing the identified barriers. The strategies may need support from others to implement.

SCENARIO 3

Many individual, social and political factors can influence mental health. Conversely, mental distress and illness can impact on employment, social organisation and the economy.

1. Identify five social factors that can influence a person's mental health.
2. For each factor discuss how that factor can be addressed.
3. Identify five social impacts of mental distress or illness.
4. For each factor discuss how the impact of mental distress or illness could be reduced.

SCENARIO 4

Rebecca is a 32-year-old woman who has been feeling increasingly tired and 'strung out' after the birth of her first child 5 months ago. When she visits her GP to ask for medication to help her sleep the GP asks a primary care nurse to interview Rebecca and assess her mood, safety and sleep. Rebecca is surprised to learn that the nurse considers she may be depressed.

1. What initial support and intervention could be considered for Rebecca?
2. What areas of assessment would you consider in interviewing Rebecca?
3. What would you consider before recommending to the GP that Rebecca is prescribed medication for her mood?
4. At what point would you consider referring Rebecca to a specialist mental health clinician for further assessment and treatment? (Refer to the outline of stepped care on page 11).

Useful websites

Australian Bureau of Statistics Mental Health Australia: https://mhaustralia.org/.

Australian Government Department of Health *PHN mental health tools and resources*: http://www.health.gov.au/internet/main/publishing.nsf/content/phn-mental_tools.

Black Dog Institute, Australia: https://www.blackdoginstitute.org.au/.

Health Navigator New Zealand: https://www.healthnavigator.org.nz/health-a-z/m/mental-illness/.

Mental Health Australia: https://mhaustralia.org.

Mental Health Commission, Australia: https://www.mentalhealthcommission.gov.au/.

Mental Health Coordinating Council: http://www.mhcc.org.au/about-mhcc/.

Mental health data and statistics (New Zealand): https://www.health.govt.nz/nz-health-statistics/health-statistics-and-data-sets/mental-health-data-and-stats.

Mental health data, Australia: https://www1.health.gov.au/internet/main/publishing.nsf/Content/PHN-Mental_Health_Data.

Mental Health Foundation of New Zealand: www.mentalhealth.org.nz.

Wellplace New Zealand: https://wellplace.nz/facts-and-information/mental-wellbeing/mental-health-in-new-zealand/.

References

Australian Bureau of Statistics (ABS), 2008. National Survey of Mental Health and Wellbeing: Summary of results. Cat. No. 4326.0. Commonwealth of Australia, Canberra.

Australian Bureau of Statistics (ABS), 2018. National Health Survey First results. Australia 2017–18. Commonwealth of Australia, Canberra.

Australian College of Mental Health Nurses, 2010. Standards of Practice for Mental Health Nursing in Australia. Canberra, Australian College of Mental Health Nursing.

Australian Government Department of Health, 2019. PHN Mental Health Flexible Funding Pool Programme Guidance: Stepped Care, Canberra: Australian Government Department of Health.

Australian Institute of Health and Welfare, 2019. Deaths in Australia. Cat. no. PHE 229. Canberra: AIHW. https://www.aihw.gov.au/reports/life-expectancy-death/deaths-in-australia. (Accessed 9 February 2020).

Balagopal, G., Kapanee, A.R.M., 2019. Lessons learnt from NGO approaches to mental healthcare provision in the community. In: Mental Health Care Services in Community Settings. Springer, Singapore, pp. 185–204.

Burns, R.A., 2016. Sex and age trends in Australia's suicide rate over the last decade: something is still seriously wrong with men in middle and late life. Psychiatry Res. 245, 224–229.

Caneo, C., Marston, L., Bellón, J.Á., et al., 2016. Examining the relationship between physical illness and depression: is there a difference between inflammatory and non inflammatory diseases? A cohort study. Gen. Hosp. Psychiatry 43, 71–77.

Chan, M.K., Bhatti, H., Meader, N., et al., 2016. Predicting suicide following self-harm: systematic review of risk factors and risk scales. Br. J. Psychiatry 209 (4), 277–283.

Cleary, M., Raeburn, T., West, S., et al., 2018. Two approaches, one goal: how mental health registered nurses perceive their role and the role of peer support workers in facilitating consumer decision-making. Int. J. Ment. Health Nurs. 27 (4), 1212–1218.

Commonwealth of Australia, 2012. Mental health statement of rights and responsibilities 2012. Canberra, Commonwealth of Australia.

Crane, D.A., Lepicki, T., Knudsen, K., 2016. Unique and common elements of the role of peer support in the context of traditional mental health services. Psychiatr. Rehabil. J. 39 (3), 282.

Damery, S., Brown, C., Sein, K., et al., 2019. The prevalence of mild-to-moderate distress in patients with end-stage renal disease: results from a patient survey using the emotion thermometers in four hospital trusts in the West Midlands, UK. BMJ Open 9 (5), e027982.

Davison, K., 2006. Historical aspects of mood disorders. Psychiatry 5 (4), 115–118.

de Munter, L., Polinder, S., Haagsma, J.A., et al., 2020. Prevalence and prognostic factors for psychological distress after trauma. Arch. Phys. Med. Rehabil. 101 (5), 877–884.

Firth, J., Siddiqi, N., Koyanagi, A., et al., 2019. The Lancet Psychiatry Commission: a blueprint for protecting physical health in people with mental illness. Lancet Psychiatry 6 (8), 675–712.

Gilbertson-White, S., Campbell, G., Ward, S., et al., 2017. Coping with pain severity, distress, and consequences in women with ovarian cancer. Cancer Nurs. 40 (2), 117.

Grech, E., Raeburn, T., 2019. Experiences of hospitalised homeless adults and their health care providers in OECD nations: a literature review. Collegian 26 (1), 204–211.

Gürhan, N., Beşer, N.G., Polat, Ü., et al., 2019. Suicide risk and depression in individuals with chronic illness. Community Ment. Health J. 55 (5), 840–848.

Harrison, J., Henley, G., 2014. Suicide and hospitalised self-harm in Australia: trends and analysis. Injury research and statistics series. Canberra: AIHW.

Inoue, M., Yamaoka, K., 2017. Social factors associated with psychological distress and health problems among elderly members of a disaster-affected population: subgroup analysis of a 1-year post-disaster survey in Ishinomaki area, Japan. Disaster Med. Public Health Prep. 11 (1), 64–71.

Islam, F.M.A., 2019. Psychological distress and its association with socio-demographic factors in a rural district in Bangladesh: a cross-sectional study. PLoS ONE 14 (3), e0212765.

Jayasuriya, D., Jayasuriya, R., Tay, A.K., et al., 2016. Associations of mental distress with residency in conflict zones, ethnic minority status, and potentially modifiable social factors following conflict in Sri Lanka: a nationwide cross-sectional study. Lancet Psychiatry 3 (2), 145–153.

Kang, S.K., Bodenhausen, G.V., 2015. Multiple identities in social perception and interaction: challenges and opportunities. Annu. Rev. Psychol. 66, 547–574.

Kolappa, K., Henderson, D.C., Kishore, S.P., 2013. No physical health without mental health: lessons unlearned? Bull. World Health Organ. 91, 3–3A.

Kurtz, D.L.M., Janke, R., Vinek, J., et al., 2018. Health sciences cultural safety education in Australia, Canada, New Zealand, and the United States: a literature review. Int. J. Med. Educ. 9, 271–285.

Laverty, M., McDermott, D.R., Calma, T., 2017. Embedding cultural safety in Australia's main health care standards. Med. J. Aust. 207 (1), 15–16.

Lubbe, J.C., Roets, L., 2014. Nurses' scope of practice and the implication for quality nursing care. J. Nurs. Scholarsh. 46 (1), 58–64.

Maybery, D., Jones, R., Dipnall, J.F., et al., 2019. A mixed-methods study of psychological distress following an environmental catastrophe: the case of the Hazelwood open-cut coalmine fire in Australia. Anxiety Stress Coping 33 (2), 216–230.

McCarthy, M.M., Whittemore, R., Gholson, G., et al., 2019. Diabetes distress, depressive symptoms, and cardiovascular health in adults with type 1 diabetes. Nurs. Res. 68 (6), 445–452.

McPhillips, R., Salmon, P., Wells, A., et al., 2019. Cardiac rehabilitation patients' accounts of their emotional distress and psychological needs: a qualitative study. J. Am. Heart Assoc. 8 (11), e011117.

Mental Health Commission of NSW, 2016. Physical health and mental wellbeing: evidence guide, Sydney, Mental Health Commission of NSW.

Ministry of Health, 2018. He Ara Oranga. Report of the Government Inquiry into Mental Health and Addiction, Wellington: Ministry of Health.

Ministry of Health, 2016. Annual Update of Key Results 2015/16: New Zealand Health Survey. Wellington: Ministry of Health.

Ministry of Health, 2017. Briefing to the Incoming Minister of Health 2017: The New Zealand Health and Disability System. Wellington: Ministry of Health.

Ministry of Health, 2019. Every life matters – He Tapu te Oranga o ia tangata: suicide prevention strategy 2019–2029 and suicide prevention action plan 2019–2024 for Aotearoa New Zealand. Wellington: Ministry of Health.

Morgan, V.A., Waterreus, A., Jablensky, A., et al., 2012. People living with psychotic illness in 2010: the second Australian national survey of psychosis. Aust. N. Z. J. Psychiatry 46 (8), 735–752.

Mortier, P., Cuijpers, P., Kiekens, G., et al., 2018. The prevalence of suicidal thoughts and behaviours among college students: a meta-analysis. Psychol. Med. 48 (4), 554–565.

Nasif, J., 2015. The emotional impact of chronic illness. J. Psychol. Clin. Psychiatry 3 (6), 00177.

Neil, A.L., Carr, V.J., Mihalopoulos, C., et al., 2014. Costs of psychosis in 2010: findings from the second Australian National Survey of Psychosis. Aust. N. Z. J. Psychiatry 48 (2), 169–182.

NiaNia, W., Bush, A., Epston, D., 2017. Collaborative and Indigenous Mental Health Therapy. Tataihono – Stories of Maori Healing and Psychiatry. Routledge, New York.

Nursing Council of New Zealand, 2011 Guidelines for Cultural Safety, the Treaty of Waitangi and Maori Health in Nursing Education and Practice. Wellington. Nursing Council of New Zealand.

O'Brien, A., 2014. Every nurse is a mental health nurse. Nurs. N. Z. 20 (8), 2.

O'Brien, A.J., DeSouza, R., Baker, M., 2017. Providing culturally safe care. In: Chambers, M. (Ed.), Psychiatric and Mental Health Nursing. The Craft of Caring. Routledge, London, pp. 419–430.

Oakley Browne, M.A., Wells, J.E., Scott, K.M., et al., 2006. Lifetime prevalence and projected lifetime risk of DSM-IV disorders in Te Rau Hinengaro: the New Zealand Mental Health Survey. Aust. N. Z. J. Psychiatry 40 (10), 865–874.

Olver, J.S., Hopwood, M.J., 2013. Depression and physical illness. Med. J. Aust. 199, S9–S12.

Perkins, D., Williams, A., McDonald, J., et al., 2017. What is the place of generalism in mental health care in Australia?: A systematic review of the literature. Australian Primary Health Care Research Institute. Available at: https://openresearch-repository.anu.edu.au/handle/1885/119238.

Prioreschi, P., 1991. Possible reasons for neolithic skull trephining. Perspect. Biol. Med. 34 (2), 296–303.

Productivity Commission, 2019. Mental Health, Draft Report, Australian Government, Canberra.

Rhodes, A., 2013. Youth suicide in Canada: distinctions among boys and girls. Healthc. Q. 16 (3), 11–13.

Summers, A., Leidman, E., Periquito, I.M.P.F., et al., 2019. Serious psychological distress and disability among older persons living in conflict affected areas in eastern Ukraine: a cluster-randomized cross-sectional household survey. Confl. Health 13 (1), 10.

Tapsell, R., Hallett, C., Mellsop, G., 2018. The rate of mental health service use in New Zealand as analysed by ethnicity. Australas Psychiatry 26 (3), 290–293.

Tauranga, M., Moore, D., 2018. Adult Māori patients' healthcare experiences of the emergency department in a district health facility in New Zealand. Int. J. Indig. Health 13 (1), 87–103.

Te Ao Maramatanga (New Zealand College of Mental Health Nurses), 2012. Standard of Practice for Mental Health Nursing in New Zealand. Auckland: Te Ao Maramatanga.

Te Pou o Te Whakaaro Nui, 2017. The physical health of people with mental health conditions and/or addiction. Evidence update: December 2017. Auckland: Te Pou o Te Whakaaro Nui.

Te Pou o Te Whakaaro Nui, 2014a. The physical health of people with a serious mental illness and/or addiction: an evidence review. Te Pou o te Whakaaro Nui, Auckland.

Te Pou o Te Whakaaro Nui, 2014b. Take action to improve physical health outcomes for New Zealanders who experience mental illness and/or addiction. A consensus position paper. Auckland: Te Pou o Te Whakaaro Nui.

Te Pou o Te Whakaaro, 2012. Talking Therapies: Where to Next? Te Pou o te Whakaaro Nui, Auckland.

Thomas, H.J., Chan, G.C., Scott, J.G., et al., 2016. Association of different forms of bullying victimisation with adolescents' psychological distress and reduced emotional wellbeing. Aust. N. Z. J. Psychiatry 50 (4), 371–379.

Tomitaka, S., Kawasaki, Y., Ide, K., et al., 2019. Distribution of psychological distress is stable in recent decades and follows an exponential pattern in the US population. Sci. Rep. 9 (1), 1–10.

Trueman, S.W., 2013. Contextualizing mental health nursing encounters in Australian remote Aboriginal communities: part 2, client encounters and interviews. Issues Ment. Health Nurs. 34 (10), 772–775.

Vicary, D., Westerman, T., 2004. That's just the way he is': some implications of Aboriginal mental health beliefs. Aust. e-J. Adv. Ment. Health 3 (3), 103–112.

Walker, E.R., McGee, R.E., Druss, B.G., 2015. Mortality in mental disorders and global disease burden implications: a systematic review and meta-analysis. JAMA Psychiatry 72 (4), 334–341.

White, J., Hemingway, S., Stephenson, J., 2014. Training mental health nurses to assess the physical health needs of mental health service users: a pre-and post-test analysis. Perspect. Psychiatr. Care 50 (4), 243–250.

Wilson, A., Reilly, R., Mackean, T., 2018. Analysis of factors associated with Aboriginal and Torres Strait Islander suicide in Australia: a scoping review. Transcult. Psychiatry Manuscript submitted for publication.

World Health Organization (WHO), 2019. Mental health. who.int/news-room/facts-in-pictures/detail/mental-health.

World Health Organization (WHO), 2014. Constitution of the World Health Organization, Geneva: WHO.

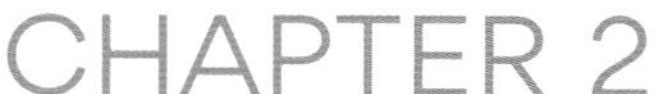

CHAPTER 2

Nursing and mental health in context

Kim Foster, Peta Marks, Anthony J O'Brien and Toby Raeburn

KEY POINTS

- Developing therapeutic relationships is the key to effective nursing practice in mental health.
- Together, nurses and mental health consumers develop therapeutic alliances as a basis for consumers' growth and recovery.
- A social ecological approach to mental health nursing practice provides a framework for holistic practice.
- Self-awareness, insight and reflexivity are fundamental skills for nursing practice in mental health.
- Nursing practice occurs in the broader context of mental health, including the social determinants of mental health.

KEY TERMS

- Caring
- Compassion
- Empathy
- Healing
- Hope
- Professional boundaries
- Recovery
- Reflection
- Self
- Self-awareness
- Self-disclosure
- Social determinants
- Social ecological
- Spirituality
- Therapeutic alliance

LEARNING OUTCOMES

The material in this chapter will assist you to:

- describe the social ecological approach to mental health nursing practice
- identify the social determinants of mental health
- describe therapeutic relationships and how they are developed in the context of a person's mental health
- describe the three components of empathy
- define self-awareness and describe a strategy for developing self-awareness.

Introduction

Mental health nursing is one of the most interesting and challenging areas of nursing practice. The challenge of mental health nursing is working with people who are experiencing mental and emotional distress and may doubt themselves, the environment and the people around them. The reward of this work is often the satisfaction of using knowledge and skill to provide a context of safety and care where trust in self and others can be re-established. Mental health nursing requires a fusion of personal characteristics, professional knowledge, experience and clinical and interpersonal skills. People with mental illnesses have complex and sometimes long-term needs. They may engage in frequent and regular encounters with the healthcare system or have a one-off experience that brings them in to contact with mental health services or providers. The long-term and cyclic nature of some mental illnesses means that the therapeutic relationships between mental health nurses and consumers can last for long periods. The relationship will also vary in intensity as consumers move along a continuum between periods of high dependence at one end (in acute phases when they are experiencing acute distress or illness) and independence at the other (when their symptoms are less troublesome or their mental illness has resolved).

This chapter outlines the social ecological framework for mental health nursing practice that frames the text. This is a holistic framework for practice and the various elements of the framework are described: therapeutic relationships and consumer–nurse partnership; personal and contextual factors influencing practice; identities including gender and culture (nurse and consumer); and the context of practice (including social determinants of health and major approaches to mental health care – recovery-oriented care and trauma-informed care). The remainder of the chapter explores the interpersonal relationship as the foundation of effective mental health nursing practice and the knowledge, attitudes and skills needed to work with people in mental distress. Key concepts and issues that are fundamental to effective and safe mental health nursing practice are introduced. Holistic and skilful mental health nursing requires a sound knowledge of human physiology, health and illness, as well as a biopsychosocial understanding of mental illnesses and their treatments, including pharmacology. In addition, to practise effectively nurses working in mental health need to be open-minded and reflective and to have developed an understanding of concepts such as compassion, empathy, spirituality and hope. Personal qualities such as responsiveness, self-awareness and insight are essential for effective therapeutic relationships. Nurses in all settings care for the mental health and wellbeing of consumers, and mental health skills are required of all nurses and can be applied in all clinical settings.

Social ecological approach to mental health nursing practice

In this text we take a social ecological approach to mental health nursing practice. A social ecological perspective refers to the dynamic interactions between a person and their environment that influence their health and wellbeing. This person–environment interaction involves a number of factors and processes. Mental health can be understood as involving a person's physical, mental, emotional and spiritual characteristics and the interactive processes that occur between them and their environment or ecology (including their social and family context). This includes being able to access available resources that help sustain their mental health (Ungar 2011) and support their recovery such as human resources and supports including family and friends, healthcare resources including nursing care and mental healthcare (hospital or community-based) and practical resources such as financial support and housing. A social ecological or holistic perspective is relevant to understanding mental health and mental health nursing practice because mental health problems can challenge people in, and are challenged by, every aspect of their life. Similarly, nursing practice is shaped by our personal characteristics and skills and the health service context we work in. This dynamic person–environment interaction involves personal and contextual factors that influence nurses' practice and their relationships with consumers.

Therefore, from an ecological perspective nursing practice includes:

- nurses' personal characteristics (e.g. their personality, interpersonal style, cultural and gender identity, and nursing knowledge, attitudes and skills)
- therapeutic relationships and interpersonal interactions between nurses and consumers
- cultural and practice context within which a nurse and consumer are based
- available people and resources that can be accessed to support consumers' recovery.

Fig. 2.1 provides a diagrammatic representation of all these elements and their interactions. The following section outlines each of the elements.

Social determinants of health

In relation to the context or environment of mental health, the social determinants of health are the social and economic circumstances within which we are born and live (World Health Organization (WHO) 2018). These determinants are shaped by the distribution of power and resources in society and can lead to health inequities because they have a direct influence on the prevalence and severity of mental health conditions, which can extend across the life course (WHO 2018).

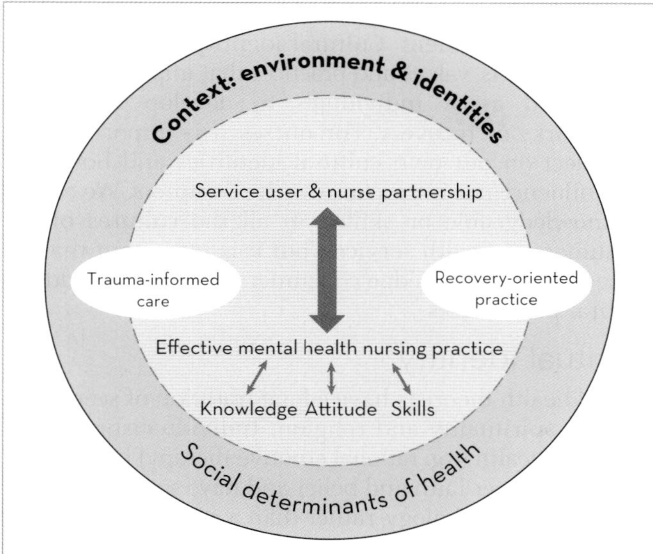

Figure 2.1
Social ecological approach to mental health nursing practice

In respect to mental health, key social determinants that directly influence health and quality of life include:

- mental health stigma
- poverty
- violence
- forced migration
- insecure living conditions including homelessness (WHO 2018).

Because mental ill health is strongly determined by these factors, mental health problems are not able to be improved by mental health treatments alone. The social factors that have contributed to these problems also need to be addressed and, wherever possible, eliminated. Social determinants can be either proximal or distal. Proximal factors are those that act directly to influence health (e.g. ongoing trauma), whereas distal factors act more indirectly (e.g. social deprivation). There is a need for targeted reduction of social determinants. To reduce the burden of mental ill health, Lund et al. (2018), using an ecological framework, identified the proximal and distal social determinants that are risk and/or protective factors for mental ill health according to five domains (see also Table 2.1):

- demographic
- economic
- neighbourhood
- environmental
- social and cultural.

An ecological approach to nursing therefore requires that nurses understand and address the social contexts within which people live. Nurses working clinically do not necessarily have the capacity to influence, prevent or intervene with all these factors, but it is vitally important when working with mental health consumers, and as relevant for the person, that these factors are taken into consideration and identified as part of history taking and assessment. As part of the work of the multidisciplinary team, a number of these factors can be directly addressed to help decrease risk and increase protection against further ill health – for example, negotiating adequate housing for consumers (and ensuring people are not discharged if they have nowhere to go), helping to build social support for consumers who are isolated and providing psychological support for the psychological impacts of trauma and associated distress such as a trauma-informed approach to care. An ecological approach to nursing also requires that nurses understand the environments within which they practice.

TABLE 2.1 Social and cultural determinants of mental disorders

DOMAIN	PROXIMAL	DISTAL
Demographic	Age Gender Ethnicity	Community diversity Population density Longevity Survival
Economic	Income Debt Assets Financial strain Relative deprivation Unemployment Food security	Economic recessions Economic inequality Macroeconomic
Neighbourhood	Safety and security Housing structure Overcrowding Recreation	Infrastructure Neighbourhood deprivation Built environment Setting Safety and security
Environmental	Natural disasters Industrial disasters War or conflict Climate change Forced migration	Trauma Distress
Social and cultural	Community social capital Social stability Cultural	Individual social capital Social participation Social support Education

Adapted from Lund et al. 2018

Contexts of mental health: environment and identities

In terms of the contexts within which nurses practise it is important for nurses to understand that the models of care and the health service approach within which they work directly influence their practice. Equally, nursing practice can influence and shape the environments within which we work. People admitted to hospitals can pose unique ethical challenges to nurses because they may experience episodes of mental ill health that necessitate compulsory admission under mental health legislation, removing part or all of their autonomy due to considerations of risk and safety. Involuntary admission often makes it difficult for nurses to apply recovery-oriented approaches that seek to provide people with choice and opportunity to develop strengths. Working in such challenging environments means that nurses need not only have an up-to-date working knowledge of health conditions and interventions but also need to be able to empathise with the difficulties consumers face as they navigate their recovery from experiences of mental ill health within what are often disconnected and under-resourced healthcare systems (Cleary et al. 2018a).

CULTURAL, SEXUAL AND SPIRITUAL IDENTITIES

The concept of identity

Identity can be thought of as an individual's enduring sense of themselves as a person. It is the answer people give to the question: 'Who am I?' Psychologists have traditionally defined identity in individualistic terms, with an emphasis on developing stable personality traits. However, identity is deeply influenced by belonging to, or difference from, significant social groups – for example, cultural groups, religious faiths and peer groups. By identifying with the values and beliefs of a social group we come to define our own unique sense of who we are. Others have argued that identity is inherently unstable, constantly in transition and made up of multiple components or identities. Some examples of identity are outlined below, but it is important to remember that individuals will have multiple identities and that these may change over the course of their lives. Nurses should not presume to know what a consumer's identities are and should not expect individuals to conform to stereotyped ideas about what a particular identity means to an individual.

Cultural identity

Cultural identity refers to a person's sense of belonging to one or more cultural groups. For indigenous Australians and New Zealanders, indigenous culture may be their most important source of identity, but they may also identify, through ancestry or association, with non-indigenous cultures. Most healthcare providers support consumers to declare their own cultural identity, and clinicians should respect this statement. Cultural identity is an important source of beliefs, values and practices that impact on mental health and assist individuals to develop their own frameworks of recovery. For nurses it is important that we reflect on our own cultural identities and how they may influence our interactions with consumers. We cannot be knowledgeable or skilled in all the cultures of the consumers of health services, but it is important that we respectfully acknowledge consumers' culture and address cultural preferences.

Spiritual identity

Mental health theorists have a long tradition of scepticism towards spirituality and religion. Individualistic models of mental health (e.g. rational emotive therapy) have valued rationalism over faith and belief and have seen spirituality as a source of pathology, rather than a resource for mental health. The increasing diversity of our communities challenges this view and leads to spirituality and religious faith being regarded as central to identity and to psychosocial functioning. While clinical support can help people manage distress and develop coping strategies, spirituality can provide a sense of hope and acceptance in the face of seemingly insurmountable life problems. Although spirituality is often associated with religious faith, many people have a non-religious worldview while still maintaining spiritual beliefs and values. Others have both religious and non-religious worldviews. As nurses we will not always share the spiritual beliefs of consumers. However, as with cultural identity, it is important that consumers feel their spiritual beliefs and values are recognised as an important part of their identities and that they are supported in maintaining their spirituality as part of their recovery.

Gender identity

Gender is another source of identity where previous mental health practice has treated difference as pathology and sought to impose compulsory treatment on individuals whose gender identity and sexual preferences did not fit dominant social norms. From being perceived as a fixed function of biology (individuals were assigned either male or female gender at birth, with no anticipation of change), gender is now seen as a fluid, socially constructed concept. A range of terms reflects the changing perspectives on gender in contemporary society, reflected in the term 'LGBTIQ+', which incorporates the range of gender identities nurses will encounter. Specific terms for gender include bisexual, trans, gay, gender diverse, queer, intersex and cis-gender. Gender should not be confused with sexual preference, which refers to an individual's gender preferences in intimate relationships. Preferences are not necessarily fixed and can change in the course of psychosocial development. As a nurse you will meet people with gender identities and sexual preferences different from your own. It is important that you become comfortable with relating to gender diverse consumers, as gender and sexuality can often be a source of distress due to stigma and prejudice.

Identity, stress and mental illness

While a strongly developed sense of who we are as a person is important to our mental health, identity can also be a source of stress for those whose identities are disvalued and subject to stigmatising views and prejudice. The term 'minority stress' (Spittlehouse et al. 2019) refers to the experience of stigma and discrimination encountered by people in relation to their identity. This can relate to culture and ethnicity, religious affiliation, gender and sexuality and other aspects of identity. Discrimination can create a hostile environment in which minority stress leads to symptoms of mental illness including depression, anxiety, suicidal ideation and harmful substance use. People who are subject to one form of marginalisation are more likely to also experience other forms of marginalisation, a concept referred to as 'intersectionality' (Grzanka & Brian 2019). Nurses encounter many consumers who experience one or more forms or marginalisation and need to be aware of how these experiences shape the person's health experience and the responses of clinicians. Supporting consumers to negotiate contested identities enhances their mental health and helps build resilience for living in an environment in which stigma and discrimination are regrettably common.

Historical anecdote 2.1: Stigma and mental illness

In his 1963 book *Stigma: Notes on the Management of Spoiled Identity*, sociologist Erving Goffman identified three types of stigma, each of which led to disvalued identity. Goffman argued that people with mental illness experience character stigma as they are perceived as weak, unreliable and possibly dangerous, and social stigma through which disvalued aspects of being labelled 'mentally ill' lead to the person being seen as associated with a disvalued group. Goffman's work led to a focus on the negative effects of stigma on people with mental illness, including the internalisation of stigma by which individuals come to believe the negative stereotypes of the dominant social group. Goffman also argued that people who work in mental health, such as nurses, are subject to 'courtesy stigma' because their identity is influenced by their association with a socially disvalued group.

Read more about it: *Goffman E 1963 Stigma: notes on the management of spoiled identity. Prentice-Hall, Englewood Cliffs*

Working within recovery-oriented and trauma-informed approaches to care

A significant amount of research has explored outcomes experienced by people with mental illness over the past 100 years. Most of these studies have used an approach to understanding recovery developed by mental health professionals referred to as 'clinical recovery' (Slade et al. 2012). This concept considers mental illness as a health condition that is in need of clinical treatment. As such, in common with recovery from most physical illnesses, working from this perspective involves the expectation that recovery should include a substantial reduction of symptoms and restoration of function in work and relationships. This conceptualisation has enabled researchers to measure recovery in terms of 'hard' data such as numbers of people who cease needing medication, avoid hospitalisation or regain paid employment. Studies that have used the paradigm of clinical recovery suggest little improvement has been made in rates of recovery over the past 100 years. For example, a meta-analysis that reviewed the results of 50 studies published between 1921 and 2010 suggested that only 13% of people with schizophrenia experience recovery (Jääskeläinen et al. 2012). Despite the poor outcomes identified in this research, people with a lived experience of mental illness (consumers) often have more hopeful stories to tell about their recovery journey.

As people with lived experience of mental illness have gained political influence over the past few decades, they have challenged the concept of clinical recovery and models of care that focus on medical treatment alone (Cleary et al. 2018b). This has led to a review of how recovery from mental illness is understood. People with lived experience have emphasised that recovery is a personal journey (i.e. personal recovery) and that many people who are labelled or diagnosed with a mental illness have a substantial history of trauma. The next section of this chapter overviews recovery-oriented and trauma-informed care approaches that have been developed to support people with mental illness in their personal recovery. These approaches are increasingly used in mental health care and can be used by nurses to support people who are experiencing mental distress or illness.

RECOVERY-ORIENTED CARE

The concept of 'personal recovery' emerged from the consumer movement that developed in the second half of the 20th century to advocate for the rights of people living with mental illness. In their view, recovery was more about a personal developmental journey rather than just a health condition in need of clinical treatment (Warner 2010). There is no single definition of mental health recovery;

however, one of the most commonly used explanations was written by Bill Anthony (1993), who described it as:

> A deeply personal, unique process of changing one's attitudes, values, feelings, goals, skills and/or roles. It is a way of living a satisfying, hopeful, and contributing life even with limitations caused by the illness. Recovery involves the development of new meaning and purpose in one's life as a person grows beyond the catastrophic effects of mental illness.
>
> Anthony 1993, p. 15

Beginning with personal accounts of recovery journeys published by people with a history of mental illness such as Deegan (1988) and Leete (1989), a large body of literature has developed describing the lived experience of mental health recovery. Personal narratives are essential to recovery-informed perspectives and for determining what is important for any individual in their journey of recovery. Case study 2.1, about the recovery of Mary O'Hagan, a prominent international consumer 'survivor', educator and consultant, illustrates the tension between what people say is important to them and what professionals and the system focus on. This tension is underscored by the fact that although many people find meaning in their 'madness', the people they turn to for support view it primarily as pathological and something to be managed and medicated. Table 2.2 draws a distinction between recovery-informed practice and traditional practice.

CASE STUDY 2.1
Mary O'Hagan's story

In common with so many people who experience mental distress, Mary describes her madness as the loss of self, the solid core of her being. While this core is not evident during times of madness, it returns stronger, renewed and ready to go again. Madness is a crisis of being that is a part of the full range of human experience. Mary explains:

> My self is the solid core of my being. It is like an immutable dark sun that sits at the centre of things while all my fickle feelings, thoughts and sensations orbit around it. But my self goes into hiding during madness. Sometimes it slides into the great nothingness like a setting sun. Sometimes it gets trampled in the dust by all the whizzing in my body and mind ... Sometimes my madness strips me bare but it is also the beginning of renewal; every time I emerge from it I feel fresh and ready to start again.

Mary had to make friends with rather than fight her madness, to get to know, understand and respect it – a complex process.

> My madness was like a boarder coming to live in my house, who turned out to be a citizen from an enemy country. Knowing I might not get rid of him meant I had to make peace with him and learn to understand his language. Once I got to know the boarder, he was no longer the stereotypical enemy, but a complex character that deserved some respect.

Mental health professionals did not find any value in helping Mary to understand the meaning in her madness. Nor did they allow her to tap into her own power, her own resourcefulness. Mary's experience of care within mental health services was one of being 'skilled in lowered expectations' – for example, repeatedly being told that things such as studying or working would be too stressful and she would not be able to do them. The way mental health care was provided to Mary encouraged passivity rather than autonomy. She found the capacity to tap into her own resourcefulness only by coming across the consumer/survivor literature that inspired her. She was then able to find and use her own power to get out of the cycle of madness. Mary went on to be appointed as a mental health commissioner in New Zealand and has been an international consultant on mental health since that time.

What was most difficult for Mary was not the symptoms but how people regarded her. In retrospect her madness was a place of beauty and difficulty, madness filled with soul. Mary talks about the terrible suffering and the desperate struggle of her madness, but she also talks about the richness in her experience that she could interpret as filled with purpose and meaning. She wanted acceptance of her reality. For Mary, the best thing people could have done was to be kind and accept her reality – a basic human response.

We encourage you to visit Mary's website at ***www.maryohagan.com*** *to learn more about her story.*

EXERCISE FOR CLASS ENGAGEMENT

Is Mary O'Hagan's experience an isolated one? Is it an 'old' story that would not happen today?

In 2012 Glover presented the stories of two women and their personal experiences of mental distress managed in Australia by involuntary inpatient admissions. The women's perceptions of their care included that they were not helped to make sense of their experiences, felt stripped of their power and were not responded to as people but as 'diagnostic categories'. Their experiences were described using the language and meaning of the professional knowledge base; their own meaning and language for their experiences were not encouraged or valued. What makes Glover's work so powerful is that while both women

TABLE 2.2 Key differences between recovery-informed and traditional practice

RECOVERY-INFORMED PRACTICE	TRADITIONAL PRACTICE
• Person is central • Driven by a human rights agenda • Connecting with and maintaining meaningful roles, relationships and community is key; many things contribute to recovery • Looks for possibilities and promotes hope • Collaborative risk management with the person • Learns from people's narratives of recovery	• Illness and symptoms are central • Driven by the medical model • Propensity for person's life to revolve around and be taken over by illness • Looks for constraints and sets limits and lower expectations • Focuses on risk control by others • Personal narratives not a focus of care
• The person has expertise gained from their experience of mental health challenges • Medication is a small part of management; types and doses are titrated for the individual • The person is the change agent • Takes a stance of 'unknowing' and curiosity to help uncover the meaning people make of their experience • Empowering for the person to be acknowledged for their expertise • Promotes self-directed care requiring the active involvement of the person • Explores what is important to the person; recognises unique experience and takes spirituality into account • Connects with the person's strengths and draws on them to overcome challenges • Choice and ability to connect with a broad range of services in community • Peer support or peer-run services are essential • Trauma-informed care asks: 'What has happened to you?'	• The professional is the expert on the person's experience • Treatment of symptoms, usually with medications, is the main form of intervention • The program is the change agent • Takes a stance of 'knowing' and looks for confirmation of symptoms to make a diagnosis • Symptoms are more important than personal meaning • Promotes passivity and compliance • Recovery primarily involves the active involvement of others • Informs people about illness and what is important to them to manage it; spirituality not taken into account • Focuses on deficits to treat and manage • Choice of services can be limited • Peer support limited or non-existent • Not trauma-informed – the background issues ('What is wrong with you?') are more important
• Recovery is moving beyond premorbid functioning towards thriving and developing a new sense of self • Non-linear process • Timeframes meaningless – ongoing process • Crisis is a time of learning how to thrive; an active recovery space	• Recovery is, at best, returning to a premorbid level of functioning • Linear process of interventions • Recovery is the end point of the process • Crisis is viewed as a relapse and failure

had very similar experiences, one story took place in 1985 and the other in 2010. The latter occurred at a time when services were promoting their model of care as 'recovery-informed', leading Glover to ask, what has actually changed in the past 25 years?

In 2011 Leamy et al. undertook a systematic literature review to identify experiences commonly associated with personal recovery. After screening more than 5,000 papers, the authors identified five processes common in personal recovery: connectedness; hope and optimism; identity; meaning in life; and empowerment (Leamy et al. 2011). Not only have experiences associated with personal recovery been well explored but the concept is increasingly incorporated into government mental health policies, including Australia's national mental health service policy and framework for recovery approaches to service provision (Commonwealth of Australia 2013) and the *Fifth National Mental Health and Suicide Prevention Plan* (COAG Health Council 2017). Concepts of recovery have also influenced mental health policy in New Zealand (Mental Health Commission 2012). In respect to mental health recovery, there are five key domains that health professionals and mental health services are expected to practise within:

- promoting a culture and language of hope and optimism
- putting the person first and at the centre of practice and viewing their life holistically
- supporting personal recovery and placing it at the heart of practice
- organisational commitment and workforce development for skilled practitioners and an environment that is conducive to recovery
- action on social inclusion and social determinants of health, mental health and wellbeing (Commonwealth of Australia 2013).

To better understand the sort of practices promoted in government guidelines, Le Boutillier et al. (2011) undertook a qualitative analysis of 30 recovery policy documents from governments in England, Scotland, Ireland, Denmark, New Zealand and the United States. The study found that the policies promoted four common practice domains including organisational commitment, supporting personally defined recovery, working relationship and promoting citizenship. Despite these findings, the authors concluded that a key challenge for mental health services is the continued lack of clarity about what constitutes service-level recovery-oriented practice (Raeburn et al. 2017). This lack of clarity has remained an ongoing knowledge gap, with researchers such as Slade et al. (2015) observing that while government policy may promote the concept of personal recovery, evidence regarding how recovery practices are implemented and whether (and how) this is achieved in practice within individual services is lacking.

Greater collaboration and co-design of services, service planning, policy and research by people with a lived experience of mental illness is required for better recovery-oriented care (Gordon & O'Brien 2018). This requires a purposeful shift away from paternalistic and authoritative ways of treating people towards more mutually respectful person-centred care (Reid et al. 2018). Consumers and carers understand the inadequacies and opportunities that exist within the health and mental health system (Banfield et al. 2018) – after all, they are the ones who are attempting to navigate it! Transforming the health and mental health system to be fully recovery-oriented requires genuine integration of lived experience perspectives, addressing discrimination and factors that inhibit consumer participation at all points in the healthcare continuum.

Trauma-informed care

An essential component of a recovery-oriented approach is to practise within a framework that recognises that many people experiencing mental health challenges have a background of trauma. A trauma or traumatic event can be described as a distressing event – for example, a severe physical injury or a specific experience that triggers mental and emotional distress. Trauma is often linked with loss and grief. Experiences of loss and grief are a universal part of human life. Loss can be described as an event where something that belongs to you and is either precious or has meaning for you has been taken away or destroyed. This encompasses a range of losses, from a 'minor' loss such as losing your wallet to a 'devastating loss' such as losing your home and all your belongings in a bushfire. Bereavement generally refers to being deprived of an object or a person – usually used in the context of losing someone you love through death. Grief has been defined as 'the response to the loss in all of its totality – including its physical, emotional, cognitive, behavioural and spiritual manifestations – and as a natural and normal reaction to loss' (Hall 2014, p. 182).

Research demonstrates clear links between trauma and the onset of a range of mental health problems (Green et al. 2018). This makes it imperative for nurses to be sensitive to the vulnerabilities and potential triggers that may give rise to re-traumatisation and to be aware that this could impede recovery.

While a single-incident traumatic event such as a severe car accident, an unexpected death of a close family member or natural disaster results in disruption to a person's life, it does not necessarily result in crisis. Such an event does, however, signal *a potential risk of impending crisis.* A person's reaction to and perception of the event and the nature of the trauma may lead to an acute crisis state when the person's ability to cope is overwhelmed. In contrast to popular ideas, research indicates that the majority of people exposed to a traumatic event recover after an initial period of destabilisation. After a period of adjustment and recovery, some people will describe positive changes such as a renewed appreciation for life and loved ones, personal growth and enhanced coping strategies (van Weeghel et al. 2019).

A large American study called the Adverse Childhood Experiences (ACE) study began in the late 1990s (Felitti et al. 1998). Participants were asked to report on adverse events experienced during childhood. Adverse childhood events included: experiencing psychological, physical or sexual abuse as a child; living with a mother who was being abused; or living in a household where there were people who abused substances, were suffering from mental illness, were suicidal or had ever been in prison. Researchers found that the more of these adverse events a child experienced, the greater the burden of physical illnesses such as chronic obstructive pulmonary disease and heart disease and mental illnesses such as depression. The researchers for the study have continued to collect data documenting the health status from these initial participants (see the useful websites list at the end of this chapter for more details). These findings have been confirmed in subsequent research, demonstrating that early adversity has lasting impacts – increasing the risk of both physical and mental illness over the course of the person's life (Javier et al. 2019). Children exposed to trauma are less likely to develop resilience and have a more than 50% increased risk of depression (Jones et al. 2018).

Despite the negative effects of trauma and mental ill health, the human brain has a remarkable ability to adapt. Research (some of which dates back more than 100 years) has demonstrated how individuals with significant brain damage arising from physiological disorders such as stroke (cerebral vascular accident) and traumatic brain injury can recover and regain function that seemed to have been lost as a result of the damage (Turolla et al. 2018). The mechanism for this process is the brain's capacity to generate new brain cells (neurogenesis) and to establish alternative neural pathways. The term 'neuroplasticity' was introduced in the 1960s as a way of understanding the reorganisation of neuronal anatomy affecting the structure and function of the brain in response to many external and internal events (Voss et al. 2017).

You will recall from your nursing education that the brain consists of three parts that develop from the bottom up. The parts 'talk' to one another via trillions of neural pathways. The 'reptilian brain' (brain stem) is responsible for the automatic functions such as breathing, heart rate and survival. The 'mammalian brain' (limbic system) is responsible for emotions and memory; it is about survival and safety. The 'primate brain' (cerebral cortex) is responsible for higher order tasks such as thinking, learning, decision making, reasoning, organising, planning, meaning making, gaining control over emotions and language. When people experience trauma and/or severe emotional stress, it can be much harder to engage the cerebral cortex. Instead they 'loop' in the limbic cortex and this builds stronger neural pathways, making it more likely they will experience distressing emotions in the future when challenges arise. The key here is the absolute necessity for people to feel safe so they can effectively engage with others in their ongoing care (Oral et al. 2016). Consider when people come into care in an inpatient unit. Personal safety is an important basis for effective nursing care. Often, people will be frightened of the inpatient environment, including acute mental health units, particularly if it is their first experience of admission to a mental health care setting. It is important to take time to find out how the person feels and what they need to feel safe and secure. It may be listening to them or helping them consider strategies they could use to increase feelings of safety – for example, calling for help if someone enters their room. Do not assume that the person experiencing mental distress will feel safe in the healthcare setting just because you feel comfortable in the environment as a nurse.

The essentials of trauma-informed care include recognising the following (Sweeney et al. 2018):

- Trauma and its effects have been historically unrecognised in the design of mental health systems. To counteract this, it is necessary to take a universal precaution approach that assumes that all people who seek mental health care may have experienced trauma.
- Services need to ensure early assessment of trauma history and supervision for staff in responding sensitively and appropriately to disclosures of trauma.
- Reiterating the necessity for the person to feel safe, nurses can respond by helping the person to lower their distressing emotions – for example: sitting, listening or walking with the person; using basic mindfulness or relaxation techniques; and ensuring a calm environment can all help. When this occurs, people are more likely to be able to engage their thinking brain and find ways that work for them to feel safe.
- Impacts of trauma can affect how people react to potentially helpful relationships. Building trust is essential so you can work with the person. Remember, trauma often occurs when a person's trust in people or situations has been severely violated. Nurses need to understand how trauma and abuse may have shaped difficulties in relationships and affect therapeutic relationships.
- Coercive interventions may re-traumatise people. Be mindful that nurses are often seen as figures of authority. Using the power that comes with this to exercise control over the person to do what you think they 'should' do will most likely be counterproductive, be seen as coercive and may even re-traumatise the person. Recognise the person's strengths and support them by collaboratively developing a care plan that affirms their preferences for care and how they can manage distress.
- Avoid interventions that may be perceived as shaming and humiliating. Nurses are responsible for maintaining the dignity and individual rights of the person at all times and providing services in ways that are flexible, individualised, culturally competent, respectful and based on best practice.
- There is a strong need to focus on what *happened* to the person rather than pathologising the person as a result of their presenting symptoms (where the focus is on *what is wrong* with the person). Nurses need to develop an understanding of presenting behaviour and symptoms in the context of past experiences.

In summary, trauma-informed services are informed by three key principles to guide practice (Muskett 2014):

- People need to feel connected, valued, informed and hopeful about their recovery from mental illness.
- Staff understand the connection between childhood trauma and adult mental health issues is understood.
- Staff practice in empowering ways with consumers and their family and friends and other services to promote consumers' autonomy.

While these principles focus on the needs of consumers and their family and friends, a trauma-informed approach to care can also provide support for managing workplace stress (Isobel & Edwards 2017). Trauma-informed practice does not replace recovery-oriented practice but is complementary and provides another perspective from which people (staff and consumers) may view recovery and therapeutic engagement.

NURSE'S STORY 2.1

Katrina's story of choosing mental health nursing

I did not start my nursing education with a plan to work in mental health nursing. Like many of my fellow students I thought about paediatric nursing, or maybe cardiac nursing. I enjoyed all my clinical placements and my greatest pleasure was talking to consumers in whatever setting they were. I found the most interesting theoretical study was of understanding people from a psychological, sociological and cultural perspective: how people came to be like they were; how they responded to health and illness and stress. My understanding about mental illness had been coloured by common community attitudes, by media depictions of psychiatric hospitals, and by the experience of an aunt being forcibly admitted for treatment. It was not really talked about in the family and I am not sure if anyone visited while she was in hospital.

There have been two 'lightbulb moments' that led me to choose to work in mental health following graduation. The first was a visiting lecturer who was a 'mental health consumer', someone who had experienced mental illness and its treatment. I left that tutorial with a mixture of feelings: sadness for the experience of stigmatisation; admiration for the bravery to speak up and for the resilience to re-establish a life that was satisfying; an awful awareness of the way my family had silenced my aunt by acting like her experience had not happened; and a new compassion for people with mental illness.

When it came to my mental health clinical placement I was rather anxious. I really did not know what to expect. My mental health clinical placement was a second 'lightbulb moment'. I found the consumers had interesting stories to tell and that they wanted to tell me about their lives. I watched the staff as they interacted with consumers. I admired their capacity to remain calm and to intervene early when someone became upset. The staff taught me a lot about how mental illness is manifest and experienced and what treatments were used. I enjoyed the interdisciplinary discussions and felt that nurses' observations about consumers were taken seriously.

I have now been working in an acute mental health inpatient unit for a year and I have found this time to be a steep learning curve. The biggest challenge has been developing an understanding of me and how I respond to various people and situations. At times I found myself getting upset or angry with consumers if things did not go according to my plan and I really needed to make sure I did not get into negative talk with other staff who were also frustrated. I attend group clinical supervision sessions every 2 weeks and this is helpful in keeping us focused on the person and their needs. The group has provided a safety net that we can use between sessions. I had a preceptor assigned when I first started and that helped with day-to-day skill development. I have an informal arrangement with a mentor who is an experienced nurse that I identified as someone I want to emulate in my practice. She has been very supportive in helping me identify knowledge that I need to gain, what further education would be helpful, where my career path might lead and what kind of clinical experience would be beneficial to me. I would like to work on one of the community mental health teams in the future.

Effective mental health nursing practice

A central element of the social ecological framework for practice is effective mental health nursing practice. To practise effectively in their roles, mental health nurses need sound theoretical knowledge of mental health and illness and associated treatments, positive attitudes towards mental illness and people living with mental illness, and effective mental health nursing skills. In their practice, mental health nurses consider the person's physical, psychological, social, cultural and spiritual healthcare needs; that is,they take a holistic or comprehensive approach.

A holistic approach to mental health nursing includes knowledge and skills in:

- preventative and early intervention strategies for mental health and mental illness
- biological processes that may underpin mental illness
- the impacts of social determinants of health on the development and course of mental illness

Historical anecdote 2.2: We were convicts

The first nurses involved in mental health care in Australia were convict nurses assigned to care for patients sent to Castle Hill and Liverpool 'lunatic asylums' in colonial New South Wales. In spite of their pioneering role, contemporary nurse historians often skip over them without any acknowledgement. Such a generalised approach to nursing history may be tied to a desire to eradicate the memory of a so-called 'convict stain' from modern nurses' professional identity. It perpetuates a tradition started in early healthcare journals that promoted the myth that nursing in Australia was 'rescued' by Lucy Osbourne and her Nightingale nurses in 1863. Nurses prior to Osbourne were characterised as 'gamps', which was a reference to the fictional character of the coarse, fat, drunken nurse 'Sarah Gamp' in Charles Dickens' novel, *Martin Chuzzlewit*. In contrast, early convict nurses such as Martha Entwistle at Castle Hill Lunatic Asylum and Mary Coughlen at Liverpool Lunatic Asylum were resilient women who overcame traumatic experiences in their own lives while caring for others in harsh colonial environments, short of adequate resources, during an era of fast-paced industrial and technological change. We should be more proud of our convict nursing roots.

Read more about it: *Raeburn T, Liston C, Hickmott, J, Cleary M 2018 Life of Martha Entwistle: Australia's first convict mental health nurse. International Journal of Mental Health Nursing 27(1): 455–63*

- the importance of social connections and relationships for mental health and illness
- spiritual belief and faith and its relationship to mental health
- cultural practices and beliefs and their relationship to mental health
- communication and interpersonal relationship knowledge and skills
- the physical health care of people with mental illness
- psychological processes associated with mental health and illness
- psychotherapeutic approaches and strategies for mitigating mental distress and mental illness
- the physiological effects and side effects of psychotropic medications and physical treatments for mental illness.

Therapeutic relationship – consumer and nurse partnership

As nurses we bring our knowledge and attitudes to mental health/illness, our identities (e.g. cultural and gender) and our values, knowledge, experience and skills in nursing. This shapes how we develop a therapeutic relationship with consumers. The therapeutic relationship is the foundation of effective mental health nursing practice (Browne et al. 2012). We consider this relationship to be one of equal partnership. Partnership involves working with the consumer and their family/carers to provide support in a way that makes sense to them, including sharing information and working with consumers and carers in a positive way to help them reach their goals (Commonwealth of Australia 2010). The therapeutic relationship is underpinned by the nurse's use of self. Key knowledge and skills for an effective therapeutic relationship include developing a therapeutic alliance, self-awareness and empathy.

Lived experience comment by Jarrad Hickmott

The framing of nursing around the therapeutic use of self and therapeutic alliance is very important. A lot of times it can be difficult to maintain these aspects in an environment where a heavily medicalised model is dominant. Discussing the very human side of nursing and the different domains of life that interplay with the mental ill health of consumers is very enriching and of great benefit.

Therapeutic use of self

Therapeutic relationships are the central activity of mental health nursing. The therapeutic relationship provides a healing connection between the nurse and consumer through a caring, emotional connection, narrative and anxiety management, and this process can have a powerful neurobiological impact on the mental health of the person (Wheeler 2011). Therapeutic relationships are the foundation upon which all other activities are based. Mental health nursing is therefore primarily an interpersonal process that uses self as the means of developing and sustaining nurse–consumer relationships. Therapeutic use of self involves using aspects of the nurse's personality, background, life skills and knowledge to develop a connection with a person who has a mental health problem or illness. Nurses intentionally and consciously draw on ways of establishing human connectedness in their encounters with service users. The process is based on a genuine interest in understanding who the consumer is and how they have come to be in their current situation – separating the person from the illness (Wyder et al. 2017). Lees et al. (2014, p. 310) describe therapeutic engagement as the 'establishment of rapport, active listening, empathy, boundaries, relating as equals, genuineness, compassion, unconditional positive regard, trust, time and responsiveness' and suggest that most of these elements need to be present for engagement to occur.

The purpose of using self therapeutically is to establish a therapeutic alliance with the service user. Service users in mental health services may not only be experiencing frightening symptoms or perhaps overwhelming mood changes or overwhelming thoughts and feelings, they may also be experiencing alienation and isolation. Service users may be fearful of talking to others about their symptoms or difficulties because they fear being rejected and seen as 'crazy', or they may have had experiences of rejection because of their mental illness that make it difficult for them to form relationships. Studies of service users' experiences of mental health services provide evidence that being understood and listened to in a thoughtful, sensitive manner confirms their humanity and provides hope for their future (Gunasekara et al. 2014). In the process of using self therapeutically, the nurse develops a dialogue with the service user to understand their predicament. Service users need to feel safe enough to disclose personal, difficult and distressing information. It is in the way in which the nurse conveys genuine interest, concern and desire to understand that a therapeutic alliance can be established. How the nurse relates to, and what prior understandings they bring to, the encounter will affect this relationship (Wyder et al. 2015).

Studies of the experiences of both mental health nurses and service users of mental health services overwhelmingly attest to the importance of therapeutic relationships. Consumers have identified the need to feel compassionately cared for, to have meaningful contact with nurses, to be listened to, and for nurses to know them as people and understand their predicament (Gunasekara et al. 2014; Lees et al. 2014; Stewart et al. 2015; Wyder et al. 2015; Wyder et al. 2017). Similarly, studies of nurses' experiences identify that they see therapeutic engagement as the hallmark of good practice in mental health settings (Cleary et al. 2012; McAndrew et al. 2014).

Empathy and therapeutic use of self

The ability to empathise with service users is underpinned by caring and compassion and is positively linked with the ability to develop therapeutic relationships and the desire to alleviate suffering. As indicated earlier, the ability to engage empathically with consumers is highly valued. Empathy is not merely a feeling of understanding and compassion. Empathy, as used in the therapeutic relationship, is linked to intentional actions that are aimed at reducing the person's distress. Empathic interactions have a number of components:

- First, empathy involves an attempt to understand the person's predicament and the meanings they attribute to their situation. This means the nurse makes a conscious attempt to discuss with the person their current and past experiences and the feelings and meanings associated with these experiences.
- Second, the nurse verbalises the understanding that they have developed back to the person. The understanding that the nurse has of the service user's situation will be at best tentative; we can never really know what life is like for another. However, the process of seeking to understand, and of conveying the desire to understand, creates the opportunity for further exploration in a safe relationship. In addition, maintaining the stance of trying to understand rather than making assumptions averts the tendency to make judgements about the person and their behaviour.
- Third, empathy involves the service user's validation of the nurse's understanding. One of the most important aspects of developing the therapeutic relationship through empathic understanding is that the nurse can convey to the person a desire to understand. This level of empathic attunement allows the service user to participate in identifying those aspects of their illness and healthcare experience that are problematic.

The therapeutic alliance

The value of a therapeutic alliance, developed through therapeutic use of self, has been clearly identified from the perspective of nurses and service users in international studies (Zugai et al. 2015). A therapeutic alliance is characterised by the development of mutual partnerships between consumers and nurses and has been linked with greater consumer satisfaction with care (Zugai et al. 2015). Several studies have indicated that a therapeutic alliance can have a significant impact on consumer outcomes and that it is possibly one of the most important factors contributing to the effectiveness of a mental health service (Cleary et al. 2012; Stewart et al. 2015). People who have a positive relationship with their clinician have better outcomes (Pilgrim et al. 2009). However, a therapeutic relationship alone may not be sufficient to sustain health improvements, and so a combination of both therapeutic relationships and the technical skill of specific therapeutic approaches may provide the best outcomes (see, for example, Smith & Macduff 2017).

Historical anecdote 2.3: Mental health nurse of the century!

Hildegard Peplau (1909–1999) has been cited as the most influential mental health nurse of the 20th century. She was trained and began her career in the United States where she was heavily influenced by psychologist Harry Stack Sullivan's work on interpersonal therapy. During World War II she moved to England where she served in an army hospital involved in the mental health rehabilitation of soldiers. After returning to North America after the war she contributed to developing the 1946 National Mental Health Act, which involved a major reconfiguration of mental health services away from asylums towards community-based care. In 1952 Peplau published an influential book titled, *Interpersonal Relations in Nursing*. In it she described the essential skills, functions and roles of mental health nurses of her era. The book is viewed as being the first systematic, theoretical framework for the practice of modern mental health nursing. Later in her career Peplau was appointed to various influential roles with the World Health Organization, the American Nurses Association and various universities in the United States and around the world.

Read more about it: *Peplau H 1997 Peplau's theory of interpersonal relations. Nursing Science Quarterly, 10(4): 162–7*

Self-awareness

The process of working together and understanding others begins with understanding the self. 'Self' is a concept that describes the core of our personality. We use the concept of self when we want to convey our uniqueness as a human being. The self has consistent attributes that pervade the way we live in and experience the world. It is awareness of these attributes of self that can enhance the way we relate to others. A strong sense of self allows us to develop resilience in dealing with the difficulties and complexities of human communication and experience. Self-awareness is about knowing how you are going to respond in specific situations, about your values, attitudes and biases towards people and situations, and about knowing how your human needs might manifest in your work. The purpose of being self-aware is to know those things in our background and our way of relating that might affect how we relate to others. The way we view people is always subjective. The lens through which we look at the world is always our own. Although there can be no true objectivity, knowledge of the things that impinge on our subjective view of the world allows us to identify how they influence our thinking. Nurses need to be aware of the belief systems and values that arise from their cultural, social and family backgrounds. Everyone develops biases that affect the way they view other people's behaviour. Behaviour that is understandable to one nurse might not be understandable to another. However, the self is not static but constantly evolving and sensitive to experience. We bring values, biases and beliefs to nursing and to our relationships with service users, and in turn those relationships offer the opportunity for self-development. It is through the process of self-reflection and the examination of particular experiences that nurses can learn and flourish (Fowler 2019).

Working in the mental health field requires the ability to listen to, respond to and empathise with people from a range of backgrounds. Unexamined belief systems can become obstacles to developing a therapeutic alliance. Lack of self-awareness can cause nurses to respond to a person's distress and behaviour in ways that may not be helpful. For example, it might cause nurses to use their power coercively in the belief that this is best for the service user. Lack of self-awareness can also lead to nurses being overly concerned, refusing to allow service users choice or overwhelming them with advice, in an attempt to protect them. Alternatively, nurses may avoid contact with particular service users or fail to respond to distress. This growing self-awareness needs to take place against a background of self-compassion, and to develop the ability to empathise with others requires 'the ability to be sensitive, non-judgemental and respectful to oneself' (Gustin & Wagner 2013, p. 182).

Hope and spirituality

There is still much that we do not know about recovery, healing and how people manage chronic health problems. Why do some people pull through a disease, while others do not? How is it that some people seem to cope well with even very invasive treatments, while others suffer terribly? How do some people with chronic mental illnesses function well in the community, while others are in and out of hospital? We know that factors such as personality, resilience, social support, general health and access to acceptable (to the service user) health services all play a crucial role in service user outcomes. But the importance and value of concepts such as hope and the role hope plays in the lives of service users and their families are areas of increasing interest. 'Hope' is a taken-for-granted term and, although it is used widely in the literature, it is seldom clearly defined. Hope is considered essential in handling illness and can be described as an act by which the temptation to despair is actively overcome. We know hope is a complex and multidimensional variable that has optimistic and anticipatory dimensions and involves looking ahead to the future. Hope has been linked to emotional healing and better adaptation to life stress (Carretta et al. 2014) and is a central component in recovery from mental illness (Slade et al. 2015).

In a study of qualitative literature related to hope in older people with chronic illnesses, Carretta et al. (2014, p. 1,211) identified characteristics of hope as including 'transcending possibilities' and 'positive reappraisal'. Transcending possibilities involve finding meaning through searching and connecting with others. The positive role of health professionals in maintaining hope is described as supporting hope and the search for meaning. Positive reappraisal depends on the ability to seek and find positives in the illness experience, and health professionals also have a role in supporting service users in this search. Hope has particular relevance to mental health nursing practice, and there is growing recognition of the concept of hope and its relationship to health, wellbeing and recovery from illness or traumatic life events (Duggleby et al. 2012). Closely linked with hope, Hemingway et al. (2014) describe therapeutic optimism in mental health nurses as a belief that they can make a difference and a belief that the people they work with can recover.

The need for further research to generate knowledge and enhance understanding about suffering, hope and spirituality in relation to mental health nursing is acknowledged in the literature (Cutcliffe et al. 2015; Schrank et al. 2008). However, the emphasis on the biomedical understanding of mental illness provides barriers to such research. The biomedical model values things that can be seen, measured and quantified. Although hope and spirituality can be felt, they cannot be seen, touched or smelt and cannot always be clearly articulated and so occupy what Crawford et al. (1998, p. 214) termed 'an embarrassed silence'. However, if we recognise that spirituality underpins the meanings that people make of illness and other life events, and that hope is a variable that has some form of healing potential, then we cannot ignore the importance of spirituality and the search for meaning in practice. Indeed, Cutcliffe et al. (2015) reinforces the importance of recognising and responding to the spiritual care needs of service users and calls for nurses to develop skills in supporting service users to understand and search for meaning in their experience. The ability to maintain hope and to make meaning of the experience of illness is central to recovery, and it is important for mental health nurses to maintain hope for consumers' recovery and to support consumers in maintaining hope and finding meaning in their experiences. This leads to the question: What skills do nurses need if we are to care for the spiritual needs of consumers? The short answer is that we need to develop effective interpersonal skills. Being open to the belief systems of other people, intuitiveness, active listening, being alert to the cues that tell us the things that matter to a person, self-awareness, spiritual awareness and reflective skills are crucial in providing spiritual care (Ramezani et al. 2014).

Compassion and caring

Compassion is a concept closely associated with and underpinning caring. Compassion is linked with sensitivity to suffering and a desire to alleviate distress (Day 2015; Gustin & Wagner 2013; Sawbridge & Hewison 2015). Gustin and Wagner (2013) suggest that compassion inspires 'the act of the conscious intention of being present in moments of another's despair' (p. 175). Compassion underpins concepts of acceptance, a non-judgemental attitude, awareness, being present and listening. To be able to provide compassionate nursing care, we need to be able to imagine what it would be like to be in the person's situation, what it would be like to experience the world as they are experiencing it and to imagine what might help.

Caring is widely considered to be central to nursing theory and practice (Hogan 2013; Schofield et al. 2013). Although the word 'caring' is simple, its use in complex healthcare situations has rendered it problematic. Following a meta-synthesis of research, Finfgeld-Connett (2008) conceptualised caring as a 'context-specific interpersonal process that is characterised by expert nursing practice, interpersonal sensitivity and intimate relationships' (p. 196). Finfgeld-Connett further elaborate on the concept to make explicit factors related to the roles of the consumer and the nurse, and to the working environment, discussing the 'recipient's need for and openness to caring, and the nurse's professional maturity and moral foundations ... [as well as] a working environment that is conducive to caring' (p. 196). Providing nursing care in mental health settings can, however, be even more complex as people with mental illnesses may not identify the need for care, or be open to caring interventions, especially in acute phases of illness. Nurse scholars have invested much time and energy in trying to explain what it is that makes nurse caring special or different from informal caring and from the caring provided by medical practitioners. There have also been many attempts to find a 'fit' between caring as a construct and the biomedically dominated and economically driven healthcare sectors within which nursing is situated. From a mental health perspective, there are even more issues to consider in relation to nurse caring. For example, there are special issues associated with caring for consumers who are compelled to accept professional care under mental health legislation.

Historically, mental health nursing was associated with custodial care and control. Godin (2000) captured the dilemma of mental health nurses when he raised questions about the *dis*-ease between the caring and coercive roles that mental health nurses assume. Godin positioned caring as 'clean' and constructed the coercive control elements of mental health nursing (a term he used for forced treatment, community orders and so on) as 'dirty' (Godin 2000, p. 1,396). While Godin's argument focused on service users and nurses in the community, many of the issues he raised (related to forced administration of medication, seclusion and detention) are still relevant to nurses in inpatient and community settings. In addition, forensic mental health units raise further challenges (Cashin et al. 2010). From the perspective of people who have been involuntarily detained for treatment, Wyder et al. (2015) found that having staff willing to listen empathically was important and that the person's involuntary legal status should not be an impediment to nurses providing compassionate care and forming therapeutic relationships. The absolute vulnerability of service users who can be detained against their will and subjected to various treatments that they may vigorously and robustly resist means that elements of the caring role, such as consumer advocacy, are critical to skilful and compassionate mental health nursing practice.

Professional boundaries

In nursing, professional boundaries are invisible yet powerful lines that mark the territory of the nurse. They define a role and allow the nurse to say: 'This is what I do. This is the purpose of my presence here.' Professional boundaries are important in all areas of health care, but in mental health nursing they have an increased importance due to the nature of the work of mental health nurses and the vulnerability of the service user population. Clear boundaries provide service users and nurses with a safe interpersonal context in which therapeutic work can take place. Over time there has been a decrease in formal divisions between staff and service users in mental health services, with the encouragement of friendliness and collaborative partnerships (Gardner 2010). However, a power imbalance is always present in clinician–consumer encounters (Henderson 2004), and there are a number of ways that boundary violations can occur. Boundary violations can involve exerting power through coercion, use of force, over-treatment or under-treatment, or inappropriate intimate relationships. Maintaining professional boundaries while being involved in therapeutic relationships is a skill that cannot be underestimated in importance. Tariman (2010) noted that social networking provided a further challenge. This medium for relationships needs to be viewed with caution when considering professional boundaries.

Mental health nurses have to be able to maintain professional boundaries while simultaneously developing close therapeutic relationships with service users based on empathy and positive connectedness. While many of the interactions and interventions of mental health nurses may appear social in nature (e.g. playing table tennis, cards or volleyball with a service user, or going for a walk or having a coffee with a service user), it is the therapeutic intent and the conscious awareness of the purpose of the relationship that put them within the professional role. It is when interventions and interactions lose their therapeutic intent and are instead primarily for the benefit of the nurse that professional boundaries are breached. Any breach of professional boundaries has the potential to cause serious harm to service users and is a violation of professional ethics.

Professional boundaries are maintained by nurses having a clear understanding of their therapeutic role, being able to reflect on therapeutic interactions and being able to document and narrate their interventions. Maintaining professional boundaries is always the responsibility of the nurse.

Self-disclosure

Mental health nurses use self-disclosure as a way of developing therapeutic relationships with service users. Many of the relationships that nurses have with service users are long term, either by repeated admissions to hospital or by continued contact in community or primary care/private practice settings, so nurses and service users may come to know each other well. In a study of nurse–consumer relationships between community mental health nurses and service users with long-term mental illness, nurses described the use of self-disclosure: 'The nurses used their own experiences of living a life to: be seen as ordinary people; be credible; illustrate aspects of being-in-the-world; allow the service users to identify with them; and to normalise the service user's fears and difficulties' (O'Brien 2000, p. 188). Service users described the nurse as 'a friend – but different ... not like other friends' (O'Brien 2001, p. 180). Service users were able to identify that the therapeutic relationship was different even though they knew things about the nurse's life (O'Brien 2001, p. 180).

However, self-disclosure should be used consciously and carefully. The boundary issue is not whether disclosure of information occurs or does not occur. The issue is the nature of the disclosure and whether the nurse burdens the service user with their own personal problems. The decision about what to disclose to service users about your life needs to be made in advance. Self-disclosure does not include unburdening your personal problems. In the above studies, the experienced nurses were able to use their own life experiences to relate in ways that were beneficial to service users without overburdening them. These experienced clinicians also made decisions about what to share with service users according to the length of the relationship and what each service user could use productively.

Chapter summary

This chapter has introduced some of the core concepts and ideas that shape and inform mental health nursing practice and outlined the social ecological approach to practice used throughout this text. Therapeutic relationships lie at the heart of mental health nursing, and a clear understanding of professional boundaries is crucial to developing and sustaining such relationships. To be effective and therapeutic in caring for others, nurses must understand concepts such as compassion, caring, hope and spirituality.

Mental health nursing is an exciting and challenging area of nursing practice. Effective mental health nursing requires the culmination of all your skills as well as your professional and life experiences, and in return it offers a stimulating and rewarding career path. As we strive to meet the complex needs of diverse communities and to provide care within increasingly restrictive economic environments, there are many challenges before us. Developing positive personal qualities such as self-awareness and fostering productive and supportive collegial relationships will help us to meet the challenges that lie ahead.

Acknowledgement

This chapter has been adapted and extended from a chapter by Louise O'Brien in the previous edition of this book.

EXERCISES FOR CLASS ENGAGEMENT

Consider the social ecological approach to mental health nursing described in this chapter.

1. What personal characteristics (including strengths) do you bring to your nursing practice?
2. How can these be used to develop an effective partnership with consumers and their family/carers?
3. In respect to social determinants of health, which determinants do you think nurses can have an influence on? How might they do this?

CONSUMER'S STORY 2.1

Therese

You are a new nurse working in an emergency department and have been assigned Therese. You are aware of the other staff's negative feelings about this consumer. Some of the staff know her from previous presentations and see her problems as self-inflicted. However, as you take the necessary observations you ask Therese about what has happened to her.

Therese then tells her own story:

> I am 28 years old and have had lots of presentations to emergency departments. I used to cut myself often or take overdoses. However, in the past 3 years I have hardly had any presentations and no admissions to hospital. I have two children aged 4 and 2 and I am trying to get my act together for them. I do not want to lose my children. My childhood was chaotic with lots of foster care. I spent time in refuges and took drugs for a while. I do not take drugs or drink alcohol now. I have had a community mental health nurse who has been seeing me regularly for more than 3 years. Tonight I took an overdose of antidepressants that I had been prescribed. I feel ashamed because it was impulsive and stupid. I can see the staff talking about me and saying all the old things. They do not think I deserve care because I inflicted this

on myself and everyone else here is physically ill or has had an accident. I just got to the end of my tether. I had a boyfriend who moved in and I didn't like how he treated the kids so he has gone now. My community nurse is on leave. I couldn't contact anyone; I just felt so alone, empty and lost. I thought the kids would be better off without me.

If my community nurse was here, she would ask me what happened, how I was feeling. She would treat me with respect without condoning what I did. She would help me identify how I can get out of this mess I have made. We would talk about the crisis plan that is on my fridge and how I can get through the next few days keeping myself and my children safe.

Critical thinking challenge 2.1

Consider Consumer's story 2.1. What are your thoughts and feelings on reading about Therese's self-harm? How do you think this might impact your relationship and nursing practice with her?

Useful websites

Professional boundaries

Australian Nurses and Midwives Council: www.nursingmidwiferyboard.gov.au/Codes-Guidelines-Statements/Codes-Guidelines.aspx

Te Kaunihera Tapuhi o Aotearoa, Nursing Council of New Zealand – Guidelines: professional boundaries: https://www.nursingcouncil.org.nz/Public/Nursing/Standards_and_guidelines/NCNZ/nursing-section/Standards_and_guidelines_for_nurses.aspx?hkey=9fc06ae7-a853-4d10-b5fe-992cd44ba3de

Recovery

National Standards for Mental Health Services – Principles of recovery oriented mental health practice: www.health.gov.au/internet/publications/publishing.nsf/Content/mental-pubs-i-nongov-toc~menta l-pubs-i-nongov-pri

Trauma

Adults Surviving Child Abuse: http://www.asca.org.au/

Adverse Childhood Experiences (ACE) study: http://acestudy.org/ and www.cdc.gov/violenceprevention/acestudy/

Australian Institute of Health and Welfare – Closing the Gap: Trauma-informed services and trauma-specific care for Indigenous Australian children: http://www.aihw.gov.au/uploadedfiles/closingthegap/content/publications/2013/ctg-rs21.pdf

Domestic Violence Services New Zealand Help for family violence: www.police.govt.nz/advice/family-violence/help

Mental Health Coordinating Council (MHCC) – Trauma informed care and practice: http://www.mhcc.org.au/our-work/resources/

NSW Service for the Treatment and Rehabilitation of Torture and Trauma Survivors (STARTTS): http://www.startts.org.au/

Phoenix Australia, Centre for Posttraumatic Health: www.acpmh.unimelb.edu.au/trauma/ptsd.html

References

Anthony, W.A., 1993. Recovery from mental illness: the guiding vision of the mental health service system in the 1990s. Psychiatr. Rehabil. J. 16 (4), 11–23.

Banfield, M.A., Morse, A.R., Gulliver, A., et al., 2018. Mental health research priorities in Australia: a consumer and carer agenda. Health Res. Policy Syst. 16, 119.

Browne, G., Cashin, A., Graham, I.W., 2012. The therapeutic relationship and the mental health nurse: it is time to articulate what we do! J. Psychiatr. Ment. Health Nurs. 19 (9), 939–943.

Carretta, C.M., Ridner, S.H., Dietrich, M.S., 2014. Hope, hopelessness, and anxiety: a pilot instrument comparison study. Arch. Psychiatr. Nurs. 28, 230–234.

Cashin, A., Newman, C., Eason, M., et al., 2010. An ethnographic study of forensic nursing culture in an Australian prison hospital. J. Psychiatr. Ment. Health Nurs. 17, 39–45.

Cleary, M., Horsfall, J., O'Hara-Aarons, M., et al., 2012. Mental health nurses' perceptions of good work in an acute setting. Int. J. Ment. Health Nurs. 21 (5), 471–479.

Cleary, M., Raeburn, T., West, S., et al., 2018a. Two approaches, one goal: how mental health registered nurses' perceive their role and the role of peer support workers in facilitating consumer decision-making. Int. J. Ment. Health Nurs. 27 (4), 1212–1218.

Cleary, M., Raeburn, T., West, S., et al., 2018b. 'Walking the tightrope': the role of peer support workers in facilitating consumers' participation in decision-making. Int. J. Ment. Health Nurs. 27 (4), 1266–1272.

COAG Health Council, 2017. The Fifth National Mental Health and Suicide Prevention Plan. Retrieved from: https://apo.org.au/sites/default/files/resource-files/2017-10/apo-nid114356-1220416.pdf.

Commonwealth of Australia, 2010. National Standards for Mental Health Services. https://www1.health.gov.au/internet/main/publishing.nsf/Content/CFA833CB8C1AA178CA257BF0001E7520/$File/servst10v2.pdf.

Commonwealth of Australia, 2013. A national framework for recovery-oriented mental health services: guide for practitioners and providers. https://www1.health.gov.au/internet/main/publishing.nsf/content/67D17065514CF8E8CA257C1D00017A90/$File/recovgde.pdf.

Crawford, P., Nolan, P., Brown, B., 1998. Ministering to madness: the narratives of people who have left religious orders to work in the caring professions. J. Adv. Nurs. 28 (1), 212–220.

Cutcliffe, J.R., Hummelvoll, J.K., Granerud, A., et al., 2015. Mental health nurses responding to suffering in the 21st century occidental world: accompanying people in their search for meaning. Arch. Psychiatr. Nurs. 29, 19–25.

Day, H., 2015. The meaning of compassion. Br. J. Nurs. 24 (6), 342–343.
Deegan, P.E., 1988. Recovery: the lived experience of rehabilitation. Psychiatr. Rehabil. J. 11 (4), 11–19.
Duggleby, W., Hicks, D., Nekolaichuk, C., et al., 2012. Hope, older adults, and chronic illness: a metasynthesis of qualitative research. J. Adv. Nurs. 68 (6), 1211–1223.
Felitti, V.J., Anda, R.F., Nordenberd, D., et al., 1998. Relationship of childhood abuse and household dysfunction to many of the leading causes of death in adults. The Adverse Childhood Experiences (ACE) Study. Am. J. Prev. Med. 14 (4), 245–258.
Finfgeld-Connett, D., 2008. Meta-synthesis of caring in nursing. J. Clin. Nurs. 17 (2), 196–204.
Fowler, J., 2019. Reflection and mental health nursing. Part one: is reflection important. BJMHN 8 (2), 68–69.
Gardner, A., 2010. Therapeutic friendliness and the development of therapeutic leverage by mental health nurses in community rehabilitation settings. Contemp. Nurse 34 (2), 140–148.
Glover, H., 2012. Recovery, Life-long learning, social inclusion and empowerment: is a new paradigm emerging? In: Ryan, P., Ramon, S., Greacen, T. (Eds.), Empowerment, Lifelong Learning and Recovery in Mental Health Towards a New Paradigm. Palgrave Macmillian, London, pp. 15–35.
Godin, P., 2000. A dirty business: caring for people who are a nuisance or a danger. J. Adv. Nurs. 32 (6), 1396–1402.
Goffman, E., 1963. Stigma: Notes on the Management of Spoiled Identity. Prentice-Hall, Englewood Cliffs.
Gordon, S., O'Brien, A.J., 2018. Co-production. Power problems and possibilities. Int. J. Ment. Health Nurs. 27 (4), 1201–1203.
Green, M., Linscott, R.J., Laurens, K.R., et al., 2018. Latent profiles of developmental schizotypy in the general population: associations with childhood trauma and familial mental illness. Schizophr. Bull. 44 (Suppl. 1), S229.
Grzanka, P.R., Brian, J.D., 2019. Clinical encounters: the social Justice question in intersectional medicine. Am. J. Bioeth. 19 (2), 22–24.
Gunasekara, I., Pentland, T., Rodgers, T., et al., 2014. What makes an excellent mental health nurse? A pragmatic inquiry initiated and conducted by people with lived experience of service use. Int. J. Ment. Health Nurs. 23, 101–109.
Gustin, L.W., Wagner, L., 2013. The butterfly effect of caring – clinical nurse teachers' understanding of self-compassion as a source of compassionate care. Scand. J. Caring Sci. 27, 175–183.
Hall, C., 2014. Bereavement theory: recent developments in our understanding of grief and bereavement. Bereave. Care 33 (1), 7–12.
Hemingway, S., Rogers, M., Elsom, S., 2014. Measuring the influence of a mental health training module on the therapeutic optimism of advanced nurse practitioner students in the United Kingdom. J. Am. Assoc. Nurse Pract. 26, 155–162.
Henderson, J., 2004. The challenge of relationship boundaries in mental health. Nurs. Manage. 11 (6), 28–31.
Hogan, K., 2013. Caring as a scripted discourse versus caring as an expression of an authentic relationship between self and other. Issues Ment. Health Nurs. 34, 375–379.
Isobel, S., Edwards, C., 2017. Using trauma informed care as a nursing model of care in an acute inpatient mental health unit: a practice development process. Int. J. Ment. Health Nurs. 26 (1), 88–94.
Jääskeläinen, E., Juola, P., Hirvonen, N., et al., 2012. A systematic review and meta-analysis of recovery in schizophrenia. Schizophr. Bull. 39 (6), 1296–1306.
Javier, J.R., Hoffman, L.R., Shah, S.I., Pediatric Policy Council, 2019. Making the case for ACEs: adverse childhood experiences, obesity, and long-term health. Pediatr. Res. 86 (4), 420–422.
Jones, T., Nurius, P., Song, C., et al., 2018. Modeling life course pathways from adverse childhood experiences to adult mental health. Child Abuse Negl. 80, 32–40.
Le Boutillier, C., Leamy, M., Bird, V.J., 2011. What does recovery mean in practice? A qualitative analysis of international recovery-oriented practice guidance. Psychiatr. Serv. 62 (12), 1470–1476.
Leamy, M., Bird, V., Le Boutillier, C., et al., 2011. Conceptual framework for personal recovery in mental health: systematic review and narrative synthesis. Br. J. Psychiatry 199 (6), 445–452.
Lees, D., Procter, N., Fassett, D., 2014. Therapeutic engagement between consumers in suicidal crisis and mental health nurses. Int. J. Ment. Health Nurs. 23 (4), 306–315.
Leete, E., 1989. How I perceive and manage my illness. Schizophr. Bull. 15 (2), 197.
Lund, C., Brooke-Sumner, C., Baingana, F., et al., 2018. Social determinants of mental disorders and the Sustainable Development Goals: a systematic review of reviews. Lancet Psychiatry 5 (4), 357–369.
McAndrew, S., Chambers, M., Nolan, F., et al., 2014. Measuring the evidence: reviewing the literature of the measurement of therapeutic engagement in acute mental health Inpatient wards. Int. J. Ment. Health Nurs. 23, 212–220.
Mental Health Commission, 2012. Blueprint II: How Things Need to Be. Mental Health Commission, Wellington.
Muskett, C., 2014. Trauma-informed care in inpatient mental health settings: a review of the literature. Int. J. Ment. Health Nurs. 32 (1), 51–59.
O'Brien, L., 2000. Nurse-service user relationships: the experience of community psychiatric nurses. Aust. N. Z. J. Ment. Health Nurs. 9, 184–194.
O'Brien, L., 2001. The relationship between community psychiatric nurses and service users with severe and persistent mental illness: the service user experience. Aust. N. Z. J. Ment. Health Nurs. 10, 176–186.
Oral, R., Ramirez, M., Coohey, C., et al., 2016. Adverse childhood experiences and trauma informed care: the future of health care. Pediatr. Res. 79 (1–2), 227.
Peplau, H., 1997. Peplau's theory of interpersonal relations. Nurs. Sci. Q. 10 (4), 162–167.
Pilgrim, D., Rogers, A., Bentall, R., 2009. The centrality of personal relationships in the creation and amelioration

of mental health problems: the current interdisciplinary case. Health (London) 13, 235–254.

Raeburn, T., Liston, C., Hickmott, J., et al., 2018. Life of Martha Entwistle: Australia's first convict mental health nurse. Int. J. Ment. Health Nurs. 27 (1), 455–463.

Raeburn, T., Schmied, V., Hungerford, C., et al., 2017. Autonomy support and recovery practice at a psychosocial clubhouse. Perspect. Psychiatr. Care 53 (3), 175–182.

Ramezani, M., Ahmadi, F., Mohammadi, E., et al., 2014. Spiritual care in nursing: a concept analysis. Int. Nurs. Rev. 61, 211–219. doi:10.1111/inr.12099.

Reid, R., Escott, P., Isobel, S., 2018. Collaboration as a process and an outcome: consumer experiences of collaborating with nurses in care planning in an acute inpatient mental health unit. Int. J. Ment. Health Nurs. 27 (4), 1204–1211.

Sawbridge, Y., Hewison, A., 2015. Compassion costs nothing – the elephant in the room? Pract. Nurs. 26 (4), 194–197.

Schofield, R., Allan, M., Jewiss, T., et al., 2013. Knowing self and caring through service learning. Int. J. Nurs. Educ. Scholarsh. 10 (1), 267–274.

Schrank, B., Stanghellini, G., Slade, M., 2008. Hope in psychiatry: a review of the literature. Acta Psychiatr. Scand. 118, 421–433.

Slade, M., Bird, V., Clarke, E., et al., 2015. Supporting recovery in patients with psychosis through care by community-based adult mental health teams (REFOCUS): a multisite, cluster, randomised, controlled trial. Lancet Psychiatry 2 (6), 503–514.

Slade, M., Leamy, M., Bacon, F., et al., 2012. International differences in understanding recovery: systematic review. Epidemiol. Psychiatr. Sci. 21 (4), 353–364.

Smith, S., Macduff, C., 2017. A thematic analysis of the experience of UK mental health nurses who have trained in Solution Focused Brief Therapy. J. Psychiatr. Ment. Health Nurs. 24 (2–3), 105–113.

Spittlehouse, J.K., Boden, J.M., Horwood, L.J., 2019. Sexual orientation and mental health over the life course in a birth cohort. Psychol. Med. 1–8. doi:10.1017/S0033291719001284.

Stewart, D., Burrow, H., Duckworth, A., et al., 2015. Thematic analysis of psychiatric patients' perceptions of nursing staff. Int. J. Ment. Health Nurs. 24 (1), 82–90.

Sweeney, A., Filson, B., Kennedy, A., et al., 2018. A paradigm shift: relationships in trauma-informed mental health services. BJPsych Adv. 24 (5), 319–333.

Tariman, J.D., 2010. Where to draw the line: professional boundaries in social networking. ONS Connect 25 (2), 10–13.

Turolla, A., Venneri, A., Farina, D., et al., 2018. Rehabilitation induced neural plasticity after acquired brain injury. Neural Plast. 2018.

Ungar, M., 2011. The social ecology of resilience: addressing contextual and cultural ambiguity of a nascent construct. Am. J. Orthopsychiatry 81 (1), 1–17.

van Weeghel, J., van Zelst, C., Boertien, D., et al., 2019. Conceptualizations, assessments, and implications of personal recovery in mental illness: a scoping review of systematic reviews and meta-analyses. Psychiatr. Rehabil. J. 42 (2), 169–181.

Voss, P., Thomas, M.E., Cisneros-Franco, J.M., et al., 2017. Dynamic brains and the changing rules of neuroplasticity: implications for learning and recovery. Front. Psychol. 8, 1657.

Warner, R., 2010. Does the scientific evidence support the recovery model? Psychiatrist 34 (1), 3–5.

Wheeler, K., 2011. A relationship-based model for psychiatric nursing. Perspect. Psychiatr. Care 47 (3), 151–159.

World Health Organisation (WHO), 2018. Social determinants of health. Retrieved from: http://www.who.int/social_determinants/sdh_definition/en/.

Wyder, M., Bland, R., Blythe, A., et al., 2015. Therapeutic relationships and involuntary treatment orders: service users' interactions with health-care professionals on the ward. Int. J. Ment. Health Nurs. 24 (2), 181–189.

Wyder, M., Ehrlich, C., Crompton, D., et al., 2017. Nurses experiences of delivering care in acute inpatient mental health settings: a narrative synthesis of the literature. Int. J. Ment. Health Nurs. 26 (6), 527–540.

Zugai, J.S., Stein-Parbury, J., Roche, M., 2015. Therapeutic alliance in mental health nursing: an evolutionary concept analysis. Issues Ment. Health Nurs. 36 (4), 249–257.

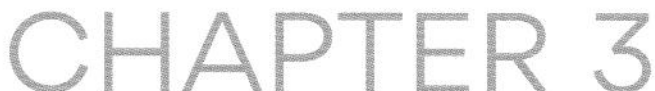

The spectrum of mental health and illness

Toby Raeburn, Peta Marks and Kim Foster

KEY POINTS

- In the course of their work, nurses frequently encounter people experiencing mental health challenges.
- Nurses need to appreciate the spectrum of mental health and illness, including stress and emotional upset, crisis, mental distress, mental disorder and mental illness, and respond according to the person's needs.
- Nurses need mental health nursing skills in every clinical setting to support the mental and emotional wellbeing of the people they work with. This will enable them to provide a platform for developing therapeutic relationships.
- Most people who experience episodes of mental ill health will experience recovery.

KEY TERMS

- Bereavement
- Coping strategies
- Crisis
- Emotions
- Grief
- Loss
- Mental disorder
- Mental health
- Mental health problems
- Stress

LEARNING OUTCOMES

The material in this chapter will assist you to:

- understand the spectrum of mental health and illness that people may experience during their lives
- distinguish between stress, crisis, loss and bereavement
- identify the various types of crisis
- describe how to take a strengths focus in practice.

Introduction

It doesn't matter where a person is from, what language they speak or how much money they have, mental health is crucial to everybody's quality of life. Research has shown that mental health affects not only individuals and families but also the social and economic fabric of whole communities, states and nations (Grech & Raeburn 2019; Maron et al. 2019).

Mental health and illness are not static states. Rather, all people experience a spectrum of mental health and illness including a wide variety of complex states that are constantly variable and open to change. In the same way that any physically healthy person may become sick or a physically sick person may become well, there is always the opportunity for a person who is mentally healthy to develop mental ill-health or for a person who is experiencing mental illness to recover and regain mental health. People can move along the spectrum of mental health and illness (see Fig. 3.1) and remain in various states for shorter or longer periods. Understanding the spectrum of mental health and illness is therefore crucial if nurses are to effectively assist the people to whom they deliver care. Mental health cannot be separated from the concept of overall health, which is defined in the constitution of the World Health Organization as:

> A state of complete, physical, mental and social well-being and not merely the absence of disease or injury.
> (World Health Organization 1947)

Unfortunately, mental health is often underemphasised by nurses and other health professionals, who often focus more on assessing people for mental illness than assisting them towards recovery. This may be compared to a football team that becomes focused on defence, forgetting to invest in training that supports them to score goals. Such services inevitably end up in an ongoing cycle of assessment, diagnosis, treatment and discharge, resulting in poor outcomes for patients and families, with high rates of relapse (Rosenberg & Hickie 2019). As discussed in Chapter 2, in this book we promote a 'social ecological' understanding of mental health nursing practice that views mental health as existing within a multifaceted environment of social, environmental, psychological and biological influences. Using this conceptualisation, mental health and illness can be described as existing on a spectrum ranging from mental health to illness. The spectrum of mental health is heterogeneous, meaning everyone experiences it differently, and it is important to acknowledge that there are a wide variety of words and concepts used to explain various stages of the spectrum. The following sections synthesise several major concepts in mental health and illness.

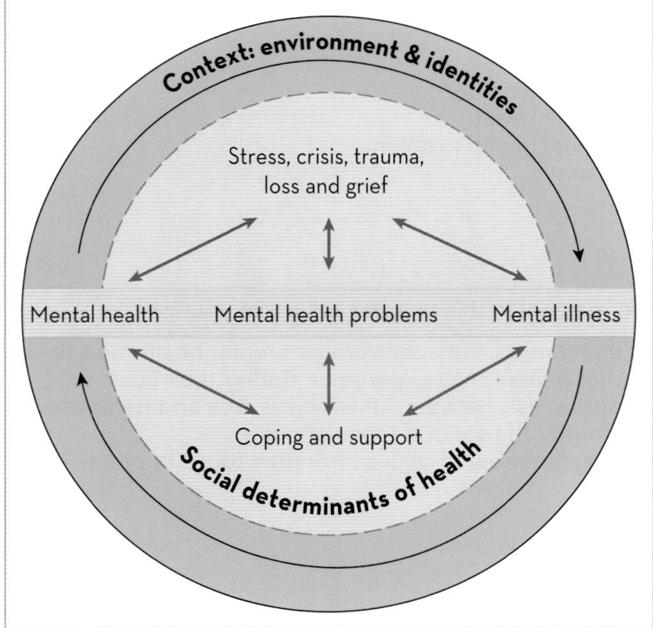

Figure 3.1
The spectrum of mental health and illness

Mental health

Mental health is a phenomenon that includes the common social and emotional experiences shared by all human beings on a daily basis. In spite of this, descriptions of mental health have differed throughout history and continue to vary in the modern era due to factors such as language, culture and the influence of particular interest groups. For example, in 2009 the Australian Government emphasised the importance of mental health to maintaining a productive and harmonious society:

> Good mental health is a crucial aspect of good general health, and underpins a productive and inclusive society.
> (Commonwealth of Australia 2009, p. 10)

Perhaps the most widely accepted modern description of mental health is the one promoted by the World Health Organization:

> Mental health is defined as a state of well-being in which every individual realizes his or her own potential, can cope with the normal stresses of life, can work productively and fruitfully, and is able to make a contribution to her or his community.
> (World Health Organization 2013, p. 38)

It is important to recognise that a mentally healthy life is not an all-perfect, all-positive life. Most societies accept a wide range of diversity, and most human beings living a mentally healthy life present a wide range of personal and social characteristics. A person who is living a mentally healthy life may present a variety of personal characteristics and social circumstances. Personal characteristics exhibited by people who are mentally healthy may mean that they appear to be: accepting or angry, hopeful or hateful, active or anxious, humble or humourless, joyful or jealous, brave or bullying, successful or sad, compassionate or conniving, flexible or fanatical, trusting or intolerable, or wise or not. Similarly, the social circumstances of people who are mentally healthy also vary tremendously. People who are single or married, gay or straight, employed or unemployed, wealthy or poor, connected or disconnected, introverted or extroverted, or with or without family and friends can live mentally healthy lives. Mental health helps a person to live a life that is satisfying to them and the community they live in. It does not matter how this is achieved or what the person's life looks like – this is of no consequence at all – as long the person and the community they live in believe that their life is satisfying.

Mental health nurses are well placed to assist individuals and communities to improve modifiable environmental, relational, psychological and physical determinants that can affect a person's mental health. Nurses can work clinically to enhance people's mental health using practices such as mental health assessment, psychotherapy, promotion of physical health care, social advocacy and promotion of ethical medication management. At the public health level nurses may work to influence the development of service models and advocate for fairer social factors that impact on mental health such as affordable housing schemes, access to education, income equality, employment and access to community resources.

In describing aspects of the spectrum of mental health, parts of consumer advocate Jarrad Hickmott's mental health journey are used for illustrative purposes. The first part of Jarrad's story is in the box below.

Jarrad's story: mental health

It seems that when things are going well and we are experiencing what is referred to as 'mental health' we tend to kind of take it for granted and don't really think much about it. Blessed with a happy childhood in a safe and loving family home, I performed well at primary school. In my final year of primary I was school captain, debating team captain, school sports representative, involved in and achieving all that I could.

Stress

Regular experiences of stress are a normal part of life. Stressors can include life events such as exams, a relationship breakdown or running late for an important appointment. A person's response to these stressors is referred to as the 'stress response', where 'stress' involves the effects of something that might threaten a person's physical and psychological homeostasis, or constant state of being (Selye 1956). Emotional distress can occur in relation to personal and social difficulties created through a range of life stressors, a crisis, trauma, loss or bereavement. For the most part, a person presenting in mental distress needs empathy, understanding and emotional support, rather than a diagnosis, treatment and medication (Middleton & Shaw 2000). Every individual responds to stressors differently, depending on factors including their appraisal of the stressor, and their existing coping strategies. Research informs us that life stress can generally be divided into four broad groups:

1. **Environment**: When human beings live in environments overwhelmed by circumstances such as unemployment, poverty, homelessness, violence, war or natural disasters such as bushfires or floods, they are more likely to experience levels of distress.
2. **Relationships:** Our family, community, living environment and culture can affect us as well. Any of these factors may in one way or another affect mental health.
3. **Psychology:** The attitudes we bring to circumstances we face, our thinking skills, our personality and the way we cope with stress can have a huge impact on whether or not we experience mental health.
4. **Physical health:** Many illnesses such as depression, bipolar disorder, schizophrenia and alcoholism can affect biochemicals that keep our body running smoothly. Vulnerability to such problems can sometimes run in families. Just as some families are predisposed to diabetes or high blood pressure, so too other families may be predisposed to mental health vulnerability.

Stress may be acute or chronic. It is different from crisis, which is an acute state where the person's usual coping strategies and ability to manage a situation has been overwhelmed.

Historical anecdote 3.1: Ancient ideas about mental health

Ancient Greek philosopher Aristotle (384–322 BC) theorised that good mental health was connected to the pursuit of happiness. He proposed two broad ways to experience happiness. The first was to cultivate good character through principled living such as caring for the poor or homeless; he referred to this as 'eudemonic' happiness. The second was seeking pleasure through wealth or sex; he referred to this as 'hedonic' happiness. Aristotle suggested that eudemonic happiness was more valuable than hedonic happiness because hedonic interests like power, wealth and sexual pleasure were generally associated with feelings that failed to last. According to Aristotle, parental guidance, good education and a moderate level of wealth were all required for people to be able to pursue eudemonic happiness, and he argued that providing the social platform for such opportunities was the role of government.

Read more about it: *Ryan RM, Huta V, Deci EL 2008 Living well: a self-determination theory. Anecdote on eudemonia. Journal of Happiness Studies 9(1):139–70*

Mental health problems

No matter if we are at home, at school, at work or in any other situation, if a person experiences an inability to cope and adapt to life stressors or crises, we are all capable of experiencing mental health problems. In this chapter mental health problems are defined as social or emotional wounds that affect a person's life but not to the extent that they seriously disrupt the person's relationships or normal daily activities. For some, the chances of experiencing mental health problems may increase at times when we feel vulnerable, perhaps on the first day in a new course of study or the first day of work, or maybe during a period of physical illness or a hospital admission. Our sense of vulnerability to mental health problems may be heightened by anxiety or fear or perhaps by feeling that we have little or no control over a situation, or over what is about to happen. Alternatively, vulnerability to mental health problems may increase for groups in society that experience particular social or political issues needing a solution – for example, those who are homeless, people seeking refuge from domestic violence, or those in prison. Mental health problems may also increase for people at risk of physical abuse or violence, thus needing measures to be put in place to keep them safe.

It is important for nurses to recognise, however, that mental health problems are not the same as diagnosable mental illness. Mental health problems can generally be understood with reference to three types of phenomena: distress, dysfunction and deviance (Rashed & Bingham 2014). Experiences of *distress* are commonly exhibited through thinking, feeling and behavioural symptoms such as anxious thoughts, low mood, isolative behaviour, memory loss (or perceptual abnormality), broken sleep, irritable behaviour or increased use of alcohol or other drugs. *Dysfunction* refers to behaviour that is negatively interpreted by others and may cause damage to a person's relationships over an extended period. *Deviance* describes behaviours that are dangerous to the person or others, including engaging in antisocial or criminal activities.

It is essential that nurses seek to assist people experiencing mental health problems on an individual basis. Keep in mind that some groups – such as infants, children and those who are unable to communicate at all due to disability, serious physical illness, frailty or extreme age – are vulnerable and need a high degree of care and support. Likewise, people arriving as refugees or seeking asylum after being exposed to war and traumatic events such as physical or sexual violence and assault, being kidnapped, tortured and seeing family members killed are extremely vulnerable and also in need of extensive care and support. However, assessing whether a person is vulnerable requires careful consideration of both personal and situational factors.

Jarrad's story: mental health problems

I don't remember much about what went on but my parents had marriage trouble towards the end of primary school and by the time high school rolled around I didn't want to attend. It remains inexplicable to me, but on my first day at high school aged 12 my mother drove me to school and I panicked about her leaving me there. A teacher had to restrain me because I was crying, kicking and screaming whilst my mother left. From that day on, high school was a difficult experience for me. I often managed to avoid school from Year 7 (age 12) to Year 10 (age 16) and the school rarely seemed to notice. When I did attend, I coasted without much attention to education. I found that being of a younger age I was able to avoid social engagements with little to no fallout or effort. When asked to attend a friend's party or event I would make excuses that I was playing sport or that I was helping a grandmother move or whatever else I could fabricate in order to avoid invitations. Not only was I trying to avoid the invitations out but also the awkwardness of a group of friends talking about something they all did on the weekend at an event I hadn't attended. People would often talk about their plans for after they graduated from high school and what universities they were planning to attend, where my only concern was just surviving the high school experience. Counselling support at our school was provided by an old Irish priest. His kind approach was that if I didn't want to go to class, I could just sit in his room in the office instead. That often involved random casual chats, which a lot of the time I found helpful to avoid the social anxiety I experienced when sitting in class.

Crisis

Nurses see people who are experiencing crisis, trauma, loss and grief in all clinical settings.

A *crisis* can be simply described as a difficult or dangerous situation that needs attention. As with life stressors, a crisis may be associated with aspects of a person's financial, social, environmental, political or personal life (see Table 3.1). In contrast to a stressful event, such as a job interview or an exam, a specific experience that the person perceives to be threatening, such as loss of employment, the death of a loved one, assault (physical, emotional or sexual) or divorce, may trigger a state of acute crisis. In this state, usual coping strategies can be seriously challenged, resulting in increasing feelings of vulnerability and rising levels of anxiety, distress and confusion. A person's usual ability to manage the demands of everyday life can be disrupted, resulting in disorganisation and disequilibrium. Without relief, such a crisis may result in severe emotional, cognitive and behavioural dysfunction, leading to a person being a risk to themselves or others (James & Gilliland 2013).

Differentiating between triggering events and an individual's response can be useful because a sense of crisis can arise from a broad range of possible incidents – from something seemingly insignificant to an outside observer, to a situation that others may view as a crisis while the person 'in crisis' does not see that there is a problem at all (Loughran 2011). You may have experienced

TABLE 3.1 Common types of crisis

TYPES OF CRISIS	DESCRIPTION
Developmental crises	Major transitions between life stages ('rites of passage'); these can be periods of significant and at times prolonged stress such as birth, adolescence, marriage, retirement or dying
Situational crises or 'accidental crises'	Crises that are situation-specific or culture-specific such as loss of employment, income or home, accidents, theft, loss of relationship, separation, divorce or domestic violence
Social crises	Arising from abuse of drugs or alcohol, criminal activities or violence
Complex crises	Not part of the everyday experience or shared accumulated knowledge, including crises associated with: • mental illness • trauma • diagnosis of a life-threatening physical illness • needing to seek asylum because of civil war, ethnic cleansing or religious persecution

a time when you felt that a particular event was catastrophic while your friends or family members had difficulty understanding 'what all the fuss was about'. Perhaps failing an exam for the first time shook your confidence in your ability to complete your study program successfully and you seriously contemplated withdrawing from your program. You may also have found yourself feeling that your future was ruined by this failure. In contrast, you may have had a friend who, from your perspective, was in a crisis situation. You'd had multiple discussions with your friend over several months about the increasing physical violence she was experiencing in her relationship. At times, you had tried to encourage her to leave the relationship and provided her with information about services for people experiencing domestic violence. Maybe your friend had come to work yet again with heavy make-up covering a black eye and you noticed bruises on her arms. While you feared for her safety, she dismissed this as 'not as bad as last time' and 'nothing to be concerned about'. Although you saw this as a crisis situation, your friend would not access support or even acknowledge the difficulty. The crisis model in Table 3.1 shows the unfolding sequence from a clearly identifiable precipitating stressor, loss or traumatic event to an acute crisis state. Considering the type of crisis can help to deepen understanding both of what may have triggered the crisis and what course of action may assist the person.

CONSUMER'S STORY 3.1
Nathan

Twenty-five-year-old Nathan presented to an emergency department distraught and overwhelmed. Several recent losses had caused him considerable grief and eroded his usual resilience and pragmatic coping style. He felt helpless to instigate any previously used problem-solving strategies. Nathan was distressed and tearful as he recounted the sequence of events that had led him to think ending his life was his best course of action. The nurse's initial assessment concluded that Nathan was displaying depressive symptoms with suicidal thoughts. Nathan had no specific plan to harm himself, but he did admit that his suicidal thoughts had scared him because he had never previously experienced such thoughts. Given his risk of self-harm, the nurse felt concerned about his ability to keep himself safe and her first inclination was to admit him to hospital, if necessary, against his will.

Slowly, Nathan calmed a little but still felt helpless and hopeless and unable to see any way through his distress. The nurse reassured Nathan that he was safe, and he agreed to continue with the assessment. As the nurse talked with Nathan, she raised her concerns and discussed how they might work together to keep him safe through this challenging time. Admission to hospital was a possible option. Although Nathan did not refuse hospitalisation, he was clearly not keen about this suggestion. Together they considered other options as the nurse attempted to tap into Nathan's strengths and to help him utilise his now disrupted coping strategies. The nurse asked Nathan what he thought he needed to overcome his distress. 'I don't know', he replied. This response is typical of a person whose thinking is affected by the emotional upset of an acute crisis. The nurse reframed the question, asking Nathan what his life and circumstances would look like if none of these events had happened. He described in some detail how life would be without such overwhelming grief and loss. Nathan rapidly became discouraged again when he could not think of how to live without feeling overwhelmed with grief and loss.

A shift in focus was needed again. Calming her own anxiety, the nurse expressed her curiosity about his efforts and past success in overcoming adversities in his life. Nathan recalled several difficult events and described how he had overcome these difficulties. The nurse reflected aloud on the strength and resilience he had demonstrated in overcoming these challenges. As Nathan acknowledged his own capacity to overcome adversity, the change in him was almost tangible. The nurse witnessed an 'aha' moment. When he realised he was already working hard to recover, Nathan's level of distress dissipated markedly and he began to think of other strategies he could employ to continue his recovery. Nathan was very thankful for the nurse's help. While the nurse accepted his thanks, at the same time she was humbled as she really hadn't worked miracles, nor did she have easy answers for Nathan. Rather it had been a process of listening (*really* listening) while taking time to allow Nathan to reconnect with his own strength and resilience. Instead of letting anxiety overwhelm her, the nurse had been able to avoid reinforcing Nathan's sense of helplessness and circumvent an admission to hospital. Nathan was able to leave with renewed strength and hope for his future. Before leaving, Nathan was happy to take an appointment for follow-up and phone numbers that he could call if he needed to talk before they met again.

Mental illness

Many people who experience mental health problems never access a mental health professional for assistance and so never interpret their problems as mental ill health. Many people access the internet, which may provide them with helpful information on how to adapt and recover a sense of mental health. However, research has also indicated that internet-based advice can lead to over analyses of problems and self-diagnoses, which can lead people to negative beliefs about their experience of problems and capacity to recover (Robertson et al. 2014).

In the same way that descriptions of mental health have varied throughout history, so too have ideas about mental illness. Modern definitions of mental illness vary considerably depending on the culture, language and interests of particular groups. For example, in Australia, the New South Wales Government emphasises 'impairment', defining mental illness in its *Mental Health Act 2007* (s. 4) as:

> ... a condition that seriously impairs, either temporarily or permanently, the mental functioning of a person and is characterised by the presence in the person of any one or more of the following symptoms: (a) delusions, (b) hallucinations, (c) serious disorder of thought form, (d) a severe disturbance of mood, (e) sustained or repeated irrational behaviour indicating the presence of any one or more of the symptoms referred to in paragraphs (a)–(d).
> (New South Wales Government 2007)

In this book when we refer to mental illness, we use the World Health Organization definition published in the 11th edition of the International Classification of Diseases:

> A syndrome characterized by clinically significant disturbance in an individual's cognition, emotion regulation, or behaviour that reflects a dysfunction in the psychological, biological, or developmental processes underlying mental functioning. Mental disorders are usually associated with significant distress in social, occupational, or other important activities.
> (American Psychiatric Association 2013, p. 20)

It is important to acknowledge that the mental health spectrum described in this chapter is an attempt to simplify exceptionally complex human phenomena. Providing simple models of understanding can be both useful and detrimental, depending on how they are applied. The reality is that, as stated above, people's emotional and psychological experiences are in a constant state of change as they react to life experiences, thereby affecting their social functioning. A person with mental illness often experiences so much distress in their thoughts, feelings and behaviours that they lose the ability to meet the expectations they have for themselves and the demands that society has for them, causing significant disruption in relationships at home and at work. The person's experience of mental illness may cause such disharmony between their pursuit of a satisfying life and society's ability to accommodate their behaviours, that society may deem them to be disabled. In line with this understanding the statement is often made that 'no one has absolute health' or is 'completely normal'. Contrary to this, however, when a person is described as experiencing mental illness, seldom does one hear or see a disavowal of the claim of absolute illness. The person is generally described as either mentally ill or not; that is, the person is identified as having a specific set of symptoms and is therefore labelled as having a specific clinical condition. Such a concrete distinction between mental health and illness, however, is overly simplistic because it fails to address the range of human experiences of everyday life. In the end, mental health and illness are complex social constructs that vary in each society and cultural group as we attempt to describe differences we perceive in life experiences.

Jarrad's story: mental illness

By age 17 my anxieties about social interactions became very pronounced. From age 16 to 18 there was a lot of added pressure to go out socially, which would make me anxious and fearful of experiencing further panic. I cared very little for academic or social pursuits; every day presented a difficulty just to get through without having a full-blown panic attack. To avoid social contact in the school yard during lunchtimes it became my habit to wander back and forth between the toilets at one end of the school and the toilets at the other end, not because I had a weak bladder but purely because I could hide away from others by sitting on the toilet.

I had been missing school, missing assessments and avoiding going to the doctors ... Eventually something had to give, and that time came halfway through Year 11. I attended a mental health service where I was diagnosed with social phobia and, on reflection, I suppose it was at that point when society labelled me with a mental illness.

Eventually the school decided that I had missed too many days and would be unable to complete the academic year and progress to Year 12. It was not a great shock to me or my family, but we didn't really have any plan for what to do for the next 6 months and how to use the time productively. My family was under the impression that it just meant that I would return the next year and do the year over again.

I spent the next 6 months in my bedroom at home with little to no engagement with the world, including my family. The only times I would leave my room would be to go to the bathroom or to eat. Rather than attend the dinner table for meals like the rest of my siblings I would instead leave my room to collect a plate of food then return to my room to eat. It was no way to live.

Looking back I view my life in those days as akin to a mouse scurrying from the safety of its dark crevice to fill its stomach, depending on the guise of night or its own agility and low profile as to not be disturbed by unwanted guests. The mouse is concerned not to cross paths with the family pet or a conveniently placed piece of food in the jaws of a trap. For me, I was trying to avoid crossing paths with members of my family and the anxieties that such interactions could cause. I had to avoid what often felt like a trap (the dinner table), which, to me, seemed like an attempt to be lured into social interaction by food.

Coping

Human beings are remarkably resilient and, mostly, people are able to cope with the life stressors they face and regain mental health relatively quickly. Coping refers to people's capacity to 'bounce back' after life stressors without experiencing ongoing problems. Individuals and groups that display good coping skills tend to possess a set of common characteristics that equip them to adapt to life's challenges. The ability to cope is not only reliant on internal psychological attitudes but on multiple external factors that contribute to each person's capacity to 'bounce back' after stressful events. Increasingly, research attention is being given to the impact of the social and cultural context on people's ability to cope. Globally, large numbers of people live in environments of extreme duress, which can stretch to breaking point the coping abilities of even the most durable individuals and communities. Situations where there is heavy loss of material resources and psychosocial supports in the context of violence markedly increase psychological distress and the risk of mental illness. Individual and community coping abilities are heavily affected in regions where ongoing war and civil conflict causes loss of life, mass displacement and the loss of even the most basic of human needs – food and safe drinking water, shelter and safety.

So why might some people cope and others struggle with what appear on the surface to be similar life stressors? It is useful to appreciate that there are a range of factors that can either protect or pose risks to a person's mental health (Fazel et al. 2012). Protective factors commonly include things such as regular physical exercise, a close relationship with a partner or parental figure; risk factors might include a lack of safe housing and biological stressors. Table 3.2 provides illustrative examples of factors that are

TABLE 3.2 Protective and risk factors

	PROTECTIVE FACTORS	RISK FACTORS
Social environment	• Safe housing • Access to education • Employment • Economic stability • Access to social welfare support if needed	• War • Poverty and crime • Political instability • Insecurity • Homelessness • Discrimination • Lack of support services
Relationships	• Positive childhood attachment • Supportive family and friends • Communication skills • Sense of personal autonomy • Community participation	• Abuse (physical, psychological, sexual, financial, spiritual) or exposure to abuse (e.g. domestic violence) • Neglect • Separation and loss • Peer rejection • Social isolation
Psychological factors	• Positive sense of self • Good coping skills • Attachment to family • Social skills • Good physical health	• Low self-esteem • Low self-efficacy • Poor coping skills • Insecure attachment in childhood • Physical and intellectual disability
Physical health	• Access to clean air and water • Adequate nutrition • Regular physical exercise • Access to quality physical health care	• Low-quality nutrition • High consumption of alcohol/drugs • Cigarette smoking • Low access to healthcare services

protective and those that are often risks across social environments, relationships, and psychological and physical health.

NEUROBIOLOGY AND NEUROPLASTICITY

The significance of distress is seen when we consider that although distress is experienced psychologically, it has profound effects on brain functioning, in some cases establishing neural pathways that predispose individuals to responses that become automatic and can be resistant to change (Yaribeygi et al. 2017). These stress responses, while they are adaptive ways of meeting the immediate challenges of the external environment, can be persistent over time, prevent new learning and become maladaptive. Chronic stress can lead to hypersensitivity of the limbic system of the brain, with the result that experiences resembling those that caused the initial stress can trigger an acute stress reaction, including the associated patterns of thinking and behavioural responses. In such cases the stress response becomes encoded in our memories and is activated automatically (Goldfarb et al. 2019). Chronic stress is mediated by the sympathetic nervous system and higher neural functions in the pituitary and hypothalamus, resulting in high levels of cortisol, which maintain a heightened sense of arousal. If you consider the case of a child raised in an environment of physical and emotional abuse, the constant exposure to high levels of psychological distress will cause a sustained stress response that becomes the child's way of living with their adverse experiences. In time they become less able to return to a non-aroused emotional baseline, and even minor stimuli such as words associated with a traumatic experience can trigger an acute stress response (Neumeister et al. 2018). Without intervention, this pattern of sustained stress response can contribute to profound alterations in emotional, psychological and social functioning, which can lead to a diagnosis of mental illness. Conversely, developing positive coping strategies has also been found to lead to changes in brain function. Resilience in adolescents who have experienced adversity is associated with changes in prefrontal structures (Burt et al. 2016), showing that the brain changes in response to both negative and positive life experiences. The concept of neuroplasticity refers to the capacity of the brain to change in response to new experiences and to develop new neural pathways that replace those that have become maladaptive or unhelpful (Voss et al. 2017). Yet the process of change can be difficult, as the brain tends to revert to established responses, however unhelpful and unwanted these are. Problems of addiction are one example of this difficulty, although other habituated behaviours such as responses to perceived threat can be equally difficult to change. Psychological interventions, in some cases supported by pharmacological interventions, can lead to changes in brain function and can help the person, over time, to sustain new responses (Solomon & Siegel 2017).

WORKING WITH PEOPLE WHO EXPERIENCE MENTAL HEALTH DISTRESS

As discussed in Chapter 2 nursing care for people who experience mental ill health needs to be both recovery-oriented and trauma-informed. In respect to mental health recovery, there are five key domains that health professionals and mental health services are expected to practise within:

- promoting a culture and language of hope and optimism
- putting the person first and at the centre of practice and viewing their life holistically
- supporting personal recovery and placing it at the heart of practice
- organisational commitment and workforce development for skilled practitioners and an environment that is conducive to recovery
- action on social inclusion and social determinants of health, mental health and wellbeing (Australian Health Ministers Advisory Council 2013).

In respect to trauma-informed care, nursing practice must involve awareness that trauma can have a significant impact on people and that mental health services and staff have a responsibility to provide emotionally and physically safe environments (Isobel & Edwards 2017). Services may re-traumatise people who have a history of trauma through using coercive practices such as seclusion and restraint, and admissions to mental health services can be potentially traumatic for people with and without a history of trauma due to loss of autonomy and control and being away from family and friends (Isobel & Edwards 2017; Muskett 2014).

In recognising these concerns, trauma-informed services are led by three key principles to guide practice (paraphrased from Muskett 2014):

- People need to feel connected, valued, informed and hopeful about their recovery from mental illness.
- Staff understand the connection between childhood trauma and adult mental health issues.
- Staff practise in empowering ways with consumers and their family and friends and other services to promote the consumer's autonomy.

While these principles focus on the needs of consumers and their family and friends, a trauma-informed approach to care can also provide support for managing workplace stress (Isobel & Edwards 2017). Trauma-informed practice does not replace recovery-oriented practice but is complementary and provides another perspective from which people (staff and consumers) may view recovery and therapeutic engagement. Implementing recovery-oriented and trauma-informed care can be challenging for both novice and experienced nurses. Research suggests that consumers often experience nurses taking a 'hands off' approach rather than working in partnership with the person (Hungerford 2014). This may be due to uncertainty about what to do. Focusing on the person driving their own recovery can be mistakenly interpreted as keeping out of the person's way. The following section aims to address these issues by providing some simple suggestions to guide your practice.

Historical anecdote 3.2: Compassionate approaches in history

The ancient Greek healer Asclepiades (129–40 BC) condemned the use of restraints on mental patients and promoted diet, soothing baths and music for mental health. Asclepiades' symbol the 'caduceus' continues to be associated with the medical profession today. Similar to Asclepiades, Roman physician Seranus (circa 250 BC) promoted compassionate approaches to people experiencing mental ill health. He believed people with mental illness required interest and understanding to protect them from fear, anger and blame. He promoted the idea that mental illness required companionship of non-threatening assistance from carers who could engage in discourse, reading, music and long walks. For Seranus, healing was contingent on a caring relationship.

Read more about it: *Horden P (Ed.) 2017 Music as medicine: the history of music therapy since antiquity. Routledge, New York*

WORK IN PARTNERSHIP

Past practices in mental health focused on the illness, to the exclusion of the person experiencing the illness. Tondora et al. (2014) described the process as follows: A person would go to a health professional for help. The professional would ask about 'the problem' (usually the symptoms they were experiencing), building a bigger and bigger picture of 'the problem'. This would lead to the person focusing more and more on 'the problem'. The problem would grow bigger and bigger and be added to by the person's family or others asking about it. Soon the person's identity would be taken over and consumed by 'the problem' or 'the illness'. Further contact with mental health professionals would reinforce this by almost exclusively focusing on asking questions about the illness. This is similar to the concept of problem saturation. Clearly, this scenario is unhelpful and disempowers people. Asking questions about the person and their experience, their strengths and how they have overcome adversity in the past promotes understanding and a sense of agency. It puts 'the problem' in context. The person retains a more robust sense of self, rather than thinking about themselves as fully integrated with the illness or problem. There is a tension between doing something for someone and encouraging people to care for themselves. There are times when fostering dependency by doing tasks for the person appears necessary, but in many cases it is counterproductive.

We know relationships are fundamentally important, from our earliest attachment experiences, for our emotional, social and physical wellbeing. Research on the outcomes of psychotherapy that are relevant to relationships in nursing has consistently found that the 'non-specifics of psychotherapy' (genuineness, empathy, warmth, positive regard, flexibility and the therapeutic alliance) are the most important in determining outcome (Nienhuis et al. 2018; Siegel 2004). Other outcome studies report 15% of outcome effect is attributed to placebo, 15% to techniques of therapy, 30% to the therapeutic relationship and 40% to client-specific factors (Nienhuis et al. 2018). Such factors revolve around what the person does outside the therapeutic relationship but also includes knowing what the person wants. When the therapeutic relationship and client factors are considered, the importance of working in partnership and considering the person's perspective of what is helpful appears to be more important than what the nurse believes might work.

Research shows that partnerships are the key to the transformation needed in recovery. An emphasis on activity and occupation as core aspects of agency determine a person's quality of life (Javed & Amering 2016; Raeburn et al. 2016; 2017). Agency is the fundamental freedom to fully participate in the community with the full rights of all citizens. It is also being active in making meaning of one's life and being an active agent by deciding to do particular activities (e.g. returning to work) or asserting one's basic human rights (Allard et al. 2018; Cleary et al. 2018a).

Jarrad's story: recovery

Things really started to change for me when I was referred to a headspace youth centre that had opened in my local area. Rather than a psychologist, I was given an appointment with a mental health nurse practitioner. Due to funding available at the time I was able to see him long term, which already was doing better than other services.

Unlike other clinicians I had seen in the past, the nurse didn't jump straight in and try and ask me what was wrong and how they could help straightaway; he seemed to realise that that approach was never going to work with me. I had sat through many appointments with psychologists previously during which I remember just staring at the ground incommunicado. I was crying and I remember the nurse trying to reach out without having to delve into anything too personal. I was wearing a black New Zealand rugby jersey and at that first appointment after receiving some brief information from my mother and asking her to leave the two of us in the room alone, the nurse began with some friendly banter about the Australian and New Zealand rugby team, which proved an easy way to get me to interact. Rather than the relationship with the nurse practitioner forming as 'expert and patient', it was almost like 'teacher and student'. The nurse practitioner taught me that my experiences were not uncommon and that they could be explained with reference to my body, brain, and various biological and social interactions I had been having. I learnt a lot about what was going on for me both mentally and physically, whereas with previous therapists I was only left with questions. This insight and knowledge helped me grow and understand, leading to better outcomes for me. Where before I would end up in situations that made me extremely uncomfortable and I had no way of explaining them, now I still felt uncomfortable but I understood why that uncomfortableness was there and why it manifested in the way it did.

A kind of partnership developed between us where I was able to have real input into my own care. There were times where I would suggest a way to move forward because I had that insight into his mindset as well as my own. There were times where I would disagree with his perspective and recommendations because I knew that it wouldn't work for me. There were times where he would suggest an approach that I would disagree with because it made me uncomfortable, but, based on mindset, he knew that it was the right choice for me. The chance to negotiate in a kind of team as I sort to recover led to far better outcomes than previous services, which had felt very prescriptive.

I also enjoyed the freedom around our sessions, not only in dialogue but also environment. There were some sessions where we would meet at the local coffee shop or some just walking around the local shops. Another great benefit was the fact that at times there would be university nursing students on placement. They were a really nice middle ground for me in that they weren't overly clinical but they also weren't completely ignorant of mental health concerns. It also changed the dynamic of the relationship to me being the expert of them. It also allowed for the exploration of different environments. Whereas before I would not buy anything at the shop, catch a train, catch a bus or basically interact with anyone, I now had the support with the students to conquer what were simple things for others but huge hurdles for me.

Not only was this nursing care a catalyst for significant progression on the social side of things but also in terms of longer term goals. Throughout our interaction the idea was put forward that university might be a reasonable goal to aspire to complete. Naturally, at first, I was quite hesitant given that my time at school had been so hard. There was a fair bit of discussion back and forth and a healthy amount of challenging, planning and discussion. In the end I ended up entering Sydney University through a mature entry scheme. The scheme saw me complete a short course for a year in preparation for entering a bachelor's degree. Naturally there were challenges, but unlike before I had that insight now so was able to work through it. I was able to better engage with peers, the content and my teachers as I had a lot more experience under my belt now compared to my schooling before. Whereas before in high school I didn't achieve that well, in this course I topped my course with high distinction-level results.

FOCUS ON STRENGTHS

The strengths model proposes that all people have goals, talents and confidence, and that all environments contain resources, people and opportunities (Deane et al. 2019). It supports Deegan's (1988) assertion that people who have experienced mental distress are more interested in focusing on what they can do to move on with their lives and live as normally as possible within their community. Focusing on strengths and personal values promotes a person's resilience, aspirations, talents and uniqueness, and how these strengths can be mobilised and built on to overcome difficulties.

A key therapeutic practice is 'reframing' from a pessimistic worldview to an optimistic one that instils hope and challenges self-stigma. For example, the nurse will want to know what the person has done in the past to overcome life's difficulties and how they can use the strengths they used previously to overcome their current challenges. Nurses are well placed to *gently* prompt people from taking a less positive view by asking about the exceptions – the times their approach *did* work and so on. It is critical here not to invalidate the person. Consider: 'I appreciate that is how you feel'; 'I wonder if there are times when things work for you?'

People overwhelmingly talk about the experience of mental distress as a transformative process where the old self is let go of and a new sense of self emerges (Deegan 2004). The intense struggle of dealing with mental health challenges leads to positive outcomes and a sense of personal agency that moves the person beyond where they would have been if they had not had the experience.

Lived experience comment by Jarrad Hickmott

This chapter expertly covers the important areas of the strengths model, recovery model and trauma-informed care. These models are the cornerstones of the lived experience and consumer movements. I very much appreciate the acknowledgement of mental distress as being a 'human experience' in that we all experience it to varying degrees and for different reasons.

NURSE'S STORY 3.1

Pamela

Sarah, a 22-year-old university student, was brought in for involuntary admission after having walked in front of traffic, unable to explain what had happened or to communicate what she was thinking or feeling. Sarah had a history of having been sexually assaulted the previous year and more recently had witnessed a woman falling in front of a train. She had also recently experienced sleeplessness and poor appetite, could not study and had great fears about herself and her family members dying. She had a very close and loving relationship with her parents and her twin brother.

Using principles of recovery-informed care, the nurse took considerable time to assist Sarah in establishing a sense of safety and control in the inpatient environment. This was achieved by allowing her family members to stay with her until she went to sleep. This involved the nurse negotiating for the hospital's visiting policy to be interpreted more flexibly, as well as negotiating with other staff to spend as long with Sarah as she required to establish a sense of safety.

Sarah had difficulty talking directly with the nurse, but talking with family members in Sarah's presence about their lives, their strengths as a family and how they had supported each other through difficult times was an approach that seemed to permit Sarah to calm herself. Eventually she was able to communicate what her family could do to help her feel in control. She was able to make arrangements for the next day with her family and asked for her belongings to be brought into the hospital and for friends to be contacted. Family members were able to tell stories of times they had overcome problems and the strengths they all brought to support each other. Sarah's admission was very brief, and she reported feeling that the nurse and her family were encouraging, reminding her of the resources she had in her family and friends and how they were there to support her. She appreciated the time the nurse took to patiently wait for her to be able to communicate.

Critical thinking challenge 3.1

- Develop a concept map that answers the question: How do people who are mentally well/healthy become mentally ill?
- Now develop a concept map that answers the question: How do people who experience mental illness become mentally well/healthy?
- Are there similarities between the two maps? What are the differences?
- What do these concept maps suggest about mental health and illness?

PROMOTE SELF-DETERMINATION

Self-determination is the basic human right to be able to make and participate in decisions about your life, having a choice in determining how you live your life and having control over your life. These are fundamental tenets in all the human rights declarations and conventions. The theory of self-determination is part of the recovery paradigm because of its centrality to a person's recovery. Self-determination theory proposes that the components of self-determination are autonomy, competence and relatedness (Raeburn et al. 2015). These are required to effectively participate in and make decisions and to have choice and control over one's life. All people need these to grow and thrive. Self-determination allows people to live a good life according to their own values and beliefs. What this looks like will vary among individuals and cultures. The consumer movement's motto 'nothing about me without me' reflects the above. Maintaining and promoting a person's right to be self-determining is a fundamental principle of mental health service standards and legislation (Australian Health Ministers Advisory Council 2013; Department of Health and Ageing 2013).

Remember that when we interact with people during times of distress or challenge, we have a skewed view of their inherent capacities. Continually reflect on the assumptions you may be making about people to keep in check the capacity we all have to act 'as if' these assumptions are true. To protect and promote a person's right to self-determine, you could consider the following:

- Maximise the person's autonomy and their ability to self-regulate by taking control of and responsibility for what they do.
- Maximise the person's capacity to make informed choices and make sure they are involved in decisions concerning them.
- Medications or other interventions may not be the person's choice. Consumer advocate Pat Deegan has attempted to address this by developing 'Common Ground' – a tool for maximising a person's autonomy and decision making within a treatment setting. Watch the short video at **www.patdeegan.com/commonground**.

People with lived experience of mental ill health can be key supports for each other in terms of recovery, self-help and responsibility. The sharing of experiences and stories of overcoming with others who have had similar experiences can be far more powerful than the support provided by workers. This is because people learn they are not alone in their experience, that there is hope and there are many different options and opportunities for recovery that may be helpful. Within Australia and New Zealand there are consumer organisations that provide advice, advocacy, support and service delivery. Many other organisations providing broader supports operate at the local level throughout Australia and New Zealand. There are also a growing number of peer workers and peer-run services emerging. Several alternative support groups have been established to support those consumers who hold firmly to their experiences, such as voice-hearing groups and groups to support people to explore unusual beliefs, without having to label their experiences in professional jargon.

Chapter summary

This chapter has provided a platform on which you can continue to build your understanding of the spectrum of mental health and illness. You now have a beginning understanding of the long-lasting impact of trauma on a person's development and the ways in which this may influence a person's response to difficulties over their lifetime. Mental distress is a part of human existence: it varies in degree, but it will happen to all of us at times. The journey of healing and recovery is salient for everyone. There is a need to talk about recovery in more humane terms because it is not something that happens to 'the other' – we are all vulnerable to mental distress under certain circumstances. Nurses need to be with people in this humane context rather than in a context of pathology, difference and a reductionist focus on symptoms and diagnosis (Cleary et al. 2018b).

We encourage you to reflect on how the principles of mental health practice are fundamental to all nursing practice, regardless of setting. We hope we have encouraged you to think about how you can participate more fully in your practice by developing your awareness of the complexities and realities of the context in which practice occurs. More specifically, we hope you appreciate how your attitudes, values and beliefs play a crucial role in your everyday practice.

Mental health nursing practice is influenced by an ever-evolving knowledge base; hence, the principles informed by this knowledge base continue to change and to evolve. Practice is time- and context-specific, making the ability to tolerate and incorporate change vital. Consequently, your thinking about your practice will be continually influenced by your developing self-awareness, your incorporation of new ideas into your practice, and your increasing professional and personal experience. The primary focus of mental health nursing practice is people with lived experience and how nurses can help facilitate recovery. Nurses can assist in this process by working in trauma-informed partnership with consumers to help them realise their potential and tap into a wide range of community resources and supports, of which mental health services are just one. Just as importantly, we hope you find the experience of mental health nursing as rewarding as we have.

EXERCISE FOR CLASS ENGAGEMENT

An idiom is a phrase or expression that means something different from the literal definition of the actual words used. Have a discussion with a fellow student who is from a different culture and identify as many idioms as possible that each of you use when you are feeling physically unwell or emotionally distressed. Extend your list to include idioms that other members of your family may use. Reflect on whether you can interpret what your colleague's idioms mean. What implications might this have for mental health assessment?

Useful websites

Mental Health Australia: http://mhaustralia.org/about-us.
Mental Health Council of Australia: http://www.mhca.org.au/.
Mental Health in Multicultural Australia: http://www.mhima.org.au/framework/mhima-website.
National Mental Health Commission: http://www.mentalhealthcommission.gov.au/.
NSW Mental Health Act (2007): https://www.legislation.nsw.gov.au/#/view/act/2007/8/whole.
NSW Mental Health Commission: Lived experience (contains consumer stories): https://nswmentalhealthcommission.com.au/lived-experience.
NSW Mental Health Coordinating Council: http://www.mhcc.org.au/about-mhcc/.
Royal Australian and New Zealand College of Psychiatrists Practice Guidelines: https://www.ranzcp.org/practice-education/guidelines-and-resources-for-practice.
SANE Australia: http://www.sane.org/.

References

Allard, J., Lancaster, S., Clayton, S., et al., 2018. Carers' and service users' experiences of early intervention in psychosis services: implications for care partnerships. Early Interv. Psychiatry 12 (3), 410–416.
American Psychiatric Association, 2013. Diagnostic and Statistical Manual of Mental Disorders, fifth ed. APA, Washington, DC.
Australian Health Ministers Advisory Council, 2013. A National Framework for Recovery-Oriented Mental Health Services: Policy and Theory. Commonwealth of Australia, Canberra.
Burt, K.B., Whelan, R., Conrod, P.J., et al., 2016. Structural brain correlates of adolescent resilience. J. Child Psychol. Psychiatry 57 (11), 1287–1296.
Cleary, M., Raeburn, T., Escott, P., et al., 2018b. 'Walking the tightrope': the role of peer support workers in facilitating consumers' participation in decision-making. Int. J. Ment. Health Nurs. 27 (4), 1266–1272.
Cleary, M., Raeburn, T., West, S., et al., 2018a. Two approaches, one goal: how mental health registered nurses perceive their role and the role of peer support workers in facilitating consumer decision-making. Int. J. Ment. Health Nurs. 27 (4), 1212–1218.
Commonwealth of Australia, 2009. Fourth national mental health plan – an agenda for collaborative government action in mental health 2009–2014, Department of Health and Ageing, Australian Government: Canberra.
Deane, F., Goff, R., Pullman, J., et al., 2019. Changes in mental health providers' recovery attitudes and strengths model implementation following training and supervision. Int. J. Ment. Health Addict. 17 (6), 1417–1431.
Deegan, P.E., 2004. Recovery: The Experience and the Evidence. National Empowerment Center/SeaRose Productions, Lawrence MA.
Deegan, P.E., 1988. Recovery: the lived experience of rehabilitation. Psychosoc. Rehabil. J. 11 (4), 11–19.
Department of Health and Ageing, 2013. National Mental Health report: tracking of mental health reform in Australia 1993–2011. Commonwealth of Australia, Canberra.
Fazel, M., Reed, R.V., Panter-Brick, C., et al., 2012. Mental health of displaced and refugee children resettled in high-income countries: risk and protective factors. Lancet 379 (9812), 266–282.

Goldfarb, E.V., Tompary, A., Davachi, L., et al., 2019. Acute stress throughout the memory cycle: diverging effects on associative and item memory. J. Exp. Psychol. Gen. 148 (1), 13.

Grech, E., Raeburn, T., 2019. Experiences of hospitalised homeless adults and their health care providers in OECD nations: a literature review. Collegian 26 (1), 204–211.

Horden, P. (Ed.), 2017. Music as Medicine: The History of Music Therapy Since Antiquity. Routledge, New York.

Hungerford, C., 2014. Recovery as a model of care? Insights from an Australian case study. Issues Ment. Health Nurs. 35 (3), 156–164.

Isobel, S., Edwards, C., 2017. Using trauma informed care as a nursing model of care in an acute inpatient mental health unit: a practice development process. Int. J. Ment. Health Nurs. 26 (1), 88–94.

James, R.K., Gilliland, B.E., James, L., 2013. Crisis Intervention Strategies, seventh ed. Brooks/Cole, Belmont, CA.

Javed, A., Amering, M., 2016. Mental health and human rights: working in partnership with persons with a lived experience and their families and friends. Indian J. Psychiatry 58 (3), 250.

Loughran, H., 2011. Understanding Crisis Therapies: An Integrative Approach to Crisis Intervention and Post Traumatic Stress. 2011. Jessica Kingsley Publishers, London.

Maron, E., Baldwin, D.S., Balõtšev, R., et al., 2019. Manifesto for an international digital mental health network. Digital Psychiatry 2 (1), 14–24.

Middleton, H., Shaw, I., 2000. Distinguishing mental illness in primary care: we need to separate proper syndromes from generalised distress. BMJ 320 (7247), 1420–1421.

Muskett, C., 2014. Trauma-informed care in inpatient mental health settings: a review of the literature. Int. J. Ment. Health Nurs. 23 (1), 51–59.

Neumeister, P., Gathmann, B., Hofmann, D., et al., 2018. Neural correlates of trauma-related single word processing in posttraumatic stress disorder. Biol. Psychol. 138, 172–178.

Nienhuis, J., Owen, J., Valentine, J.C., et al., 2018. Therapeutic alliance, empathy, and genuineness in individual adult psychotherapy: a meta-analytic review. Psychother. Res. 28 (4), 593–605.

New South Wales Government, 2007. Mental Health Act. Retrieved from: https://www.legislation.nsw.gov.au/#/view/act/2007/8/whole.

Raeburn, T., Schmied, V., Hungerford, C., et al., 2017. Autonomy support and recovery practice at a psychosocial clubhouse. Perspect. Psychiatr. Care 53 (3), 175–182.

Raeburn, T., Schmied, V., Hungerford, C., et al., 2016. The use of social environment in a psychosocial clubhouse to facilitate recovery-oriented practice. BJPsych. Open 2, 173–178.

Raeburn, T., Schmied, V., Hungerford, C., et al., 2015. Self-determination theory: a framework for clubhouse psychosocial rehabilitation research. Issues Ment. Health Nurs. 36 (2), 145–151.

Rashed, M.A., Bingham, R., 2014. Can psychiatry distinguish social deviance from mental disorder? Philos. Psychiatr. Psychol. 21 (3), 243–255.

Robertson, N., Polonsky, M., McQuilken, L., 2014. Are my symptoms serious Dr Google? A resource-based typology of value co-destruction in online self-diagnosis. AMJ 22 (3), 246–256.

Rosenberg, S., Hickie, I., 2019. No gold medals: assessing Australia's international mental health performance. Australas. Psychiatry 27 (1), 36–40.

Ryan, R.M., Huta, V., Deci, E.L., 2008. Living well: a self-determination theory. Anecdote on eudemonia. J. Happiness Stud. 9 (1), 139–170.

Selye, H., 1956. The Stress of Life. McGraw-Hill, New York.

Siegel, D.J., 2004. Attachment and self-understanding: parenting with the brain in mind. J. Prenat. Perinat. Psychol. Health 18 (4), 273.

Solomon, M., Siegel, D.J., 2017. How People Change: Relationships and Neuroplasticity in Psychotherapy. WW Norton & Company, New York.

Tondora, J., Miller, R., Slade, M., et al., 2014. Partnering for Recovery in Mental Health: A Practical Guide to Person-Centered Planning. John Wiley & Sons, Chichester.

Voss, P., Thomas, M.E., Cisneros-Franco, J.M., et al., 2017. Dynamic brains and the changing rules of neuroplasticity: implications for learning and recovery. Front. Psychol. 8, 1657.

World Health Organization, 1947. Constitution of the World Health Organization. WHO, Geneva.

World Health Organization, 2013. Mental Health Action Plan 2013–2020. WHO, Geneva.

Yaribeygi, H., Panahi, Y., Sahraei, H., et al., 2017. The impact of stress on body function: a review. EXCLI J. 16, 1057.

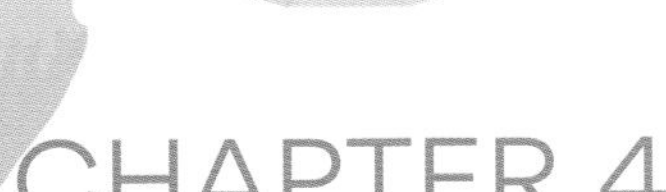

CHAPTER 4

Safety in care, safety at work

Scott Brunero and Scott Lamont

KEY POINTS

- Creating safety in care and a safe work environment is essential in the context of mental health.
- Challenges to safe care and work can occur in the context of staff knowledge, skills and attitudes, and in consumer distress, anxiety and past experiences of mental health care.
- Behaviours associated with a safe caring and work environment include empathy, compassion, reflective practice, high-level de-escalation skills, violence prevention, behavioural risk assessment and management.
- Nurses need to practise reflectively and be mindful of their own behaviour.

KEY TERMS

- Difficult behaviour
- Empathy
- Legal issues
- Limit setting
- Manipulation
- Person-centred care
- Reflection
- Risk analysis
- Safe care
- Safe work
- Self-harm
- Trauma

LEARNING OUTCOMES

The material in this chapter will assist you to:

- develop and maintain therapeutic relationships with consumers
- understand nursing staff, consumer and environmental factors contributing to safety in care and safety at work
- understand risk in the context of safe care and work
- understand general principles of creating a safe care and work environment
- identify specific approaches to managing behaviour that challenges a safe care and work environment.

Introduction

The nurse–consumer relationship is central to nursing care. Nurses in general are in continuous and direct contact with consumers and, as such, spend extended periods of time with them. Continuous contact places nurses in a unique position to develop therapeutic relationships with consumers through processes of collaboration, inclusiveness, mutuality and respect. However, there may be times when the relationship nurses have with consumers is tested, placing nurses in a difficult position and facing behaviours that challenge safe care and work (Gerace et al. 2018; Stein-Parbury 2016).

Behaviours that challenge safe care and work include aggression, manipulation, self-harm, suicide and psychosis-related behaviour. These types of behaviour occur in inpatient units, community settings, emergency departments, general hospitals and primary care settings.

This chapter will help you to engage in healthy relationships with consumers and to understand the most common types of behaviour that challenge safe care and work encountered by nurses. It will make you more aware of the antecedents of challenging behaviour, help you to recognise when they are present and guide you in developing responses and strategies. Finally, it will help you understand what people mean when they engage in these behaviours and become self-aware regarding your own emotions and care needs.

Types of behaviour that challenge safety in care and safety at work

A key skill of mental health nurses is to interpret and understand consumers with high levels of distress, to assist them in their navigation of healthcare systems, to monitor and manage their own distress and to manage conflict in interpersonal relationships (Stein-Parbury 2016). Knowing whether behaviour is a challenge or not can be subjective and individual; it may depend on the skill of the nurse or the social setting the nurse is in. Commonly encountered behaviours that challenge safe care and work reported in the literature include:

- aggression (verbal and physical threats, shouting, conflict, non-adherence, absconding)
- manipulation ('splitting' or demanding attention or that special conditions are met)
- self-harm and suicidal behaviour (cutting, ingesting poisons, overdose).

These behaviours are not mutually exclusive – they may occur in combination, or all at once, frequently or infrequently, and can be seen across the diagnostic groups in mental health settings. Nurses working within the mental health setting will experience some or a range of these behaviours in the course of their clinical practice. Responding requires a wide range of nursing skills. It is therefore essential to understand the social context and circumstances in which they occur (Llor-Esteban et al. 2017; Ritter & Platt 2016).

Historical anecdote 4.1: Gone battie?

William Battie (1703–1776) was a pioneer in the care of mental health patients. As a physician of high repute with a scientific background and distinguished social position, he helped turn mental health care into a respectable medical specialty. While observing patients Battie noted that some would recover without treatment or only after treatment had been stopped. This observation led him to consider the powerful therapeutic effects of a caring environment. He was one of England's first public figures to recognise that carers in 'mental asylums' needed to be specially selected and trained. Considering all the good he did for people with mental health problems, it is ironic that the modern derogatory term 'gone batty' was derived from his name!

Read more about it: *Bynum WF 1974 Rationales for therapy in British psychiatry: 1780–1835. Medical History, 18(4): 317–34*

Understanding the context of safety in care and safety at work

An understanding of the social context within which safe care and work occurs is essential in identifying the numerous factors that precede and influence safety. For example, staff and consumers often have different perceptions of why a safe work environment is challenged; while staff may cite consumer factors, consumers may cite staff factors. The reality is that a range of socially determined factors including staff, consumer, environmental, cross-cultural and social factors act as precipitants that can challenge a safe care and work environment (Affleck et al. 2018; SICSAW 2019).

Staff factors

A safe care and work environment often occurs as a result of what we as nurses do or, in some circumstances, don't do. We may not always be conscious of how we are perceived by consumers, or how our behaviour influences the behaviour of consumers. Our knowledge, skills and attitudes and subsequent behaviours become an important aspect of preventing, mitigating and managing how we deliver care.

Developing therapeutic relationships with consumers is essential in maintaining safety at work. This requires commitment from you as a nurse to engage purposefully with consumers in a person-centred manner: developing intimate knowledge of the consumer as a person; showing respect and being courteous; actively listening to concerns, fears and frustrations; responding in an empathic way; looking for meaning behind the behaviour (anger is directed at me but seems to be coming from being locked up in hospital!); and communicating a genuine desire to help. Nurses who are unable or unwilling to facilitate effective therapeutic relationships are likely to encounter difficulties in delivering care (Stein-Parbury 2016).

Developing therapeutic relationships can be easier said than done and may be compromised by a range of personal factors. For example, nurses may have personal issues that compromise their ability to engage therapeutically. This includes the nurse's own mental health and personality style, current stressors in the nurse's life, previous experience (or inexperience), tiredness and illness. Any of these factors can contribute to an interaction style that leads to a perception that nurses are not interested or are simply ignoring the needs of consumers. Furthermore, nurses who are impatient, controlling, authoritarian or coercive in their interactions with consumers are less likely to build positive relationships and to achieve desirable outcomes in care (Dickens et al. 2016; McAllister & McCrae 2017).

Consumer factors

Mental illness and disorders can influence a consumer's ability to engage purposefully in the health care that nurses provide. Such conditions include: psychotic disorders; adjustment disorders; mood, anxiety and personality disorders; organic disorders; drug and alcohol intoxication or withdrawal; intellectual disability; brain injury; being stigmatised or marginalised; or experiences of trauma or trauma-related mental health care.

A range of experiences associated with psychotic disorders may increase the likelihood of difficulties with consumers engaging in safe care delivery. These experiences can include thought disorder, hallucinations and delusions – in particular, where consumers may be paranoid, suspicious, fearful or frightened. Consumers who are cognitively compromised may present with anxiety, confusion and disorientation. Behaviours that challenge accepting care have been linked to the increased energy, disinhibition and irritability associated with mood disorders (mania), making care delivery challenging. This may lead to frustration, helplessness or catastrophic thinking and to difficulties engaging with consumers. Consumers with a low mood typically seen in depressive disorder may be difficult to engage in their own self-care and other daily activities, which may require constant prompting from the nurse. Consumers at risk of self-harm behaviours may need close monitoring and observations of behaviour, with constant efforts to engage in dialogue. Consumers with personality vulnerabilities may have a heightened perception of rejection or humiliation, particularly when healthcare concerns or requests are ignored or dismissed. Some consumers may have poor impulse control as a feature of their personality, while consumers with narcissistic personality styles may present with excessive demands or entitlement of nurses' time. Factors such as fatigue, pain and physical comorbidities influence consumers' quality of life and subsequently their psychological and emotional wellbeing.

If consumers are not involved in planning and discussions about their care, they will be unaware of what is expected of them. Mental health problems often adversely influence a person's control over aspects of their life; therefore, processes of partnership, inclusion and engagement can help mitigate some of the consumer factors mentioned in this section.

Environmental factors

Health staff in general are often unaware of the effect of the environment on the wellbeing of consumers. Environmental factors become part of our contextual understanding of a safe workplace. However, the physical environment should not be viewed in isolation from system or operational aspects such as the infrastructure, policies and procedures that govern its operation. Coercive or restrictive processes that limit inclusion and choice for consumers, suboptimal communication with unclear care plans, and staff caught in a reactive bind because of busy workloads and competing systemic demands are likely to experience increased frustration.

Many aspects of the environments in which nurses work are beyond our control: we may practise in ageing facilities that are no longer commensurate with modern care, and capital works funding may be scarce in relation to maintenance, improvement and renovation. Frustration, high expressed emotion and anger are more likely to be present in poorly structured environments that are aesthetically unappealing, noisy and crowded, too hot/too cold, devoid of natural light and lacking in private space (dormitories versus single rooms) (Hui 2016). There is a need to balance the design of inpatient wards so as not to overstimulate aroused or agitated consumers while not understimulating withdrawn or depressed consumers. Person-centred design using the aforementioned attributes can lead to better cognitive, motivational and emotive processes in both consumers and staff. Sensory modulation or using specific equipment and modifying the physical and social environment have been shown to assist consumers in reducing their high expressed emotions (West et al. 2017).

Cultural factors

Diverse cultures have behavioural and communication nuances that may be interpreted variously by nurses from different cultural backgrounds. Behaviours that appear challenging within one culture may be acceptable within another. Therefore, the need to be culturally aware has significant implications for nurses in the context of safe care and work (Holland 2017). In some Asian societies it is not culturally appropriate to show overt emotional reactions in public, and in some Arab cultures, women may not be allowed in the same room as a man unless accompanied by a relative. Both situations, if poorly managed by nurses, may be precursors to a conflicted work environment. Within the local context Indigenous Australians' experience of mental health services, and in particular their experience of seclusion, suggests that there is a need for social and cultural factors to be considered when engaging in these practices (Brophy et al. 2016). Indigenous Australians may have had historical traumatic experiences of governmental control and coercion and their perception of care may be influenced by this. Nurses need to be aware of their own cultural biases and potential misconceptions and tendency to subscribe to myths about particular cultural groups. Providing culturally congruent care may give the nurse an opportunity to understand why someone is behaving the way they are, to prevent the behaviour escalating, and the knowledge to approach the behaviour with confidence. Factors related to cultural and gender identity are further explored in Chapter 2.

Social factors

Mental illness in our society has been impacted by the media and public perceptions, and this has resulted in labelling consumers with mental illness as at risk, dangerous, difficult, absconders and/or frequent flyers. The power of these negative labels can influence how we as professionals engage with people. When labels are attributed to people, they can consequently be adopted by them, and individuals may therefore engage in behaviour that perpetuates these labels (Brunero et al. 2018). As nurses we must be mindful of the language we use when relating to consumers and how we engage them, by not proliferating negative labels that exist more broadly in society about mental illness.

Models of care

Care cultures that are risk-focused, coercive or restrictive in nature are likely to lead to negative interpersonal relationships and dynamics. Being aware of your own identity and practice within such cultures is essential to achieving optimum care outcomes (Slemon et al. 2017). Consumer-focused frameworks adopt strengths-based approaches to care. Models underpinned by such a framework seek to actively involve consumers as partners in all aspects of care provision and not as passive recipients of care. Thus, shared decision making and consumer-led decision making enhance goal planning, care options and subsequent outcomes. Known variously as 'person-centred' or 'patient-centred', such models are proposed as being 'underpinned by values of respect for persons, individual right to self-determination, mutual respect and understanding' (McCormack et al. 2013, p. 193).

Consumer-focused models of care operate on the premise that only consumers can understand the real experience and journey of being a consumer, therefore they are the key stakeholders in planning and discussions about care and so need to be active, valued and empowered throughout. Studies exploring strengths-based approaches have identified that these approaches are associated with improvements in quality-of-life indicators, confidence, self-esteem, self-advocacy and self-care. Strengths-based approaches focus unsurprisingly on strengths, abilities and empowerment – a shift from traditional problem-based care approaches, which largely ignore strengths and positive abilities that help fulfil wellbeing. Strengths-based approaches effect more purposeful engagement with consumers, help maintain a sense of control over their decision making and lead to more positive experiences of care.

There are various specific consumer-focused models:

- **The recovery model** (or recovery approach) adopts an approach whereby the consumer's potential for recovery is paramount and supported by a network of personal and professional relationships. Recovery has less of an emphasis on outcomes and instead focuses on the consumer's personal journey, instilling and maintaining hope, a positive sense of self and meaning, a secure base and social inclusion within a paradigm of empowerment and flourishing (Cusack et al. 2017).
- **The tidal model** focuses on the ebb and flow of personal human experience and aims to empower consumers in their own recovery with an emphasis on the power of their own self and wisdom, as opposed to health professionals directing this (Barker 2001; Barker & Buchanan-Barker 2010; Savaşan & Çam 2017).
- **Solution-focused (brief) therapy** is a goal-directed psychotherapeutic partnership that focuses on what consumers want to achieve in the here and now and in the future. While the relevance of past experience is not ignored, it is not an emphasis or focal point of care (Smith & Macduff 2017).
- **Trauma-informed care** adopts the principle that only a consumer who has experienced trauma can truly understand the journey of healing. The unique skills, attributes and resilience that have enabled trauma survivors to survive are emphasised within a strengths-based framework and supported by health professionals (Isobel & Delgado 2018).

These consumer-focused frameworks can be adopted as collaborative models of care or as individual philosophical frameworks for interpersonal relationships with consumers. Nurses must be mindful that to engage purposefully with consumers, they must engage in activities that promote self-care in themselves to achieve desired outcomes.

Case study 4.1, by Irene Gallagher, reflects the importance of looking beyond the external behaviour. Note the interactions between the people in Irene's story, how the nurse moved beyond the initial 'labels' given to the consumer and how the nurse was able to use objects in the environment to develop a social bond or therapeutic rapport. Adaptive and flexible frameworks of care will enhance relationships with individual consumers.

CASE STUDY 4.1

Irene Gallagher: the importance of therapeutic engagement

As a peer worker, I place great value on supporting a person with lived experience of mental distress with their own personal recovery journey, which may include fostering hope, self-determination, choice and intrinsically supporting them to connect with others in developing trusting relationships. Some may proclaim this to be the essence of the peer-to-peer relationship as mutuality and reciprocity. Having said this, I don't see that fostering relationships which support an individual's personal recovery journey belongs solely to peer workers; in fact, I have both personal experience as well as having been witness to seeing the wonderful connections that begin and unravel in the therapeutic relationship.

One such therapeutic engagement which comes to mind is a client who had been labelled by the system as being challenging and hard to engage with – lost in their own world of what the medical profession would label as 'delusional'. This individual was in fact difficult to engage with, loud and verbally abusive to everyone around them. No one wanted to engage with this person, staff or clients, for fear of verbal backlash or perhaps a fear of not knowing what approach to use with someone in this situation.

However, one nurse chose to find a way of working with and connecting with this person on some different level. Curiously, I asked the nurse how she had established these connections, how was it that she was able to communicate and work with this person. Interestingly, the nurse responded by noting that she had worked out that the client liked to have their hair brushed, and when the nurse brushed the client's hair the client would come into 'our' reality. From there, the two were able to communicate in a way that they were previously unable to. Similarly, the nurse discovered that a gentle touch on the client's forearm had a similar effect and they were able to have meaningful discussions such as talking about the client's hope and dreams for their future and what treatments worked and did not work for them during their hospitalisation.

Those around perhaps put this positive alliance down to luck; however, the reality was that this nurse had taken the time to connect with the client, to spend quality time getting to know the individual, using the therapeutic relationship to actively engage and involve the client in their own care. Time was taken to listen intently, to explore the client's values and what made meaning for them, while supporting the individual to participate in their recovery journey.

Engaging in reflective practice with the nurse supported how much the nurse had gained from working in this way and prioritising the development of the therapeutic relationship for all it holds: working from an empathic approach, developing rapport and trust, and approaching the collaborative work ahead as a team with mutual understanding and respect. Everyone has that connection waiting to be found – and in this scenario, one nurse found it.

Preparedness for creating safety in care and safety at work

Professional boundaries

Nurses are bound by professional practice guidelines through their nurse registration bodies. Professional boundaries can be thought of as the space between the professional's power and the consumer's vulnerability. This space needs to be observed and maintained to ensure a beneficial outcome for the consumer. Table 4.1 outlines some of the differences between social and professional relationships.

So, what occurs within professional relationships that makes a safe and effective practitioner? An expectation of the nurse is that they have a professional body of knowledge, skills and attitudes that can be used to improve the consumer's health status. The following elements could describe a poor professional relationship: cynicism, judgemental attitudes, personal intimacy, being patronising, developing dependency, showing favouritism, playing one person off against another ('splitting'), showing minimal care, neglect or punitiveness (Stein-Parbury 2016). Nurses need to emphasise on creating safe, therapeutic relationships with consumers based on openness, collaboration, respect and trust.

Nurses' self-care

It may come as no surprise that for nurses to engage therapeutically in relationships with consumers, they must be aware of and take care of their own emotional and psychological wellbeing. The stressful nature of nursing

TABLE 4.1 Difference between social and professional relationships

SOCIAL RELATIONSHIPS	PROFESSIONAL RELATIONSHIPS
Open-ended time period	Restricted to period of care
Personal choice	Restricted choice
Both parties' needs considered	Consumer's need predominant
Multipurpose	Primary purpose is care
Sympathy	Empathy
Confiding	Confidential
Tolerant to personal limit	Professional tolerance
Inconsistent	Consistent
Judgemental	Non-judgemental
Unstructured	Structured
Personal responsibility	Professional responsibility
Personal boundaries	Professional boundaries

in general is well recognised and may be more prominent when attempting to create a safe work environment.

Evidence within acute generalist settings has highlighted that nursing in general can have psychological and emotional consequences for nurses. For example, a study of 382 generalist nurses by Perry et al. (2015) highlighted that 14% (n = 53) reported having a history of common mental disorders (stress, anxiety, depression). In the same study, there was high prevalence of symptoms potentially indicative of mental health-related issues, with 248 (65.1%) reporting they had experienced symptoms such as headaches, severe tiredness, anxiety, sleep problems and depression sometimes or often in the previous 12 months.

Being self-aware and able to evaluate your own actions and behaviours will help you to engage therapeutically with consumers. This may be easier said than done, however, as we are often unaware of the emotional labour and stress that the competing demands involved in contemporary mental health care place upon us. Some individuals naturally engage in reflective thinking to enhance self-awareness while others require some formal structure to engage in this practice. It may be that as mental health nursing is your chosen specialty, you have a natural tendency for critical thinking, challenge and reflection.

The following workload practices can help in maintaining psychological and emotional wellbeing: working collaboratively where the workload is shared and delegated appropriately; being honest and transparent about your limitations (we all have bad days) but also maintaining professional conduct; and engaging in more formal, structured processes of reflective practice and clinical supervision. Clinical supervision within mental health is a practice endorsed across all professional groups, particularly nursing. The process has a focus on personal and professional development in the context of safe and effective consumer care. Although there is a dearth of research within this area, attention to its effects and benefits is growing and is proposed as a key feature in reducing the emotional labour associated with nursing practice. Central to clinical supervision is the opportunity for protected 'time out' from clinical activity spent with an experienced nurse who supports and guides processes of reflection and structured discussion. Reflection involves processes of enlightenment as to what nurses do and how we behave. During these processes the nurse may reflect on what they did, why they did it and implications for consumers, colleagues and wider professional and ethical practice (Cutcliffe & Sloan 2018). There is a role for nurses to engage each other about the emotions evoked in them: the more transparent we are about these emotions, the more adaptive and self-aware we become.

How nurses behave

As nurses, we need to be aware of our own expectations of a consumer's behaviour. Having high levels of expectation that a consumer will change their behaviour completely and quickly and/or express gratitude for your help may be unhelpful to you. How you respond can have a significant impact on the outcome of the strategies employed to help consumers change these behaviours. Unhelpful nursing responses include avoiding the consumer and minimising the issue. Such responses may be seen with consumers who are demanding of care, constantly approaching the nurse's office space or persistently phoning a nurse in a community setting. Taking the avoidance approach often leads the consumer to escalate their behaviour as they feel that their needs are not being met. While nurses may not want to encourage some behaviours, there is still a need to engage the consumer in this instance. If you respond to anger from a consumer by being angry yourself or respond to manipulative behaviour by being punitive in return, these responses are unhelpful. Therefore, being aware of your own emotional responses to consumers is an integral part of creating a safe work environment (Edward et al. 2017).

How to manage your own emotions

In any relationship you will need to be able to make sense of and manage your own emotions and behaviour. The natural response we have, known as the 'fight or flight response', is often evoked when people are threatening, angry and/or manipulative, resulting in an immediate natural response to defend yourself (Beattie et al. 2018). Nurses should be aware that the fight or flight response is normal, and you should expect it to occur. Some of the physical signs that you may experience include:

- increased pulse rate and blood pressure
- shallow, rapid respirations
- muscular tension
- dry mouth
- excessive perspiration.

There are also a range of psychological symptoms that you may experience following a fight or flight response:

- irritability and impatience
- frequent ruminating, worry and anxiety
- moodiness
- feeling sad or upset
- poor concentration, memory lapses
- ambivalence and feeling overwhelmed, or inability to face even minor problems.

To assist you in managing your fight/flight response, a self-management plan can be helpful. For example, concentrating on your breathing or counting to five before you engage someone may help you to respond in a calm and measured way. Inner dialogues are also posited as a strategy for successfully approaching challenging situations. For example, if you approach a situation with a negative attitude that things are not going to go well, this will probably influence your behaviour and resulting outcome. Be aware of what you are telling yourself or thinking to yourself. Thinking the worst, or catastrophic thinking, can lead you to behave in a negative way (e.g. 'This patient will never change' or 'I can't nurse this patient anymore').

Conversely, having an inner dialogue that you can negotiate a successful resolution to a challenging situation will likely help you to utilise skills and resources in doing. You can also take time out for a few minutes to reflect on your own behaviour: 'Am I being too angry here?' or 'Do I need to calm myself down before interacting with this consumer again?'. In addition, conveying how you feel and reflecting on your behaviour with a colleague can be helpful.

Principles for engaging consumers in safe care

It is important to understand some general principles in creating safety in care and work (McAllister et al. 2019).

Verbal interactions

How we say things can often be more important than what we say. Using an appropriate tone of voice, the rate at which you talk and the volume and pressure in your speech can influence how you engage consumers. You need to make adjustments to the 'how' of speaking. Ask yourself 'Am I speaking loud enough?', 'Am I too loud, and am I sounding threatening?' You will need to finetune your tone of voice as the interaction with the consumer occurs, testing and retesting your approach. Linking your words with actions can give the consumer a sense that you are interested in the engagement and can help maintain therapeutic rapport. Alternatively, if you show incongruence between your words and actions, the consumer and others may interpret this as you being untrustworthy and lacking authenticity.

Non-verbal interactions

Your non-verbal communication, how you hold yourself or behave, is an important aspect of engaging consumers. Through body language we constantly (and sometimes unconsciously) send and receive non-verbal signals. Awareness of the non-verbal signals you are sending may be particularly useful. Your words might convey one message but the movements and gestures you make might convey another, potentially creating confusion, misunderstanding and an array of negative feelings. The following are some ways of non-verbally responding:

- While you are talking, try to be aware of how you are sitting or standing, the expression on your face and what your hands and legs are doing.
- Allow the consumer to determine the distance between yourself and them. This may help the consumer to feel some sense of control. Personal space or distance can vary according to cultural or personal nuances.
- Keeping a relaxed open posture with your hands visible at either waist height or below can make you appear less threatening.
- The way you make eye contact can help. It is helpful to make intermittent eye contact and to avoid prolonged staring.
- Using appropriate facial expressions for the situation can be important – seek a balance between smiling and looking concerned. Expressions of warmth and acceptance can help. Be mindful that your position, movements and gestures may need to vary depending on the clinical situation.

Being flexible

Nursing requires the ability to be flexible and engage in different approaches. Nurses are often tempted to take control, when a more helpful approach is to consider how you can help the consumer to maintain or regain internal self-control – care versus control is a good mantra to keep in mind. You may be required to restructure requests and allow time for information to be processed. This requires qualities such as being patient and empathic, as well as skills in redirecting and negotiating.

Active listening

Mental health nurses use active listening skills in most of their daily work with consumers. Active listening shows that we are attending to someone's needs. The act of active listening starts a process of being empathic and may give you more time to formulate your response. Reflecting what the consumer is saying while taking a position of not offering advice but expressing acceptance without agreeing may offer the consumer a more comfortable position to reflect on their behaviour. Active listening demonstrates the presence of empathy and helps consumers to acknowledge their emotions while enabling consumers to talk about them as opposed to negatively acting upon them (Stein-Parbury 2016).

Empathy

A sense of openness can be developed by disclosing our concerns and issues with the consumer openly and honestly. Being empathic or entering into the feelings of the consumer and trying to appreciate their point of view gives the consumer a sense that you are acknowledging their concerns and trying to connect with them (Gerace et al. 2018). Respecting different points of view does not mean you agree with them; for example, 'I understand that you would like to visit your family tonight, and I can see that you are angry about not being able to do that'. This position demonstrates that you can accept someone's experience, without the need to agree with it (Gerace et al. 2018).

Assertiveness

Being assertive is a skill that requires careful consideration so as not to appear punitive or indeed aggressive. Being assertive may involve reflecting your own experience simultaneously setting expectations about behaviour from others. This approach involves displaying high levels of empathy while setting clear limits or boundaries. The following are examples of assertiveness statements that demonstrate showing empathy and setting limits in a way that is non-judgemental and therefore humanistic:

- 'You are speaking very loudly, and I am finding it hard to understand how I can help you.'
- 'You seem distressed and angry. Can we talk more when you are ready?'

Combining these assertiveness statements with statements such as 'I realise you don't want to do this' and 'I appreciate you are trying' can also be helpful. It is important to avoid argument, conflicting advice and long-winded explanations. Some situations may also require a firm and concise request about what needs to happen; for example:

- 'I appreciate you want your visitors to stay after hours but unfortunately it is hospital policy that they leave by 7.30.'
- 'I need you to spend some time in this area because your behaviour is upsetting some people.'

Initially, a consumer may continue with the same behaviour but as you repeat your expectations your message is reinforced. Provided that your demeanour is not aggressive, and your response is consistent, this offers the best opportunity to change the problematic behaviour. Be mindful to acknowledge any satisfactory outcome – saying 'thank you' and showing humility are extremely powerful tools in any nurse–consumer relationship.

Critical thinking challenge 4.1

Think about a situation of conflict that you were involved in or observed that was approached safely or you believe could have been treated differently. Write down some notes to the following questions:

1. What was the context preceding the situation?
2. What were the safety issues? Who was involved and what was each person's role? What was the outcome?
3. Could the situation have been approached differently from a safety point of view? If so, how?
4. What are the safety implications for the consumer or other consumers?
5. What safety issues have you learned from this situation? Have you identified any learning needs?
6. How can you incorporate your new learning into future practice?

Safety in care during aggression

Nurses often use the word 'agitated' to describe some of the behaviours they see. Agitation is a signal that something is wrong. It can be a consumer's reaction to an extremely abnormal situation (Renwick et al. 2016). Aggression or aggressive behaviour is frequently perceived to be hostile, injurious or destructive and is often caused by frustration. Sometimes, despite our best attempts at being empathic and actively listening, consumers become frustrated and agitated. While the anger may be directed at you as the nurse, it is not directed at you as a person. Although this difference appears subtle, the implications can be significant. By not personalising the behaviour, but rather seeing it through the eyes of your professional role, this will help you to remain objective. When someone is angry, they are often unaware of their own emotional state (Lavelle et al. 2016). An integral part of mental health nursing is the observation of consumers' demeanour and interactions with others. Some physiological observations that may require early intervention include:

- flushed or red face
- gritted teeth, tense facial features
- increased muscle tone such as clenched fists
- increased motor activity such as pacing or shuffling
- prolonged eye contact or staring.

Consumers who are frustrated or agitated may refuse to communicate or even withdraw from you. It is on these occasions that you may be required to intervene to prevent these physiological observations from escalating.

Safety in care and de-escalation techniques

De-escalation aims to bring about resolution through effective communication techniques (not force) and its success is underpinned by an empathic, respectful and collaborative approach by the nurse (Price et al. 2018). This approach involves understanding common signs of escalating behaviours and an ability to use communication skills to purposefully engage anxious, emotionally aroused or agitated individuals. Several elements of de-escalation have been identified from the literature that may be helpful in preparing you to de-escalate situations. These primary elements of de-escalation are outlined in Table 4.2.

Critical thinking challenge 4.2

What might be your emotional response when someone is aggressively shouting, intimidating and demanding your attention? Can you describe in words how you would feel? What physical reaction would you have? What thoughts would go through your mind? How could you approach the situation in a safe manner?

Variously known as 'talking down', de-fusion or diffusion, de-escalation is widely considered a first-line intervention for escalating behaviour. General principles involve non-provocatively engaging someone using short-term psychosocial interventions that minimise restriction and enable a mutually satisfactory outcome for both parties (Hallett & Dickens 2017).

THEMES, PRINCIPLES AND ATTRIBUTES OF DE-ESCALATION

A multitude of techniques, domains, themes and validated scale items have been identified within the international literature suggesting the principle components of de-escalation. However, a recent concept analysis of de-escalation in healthcare settings, which included 79 studies, has attempted to resolve concerns over clarity by proposing the following theoretical definition:

> ... a collective term for a range of interwoven staff-delivered components comprising communication, self-regulation, assessment, actions, and safety maintenance which aims to extinguish or reduce patient aggression/agitation irrespective of its cause, and improve staff-patient relationships while eliminating or minimising coercion or restriction.
>
> (Hallett & Dickens 2017, p. 16)

This definition arguably provides the most comprehensive understanding of de-escalation as a concept and provides an opportunity to explore theory–practice translational aspects of de-escalation. Successful de-escalation, therefore, comprises a complex set and interaction of skills and behaviours, which can be helpful in addressing challenging behaviour and workplace violence exposure, and may prevent the need for more restrictive practices such as sedation and restraint.

Restraint and seclusion

There may be occasions when your attempts to de-escalate are unsuccessful and consequently a decision is made to physically intervene. It should be emphasised that physical restraint of consumers is an intervention of last resort and should be carried out only by health professionals trained in safely facilitating this. Programs such as 'Safewards' (www.safewards.net) have been developed to minimise the use restraint and seclusion in mental health units (Bowers 2014; Fletcher et al. 2017). You should always consider whether any alternative strategies are available and, if so, have these been exhausted? Also, what would happen if you did nothing? These questions may be asked in the context of alleged assault when considering whether reasonable force was applied, either in a consumer's best interests or as a basis for self-defence. Restraint carries with it significant risks of injury to consumers and staff and, in some cases, even death (Kennedy et al. 2019). Seclusion also carries with it significant trauma and distress for consumers and staff alike. Some guiding principles for use of safe restraint and seclusion are summarised in Box 4.1 (Al-Maraira & Hayajneh 2018; Bowers et al. 2015; SICSAW 2019).

Nurse's story 4.1, by Natalie Cutler, illustrates the complexities and emotional and psychological issues associated with using consumer restraint and seclusion. Narrated by an experienced mental health nurse who reflected upon her early beginnings in mental health nursing, the story depicts a powerful representation of trauma associated with human interaction within the mental health specialty.

Deliberate self-harm and suicide

Deliberate self-harm can be an extremely confronting and challenging. Consumers who harm themselves often do so in the context of a situational crisis or in relation to their lived experience of trauma, and consumers often describe how deliberate self-harm is a means of managing distressing emotions. Self-harming behaviour can include injury that is either external or internal. External behaviours such as cutting, scratching, burning, picking and head banging are more common. However, internal behaviours such as swallowing objects and substances may also be seen in clinical practice. Trying to understand someone's motivations, emotional state and/or triggers for self-harming behaviour is essential. Assessing impulsiveness, the wish to control oneself or the effort to stop oneself is also important.

Traumatic experiences

Physical and sexual trauma histories strongly predict and underpin self-injury. Dissociative states or feelings of detachment from physical and emotional experience

TABLE 4.2 De-escalation, themes, principles, attributes and interventions

THEMES AND PRINCIPLES	HOW YOU COULD DO THIS	WHAT YOU COULD SAY
Communication		
Establish contact early in escalation	One person should engage in a calm and measured way because it can be confusing and counterproductive when more than one person is speaking. Use the person's name and yours, and use tactful language and humour sensitively (only if you feel it safe to do so).	*'Hello, John. My name is Jane. That looks painful. Can I take a look at it?*
Non-provocative engagement	Display a calm demeanour and appropriate tone of voice and engage assertively (not emotively or confrontationally). Eye contact should be intermittent to avoid staring. Awareness of one's own body language and adoption of an open, non-threatening posture with arms visible (not folded or behind back). Humour can help but only when appropriate.	Avoid saying: *'You need to calm down'*, *'Don't speak to me like that'* or *'You're upsetting other people'*. Try: *'Let's sit down and talk so I can understand what's happening'*
Identify wants and feelings	Violent behaviour is a primitive form of communicating that something is wrong or a need is not being met. Look beyond the external manifestation of this and ask how you can help.	*'I understand you're frustrated. Let's sit down and discuss that'* or *'We're here to help you. How best can we do that?'*
Active listening	Convey through body language and verbal acknowledgement that you are interested and repeat back (paraphrasing) that you understand. Be congruent in actions and words. Silence can allow a person time to clarify their thoughts.	*'You said that you want...?'* or *'Am I correct in saying...?'*
Display empathy	Demonstrate empathy in verbal and non-verbal communication. Listen and offer understanding (not sympathy) while acknowledging the person's feelings/situation.	*'That would frustrate me, too'* or *'I can appreciate how this is affecting you'*
Be concise	A person's ability to concentrate is compromised when in an emotionally aroused state. Avoid jargon or medical terminology. Speak clearly and slowly; information may have to be repeated several times.	*'Let's sit down and discuss your pain'* or *'We're concerned about your health and your safety'*
Agree or accept	Validate concerns where relevant and accept that concerns are distressing for the person (even if you may not agree with them). Concentrate on opportunities for agreement.	*'I'm sorry this has happened to you, it's unacceptable'* or *'I would feel angry too if I had to wait this long'*
Offer choices and optimism	Offering choice, where relevant, is empowering and can enable a sense of internal control while providing an acceptable 'out' from challenging behaviour. Also offer things perceived as acts of kindness, where relevant, such as food/drink or pain relief. Be honest and don't make promises that can't be kept or that compromise others.	*'Can I get you some water and medication for your pain? Then we can discuss this'* or *'I'm sorry, but I'm unable to do that. What I can do is help you with...'*
Self-regulation		
Self-control / remain calm	Appearing fearful may make someone feel unsafe or may escalate behaviour in the context of manipulation. Maintain emotional regulation, self-control and confidence. Concentrate on your breathing; count to three before engaging. Having positive inner dialogues that you can successfully negotiate and de-escalate can contribute to effective self-control plans.	Say to yourself: *'I'm confident I can connect with [person's name] and successfully de-escalate the situation'* or *'This will resolve with everyone safe'*
Non-judgemental approach	Separate your feelings about the person and the problem. Avoid making judgements about the person and don't personalise any challenging behaviour.	*'I don't think that of you at all'* or *'I'm sorry you think that of me'* or *'I didn't mean to give you the wrong impression'*

Continued

TABLE 4.2 De-escalation, themes, principles, attributes and interventions—cont'd

THEMES AND PRINCIPLES	HOW YOU COULD DO THIS	WHAT YOU COULD SAY
Self-reflection	Personal reflection following an incident allows you to consider and make sense of what went well or not so well. This enables consistency or modification of engagement/intervention strategies.	Ask your colleague: *'How did I do?'* or *'Could I have done anything differently?'*
Assessment		
Is it safe to intervene?	Assess the risks associated with any intervention. Early intervention is always recommended for escalating behaviour, but patience and caution, if safe, may be more prudent when assessing benefit–harm ratio. Ask yourself what would happen if you did nothing or waited for support.	*'Can we take a minute, then I'll attend to that?'* or *'I need you to put that blade down before I can treat that'* or *'Do you mind if we wait for my colleague? He has something that can help with your pain'*
Here and now	Assess the person's emotional state or the immediate situation in relation to safety for all. Other aspects of assessment and intervention can wait.	*'You look distressed (or angry). Can you talk to me about it?'*
Escalating aggression	Observe for and recognise known early-warning signs of violence such as pacing, clenched-fists, kicking objects, loud voice, staring, tense facial expressions, posturing or ignoring requests.	*'I need you to sit down so I can attend to your...'*
Actions		
Positional imitation	Stand if the person is standing (personal safety); sit if they are sitting. This reflects a sense of equity required for successful de-escalation.	*'Do you mind if I sit down?'* or *'Do you mind if I join you?'*
Reduce stimuli; create a safe space	Decrease environmental stimuli and encourage private interaction free from any potential triggers or antagonists. Attempt to remove the person, or others, from the situation, thus creating a safe space for engagement and intervention.	*'Can we move over here and talk in private?'* or *'Can we sit in the ambulance so we can attend to...?'*
Distraction	Redirect the person's attention from escalating behaviour. Bringing in a different person to interact with the individual may change the dynamic of unsuccessful de-escalation.	*'Is there anyone you'd like me to call to let them know you're safe or where you are going?'* or *'This is my colleague, Jane. Do you mind if she attends to you while I get you something for the pain?'*
Set limits	Be clear about what you would like to happen and that you want to help, in a non-confrontational and respectful way. A discussion of behavioural expectations may help if safe to do so. Acknowledge if you are feeling uncomfortable – humility is a very powerful tool!	*'When you're shouting, I find it hard to understand how I can help you'* or *'I can't attend to your needs while you're threatening me'*
Therapeutic treatment	Identifying and alleviating causes of escalating behaviour such as pain or confusion can quickly inform de-escalation strategies and required treatments.	*'Can I give you something to help with the pain?'* or *'Can I give you some medication to help take your mind off it?'*
Maintaining safety		
Situational awareness	Situational awareness is being aware of what is happening around you in terms of where you are, whether anyone or anything around you is a threat, and what supports may be available. It is essential to remain vigilant. Awareness of the environment in terms of isolation, quick egress and exit routes and removal or moderation of potential weapons, dangers and triggers is paramount.	*'Can we talk somewhere else?'* or *'Do you mind if I sit here?'* or *'If you could put the syringe down I'll attend to that'*

TABLE 4.2 De-escalation, themes, principles, attributes and interventions—cont'd

THEMES AND PRINCIPLES	HOW YOU COULD DO THIS	WHAT YOU COULD SAY
Situational support	Communication with colleagues is essential. Identify availability of backup should it be needed while being mindful that an excessive show of force can escalate a person's behaviour.	*'No one's in trouble. The police are here for everyone's safety'* or *'I need to contact someone to let them know we'll be longer than expected'*
Approach with caution	Approach in a measured way, careful to avoid sudden movements. Avoid being too close to someone fearful or confused (this may appear threatening) while maintaining a distance that protects from a potential punch or kick until you feel it safe for close proximity.	*'Can we take a look at that injury?'* or *'Someone phoned because they are concerned about your safety'.*
Respect personal space	Acknowledge that more personal space than usual may be required while being mindful not to appear fearful or disinterested.	*'Do you mind if I have a look at that?'* or *'I won't come any closer, I just want to chat'*
Debrief all involved	Debriefing helps maintain therapeutic aspects of a relationship. It is important that a person does not feel isolated following resolution, irrespective of how this is achieved. Debriefing with colleagues ensures that psychological first aid can be administered. Bystanders may also require debriefing if witnessing potentially traumatic events. Debriefing allows learning from situations that may prove useful in future crises.	To the patient: *'I'm sorry we did that, I know you didn't want to. We did this because...'* To a bystander: *'That must have been very difficult to witness. Are you okay? Can I contact someone to take you home?'* To a colleague: *'How do you think that went? Should we do anything differently next time?*

Adapted from Lamont & Brunero 2019

Box 4.1 Guiding principles for safe restraint

1. Restraint is the option of last resort; it is to be used when other less coercive interventions are unsuccessful or inappropriate.
2. Any restriction to a consumer's liberty and interference with their rights, dignity and self-respect should be kept to a minimum and should cease as soon as the consumer has regained self-control.
3. Restraint and seclusion should never be used as a method of punishment. All actions undertaken by staff must be justifiable and proportional to the consumer's behaviour, with the least amount of force necessary.
4. Staff must exercise reasonable care and skill to ensure the safety, comfort and humane treatment of consumers in restraint or seclusion.
5. Communication and engagement with the consumer should be maintained at all times, with all opportunities taken to de-escalate the situation.
6. Pain compliance should never be used when restraining someone, and any direct pressure on the neck, abdomen, thorax, back or joints is to be avoided.
7. The consumer's physical condition should be continuously monitored, with any deterioration, in particular to the airway, noted and managed promptly.
8. All episodes of restraint should have an appointed leader throughout the restraint to maintain safety.
9. Face-up restraint (supine) should be used where it is safe to do so. Face-down restraint (prone) should be used only if it is the safest way to protect the consumer and staff. Prone restraint should be used for only the minimum amount of time necessary to administer medication and/or move the person to a safer environment.
10. A post-restraint/seclusion debrief for the consumer, staff and any relevant others should be undertaken in all situations.

Adapted from Clinical Excellence Commission 2015

NURSE'S STORY 4.1

Natalie cutler

I've been a nurse for more than 20 years, specialising in mental health. Two things drew me to mental health: firstly, that it was a 'frontier' with little research happening and lots waiting to be discovered. Secondly, and most importantly, I could see 'mental health' everywhere. From my previous experience as a dental nurse, I was familiar with the fear and anxiety people experienced. I became aware of how powerful human interactions could be in making people feel safe. I'd say that was my beginning as a mental health nurse, well before I'd completed any training.

Something that resonated powerfully with me when I was undertaking nurse training was the concept of the nurse as advocate. The more I learned about this, the more determined I became to actively advocate for people with mental health problems wherever I could. As a clinician, and later as an educator and manager, this has been my most valued role.

To be an effective advocate, it is important to understand one's own motivations and be vigilant to the fine balance between seeking to build another's strength versus disempowering them by seeking to 'rescue'. Continuous reflection on whose needs are being met is the key. Advocacy requires being a resource for the other person to help them achieve their goals. If assertive advocacy is required, this should ideally be activated on the request or with the consent of another person. In addition to considering the needs of people with lived experience of mental illness, mental health nursing also encompasses an awareness of one's own needs. Self-advocacy and peer advocacy thus provide the foundation for safe and sustainable practice.

Being an advocate is not always easy. This is reflected in a scenario from my early career. As a new graduate nurse, my very first placement was in an acute mental health inpatient unit. Returning from a meeting on my second day, I walked into the lounge area in time to see a large male being held on the ground by several of my colleagues. Other consumers in the area looked frightened. I did not have time to process what was happening before I was commanded to 'hold his foot'. For the next 25 minutes, I was part of a team involved in restraining, medicating and ultimately secluding this man. I had no idea what had happened, why we were doing this or what I was expected to do. None of my university training had prepared me for this. I was shocked and inwardly distressed.

Shortly after, my colleagues resumed their usual activities and not much was said about the incident. What appeared routine to my colleagues left me completely bewildered. Nothing in my private life or training had prepared me to be involved in holding another person on the ground against their will. I found it hard to reconcile this 'security' function with my beginning identity as a nurse, and an advocate. This confusion has stayed with me to this day. However, it also started a career-long reflection on questions such as 'What is a nurse?' and 'Who am I as a nurse?' It also made me determined never to see restraint and seclusion as 'normal' parts of being a nurse. Consequently, I have moved towards roles that allow me to engage with consumers as equals. Wherever possible I try to challenge 'the way we do things round here'. For me, being a nurse means being brave and self-aware, and providing a platform for others to have a voice.

are commonly described by consumers who self-harm. There may be several mediating factors in consumers who self-harm, including the type of trauma, affective dysregulation, dissociation, poor modulation of aggression and/or poor impulse control. Confusion may arise when differentiating between deliberate self-harm and suicidal behaviour. Deliberate self-harm is not necessarily suicidal behaviour as there is rarely an intention to die. The behaviour may be intended as a relief from anxiety or tension or as an escape from distressing emotions rather than an attempt at suicide. The complexity is that people with self-harming behaviour may also be suicidal. Assessing suicidality in a consumer who also self-harms is difficult because people often feel dysphoric with depressed mood. An issue of concern when managing deliberate self-harm is not being complacent about it; for example, this behaviour carries extensive risks, even when there is no intention to die or when a consumer may have been engaging in this type of behaviour for many years (Smith et al. 2015).

Interventions

As with most of the focus in this chapter, having empathy in exploring meanings of behaviour for the consumer is the best place to start. Understanding the pain during the act of self-harm and what this means to the person may help engage them in a therapeutic relationship with you. Going beyond what is in front of you (i.e. the wound or cut on the arm) and exploring the meaning and significance of the act will help you to engage the consumer therapeutically. Obtaining details of incidents, thoughts, feelings, precipitating events and other ideas that occur during the self-harming behaviour demonstrates a willingness to work collaboratively with the consumer. Intolerant or dismissive approaches by nursing staff often cause an increase in self-harming behaviours because the emotional distress that underpins them is not being engaged or validated.

General strategies include the consumer learning distress management techniques including relaxation and other distraction strategies such as pinging rubber bans on the wrist when distressed, ice cubes, throwing or hitting soft objects and/or exercising when thoughts of self-harm occur. Consumers may learn about their early warning signs and make plans for potentially stressful or difficult situations they may encounter. Encouraging consumers to articulate these experiences into words, drawings or stories may help them to understand how they are relating to the world around them. An ongoing emphasis should be placed on developing alternatives to self-harm. Deliberate self-harm is a complex issue and treatment processes can be prolonged and unpredictable. Generally, psychotherapy is the most common treatment, with dialectical behaviour therapy having dominance in this area more recently (Toms et al. 2019).

Manipulation

Manipulation generally refers to behaviours that someone exhibits to get their needs met. This may include the following types of behaviours and actions: attempting to maintain control and power over others; playing one staff member off against another ('splitting'); evoking guilt and shame in others; attempting to get others to take responsibility for one's actions; and attempting to gain an advantage in interactions. Manipulation can be used by both nurses and consumers. The meaning behind the word 'manipulative' is negative, suggesting that the consumer is bad or difficult rather than just the individual behaviour. As nurses we need to be careful how we label behaviour and the meanings that arise out of those labels (Valente 2017).

Influence versus manipulation

Generally speaking, as a nurse, you hold the power in the therapeutic relationship. As such, you need to be aware of how you exercise that responsibility. Consumer–nurse collaboration and positive outcomes are more likely to be achieved by using influence rather than manipulation. The goal is encouragement and negotiation rather than coercion or manipulation, and consumer involvement in decision making will provide the best opportunity for engaging someone in safe care. Provide balanced not biased information and consider the needs and concerns of the consumer, not just your own needs and concerns. Identify the manipulative behaviour and communicate this with your colleagues. It is important to maintain communication and consistency. Comprehensive documentation is important, and minimising the number of staff involved with the consumer may help. Be clear and direct when setting limits on behaviour; enforce the limits but also reward and praise positive behaviour. Collaborative care plans should communicate clearly what you expect from the consumer and what the consumer can expect from you. A written plan may contain a set of simple statements of what you will do and what the consumer will do. It may even be signed by both parties to demonstrate an agreement, but it should not be considered as a contract. It is simply a negotiated agreement with another person (Bee et al. 2015).

Critical thinking challenge 4.3

A consumer is displaying 'splitting' behaviour, describing one staff member as their favourite while others are the worst they have met.

1. What would you say to the consumer?
2. What would you say to the team?
3. How would you behave with the consumer and the clinical team?
4. What would be your safety plan?

Understanding safety risks in care and at work

There is increasing pressure on nurses and other professionals to assess, predict and manage the risk of adverse events (Slemon et al. 2017). It is unfortunate that high-profile, yet rare, events involving staff and consumers and subsequent media interest lead to heightened community concern around the safety of consumers and others, often laying the blame on inadequate or inefficient mental health care. This has led to the expectation that nurses become proficient in assessing and managing risk and in justifying their actions in terms of their risk implications and preventing adverse events. Risk therefore pervades the research literature, health service policy and practice, media and public debate, and even healthcare legislation (Iozzino et al. 2015).

As a nurse, you will be expected to provide assessment in relation to some specific forms of risk. Typically, this may involve but is not limited to:

- aggression and violence
- suicide and self-harm (risk of further attempts and death)
- severe self-neglect (risk of poor physical health, infectious disease)
- sexual safety (risk of sexually transmitted infection, assault and trauma)
- exploitation/reputation (risk of harm to reputation, financial loss)
- fire safety (risk to personal safety and belongings)
- absconding (risk of further harm, prolonging hospital admission)
- noncompliance with medications (risk of relapse).

Risk has become an integral component of mental health care; however, there remains much controversy and debate around minimum expectations in practice, how best to facilitate risk assessment and management processes, and even whether the outcomes of processes are commensurate with our time and efforts.

The risk assessment processes

The search for reliable methods of risk assessment has led to a plethora of risk tools, instruments and algorithms that attempt to measure or predict risk behaviours. It is estimated that more than 150 structured tools exist for assessing the risk of violence alone, yet these instruments have a reported low reliability in determining a consumer's risk level (Douglas et al. 2017). Other instruments focus on suicide and self-harm. Research suggests that more than 60% of general psychiatric consumers are assessed routinely for violence risk, which reflects the scale of risk assessment practice (Fazel et al. 2012; Hurducas et al. 2014). Notwithstanding, three methods of risk assessment have been prominent throughout:

- **Unstructured clinical judgement** involves a subjective clinician assessment on what factors the individual assessor believes are relevant or important in relation to a risk. Critics of this unstructured approach relate the lack of consistency and inter-rater reliability of such assessments, as individual assessors have different levels of experience, exposure to risk, values and interpersonal skills. These factors may influence the overestimation or underestimation of risk, which is obviously suboptimal to care provision.
- **Actuarial risk assessment** methods are known variously as mathematical, mechanical or statistical prediction, where individual factors that have been statistically associated with specific risks are measured. Therefore, individual clinical judgement is replaced by a score based on a formulaic equation, but this ignores the dynamic factors that are associated with risks eventuating (e.g. staff wellbeing, consumers' experiences, ward environment). Another limitation is that actuarial methods stop at prediction and ultimately fail to inform prevention and management. It must be noted also that any statistical significance attached to actuarial methods may be associated with specific validation samples and identified risks.
- **Structured professional judgement** essentially integrates clinical and actuarial methods in an attempt to minimise the limitations of both methods. This approach combines empirically validated risk factors, professional experience/judgement and contemporary knowledge of a particular consumer. As this approach incorporates idiosyncratic and dynamic risk factors, it is argued to have transferability across different populations and offers provisions within the framework for prevention and management.

Positive risk taking

The term 'positive risk taking' is used in this context to represent professional readiness to respect and respond to service users' own recovery goals or preferences for care. Such opportunities are perceived to be under-realised in practice, exacerbating existing power differentials between service users and professionals, and sanctioning professionals to have the 'final say' (Higgins et al. 2016; Morgan 2004).

Recovery-oriented practices adopt a position where consumers take ownership of their own personal journey and, with it, ownership of associated risks. Top-down, risk-averse cultures challenge the integrity of consumer engagement, involvement and empowerment (Bee et al. 2015; Slemon et al. 2017). It is argued that such practices are currently under-realised within mental health practice, in turn maintaining power differentials and coercive practices. As such, cultures that do not embrace consumer ownership and empowerment via philosophical frameworks and practices such as positive risk taking will probably experience challenges to safe care and work as a result of consumer disempowerment and a lack of hope.

Consequently, the concept of positive risk taking has been catapulted to the forefront of our decision making. Positive risk taking involves a process of reasoning within a framework of weighing up potential benefits and harms of one choice over another. It is argued that positive risk taking is not a negligent practice where risks are ignored or minimised; rather, situations and their potential consequences are logically and carefully considered in the context of any course of action.

A pervasive negative focus on risk can lead to defensive practices that in turn lead to often costly unnecessary interventions and care, for fear of legal recourse (Slemon et al. 2017). By contrast, positive risk taking involves accepting risk as part of everyday life and health care. Examples of positive risk taking include: discharging consumers from supervised inpatient care to community follow-up; unescorted leave from inpatient stays previously perceived to be too risky; pharmacology-free trials as a result of severe side effects; non-admission following presentation in crisis to an emergency department; or a crisis team visit at home. These are all examples of everyday positive risk taking where, as nurses, we accept that risks are omnipresent.

Ultimately, we take risks and utilise the knowledge gained following successes or mistakes for growth and empowerment. As discussed within many chapters of this text, consumer engagement, partnership and co-planning of care will enable better, safer outcomes when positively taking risks. The ability to flourish is a fundamental human right, and should be supported and advocated for by nurses, as opposed to legislation, policy and practice where fear of failure and adverse events pervades.

Community settings – safety and situational awareness

Creating a safe care and work environment in community settings poses different challenges. The community setting can be dynamic, requiring quick assessment of safety, with limited information and resources compared with the inpatient setting. As a result, it is an expectation that community nurses become situationally aware of risks and safety and are proficient at assessing risk. This will require you to:

- look for hazards
- consider retreat options and exits
- approach situations cautiously
- avoid placing yourself or others (consumer and families) at risk (e.g. intervening in a violent incident)
- observe for potential weapons
- consider additional resources required to safely assess and/or treat.

Table 4.3 outlines some specific safety and risk mitigation factors you should consider before arrival, upon arrival, during assessment/treatment and following your return to a community health centre.

Summary of risk in mental health settings

The assessment and management of risk are inextricably linked to providing mental health care. While exact predictions are not possible, this area of practice is not one in which nurses should become complacent. There is no doubt that a sense of perspective and realistic expectation is required among legislators, administrators, health professionals and the wider community. However, despite ongoing debate, there remains a community, professional and moral expectation that we engage with consumers around identified needs and potential risks, and attempt to mitigate against these. A collaborative, dynamic and continuous process of engagement and planning can support nurses when there is increased risk of adverse events, thus removing the perceived or actual burden of individual scrutiny. Box 4.2 summarises principles for working with risk (Morgan 2004, p. 18).

The legal context

Nurses need to be aware of the ethical and legal contexts in which subsequent actions and interventions are considered. Some fundamental human rights underpin

TABLE 4.3 Safety and situational awareness during community visits

PRIOR TO COMMUNITY VISIT	ARRIVAL AT COMMUNITY VISIT	ASSESSMENT/ TREATMENT	OTHER ISSUES
• Recognise that risk is dynamic and that a low-risk person or situation can change at any time • Obtain as much information as possible about the patient and others (where relevant) • Obtain information about the location: Is it in a high crime area? Isolated? Does it have reduced accessibility to or availability of police? Some addresses may be listed as 'no go' or 'locations of interest'. If so, consider police backup. • Gather specific information about the premises (if relevant): Is there security access? Stairs? External lighting? Hiding places? Are the premises modern? In good repair?	• Park the car facing the way you will be exiting and make sure you cannot be blocked in • Do not attempt to enter premises if there are any potentially aggressive animals and they are not restrained • When entering buildings check lighting and stairwells where no lift is available • If you are concerned about location or access to premises ask a family member to meet you and escort you to the client • Always check the locking mechanism on the gate so you can leave quickly if necessary • Before knocking or ringing the doorbell, listen for any arguments or other unexpected voices or anything that may make the situation unsafe (these are reasons to reassess the situation)	• Be cautious when entering a person's home • If at any time your professional instinct tells you something is wrong, leave immediately (even if you cannot work out what is wrong) • Leave immediately if you see any firearms or weapons (police need to be informed) • Be aware of all exits • Do not sit in deep-seated chairs because it is difficult to get out of some chairs in a hurry (ask for an upright chair) • Always sit between the client and the door but without blocking the client's way out • Keep your keys handy so you do not waste time searching for them at the bottom of your bag • Only take in what you need	• Always report to base at regular intervals • Always report 'near misses' where aggression became a present risk but did not eventuate • Ensure your workplace has a policy and response if you do not return on time such as activating a police response • Ensure you attend all workplace violence prevention and personal safety training offered by your service

Adapted from Lamont & Brunero 2019

Box 4.2 Principles for working with safety risks

- Risk is an everyday experience.
- Risk is dynamic and constantly changing in response to varying circumstances.
- Assessment of risk is enhanced by accessing multiple sources of information.
- Sources of information may be incomplete.
- Some sources of information may be inaccurate.
- Identification of risk carries a responsibility to do something about it – that is, risk management.
- An integral component of good risk management is risk taking.
- Decision making can be enhanced through positive collaboration.
- Risk can be minimised but not eliminated.
- Organisations carry a responsibility to meet reasonable expectations for encouraging a no-blame culture while not condoning poor practice.

Adapted from Morgan 2004

our ethical conduct, common law and relevant statutes within this context (see also Chapter 8).

Human rights

Several United Nations treaties have shaped domestic and international law in relation to healthcare rights. The *Universal Declaration of Human Rights* (United Nations 1948) is an international document that states basic rights and fundamental freedoms to which all human beings are entitled. It consists of 30 Articles, some of which have direct relevance to healthcare provision:

- Article 3: Everyone has the right to life, liberty and security of person
- Article 9: No-one shall be subjected to arbitrary arrest, detention or exile
- Article 13: Everyone has the right to freedom of movement and residence within the borders of each state.

Australia and New Zealand are signatories to the Principles for the Protection of Persons with Mental Illness and for the Improvement of Mental Health Care (United Nations General Assembly 1991), which were adopted by the United Nations General Assembly in 1991. With the underpinning aim to provide a framework for improving mental health care globally, UN91 (as it became known) sets out basic rights-based standards for providing care for people with mental illness. Since its inception, UN91 principles have received criticism for not influencing the suboptimal standards of mental health care provision enough, with some principles offering more protection than others. Consequently, UN91 should now be read and understood in the context of the United Nations *Convention on the Rights of Persons with Disabilities* (Szmukler & Bach 2015; United Nations 2006).

These frameworks set in place obligations on member states within common and legislative law for protecting others and act as a reflective guide for actions. When engaging consumers in any course of action that may impinge on these rights, nurses must be aware of where the law positions itself in relation to any subsequent interventions (Mezzina et al. 2019).

Common law issues

Failure in duty of care and negligence are common law torts (civil wrongs) that nurses need to familiarise themselves with. All health professionals must be aware that they owe a duty of care to consumers and that this involves acting in a manner that accords with competent professional practice. Negligence arises when health professionals are deemed negligent in fulfilling their duty and where such a breach directly causes damage to a consumer. This duty pervades throughout all care provision and is not something that is invoked by specific consumer behaviours. Duty of care within this context involves maintaining safety for all and, in doing so, being aware that other torts are not being committed.

The common law tort of trespass comprises three potential trespasses to the person: assault – an intentional act by someone that creates fear in another of an imminent harm; battery – a harmful or offensive touching of another (thus a distinction is created whereby assault is associated with no contact whereas battery requires contact); and false imprisonment – the illegal confinement of an individual against their will that impinges the individual's right to freedom of movement (Staunton & Chiarella 2013). Nurses may be open to scrutiny and sometimes litigation in the course of their work, particularly when engaging in restrictive or coercive care that is unsolicited or not consented to by the consumer and when the consumer has a voluntary status. Involuntary status under the relevant mental health statute or substitute consent under the guardianship statute in general offers protection to nurses. However, this protection is not absolute, and the above torts may still apply if the nurse's actions are outside the relevant legal framework.

The common law doctrine of necessity sometimes referred to as 'emergency powers' allows nurses to act and administer care/treatment in any situation where a consumer lacks capacity and the provision of treatment is immediately necessary to prevent serious injury or even death: see *Re T (adult: refusal of medical treatment)* [1992] 4 All ER 649. Again, such practice is potentially challengeable and should be used in emergencies only, not in a consistent or planned way.

Legislative frameworks

Mental health legislative frameworks irrespective of geographical location will generally be underpinned by similar philosophies and principles. These may include least restrictive care or minimising any restrictions on civil liberty, rights, dignity and self-respect, and the right to appeal (Lamont et al. 2015). If engaging in non-consensual restrictive or coercive management of consumers, mental health legislation may have to be applied to do so lawfully. This not only offers protection for care and treatment that consumers may not agree with, but more importantly also affords consumers with a right to appeal via independent arbitration (e.g. mental health review tribunals). Relevant guardianship legislation can also be used in this manner when protecting the health rights of consumers with disabilities. Again, similar procedural requirements and criteria must be met within the various geographical jurisdictions. These procedures are essential if engaging in processes that effectively impinge on a consumer's freedom of movement. Without wishing to single out any particular intervention, one such intervention that becomes prominent and requires attention within a legal context is consumer restraint.

Reasonable force

Nurses often ask what constitutes the legal definition of reasonable force in situations of consumer safety. There is no simple explanation for this. Reasonable force is essentially context-specific and is the amount of force deemed necessary at the time in relation to the risk presented. A unique set of conditions exists in each situation and essentially requires a professional judgement to be made. This judgement is quite rightly open to challenge and scrutiny by consumers and therefore any actions pursued by you as a nurse must be commensurate with the perceived risk. Potential alternative courses of action may be put forward when considering whether any force was reasonable and justified, in keeping with least restrictive principles of human rights and mental health legislation.

Notwithstanding the above, there will be occasions when as a nurse you feel there is no other option but to engage in physical contact and potential restraint of a consumer (person-to-person, mechanical or chemical), either because the perceived risk is too great for verbal engagement or when this is unsuccessful. However, you must be aware of the principles outlined above when using restraint, as this practice should always be considered a last resort because of the danger to both the consumer and staff (Cusack et al. 2018).

Chapter summary

What differentiates mental health nursing from other areas of nursing is caring for consumers who at times in their lives are unable to see the need for care. The skills you develop will take you beyond seeing these challenges to safe care and work as difficult or deliberate. Being aware of your own emotional responses to your work will allow you to de-personalise the effects that workplace challenges bring. Being able to stand back and see the wider picture of the social context that someone is in and seeing past the behaviours you are confronted with will enable you to see the person within. Achieving this level of engagement with someone indicates that you are heading towards mastery of the skills mentioned in this chapter.

EXERCISES FOR CLASS ENGAGEMENT

1. The following link has four case scenarios that you may face in your clinical practice, which you can work through to further develop your skills (Lamont & Brunero 2013; 2014): www.inkysmudge.com.au/eSimulation/mhl.html.
2. In your class group, recall a situation where a risk was identified with a consumer. Complete the safety in care and safety at work plan below from a group discussion (Morgan 2004).

SAFETY IN CARE, SAFETY AT WORK PLAN

Categories of safety risk identified (single or multiple – tick relevant boxes):

- ☐ Aggression and violence
- ☐ Severe self-neglect
- ☐ Exploitation/reputation
- ☐ Absconding
- ☐ Suicide and self-harm
- ☐ Sexual safety
- ☐ Fire
- ☐ Other (specify)

Detail any historical information that may indicate the potential for a safety risk (e.g. previous history of risk behaviours/threats/ideation).

____

____

Detail any health-related factors that may contribute to the potential for a safety risk (e.g. mental health symptoms, personality factors, physical disabilities, substance abuse).

____

____

What environmental safety factors may contribute to risk (e.g. arousal in official professional settings, access to drugs/alcohol, rejection by others, access to weapons)?

____

____

Is there any current evidence to suggest 'planned intent' to engage in risk-related behaviour?

____

____

Are there any safety risk factors that indicate preferred staff allocation (e.g. danger to women, intimidated by men, need for two workers)?

____

____

What strengths and opportunities can you identify, from the consumer and/or services, as resources to support this plan?

____

____

What barriers may hinder the implementation of this plan?

____

____

State specifically the identified risk:

____

____

Presents a risk of:

____

____

Through (behaviours/cognitions/affect):

____

____

In the context of (situations):

____

____

Early intervention signs are:

____

____

Interventions for the above circumstances:

____

____

Has this plan been discussed with the consumer?

____

____

Has this plan been discussed with the multidisciplinary team?

____

____

Frequency of review:

____

____

Additional comments (if discontinuing, specify reasons):

____

____

Useful websites

Mental Health eSimulation: http://www.inkysmudge.com.au/eSimulation/mhl.html

Safewards: https://www.facebook.com/groups/safewards/ and http://www.safewards.net/

SICSAW – Safe in Care, Safe at Work: http://www.acmhn.org/

References

Affleck, W., Carmichael, V., Whitley, R., 2018. Men's mental health: social determinants and implications for services. Can. J. Psychiatry 63 (9), 581–589.

Al-Maraira, O.A., Hayajneh, F.A., 2018. Use of restraint and seclusion in psychiatric settings: a literature review. J. Psychosoc. Nurs. Ment. Health Serv. 57 (4), 32–39.

Barker, P., 2001. The Tidal Model: developing an empowering, person centred approach to recovery within psychiatric and mental health nursing. J. Psychiatr. Ment. Health Nurs. 8 (3), 233–240.

Barker, P., Buchanan-Barker, P., 2010. The tidal model of mental health recovery and reclamation: application in acute care settings. Issues Ment. Health Nurs. 31 (3), 171–180.

Beattie, J., Innes, K., Griffiths, D., et al., 2018. Healthcare providers' neurobiological response to workplace violence perpetrated by consumers: informing directions for staff well-being. Appl. Nurs. Res. 43, 42–48.

Bee, P., Brooks, H., Fraser, C., et al., 2015. Professional perspectives on service user and carer involvement in mental health care planning: a qualitative study. Int. J. Nurs. Stud. 52 (12), 1834–1845.

Bowers, L., 2014. Safewards: a new model of conflict and containment on psychiatric wards. J. Psychiatr. Ment. Health Nurs. 21 (6), 499–508.

Bowers, L., James, K., Quirk, A., et al., 2015. Reducing conflict and containment rates on acute psychiatric wards: the Safewards cluster randomised controlled trial. Int. J. Nurs. Stud. 52 (9), 1412–1422.

Brophy, L.M., Roper, C.E., Hamilton, B.E., et al., 2016. Consumers and their supporters' perspectives on poor practice and the use of seclusion and restraint in mental health settings: results from Australian focus groups. Int. J. Ment. Health Syst. 10 (1), 6.

Brunero, S., Ramjan, L.M., Salamonson, Y., et al., 2018. A constructivist grounded theory of generalist health professionals and their mental health work. Int. J. Ment. Health Nurs. 27 (6), 1816–1825.

Clinical Excellence Commission, 2015. Principles for Safe Management of Disturbed and /or Aggressive Behaviour and the Use of Restraint. Ministry of Health, Sydney. Retrieved from: http://wwwo.health.nsw.gov.au/policies/pd/2015/pdf/PD2015_004.pdf.

Cusack, E., Killoury, F., Nugent, L., 2017. The professional psychiatric/mental health nurse: skills, competencies and supports required to adopt recovery-orientated policy in practice. J. Psychiatr. Ment. Health Nurs. 24 (2–3), 93–104.

Cusack, P., Cusack, F.P., McAndrew, S., et al., 2018. An integrative review exploring the physical and psychological harm inherent in using restraint in mental health inpatient settings. Int. J. Ment. Health Nurs. 27 (3), 1162–1176.

Cutcliffe, J.R., Sloan, G., 2018. Competences for clinical supervision in psychiatric/mental health nursing. In:

Santos, J.C., Cutcliffe, J.R. (Eds.), European Psychiatric/ Mental Health Nursing in the 21st Century. Springer, Cham, Switzerland, pp. 123–139.

Dickens, G.L., Hallett, N., Lamont, E., 2016. Interventions to improve mental health nurses' skills, attitudes, and knowledge related to people with a diagnosis of borderline personality disorder: systematic review. Int. J. Nurs. Stud. 56, 114–127.

Douglas, T., Pugh, J., Singh, I., et al., 2017. Risk assessment tools in criminal justice and forensic psychiatry: the need for better data. Eur. Psychiatry 42, 134–137.

Edward, K.L., Hercelinskyj, G., Giandinoto, J.A., 2017. Emotional labour in mental health nursing: an integrative systematic review. Int. J. Ment. Health Nurs. 26 (3), 215–225.

Fazel, S., Singh, J.P., Doll, H., et al., 2012. Use of risk assessment instruments to predict violence and antisocial behaviour in 73 samples involving 24 827 people: systematic review and meta-analysis. BMJ 345, doi:10.1136/bmj.e4692.

Fletcher, J., Spittal, M., Brophy, L., et al., 2017. Outcomes of the Victorian Safewards trial in 13 wards: impact on seclusion rates and fidelity measurement. Int. J. Ment. Health Nurs. 26 (5), 461–471.

Gerace, A., Oster, C., O'Kane, D., et al., 2018. Empathic processes during nurse–consumer conflict situations in psychiatric inpatient units: a qualitative study. Int. J. Ment. Health Nurs. 27 (1), 92–105.

Hallett, N., Dickens, G.L., 2017. De-escalation of aggressive behaviour in healthcare settings: concept analysis. Int. J. Nurs. Stud. 75, 10–20.

Higgins, A., Doyle, L., Downes, C., et al., 2016. There is more to risk and safety planning than dramatic risks: mental health nurses' risk assessment and safety-management practice. Int. J. Ment. Health Nurs. 25 (2), 159–170.

Holland, K., 2017. Cultural Awareness in Nursing and Health Care: An Introductory Text. Routledge, New York.

Hui, A., 2016. Mental health workers' experiences of using coercive measures: 'You can't tell people who don't understand'. In: Völlm, B., Nedopil, N. (Eds.), The Use of Coercive Measures in Forensic Psychiatric Care: Legal, Ethical and Practical Challenges. Springer, Cham, Switzerland, pp. 241–253.

Hurducas, C.C., Singh, J.P., de Ruiter, C., et al., 2014. Violence risk assessment tools: a systematic review of surveys. Int. J. Forensic Ment. Health 13 (3), 181–192. doi:10.1080/14999013.2014.942923.

Iozzino, L., Ferrari, C., Large, M., et al., 2015. Prevalence and risk factors of violence by psychiatric acute inpatients: a systematic review and meta-analysis. PLoS ONE 10 (6), e0128536.

Isobel, S., Delgado, C., 2018. Safe and collaborative communication skills: a step towards mental health nurses implementing trauma informed care. Arch. Psychiatr. Nurs. 32 (2), 291–296.

Kennedy, H., Roper, C., Randall, R., et al., 2019. Consumer recommendations for enhancing the Safewards model and interventions. Int. J. Ment. Health Nurs. 28 (2), 616–626.

Lamont, S., Brunero, S., 2019. Managing challenging behaviour and workplace violence. In: Hains, D. (Ed.), Mental Health for Paramedics. Elsevier, Sydney.

Lamont, S., Brunero, S., 2014. 'eSimulation' Part 2: evaluation of an interactive multimedia mental health education program for generalist nurses. Collegian 21 (1), 3–9.

Lamont, S., Brunero, S., 2013. 'eSimulation' Part 1: development of an interactive multimedia mental health education program for generalist nurses. Collegian 20 (4), 239–247.

Lamont, S., Brunero, S., Sharma, S., 2015. Application and implications of Mental Health Act 2007 (NSW) certificate use in acute generalist settings. Aust. Health Rev. 40 (2), 219–224.

Lavelle, M., Stewart, D., James, K., et al., 2016. Predictors of effective de-escalation in acute inpatient psychiatric settings. J. Clin. Nurs. 25 (15–16), 2180–2188.

Llor-Esteban, B., Sánchez-Muñoz, M., Ruiz-Hernández, J.A., et al., 2017. User violence towards nursing professionals in mental health services and emergency units. Eur. J. Psychol. Appl. Leg. Context 9 (1), 33–40.

McAllister, S., McCrae, N., 2017. The therapeutic role of mental health nurses in psychiatric intensive care: a mixed-methods investigation in an inner-city mental health service. J. Psychiatr. Ment. Health Nurs. 24 (7), 491–502.

McAllister, S., Robert, G., Tsianakas, V., et al., 2019. Conceptualising nurse–patient therapeutic engagement on acute mental health wards: an integrative review. Int. J. Nurs. Stud. 93, 106–118.

McCormack, B., Manley, K., Titchen, A., 2013. Practice Development in Nursing and Healthcare. John Wiley & Sons, Oxford.

Mezzina, R., Rosen, A., Amering, M., et al., 2019. The practice of freedom: human rights and the global mental health agenda. In: Javed, A., Fountoulakis, K.N. (Eds.), Advances in Psychiatry. Springer International Publishing, Cham, pp. 483–515.

Morgan, S., 2004. Positive risk-taking: an idea whose time has come. Health Care Risk Report 10, 18–19.

Perry, L., Lamont, S., Brunero, S., et al., 2015. The mental health of nurses in acute teaching hospital settings: a cross-sectional survey. BMC Nurs. 14 (1), 15.

Price, O., Baker, J., Bee, P., et al., 2018. Patient perspectives on barriers and enablers to the use and effectiveness of de-escalation techniques for the management of violence and aggression in mental health settings. J. Adv. Nurs. 74 (3), 614–625.

Renwick, L., Stewart, D., Richardson, M., et al., 2016. Aggression on inpatient units: clinical characteristics and consequences. Int. J. Ment. Health Nurs. 25 (4), 308–318.

Ritter, S., Platt, L.M., 2016. What's new in treating inpatients with personality disorders?: dialectical behavior therapy and old-fashioned, good communication. J. Psychosoc. Nurs. Ment. Health Serv. 54 (1), 38–45.

Savaşan, A., Çam, O., 2017. The effect of the psychiatric nursing approach based on the tidal model on coping and self-esteem in people with alcohol dependency: a randomized trial. Arch. Psychiatr. Nurs. 31 (3), 274–281.

SICSAW, 2019. Ensuring Safety in Care and Safety for Staff in Australian Mental Health Services. Canberra. http://www.acmhn.org/.

Slemon, A., Jenkins, E., Bungay, V., 2017. Safety in psychiatric inpatient care: the impact of risk management culture on mental health nursing practice. Nurs. Inq. 24 (4), e12199. doi:10.1111/nin.12199.

Smith, M.J., Bouch, J., Bradstreet, S., et al., 2015. Health services, suicide, and self-harm: patient distress and system anxiety. Lancet Psychiatry 2 (3), 275–280.

Smith, S., Macduff, C., 2017. A thematic analysis of the experience of UK mental health nurses who have trained in Solution Focused Brief Therapy. J. Psychiatr. Ment. Health Nurs. 24 (2–3), 105–113.

Staunton, P., Chiarella, M., 2013. Law for Nurses and Midwives. Elsevier, Sydney.

Stein-Parbury, J., 2016. Patient & Person Interpersonal Skills in Nursing, sixth ed. Elsevier, Sydney.

Szmukler, G., Bach, M., 2015. Mental health disabilities and human rights protections. Glob. Ment. Health (Camb) 2, 1–9.

Toms, G., Williams, L., Rycroft-Malone, J., et al., 2019. The development and theoretical application of an implementation framework for dialectical behaviour therapy: a critical literature review. Borderline Personal. Disord. Emot. Dysregul. 6 (1), 2.

United Nations, 2006. Convention on the Rights of Persons with Disabilities. Retrieved from: http://www.un.org/disabilities/convention/conventionfull.shtml.

United Nations, 1948. The Universal Declaration of Human Rights. Retrieved from: http://www.un.org/en/documents/udhr/.

United Nations General Assembly, 1991. Principles for the protection of persons with mental illness and for the improvement of mental health care. Retrieved from: http://www.un.org/documents/ga/res/46/a46r119.htm.

Valente, S.M., 2017. Managing professional and nurse–patient relationship boundaries in mental health. J. Psychosoc. Nurs. Ment. Health Serv. 55 (1), 45–51.

West, M., Melvin, G., McNamara, F., et al., 2017. An evaluation of the use and efficacy of a sensory room within an adolescent psychiatric inpatient unit. Aust. Occup. Ther. J. 64 (3), 253–263.

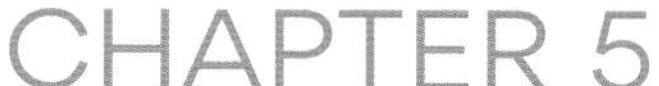

CHAPTER 5

Working with families in mental health

Kim Foster, Sophie Isobel and Kim Usher

KEY POINTS

- A person's mental illness and distress affects all members of their family.
- Supporting consumers in their personal recovery includes recognising that their family members are also in recovery.
- Nurses play a key role in preventing intergenerational mental illness and improving wellbeing and outcomes for families through partnering with and supporting families in the process of recovery.
- Family-focused practices in mental health include identifying the family system, providing information and support, and providing specific strategies and interventions to strengthen family capacity, build family resilience and support family recovery.

KEY TERMS

- Allostasis
- Carers
- Family-focused practice
- Family of origin
- Family of procreation or choice
- Family recovery
- Family resilience
- Intergenerational mental illness
- Relational recovery
- Strengths-based approach

LEARNING OUTCOMES

The material in this chapter will assist you to:

- define the key terms related to working with families in mental health
- outline a strengths-based approach to working with families when a person has mental illness
- describe key family assessment and family-focused practices when working with families in mental health
- understand the family and relational recovery process when a family member has mental illness
- identify how nurses can support family wellbeing, resilience and recovery through prevention and intervention strategies.

Introduction

We live within the context of our relationships with others, particularly our family and friends. When a person develops an illness such as mental illness, their experiences of the illness, recovery and treatment will inevitably affect the people with whom they are most connected. Mental illness affects the entire family. Recognising the vital importance of mental health consumers' relationships to their wellbeing, this chapter focuses on how nurses can provide effective care to consumers that is inclusive of the needs of the whole family – the consumer and their children and/or adults with whom they live and love.

Defining 'family'

For the purposes of this chapter, the notion of 'family' and who is included in a 'family' is understood to be defined by its members. That is, the family themselves determine who is 'family'. This approach acknowledges the many types of family relationships that may not be biological or necessarily resemble more traditional views of 'family' such as the nuclear family of mother, father and child/ren. 'Family' for some people may be families of their own making, which include close friends or extended family members.

We refer to two broad types of family. The first is 'family of origin'. This refers to the family a person is born into, where the family includes parents and siblings of a child or an adult with mental illness. We all have a family of origin. The second is 'family of procreation' or 'family of choice', where the family involves relationships chosen as an adult (e.g. a romantic partner). Family of procreation includes any children an adult has. These may or may not be biological – for instance, being a stepparent. Many of us have a family of choice or procreation. Both family of origin and family of procreation include other family members such as grandparents, extended family, caregivers and others who are considered 'family' by the family members.

You will note that in mental health services, and in the literature, families of people with mental illness are also commonly referred to as 'family carers', 'carers' or 'caregivers'. The terms 'family' and 'carer' are often used interchangeably. The term 'carer' recognises the crucial role that many family members play in providing informal or non-professional unpaid care for their loved one. However, not all family members play a caregiving role or consider themselves caregivers or wish to be identified as carers, and not all carers are family members. Therefore, throughout this chapter we mainly use the term 'family member' or 'family carers' and discuss the practical and emotional caregiving that many family members provide for their loved one.

Why work with families? Introducing a strengths-based approach

Over the past decades, deinstitutionalisation has seen the care of people with mental illness shift increasingly from large psychiatric institutions out into the community. This marked change to service provision has led to growing numbers of people with mental illness living with their families and carers in the community. Family members now provide vital informal caregiving; without this, there would be a greater risk of adverse outcomes and diminished quality of life for mental health consumers. However, a person's illness affects not only them as an individual but also those who love them, and mental illness can be understood as existing first and foremost within the context of family and the broader community (Foster et al. 2016).

The high level of care provided by many families for their family member with mental illness means they have an increased need for information and support in their caregiving roles. Despite their pivotal roles, family carers have consistently reported difficulty in gaining information about their loved one's mental illness. Family carers report that often mental health professionals, including nurses, are either not aware of their needs or are preoccupied with addressing the needs of the consumer. Family carers express a need for health professionals to listen to them with non-judgemental attitudes, respect their concerns, recognise their needs, acknowledge their strengths and include them when appropriate in decisions made about the care of their family member or loved one (Foster 2010; 2011).

In acknowledgement of the changing needs of families, there has been a paradigm shift in some areas of service provision so the focus of care provided to families has moved to a strengths-based approach rather than the previous deficit approach. A deficit approach to health care focuses on what is going wrong or what is lacking. A strengths-based approach, however, focuses on what is working well in a family and can be further enhanced. Being strengths-based includes being open to recognising the positive attributes and resources of families. A strengths-based approach acknowledges that it is more constructive to consider the strengths that a family has and to foster further positive growth and development for family members than to continue focusing only on the difficulties they face (Power et al. 2015). Importantly, this approach does not dismiss the consumer's and family's problems but focuses on the capacities and resources the family have that can be strengthened and used to support them in addressing their challenges. A strengths-based approach will be used as the framework throughout this chapter for communicating and working with consumers and their families/carers. This approach means that when we work with a consumer, we also recognise the need to assess their family's needs and the context within which they live. Further, a family and relational recovery lens and an emphasis on developing and sustaining resilience with families will inform discussion on working with families.

A strengths-based approach includes the principles that the problems and challenges families with mental illness have are addressed within a framework of understanding that:

- families have strengths and limitations and the capacity to be resilient
- the family as well as the consumer goes through a process of recovery following mental illness
- as mental health professionals we need to attend to the diversity of individual and family responses to the challenges of living with mental illness.

A strengths-based approach also acknowledges that, while problems exist, families are the best judge of their circumstances and can be supported by health professionals to find their own solutions and ways of coping. A strengths-based approach assists us as nurses to work with families, focusing on their strengths, competencies and the resources they need to deal with the particular issues they face. So, using a strengths-based framework moves us away from the idea of trying to 'fix' individual or family deficits and towards recognising their existing protective attributes and abilities. This approach encourages development of further skills in managing and finding solutions to their own situation. This in turn encourages nurses to view families as active agents and decision-makers in their own care rather than as passive recipients of the services we provide. Throughout the chapter, in addition to identifying potential problems that families may face when a person has mental illness, it is important to also keep in mind the existing strengths the family has that can be harnessed to support them in times of challenge.

Historical anecdote 5.1: Families have always been important

Families have been at the heart of mental health care since ancient times. In ancient Greece the philosopher Plato (circa 427 BCE) wrote, 'If a man is mad he shall not be at large in the city, but his family shall keep him'. In those days, managing mental illness was the responsibility of family and it has remained that way in many parts of the world in the modern age. British Law began to shift responsibility from family to government in 1300s during the reign of King Edward I, who instructed that: 'The King shall have the Custody of the Lands of Natural Fools, taking the profits of them without Waste or Destruction'. So, although the king claimed the property of the person with mental illness, the family was still expected to provide care and custody.

Read more about it: *Kleisiaris CF, Sfakianakis C, Papathanasiou IV 2014 Health care practices in ancient Greece: the Hippocratic ideal. Journal of Medical Ethics and History of Medicine, 7: 6*

Potential challenges for families when a person has mental illness

Families can be a major source of support for people during periods of illness. For many families, they have access to and existing mechanisms of support and coping that help them support their loved ones through acute or sustained illness. However, families are affected by the experiences of their members, and families can face a number of challenges when a family member has mental illness. For example, family members of people with mental illness can provide a significant amount of daily care to their relatives. The Australian Bureau of Statistics (2016) has outlined the level of informal caregiving provided by family members. The survey revealed that almost 2.7 million unpaid carers provided care for family members, representing 11.6% of the population, with more than a third of carers living with a disability themselves.

As a result of this caregiver role, family members can experience a level of burden that, over time, places them at greater risk of physical and psychological health challenges (McCann et al. 2015). In a study of caring for an older parent with mental illness, McCann et al. (2015) reported that the caregiving experience has a negative impact on the physical health of the family member, where they are more susceptible to physical illnesses and take longer to recover. The experience of caregiving in families has been linked to a concept referred to as 'burden of care' – 'burden' or overload as an outcome affects people in many ways including physical, emotional, social, financial and in making important life choices such as whether to continue working, career decisions and whether to have another child (Von Kardorff et al. 2016). Despite the 'burden', many families value their roles in caregiving and are committed to ongoing support of their loved ones. The extent of the 'burden' is individual to each family and each of its members and can change over time. Despite valuing these roles, it is also important to acknowledge that, while informal carers, who mostly care for family members, make a significant contribution to providing health care, this comes at a cost to the individual(s) providing the care. The impact of caregiving is experienced not only by the primary caregiver but also by the entire family (Kenny et al. 2012).

As well as managing their relative's symptoms and dealing with the health system, Richardson et al. (2013)

explain that family members can experience financial hardship, relationship problems, social isolation, stigmatising attitudes from others, altered daily routines, frustration and exhaustion. Caregiving can markedly reduce the time available for socialising with others and in engaging in hobbies and self-care such as exercise (Foster 2011). Many family carers report feeling isolated from others, often including other family members (McCann et al. 2015), leaving them without others with whom they can discuss concerns (Digiacomo et al. 2013). McCann et al. (2015) found that the stress of caregiving can have a serious negative impact on family relationships, especially where other family members are critical of the care delivered. Family members may feel guilty about discussing their own challenges related to caregiving out of loyalty to their loved one, not wanting to add to family burden and taking pride in their caring role. But at the same time, they may be experiencing a lack of opportunities to access support and/or fear of others misinterpreting their experiences as an unwillingness to continue in their caring role. It is important for nurses to understand these issues and to support family members to share their concerns, as well as acknowledge their strengths and commitment to the unwell family member.

NURSE'S STORY 5.1

Felicity

As a nurse, I've always worked with families. Everyone comes from a family and I think I've always been aware of the importance of connection and relationships. Currently I work with families within an adult mental health service, promoting awareness of families and offering support to families when someone is unwell. When one person has a mental illness, there's a ripple effect, it doesn't just affect them, but it affects the people around them and everybody feels it.

Families are a bit like a baby's mobile. Mental illness can cause a lot of anxiety within the family. When one bit of the mobile shakes, the whole thing shakes. The mobile can shake from any change, a change of role or a move or sickness. A mental illness in the family can cause the mobile to vigorously shake and we are often working with families to find some calm and balance again. When mental illness happens, families can feel grief, sadness, guilt or fear. There is still so much stigma and shame. Some families can be very supportive and get into patterns that work for them. Other times the mental illness can dominate the whole family and people forget to look after themselves. I remind people that in an aeroplane you have to put your own oxygen mask on first before you help others. Sometimes people don't know they are allowed to do that.

Other people may not want their family involved or their family might be disconnected or live far away. Mental illness can cause tension within a family and conflicts within relationships. Sometimes the tension was there already, and everything gets attributed to the person with the illness. But illness in any family is a stressor. You see so much more about people when you see them with their family or you see them in their home – the environment, the dynamics – things that we don't see if we just see someone in the clinic or hospital. People are different around their family; we all are, because of the emotional investment.

As a mental health nurse, if we go to someone's home, we are always a guest and we have to be respectful of people's lives and spaces. I try to be curious, ask people about their family, and make time to listen and talk to them about what help they may want. I show kindness and empathy, which helps build trust. I also ask families what brings them joy and satisfaction and I tell them what I observe as their strengths; sometimes they can't see the strengths they have. There is usually a lot of love in families, even if they are having trouble showing it. In mental health we see so many different families, there is no 'usual' family. Every family is different, every family has struggles. We need to offer hope for families that things will get better than they are right now; it might take some time, but they will. Sometimes families feel stuck or feel like things won't ever change. Families are very attuned to judgement from services and clinicians. We have to be very aware of this and focus on strengths and help them find a way forward. It's a privilege to see into people's everyday lives.

Children and families where parents have mental illness

Children and young people can be overlooked when considering the impacts of mental illness on families. Children and young people in families where there is mental illness are often called on to provide care, including for their parents. Usually the person requiring care is an older adult who is cared for by their adult child. However, 12–45% of mental health consumers in adult mental health services have children under the age of 18 years (Maybery & Reupert 2018). Some of these children need to provide physical and/or emotional care for their parent and/or for their siblings. Their caregiving role may continue into adulthood, where many adult children of parents with mental illness provide care for their ageing parents (Foster 2010). Even if they don't provide direct care, children and young people can experience a range of impacts of mental illness in their families. For some children and young people, parental or family mental illness is a part of their family experience but, with enough explanation about what is happening and other protective factors such as support from other family members and/or from health professionals, the impacts can be minimal.

The impact on children and young people is influenced by their child's age at the time of the parent or family member's diagnosis or episodes of illness (Reupert et al. 2012), the severity of the illness and the impact of chronicity, and the presence of other disorders (such as substance abuse). Children and young people may be faced not only with changing parental behaviours but also a lack of other family members being available to assist with the emotional needs of the child (Murphy et al. 2014). Children in families where a parent has mental illness can be at a higher risk of developing mental and emotional problems, but this relationship is complex and related to a number of contributing factors including other supportive adults, school engagement (Reupert et al. 2012) and episodes of separation during hospitalisation (Foster et al. 2018). While children and young people may experience social, psychological and practical challenges across their lives as a direct result of their family member's illness and will benefit from support, it is important to also note that the experiences of children and adults within families can be varied.

Parents caring for a child or young person with mental illness

Parents caring for a child or young person with mental illness can also experience challenges. Many parents worry for their children's future and experience guilt or fear. Many also experience numerous losses. Parents in one study (Richardson et al. 2013) reported losses associated with their perceptions of the child's lost expectations, uncertainty for the future, loss of financial stability and loss of social and career opportunities. The parents reported experiences such as anger, disappointment, hopelessness, sadness, shock, worry and denial related to the diagnosis of mental illness, and the many challenges faced in the caregiver role. Practically, parents may lose income and social connection through increased time spent caring for, or facilitating care for, their child.

Stigma and families

While the challenges for children, parents, adults and families associated with mental illness are often related to their own experiences and social impacts, many also experience stigma associated with having a relative with mental illness. This involves prejudice or discrimination from others. This form of stigma has been referred to as 'family stigma'. It can include, for example, blaming mental illness in a child or young person on poor parenting or blaming family members for not helping their relative adhere with medications (Corrigan et al. 2014). Stigma may make it harder for family members to accept their relative's illness and, in some cases, they may experience guilt related to the shame they feel about their relative's illness or behaviour. This can be understood as 'self-stigma', where family members endorse negative social views of people with mental illness (Corrigan et al. 2014).

Families of people with mental illness report being subjected to daily discrimination and stigma; this stigma may come from the community, extended family members or health professionals (van der Sanden et al. 2016). As a result, families can withdraw from wider social situations and connections (Murphy et al. 2014). One study of stigma experienced by family members of people diagnosed with mental illness (McCann et al. 2011) found that being open about the situation was a strategy that helped caregivers to manage the stigma and enabled support from family and reduced social isolation. However, the study also revealed that families from a range of cultural backgrounds were likely to be secretive about a family member's mental illness and hence were considered more vulnerable to the impact of stigma.

Historical anecdote 5.2: Families blamed?

In the past, families were often blamed for causing mental disorder. American psychiatrist Frieda Fromm-Reichmann even went so far as to define a so-called 'schizophrenogenic mother' in 1948, who she asserted could cause schizophrenia. This type of mother was described as being emotionally cold, rejecting and emotionally disturbed; a perfectionist, domineering and lacking in sensitivity; rigidly moral but seductive; and overprotective of the child who she kept in a dependent state so she could exert control. This parent would in theory so confuse the child with contradictory standards and expectations, or 'double-binds', that the child grew up bewildered by society's demands and unable to decipher reality, or how to react to it. Research by Australian psychiatrist Gordon Parker reviewed the schizophrenogenic mother research in 1982 and concluded that, although such people existed, they were not responsible for the development of schizophrenia.

Read more about it: *Johnston J 2013 The ghost of the schizophrenogenic mother. AMA Journal of Ethics 15(9): 801–5*

Addressing challenges and building strengths – family resilience

While it is apparent that family members can face many challenges when a relative has mental illness, there is also evidence that many families develop strengths that can enable them to address these challenges effectively. Overcoming these challenges or adversities can be understood through the lens of allostasis and resilience.

Stress and allostasis

As described previously, living in a family where a person has mental illness, particularly if the family does not have adequate support from others, can be challenging for many family members. The concept of 'allostasis' can be useful in understanding how stress in childhood or adulthood may impact on a person. Family members, especially children, may experience a range of stressors or traumatic events that can exert a negative effect on their emotional and physical health and wellbeing over time. These stressors include conflict or aggression in the family, lack of nurturing, and emotional, physical and/or sexual abuse or neglect. They may also include the impact of mental illness on family members.

Allostasis refers to the adaptation process of a person's physiological system to psychosocial, environmental or physical stressors (Logan & Barksdale 2008). The immune system and the stress response (the hypothalamic–pituitary–adrenal axis) are the two main mediators in allostasis (Repetti et al. 2011). 'Allostatic load' refers to long-term outcomes of unsuccessful adaptation and the cumulative physical damage that results from repeated physical responses to stress. The impact of these stressful experiences over time negatively affects an individual's health, resulting in illness or disease (Repetti et al. 2011).

Repetti et al. (2011) use the metaphor of meshed gears to illustrate the interrelated links between repeated short-term responses to stress or trauma and the long-term impacts of this. In a family environment, the smallest gear can be seen to represent stressful events, a child's immediate response to this as one turn of the middle gear, and their long-term health outcomes as one turn of the largest gear (see Fig. 5.1).

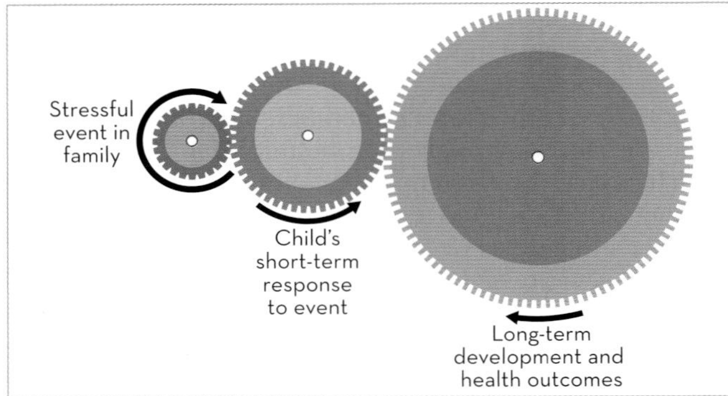

Figure 5.1
Gears as a metaphor illustrating connections between repeated short-term reactions and their long-term outcomes.
Source: Repetti et al. 2011

Resilience

Resilience has been variously defined but, in this context, it is a process that refers specifically to risk or challenge and individual or family adaptation. Resilience is a dynamic process that involves being able to adapt positively to stress or adversity and to maintain or restore wellbeing using internal and external resources, including protective factors (Foster & Robinson 2014). In this way, resilience can be understood to represent allostasis or positive adaptation. Promoting the resilience of children and families living with challenging situations such as mental illness can lead to better physical and mental health outcomes for individuals and the family as a whole and support the family's recovery.

Family resilience can be distinguished from individual resilience because it refers to the wellbeing of multiple individuals within a family system and the relationships between them, as well as the key family processes that support their resilience (Power et al. 2015). Box 5.1 outlines the key processes in family resilience. From a family resilience perspective, families are viewed as a unit with fundamental strengths and resources and potential for growth (Zauszniewski et al. 2015). In families living with mental illness, resilience has been found to involve keeping a balance between stress and distress and maintaining family members' strength and optimism (Power et al. 2015).

Box 5.1 Key processes that support family resilience

- Communication and discussion about mental illness between family members
- Maintaining rituals and routines such as family dinners, family holidays or recreational events
- Family bonding and positive relationships between family members

Adapted from Power et al. 2015

Personal factors that promote resilience for family members of people with mental illness include: hardiness; having hope and acceptance, a sense of self-efficacy, coherence and mastery; and being resourceful. Family members who have these characteristics seem better able to deal with the challenges they face (Zauszniewski et al. 2015). Individuals within families can have resilience and that may benefit the family unit; however, other resources such as warm and positive relationships and connections between family members are integral resilience factors in maintaining the family unit's ability to recover from adversity (Walsh 2006).

Family and relational recovery

In the context of mental illness, resilience and recovery can be understood to be interrelated. Resilience is a process that involves overcoming adversity and building strengths, and recovery is a process that involves transformation in the face of challenges such as mental illness. Recovery is addressed further in Chapter 2.

In mental health services, there has been a growing emphasis on providing care that supports the personal recovery of consumers. Personal recovery has been defined as 'a deeply personal, unique process of changing one's attitudes, values, feelings, goals, skills and/or roles. It is a way of living a satisfying, hopeful and contributing life even with the limitations caused by [mental] illness' (Anthony 1993, p. 13). Implicit in this is the concept that consumers define and assume responsibility for their own recovery (Wyder & Bland 2014). In personal recovery, people with mental illness can be understood as journeying through several processes. These include building *c*onnectedness with others, having *h*ope and optimism about the future, developing positive *i*dentity, finding *m*eaning in life and having *e*mpowerment (also known as CHIME) (Leamy et al. 2011).

Although there has been an increasing understanding and focus on individual consumer recovery in mental health service provision, there has been minimal corresponding identification of the recovery process that families can experience as they journey alongside their family member with mental illness or distress. Yet just as a person with mental illness can experience recovery, so too can family members. These processes overlap with the personal recovery processes of the person with mental illness (Spaniol 2010), and recovery can be understood as a family process (Nicholson et al. 2014). Family recovery draws on the strengths of all members of the family, is informed by an understanding of life events and the impact of trauma and is driven by the family and their goals and needs (Nicholson et al. 2014).

Spaniol (2010) identifies four phases in the process of family recovery. Fig. 5.2 provides a visual framework of this process.

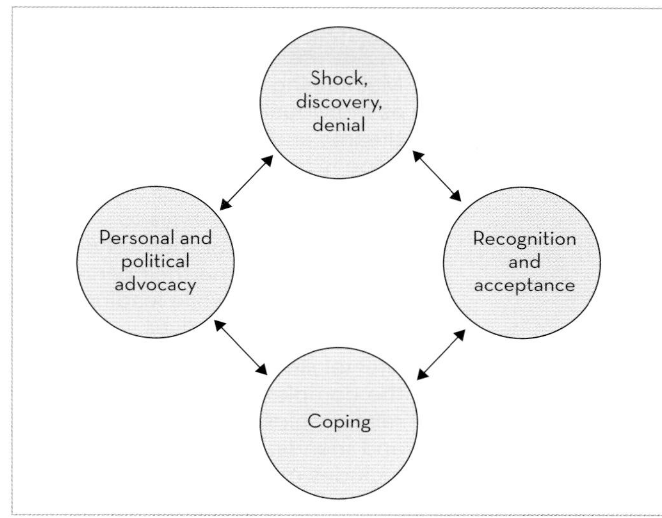

Figure 5.2
Family recovery process
Source: Spaniol 2010

1. **Shock, discovery, denial:** An individual's acute mental illness can often be shocking for family members. Changes they may observe in the person can be difficult to understand. Family members may explain these away and not believe the illness is serious. Denial may persist throughout the early phase of the illness.
2. **Recognition and acceptance:** Family members may gradually gain awareness that their relative has a mental illness. This can be accompanied by a sense of hope that health professionals know how to treat it, as well as feelings of guilt, embarrassment or even self-blame or responsibility for the illness. As part of the acceptance process, family members may feel a sense of loss for the life they had previously hoped for with their family member. Through grieving, over time they may come to accept this loss. Through a changing awareness of themselves, their relationships and life, family members can be transformed.
3. **Coping:** Initially, family members can struggle with the challenges of mental illness without adequate knowledge or skills. Later, family members learn to carry on with their lives and identify how they can support their relative. Coping begins to replace grieving. Family members may become more assertive or angry as they question the care their relative is receiving. They may ask for additional support. Over time, the family's knowledge, confidence and coping skills may grow and they may come to view professionals as a necessary but not complete part of their ability to cope.
4. **Personal and political advocacy:** In the recovery process, family members slowly come to a new awareness of themselves. This may include a stronger sense of confidence and personal advocacy. They let go of self-blame and focus on new roles and ways of working with professionals that are more collaborative. For some family members, political advocacy and working to influence and change the system becomes more important.

Wyder and Bland (2014) have contributed to our emerging understandings of the interrelationship between personal and family recovery through applying personal recovery frameworks to the family's tasks of supporting their relative and engaging in their own journey of recovery (see Table 5.1 on the next page for a summary). They

TABLE 5.1 Tasks for families in recovery

1. Maintaining hope	Maintaining hope for themselves as individuals and their own dreams and aspirations. Holding hope is complex. Families may need to hold hope for their loved one. As they find ways to maintain hope for themselves, they can continue their caring responsibilities while leading their own fulfilling lives.
2. Reconnecting	Mental illness emerges within the complex network of close relationships that includes family and friends. Reconnecting includes maintaining or re-establishing relationships and support from others, being part of peer support and support groups, and being part of the community.
3. Overcoming secondary trauma	Families can experience secondary traumatisation and share the trauma, isolation and stigma associated with mental illness. This can include feeling powerless to control their lives, feeling abused by the treatment system, experiencing guilt, feeling traumatised when their loved one is subjected to trauma and experiencing chronic grief and loss.
4. Journeying from carer to family	Families are often defined by their carer role. A family's journey is also an integral part in recovery. When families can let go of their caring role to achieve a mutually supportive role with their loved one, this ultimately enables not only their own but also their loved one's recovery.

Adapted from Wyder & Bland 2014

conclude that the family's recovery from mental illness is an active and multidimensional process rather than limited simply to the role of caregiving.

A more recent and alternate understanding of recovery that relates to families is relational recovery. This approach considers that family are important relationships in peoples' lives. Relational recovery emphasises that people are interdependent, that their lives can't be separated from the social context within which they live, and that recovery occurs in the context of relationships. Family relationships can therefore be understood to be at the heart of personal recovery and affect all aspects of a person's recovery from mental illness (Price-Robertson et al. 2017). From this perspective, recovery cannot be separated from consumers' relationships and connections with their families. As nurses, understanding that recovery is grounded in relationships is important for our practice. It means that to support a person's recovery from mental illness, we need to be inclusive of their family and supportive of family relationships and connections.

Critical thinking challenge 5.2

1. Consider the personal recovery processes (CHIME) (Leamy et al. 2011) and the tasks for families in recovery (Wyder & Bland 2014). What are the similarities and differences between them? How can nurses support individuals and families in their recovery processes?
2. For each of the tasks for families in recovery outlined in Table 5.1, consider how nurses can support families in working through these tasks. Identify at least one strategy that nurses can use in supporting families in each family task.

CONSUMER'S STORY 5.1
Jane

My daughter has had a mental illness for nearly 20 years now. We've had a lot of contact with services and always been very involved in her care. It's been very stressful and hard but she's our daughter and we love her. Experiences with services are so varied. People can't really imagine what it's like to have your daughter in a psychiatric ward and how that feels. I visit every day when she is in hospital. I had a really brilliant experience a couple of years ago in an inpatient unit. My daughter was very sick. It was very late at night when she was admitted. This really nice nurse welcomed us properly and didn't rush me out even though it was late and was happy to settle both of us and make sure my daughter was comfortable, and then she even rang me later when I had gone home to let me know how my daughter was. It's unusual to get that follow-up. She really cared for us all the way through the admission. It was like she was our guardian angel. It changed my experience and my daughter's experience. It affected my daughter enormously because she didn't feel patronised; it felt like an equal relationship and that she and the nurses were partners in her recovery.

Nurses can really affect the whole experience of care for families. Sometimes in hospital there are no nurses out on the floor. I know there's a lot of paperwork to be done but it feels to me as a family member like they might be hiding in the office. Sometimes I've felt like the nurses aren't engaged with us as a family or even with my daughter. How people treat my daughter affects me. It's been great when nurses have shared information with me, told me how my daughter is doing and even spoken to me on my own to see how I am. It makes me feel like she is being looked after properly and it's easier to go home and feel less worried.

There are always going to be some staff who are better than others. You get quite good at recognising who is going to be good. I've probably become one of those parents who are really pushy, but in a way, you have to be. I've learnt that because it can be the only way to make sure she gets the right care. I will ring as many times as I have to because I know her, and I know when she's not well. I know about her medication and what works, but sometimes staff don't listen to me or believe me. Staff think they are the experts, but I've known her for her whole life. In hospital, all the parents and carers you meet know a lot, but we are often dismissed. I've called before and told the mental health worker that my daughter was getting unwell and they didn't believe me and then things got a lot worse and we had to manage it at home. It's simple really, you just want staff to listen and care and have respect for our expertise as family.

EXERCISE FOR CLASS ENGAGEMENT

Read Consumer's story 5.1

1. What strengths do you think this family has?
2. Using the framework of family recovery by Spaniol (2010), identify the relevant aspects of the family recovery process in this story.
3. What elements of mental health service delivery were effective and ineffective in supporting this family's recovery?
4. In what ways can mental health service delivery be changed or improved to provide greater support for family recovery for all family members?

Working with families: family-focused practices

As noted earlier, many mental health services continue to approach the care of people with mental illness through an individual lens. The focus is primarily on caring for the individual consumer and managing their symptoms. If family are considered, it is often through the lens of how they can assist and support the person in their recovery, rather than from the perspective of seeing the family as intertwined with the individual and their experience of illness and a crucial context for recovery. Families need to be involved in decisions about their family member's care (Foster et al. 2016). There is need for greater recognition of family in service provision and the consequences/outcomes for family when this is not the case. An approach that focuses only on the individual and does not take into account the perspectives and needs of the people who love and care for them is an approach that fails to address the crucial family context of the lived experience of mental illness. As part of their model of care for consumers, services need to provide information for families about key issues such as the consumer's right to confidentiality, the consumer's verbal or written consent for carers to have information about their illness and treatment, and acknowledgement of carers' own needs for information about mental illness and available treatments (Rowe 2012). Of course, it also needs to be acknowledged and respected that there are times that people don't want their family involved in their care.

From an international perspective, best practice for working with consumers and family includes clinical care and communication that is empathic to carers (Rowe 2012), that is provided in collaboration with the consumer, family and clinicians, and where the path to recovery includes attention to financial, housing and social aspects of consumers' and family members' lives (Wallcraft et al. 2011). Involving the family, including children, is a recommended standard of practice for adult mental health services in Australia and New Zealand. Having clear standards for practice in mental health services can improve the quality of family participation in mental health care and result in increased family involvement in family care planning and improved contact between clinicians and family (Goodyear et al. 2015).

In mental health, family-focused practice is an approach to care that takes a 'whole of family' perspective and identifies the relationships between a mental health consumer and their 'key others'. Family-focused practice involves systematically incorporating family members'/carers' health and wellbeing and the role of parenting into a family plan of care. In attending to all the family, family-focused practice can be considered a form of preventive intervention that addresses the impact of intergenerational mental illness on family members (including children) and supports family recovery and resilience (Foster et al. 2016).

Four key principles underpin family-focused practice. These are a belief that:

- consumers' (children's or adults') families play a vital role in their recovery
- both consumers and their families can be empowered to address and meet their needs
- it is possible to support consumers via their family
- relationships between clinicians and consumers, clinicians and families, and between consumers and family members are key to enabling a 'whole of family' approach to care (Foster et al. 2016).

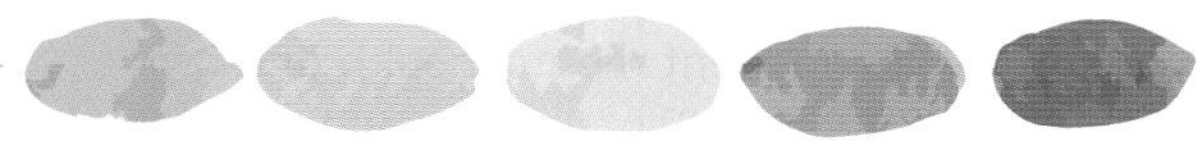

NURSE'S STORY 5.2

Sophie

Everybody comes from a family and many people hold roles in families, including parenting, which forms an integral part of their self. In adult mental health services, there is an increasing push to recognise the relationship between these family roles and mental health and recovery. When a parent has a mental illness, children are often not provided with any information or support to make sense of their world and are usually not included in care planning or delivery. Advocating for family-focused practice in mental health services is hard work, yet the opportunity to work with children and families has provided me with endless inspiration and motivation to continue. Many mental health services have dedicated positions such as mine that exist to improve the inclusion of families in care. A big part of my role is promoting awareness of children and families at the systems level and educating clinicians about ways to work with families in the care they provide to individuals. But the role has also included running parenting programs for parents with mental illness, organising children's activity programs, running support groups and coordinating playgroups specifically for families affected by mental illness, as well as large amounts of conversations, family sessions and support provided to many children, parents and families.

My role varies on a day-to-day basis. You never quite know what might happen, what projects might be started or what a referral might entail. Most referrals come from mental health clinicians, but often schools, families, early childhood and other services also seek advice or resources. There are increasing amounts of good resources and books about mental illness for families but none of them replaces a conversation with someone exploring your experiences and questions. Conversations about mental illness can occur with parents, children, young people and family members during home visits or in hospitals or health centres. Parents can often be understandably reluctant to engage in conversations about their parenting or refuse to have a professional talk to their children about their illness, so a lot of time and thought needs to be spent building rapport and including all family members in discussions where possible. While all parents have worries about their parenting roles and can benefit from parenting support, mental illness is an additional challenge that can be stressful for all members of a family.

No two days are the same in this work. One day you may find yourself walking with a teenager discussing what mental illness is, how it affects their parent and answering questions about how to tell their friends or whether they will get it too. The next you might be advocating for a parent in a family meeting on an inpatient mental health unit or navigating complex family dynamics in a home visit. Some days you might find yourself colouring in with a child and talking to them about what makes them feel worried or talking with schools or other agencies about how they can support a child or family. A lot of time is spent supporting mental health clinicians to address the needs of all family members within their care planning.

Conversations with parents might focus on what their illness stops them being able to do as a parent, what they think their children may have noticed when they were unwell, how they can explain their mental illness to their child and what children need to feel safe and secure. Often parents are concerned that they are being judged as a bad parent or may find it difficult to engage in wider parenting supports. Conversations with children need to be appropriate to their age and circumstance and context. Sometimes children want lots of information, and other times conversations may focus on other stressors, supports and worries. Conversations may include who the child can talk to if they need to, what understanding they have of their parent's illness and reassurance about the future. Children often think their parent's illness is their fault. It is also important to make plans for periods of separation or hospitalisation and offer truthful and simple explanations. Both children and parents are open to detailed discussions about the brain and what is known and understood about mental illness, including treatment and prognosis.

Children often notice more than we realise, and their questions can be quite poignant and challenging. I generally just try to be honest and thoughtful in my answers and admit what I don't know. Children can also be very accepting, so often something I am worried about talking about is not such a big deal once I start. An awkward conversation is always better than no attempt at all. Education to other nurses on talking to children and families can be rewarding as they realise how much of it is about being willing to put aside their own fears and have a go at tricky conversations about topics like depression, psychosis or suicide that may make us as adults feel uncomfortable. There is a privilege in stepping into the lives of families and looking at mental illness as a part of a wider structure that affects and is affected by all its members.

Range of family-focused practices

In working with families, nurses may feel they lack specific knowledge about the needs of children, parenting or the family as a whole. While there are a range of practices that are important for supporting families, it is not always feasible or necessary for nurses to provide all of them. Family-focused practice can be understood as comprising a continuum or range of intensity that moves from fundamental strategies through to more advanced or intensive approaches, including family therapy.

When working with families of procreation, Foster et al. (2012) recommend a minimum level of practice:

- identifying consumers' parental status (as relevant) when they enter a service

- identifying the number, age, wellbeing and location of their dependent children
- supporting consumers' and children's needs to maintain contact with each other
- providing relevant mental health information and resources including parenting information to consumers, children and family members
- referring children and family members to family workers or services as appropriate (see Fig. 5.3).

For all families, there are a range of practices that nurses and other health professionals can engage in to address the needs of all family members. A systematically conducted review of international literature on family-focused practice identified six core practices when working with families of origin or procreation (see Table 5.2). Box 5.2 on the next page outlines assessment areas for families on intake into a service. As part of the family assessment process it is common to develop a genogram (visual display) of the family structure and key relationships. See Fig. 5.4 for an example of a genogram. The genogram is a graphic representation

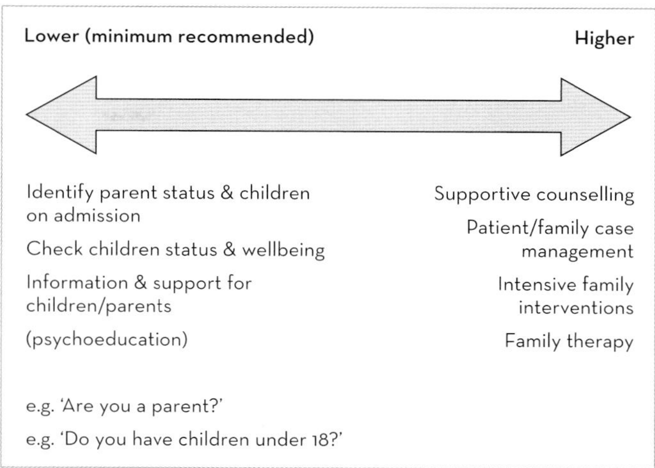

Figure 5.3
Continuum of intensity of family-focused practice
Source: Foster et al. 2012

TABLE 5.2 Family-focused practices

CORE PRACTICE	EXAMPLES OF PRACTICE
1. Assessment of family members and family functioning	Ranges from questions about family relationships at intake to service, to assessing parenting competency and/or family circumstances, the impact of family member's illness on other family members, and the level of mental health literacy in family members.
2. Psychoeducation	Information and education on mental illness and treatment (including medication) that aims to improve family members' mental health literacy. Ranges from informal discussion and providing written or online resources to evidence-based manualised family interventions.
3. Family care planning and goal setting	Collaborative care planning including crisis plans with family. Assisting family members to set goals in relation to the consumer's recovery and their own and other family members' wellbeing.
4. Liaising between the family and services	Liaising on behalf of the family between services and the family. Acting, or encouraging actions, with services to achieve better outcomes for the family.
5. Instrumental (I), emotional (E) and social (S) support	Referring family to another service and organising practical support (I). Showing empathy and compassion to family members (E). Empowering family and encouraging them to expand social connections and networks with others (S).
6. Coordinated system of care between the family and services	Coordinated system of care involving collaboration and partnership with family members, clinicians and other services. Commonly involves wraparound care for the family that includes developing a partnership between the family and service providers in a synchronised way. Ranges from a general approach involving coordinating services to defined types of service (e.g. 'wraparound') with a specific model of care.

Adapted from Foster et al. 2016

Box 5.2 Key areas of family assessment on the consumer's entry to a mental health service

- Identifying who the consumer lives with and which, if any, family members or loved ones provide emotional or practical support for them
- Identifying and documenting, as relevant, parent status and dependent child/ren (under 18 years) status
- If the consumer is a parent of dependent children, asking about the child/ren's care arrangements
- Identifying the family structure (family of origin and procreation/choice)* and the nature of key family relationships (e.g. parent(s), sibling(s), partner, children and other key family members as identified by the consumer)
- Identifying recent or longstanding family-related stressors (e.g. illness or death in the family; substance use; domestic violence; divorce/ relationship breakdown; unemployment and financial stress; relocation; transfer of schools; lack of housing)
- Identifying the consumer's and family's strengths (resources including strong family relationships/ supports and community support) and areas of vulnerability or need (stressors, current illness)

**See Fig. 5.4 for an example of family structure in a genogram for Marcia from Case study 5.1.*

of the family and its patterns across generations. The genogram is drawn up with the involvement of the family, helping to engage all family members, as the mapping process seeks input from everyone. Enduring and broken relationships, illegitimate and legitimate children, blended and nuclear family relationships are all depicted on the same page, revealing the emotional processes of the family to both the clinician and family members.

Family therapy

On a continuum of intensity of family-focused practices, family therapy is considered a more advanced or intensive family approach. Family therapy developed in the 1950s from the belief that the family was responsible for causing schizophrenia. In particular, it was believed that certain communication styles within families were responsible for causing the illness (the skewed and schismatic families). A further belief centred on the communication style of the mother – the so-called schizophrenogenic mother (see Historical anecdote 5.2). Although these ideas have long since been rejected, a group of interventions known as family therapy had been born (Goldenberg & Goldenberg 2000). Family therapy shifted the focus on therapy directed at unconscious material (psychotherapy) 'to a focus on the interpersonal process – that is, how family members interact with each other' (Kadis & McClendon 1998, p. 6).

Family therapy is an approach to treatment that is based on the fundamental premise that when a person has a problem, it usually involves the whole family. Family interactions might be causing the problem or prolonging the problem for the identified client, or the problem or behaviours of the client might be affecting other members of the family. Family therapists aim to effect change in the entire family system. Family therapy usually involves multiple family members, not necessarily the same family members each time, or therapy might involve a single family member.

Even when therapy involves a single individual, its impact will be experienced by the wider family. This might be demonstrated through an improvement in family functioning and/or through alleviating symptoms. Families who receive therapy are far more likely to experience improvements compared with those without therapy (Carr 2014). Unlike some therapists who believe that problems reside within an individual, family therapists believe that 'the dominant forces within our lives are located externally, within the family' (Nichols & Schwartz 2001, p. 6). Therapy concentrates on the family and the way it is organised. Ultimately, this affects the lives of each family member in some way. That is, the whole system is affected (see, for instance, Case study 5.1).

Carr (2014) reports that family therapy has been found effective in working with children who are having problems. This is because they are strongly influenced by the family and must remain within its influence. Marital problems, family feuds and difficulties that develop in people when there has been a major family transition are also amenable to family therapy. Family therapy has been found to be very useful in treating gambling issues (Mladenovic et al. 2015) and eating disorders (Gelin et al. 2015), and in changing the behaviours of young people who break the law (Dakof et al. 2015). The role of family therapists is to understand the dynamics that occur within families and to help the family members to reconsider the ways in which they interact with each other. The therapist then motivates the family members to change.

When working with families, the problem is viewed as dysfunction in the relationship between family members. The relationship therefore becomes the focus of attention. Sometimes the person identified as 'the problem' behaves in that way in order to hold the family together. For example, consider a child who misbehaves when her parents begin fighting. The misbehaviour distracts the parents from their conflict and so further fighting is averted. The parents then work together to manage the child's problem behaviour. Ultimately, the problem is not with the child but with the marital relationship.

The two-way mirror is a useful tool in family therapy. While there is a therapist in the room with the family, other members of the therapy team observe the session unobtrusively from behind the mirror. This allows immediate feedback, as the observers call in to the therapy room by telephone to give feedback or direction to the therapist and/or family. Observers may see things (communication styles, body language) that the therapist does not, so these can be communicated during the session rather than following it.

Critical thinking challenge 5.1

In relation to Case study 5.1 about Marcia:

1. What risk factors or challenges can be identified for Marcia, Michael, the children and the family as a whole?
2. What strengths or resources does the family have?
3. How can mental health clinicians support the family's resilience?

CASE STUDY 5.1
Marcia

Marcia and her husband, Michael, have two daughters: Nina, aged 7, and Rosie, aged 3. They came to Australia from Eastern Europe 6 years ago and have no other family in Australia. Marcia's parents are divorced, and Michael's father died 3 years ago. Marcia had an admission to a mental health inpatient unit following the birth of Rosie, with a diagnosis of postpartum psychosis, and a recent 2-week admission for a further psychotic episode. She was then transferred to a private hospital and after discharge has been followed up by her GP.

Michael works full-time to support the family. Nina attends Year 1 at a local primary school, while Rosie stays home with Marcia. The children did not visit their mum in hospital; Michael had explained to them that Marcia was sick and needed a break. Marcia has not returned to work since the first episode of her illness 3 years ago. She has limited social supports, with few friends and no family members in Australia.

Michael has rung the community mental health team with concerns that Marcia has been keeping Nina home from school. He thinks Marcia has stopped taking her antipsychotic medication, but she is refusing to see the GP. Marcia has told him that she does not need help and became angry when he told her about planning to call the mental health team.

Recent financial stress has meant Michael has been working extra hours and they have been arguing. He describes that the children are well cared for, but Nina has been teary and sleeping in their bed since Marcia was in hospital.

Planned approach to care:

- joint home visit with the mental health team to assess the family, Marcia, the children and the environment; assessment to include family dynamics, strengths, difficulties, observation of children and parent–child interactions, the state of the house and Marcia's mental state
- assess the impact of recent stressors on parents and children
- talk to both parents about their parenting concerns and the children
- talk about the impact of Marcia's hospitalisation on the children; what explanations, support and reassurance their daughters may require; what fears the children may experience; and the impact of separation and Marcia's illness
- discuss Marcia's medication and its impact on her parenting (e.g. drowsiness) with her and Michael
- talk to Nina and Rosie about Marcia's illness and its effects, including reassurance and key messages that it isn't their fault, that she is not going to go away again unexpectedly
- consider making safety plans for the children and parents for managing any further episodes of separation due to Marcia's illness
- identify social and community supports for all members of the family including local playgroups or preschools, social groups, teachers, family support organisations, friends
- link Marcia to parenting support, including local groups or services
- discuss the importance of schooling with the parents and children
- talk to the school and develop a plan to support the family (parents may be reluctant to talk to schools but schools can be an immense support to children; information can be provided to schools without parent consent but supporting Marcia and Michael to engage with the school and any potential supports for their daughter would be a more desirable option)
- talk to Marcia about liaising with her GP about medications and ongoing follow-up
- identify other family strengths and needs and develop a collaborative care plan with Marcia and Michael.

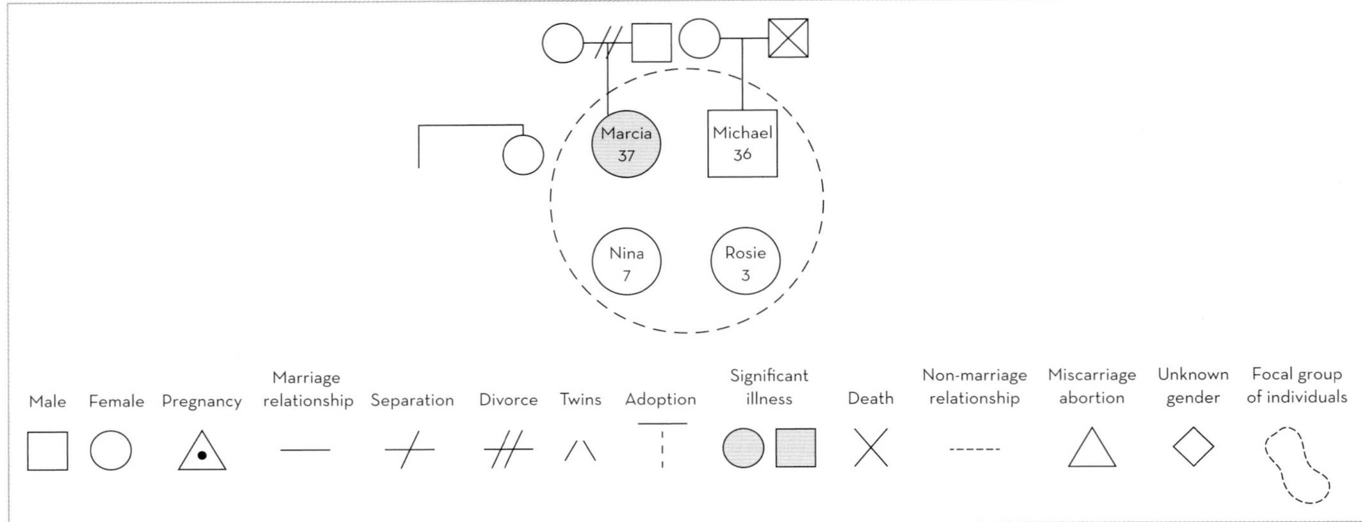

Figure 5.4
Genogram of Marcia's family
Source: Sophie Isobel

Chapter summary

This chapter has focused on the issues family members face when a relative has mental illness and the role nurses can play in supporting families through the recovery process and in building the family's resilience. Understanding the needs of and challenges faced by family members when someone they love has mental illness can inform more relevant support provision from mental health nurses. These include the need for adequate information about mental illness, its causes and treatments, and the potential for negative impacts on their own physical and mental health, the risk of stigma, and economic hardship, social isolation and relationship problems. Focusing on building family strengths and resources, and on supporting family relationships, has potential to help prevent intergenerational transmission of mental illness and enable families to journey through family and relational recovery, and to develop resilience and wellbeing.

Useful websites

Carers Australia: www.carersaustralia.com.au.
Carers New Zealand: http://carers.net.nz/.
Emerging Minds – training, programs and resources for health professionals, children and their families: https://emergingminds.com.au/our-work/.
Mental Illness Fellowship of Australia (MIFA): https://www.mifa.org.au/en/.
Mind Australia – information and advocacy for mental health carers: https://www.mindaustralia.org.au/.
Supporting Families in Mental Illness NZ: https://supportingfamilies.org.nz/.

References

Anthony, W.A., 1993. Recovery from mental illness: the guiding vision of the mental health service system in the 1990s. Psychiatr. Rehabil. J. 16 (4), 11–23.
Australian Bureau of Statistics, 2016. Disability, Ageing and Carers, Australia: Summary of Findings, 2015. Available: https://www.abs.gov.au/ausstats/abs@.nsf/mf/4430.0.
Carr, A., 2014. The evidence base for family therapy and systemic interventions for child-focused problems. J. Fam. Ther. 36, 107–157.
Corrigan, P.W., Druss, B.G., Perlick, D.A., 2014. The impact of mental illness stigma on seeking and participating in mental health care. Psychol. Sci. Public Interest 15 (2), 37–70.
Dakof, G.A., Henderson, C.E., Rowe, C.L., et al., 2015. A randomized clinical trial of family therapy in juvenile drug court. J. Fam. Psychol. 29 (2), 232–241.
Digiacomo, M., Delaney, P., Abbott, P.A., et al., 2013. 'Doing the hard yards': carer and provider focus group perspectives of accessing Aboriginal childhood disability services. BMC Health Serv. Res. doi:10.1186/1472-6963-13-326.
Foster, K., 2011. 'I wanted to learn how to heal my heart': family carer experiences of receiving an emotional support service in the Well Ways program. Int. J. Ment. Health Nurs. 20 (1), 56–62.
Foster, K., 2010. 'You'd think this roller coaster was never going to stop': the experience of being the adult child of a parent with serious mental illness. J. Clin. Nurs. 19, 3143–3151.
Foster, K., Maybery, D., Reupert, A., et al., 2016. Family focused practice in mental health care: an integrative review. Child Youth Serv. 37 (2), 129–155.

Foster, K., O'Brien, L., Korhonen, T., 2012. Developing resilient children and families where parents have mental illness: a family-focused approach. Int. J. Ment. Health Nurs. 21 (1), 3–11.

Foster, K., Robinson, T., 2014. Educating for emotional resilience in adolescence. In: Hurley, J., Linsley, P., Van der Zwan, R. (Eds.), Emotions in Education Settings. Primrose Publishing, London, pp. 56–70.

Foster, K.P., Hills, D., Foster, K.N., 2018. Addressing the support needs of families during the acute hospitalization of a parent with mental illness: a narrative literature review. Int. J. Ment. Health Nurs. 27, 470–482.

Gelin, Z., Fuso, S., Hendrick, S., et al., 2015. The effects of a multiple family therapy on adolescents with eating disorders: an outcome study. Fam. Process 54 (1), 160–172.

Goldenberg, I., Goldenberg, H., 2000. Family Therapy: An Overview, fifth ed. Wadsworth Publishing Company, New York.

Goodyear, M., Hill, T.L., Allchin, B., et al., 2015. Standards of practice for the adult mental health workforce: meeting the needs of families where a parent has a mental illness. Int. J. Ment. Health Nurs. 24 (2), 169–180.

Johnston, J., 2013. The ghost of the schizophrenogenic mother. Virtual Mentor 15 (9), 801–805.

Kadis, L.B., McClendon, R., 1998. Concise Guide to Marital and Family Therapy. American Psychiatric Press, Washington, DC.

Kenny, C., Sarma, K.M., Egan, J., 2012. An interpretive phenomenological account of the experiences of family carers of the elderly. Ir. J. Psychol. 33, 199–214.

Kleisiaris, C.F., Sfakianakis, C., Papathanasiou, I.V., 2014. Health care practices in ancient Greece: the Hippocratic ideal. J. Med. Ethics Hist. Med. 7 (6).

Leamy, M., Bird, V., Le Boutillier, C., et al., 2011. Conceptual framework for personal recovery in mental health: systematic review and narrative synthesis. Br. J. Psychiatry 199, 445–452.

Logan, J.G., Barksdale, D.J., 2008. Allostasis and allostatic load: expanding the discourse on stress and cardiovascular disease. J. Clin. Nurs. 17, 201–208.

Maybery, D., Reupert, A.E., 2018. The number of parents who are patients attending adult psychiatric services. Curr. Opin. Psychiatry 31, 358–362.

McCann, T.V., Bamberg, J., McCann, F., 2015. Family carers' experience of caring for an older parent with severe and persistent mental illness. Int. J. Ment. Health 24, 203–212.

McCann, T.V., Lubman, D.I., Clark, E., 2011. Responding to stigma: first time caregivers of young people with first-episode psychosis. Psychiatr. Serv. 62, 548–550.

Mladenovic, I., Lazetic, G., Lecic-Tosevski, D., et al., 2015. Treatment of pathological gambling: integrative systemic model. Psychiatr. Danub. 27 (1), 107–111.

Murphy, G., Peters, K., Jackson, D., 2014. A dynamic cycle of familial mental illness. Issues Ment. Health Nurs. 35, 948–953.

Nichols, M.P., Schwartz, R.C., 2001. Family Therapy: Concepts and Methods, fifth ed. Allyn & Bacon, Boston.

Nicholson, J., Wolf, T., Wilder, C., et al., 2014. Creating options for family recovery: a providers' guide to promoting parental mental health. Available: www.employmentoptions.org.

Power, J., Goodyear, M., Maybery, D., et al., 2015. Family resilience in families where a parent has mental illness. J. Soc. Work. doi:10.1177/1468017314568081.

Price-Robertson, R., Obradovic, A., Morgan, B., 2017. Relational recovery: beyond individualism in the recovery approach. Adv. Ment. Health 15 (2), 108–120.

Repetti, R.L., Robles, T.F., Reynolds, B., 2011. Allostatic processes in the family. Dev. Psychopathol. 23, 921–938.

Reupert, A.E., Mayberry, D.J., Kowalenko, N.M., 2012. Children whose parents have a mental illness: prevalence, need and treatment. Med. J. Aust. 1 (1), 7–9.

Richardson, M., Cobham, V., McDermott, B., et al., 2013. Youth mental illness and the family: parents' loss and grief. J. Child Fam. Stud. 22, 719–736.

Rowe, J., 2012. Great expectations: a systematic review of the literature on the role of family carers in severe mental illness, and their relationships and engagement with professionals. J. Psychiatr. Ment. Health Nurs. 19, 70–82.

Spaniol, L., 2010. The pain and the possibility: the family recovery process. Community Ment. Health J. 46, 482–485.

van der Sanden, L.M., Pryor, J.B., Stutterheim, S.E., et al., 2016. Stigma by association and family burden among family members of people with mental illness: the mediating role of coping. Soc. Psychiatry Psychiatr. Epidemiol. 51 (9), 1233–1245.

Von Kardorff, E., Soltaninejad, A., Kamali, M., et al., 2016. Family caregiver burden in mental illnesses: the case of affective disorders and schizophrenia – a qualitative exploratory study. Nord. J. Psychiatry 70 (4), 248–254.

Wallcraft, J., Amering, M., Freidin, J., et al., 2011. Partnerships for better mental health worldwide: WPA recommendations on best practices in working with service users and family carers. World Psychiatry 10, 229–236.

Walsh, F., 2006. Strengthening Family Resilience, second ed. Guildford Press, New York.

Wyder, M., Bland, R., 2014. The recovery framework as a way of understanding families' responses to mental illness: balancing different needs and recovery journeys. Aust. Soc. Work 67 (2), 179–196.

Zauszniewski, J.A., Bekhet, A.K., Suresky, J., 2015. Indicators of resilience in family members of adults with serious mental illness. Psychiatr. Clin. North Am. 38 (1), 131–146.

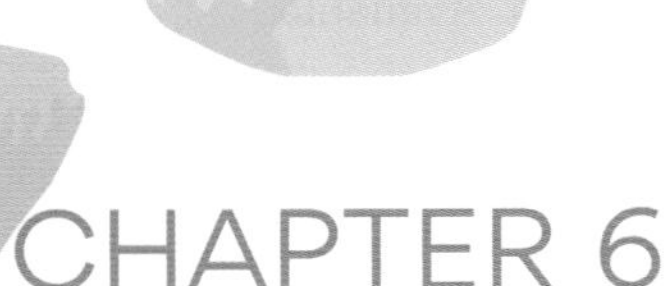

CHAPTER 6

Professional self-care

Julie Sharrock

KEY POINTS

- Self-awareness and holistic self-care are essential for mental health nurses to provide compassionate care to consumers and carers, to maintain productive working relationships with colleagues, to manage the demands of mental health nursing practice and to sustain a rewarding career.
- Holistic self-care includes physical, psychological, social and spiritual strategies.
- Lifelong learning and ongoing professional development are essential to maintaining skills and knowledge in the ever-changing world of health care.
- There are a multitude of career opportunities for mental health nurses in clinical, education, managerial and/or research roles.

KEY TERMS

- Burnout
- Clinical supervision
- Compassion fatigue
- Emotional labour
- Holistic self-care
- Professional development
- Resilience
- Workplace stress

LEARNING OUTCOMES

The material in this chapter will assist you to:

- understand the challenges, workplace stressors and health risks associated with mental health nursing
- understand how self-awareness and holistic self-care can help maintain your wellbeing in mental health nursing
- review your own self-care and health maintenance strategies to lay the groundwork for a sustainable career in mental health nursing
- develop awareness of different professional development strategies, in particular the role clinical supervision plays in maintaining practice
- consider strategies for professional development and career choices within mental health nursing.

Introduction

All nurses, including mental health nurses, need to have strategies for self-care in place throughout their careers to maintain their health and wellbeing, to provide compassionate care to consumers and carers, to maintain productive working relationships with colleagues and to manage the demands of mental health nursing practice. Holistic self-care includes physical, psychological, social and spiritual strategies to maintain our therapeutic selves so we can sustain our therapeutic work without sacrificing our own health.

The focus of this chapter is on the importance of caring for self as a nurse in the context of the rewards and demands of nursing, particularly mental health nursing. Ongoing learning and professional development is included as an essential element of career progression and work satisfaction. This chapter also presents information on the multiple career options for nurses who are planning to go into mental health.

Therapeutic use of self

As discussed in Chapter 2, the therapeutic relationship is the central activity of mental health nursing practice and is the foundation upon which all other nursing interventions are based. Actively participating in therapeutic relationships requires cognitive, emotional and behavioural work on the part of the mental health nurse. This is done through intentionally and consciously drawing on your personality, background and life skills as well as your interpersonal skills and professional knowledge as a way of establishing human connection with another person. The aim of this connection is to alleviate that person's distress and suffering in the moment and to support their healing and recovery in the long term.

The therapeutic relationship is a privileged relationship for both the consumer and the mental health nurse, but it is the responsibility of the nurse to maintain professional boundaries (Zugai et al. 2018). Maintaining professional boundaries within the nurse–consumer relationship is essential for it to be therapeutic and it is a skill that cannot be underestimated. Of particular importance to mental health nurses in maintaining boundaries is being able to regulate their emotional state through self-monitoring and self-awareness to minimise reactivity when working closely with consumers (Gardner & McCutcheon 2015). Being self-aware is essential if the mental health nurse is to intentionally use their self to develop relationships with consumers that are therapeutic and safe.

Self-awareness

Self is a complex concept that has received much attention in our attempts to understand human psychology and behaviour (Leary & Price Tangney 2012). When we pay attention to ourselves (reflect, think, see ourselves in the mirror or on video, hear our voice), we recognise our *self* and this helps us to distinguish our self from others. The self is our uniqueness as a human being and consists of attributes that pervade the way we live in and experience the world (Leary & Price Tangney 2012). The lens through which we look at the world is always our own. Although there can be no true objectivity, knowledge of the things that impinge on our subjective view of the world allows us to identify how they influence our thinking.

Awareness of self is to understand how our subjective view of the world is influenced by our background and how it affects the way we relate to consumers and carers. Nurses need to be aware of the belief systems and values that arise from their cultural, social and family backgrounds. Everyone develops biases that affect the way they view the behaviour of another (Pinel & Bosson 2013). Behaviour that is understandable to one nurse might not be understandable to another.

Mental health work requires the ability to listen to, respond to and empathise with people from a range of backgrounds. Unexamined belief systems can become obstacles to developing a therapeutic alliance with a consumer (Gunasekara et al. 2014). Lack of self-awareness can cause nurses to respond to consumer distress and behaviour in ways that may not be helpful. For example, it might cause nurses to use their power coercively in the belief that this is best for the consumer. Lack of self-awareness can also lead to nurses being overly concerned, refusing to allow consumers choice or overwhelming them with advice in an attempt to protect them against their own anxieties. Alternatively, nurses may avoid contact with particular consumers or fail to respond to distress as a result of their inability to tolerate their distress.

It is through the process of self-reflection and examination of experiences that nurses can learn and enhance the way they understand and relate to others. Self-awareness or being an 'expert of self' (Prosser et al. 2017) and having a strong understanding of your own personal experience, skills, knowledge, strengths and limitations (Foster et al. 2019a) has been associated with increased resilience.

Reflection

A key component of self-awareness is the ability to reflect. Reflection includes critically reviewing practice so it can be learned from and positively inform future practice (Bulman et al. 2014). It assists in integrating theory and practice and generating knowledge from practice (Sweet et al. 2019). Studies of reflective practices indicate that nurses who participate in reflective practice report increased self-awareness and confidence in decision making (Caldwell & Grobbel 2013). Reflection supports learning from experience, enables the integration of theory and practice and is essential for autonomous and accountable practice (Sweet et al. 2019).

It is particularly important that nurses reflect on what brings them to a helping role. Hawkins and Shohet (2012) argue that it is essential that those who enter the helping professions honestly reflect on the complex motives that led them to their current profession and role. To do this they suggest considering the 'positive' motives as well as the 'shadow' motives. The shadow motives are how we get our own needs met through helping others. For example, when we fix things or reduce suffering, we feel a strong sense of satisfaction; or when we help others, we feel useful or worthwhile. These motivations are not wrong, but if they are out of our awareness, they may affect not only the way we relate to consumers but also our ability to self-care. Exploring these aspects of our professional selves can be challenging but it is essential to maintain our capacity to be a functional helper. Clinical supervision is one of the places where such exploration can be undertaken in a safe and trusting relationship (Hawkins & Shohet 2012).

Self-awareness needs to take place in tandem with self-compassion. Self-compassion involves accepting our common humanity including our own suffering, frailties and wisdom. It is about being kind to ourselves in a mindful, caring and non-judgemental way (McCann et al. 2013). Self-compassion is a necessary element of being able to demonstrate empathy and compassion to others (Mills 2018; Wiklund Gustin & Wagner 2013). Accepting our own humanness, frailties and strengths enhances our ability to be with others in their own humanness, living with their frailties and strengths. Self-awareness also supports us when we experience workplace challenges.

Professional challenges

It is well recognised that working in health care can be challenging (Safe Work Australia 2018). Despite working within the health industry, the health of nurses generally is not good (Kelly et al. 2016), and it has been said that many nurses would fail their own health checks (Larter 2014). Stress levels and rates of depression and anxiety are high among nurses (Chiang & Chang 2012; Lim et al. 2010). Substance misuse is equivalent to or higher than the general population (La Trobe University 2019; Monroe & Kenaga 2011). Obesity, diabetes, musculoskeletal conditions, arthritis and back pain are common (Larter 2014). The suicide rate in male nurses is higher than their non-nursing counterparts, and the suicide rate for female nurses is significantly greater than the general female population (Milner et al. 2016). Compassion fatigue and burnout is also high (Zhang et al. 2018). Some of the complex factors associated with the poor health of our workforce are discussed in the following section.

Workplace stress

Stress is when we feel that the demands placed on us exceed the resources needed to respond to those demands. When a person experiences stress their sense of balance is disturbed. Physiologically a stress response is activated within the body. Any foundational anatomy and physiology textbook can provide details of the stress response, but for the purposes of this chapter it is enough to understand that the response involves the release of substances into the blood that cause a range of physiological changes, including changes to heart rate, blood pressure and the gastrointestinal tract. Prolonged stress can be harmful and can have a negative effect on physical and mental health. It is important to learn to monitor and manage your own stress because unchecked stress can become chronic and result in burnout (Hunsaker et al. 2015). Stress is often thought of as a negative experience. However, stress can have positive effects, as can be seen later in the chapter when talking about career transitions, in that it can be a catalyst for a person to make changes or a stimulant to positive action.

Workplace stressors in mental health nursing primarily arise from the interpersonal work with consumers, carers and colleagues within the demanding organisational context of the health system (Foster et al. 2018b). The nature of nursing work involves a high level of close contact with people at the extremes of human experience when a person or a loved one is experiencing life-changing health crises. Nurses are in contact with the best and worst of human nature, and everything in between. Consumers with acute or chronic mental illnesses have complex and perhaps long-term needs, and can have frequent and regular encounters with the healthcare system. The long-term and cyclic nature of some mental illnesses means that the therapeutic relationships between mental health nurses and their consumers can last for long periods. They can also vary in intensity as consumers move along a continuum between periods of high dependence at one end (in acute phases when they are experiencing symptoms of their illness) and independence at the other (when their symptoms are less troublesome or their mental illness has resolved).

Mental health nursing can involve long periods of working in intensely stressful situations, which can be exacerbated by shift work (Leyva-Vela et al. 2018). Ethical concerns (Salzmann-Erikson 2018) and the legal aspects of mental health care (Johnson et al. 2018) add a further layer of complexity, where compulsory treatment presents additional challenges for mental health nurses (Muir-Cochrane et al. 2018).

A recent Australian study described the most challenging workplace stressors for mental health nurses and grouped them according to how frequently they were reported:

1. *organisational* stressors including inadequacies in organisational policy, staffing and work environment, lack of managerial support, organisational responses to critical incidents and consumer throughput and management
2. *consumer/carer* issues in terms of addressing the needs of consumers and carers, challenging or confrontational behaviours and nursing interactions

3. *role* challenges such as practice-related concerns in performing the nursing role and maintaining standards of practice while managing personal wellbeing
4. *colleague-related* stressors such as negative staff interactions, poor communication, conflict, challenging behaviours and negative team culture (Foster et al. 2019b).

Some or all of these stressors are likely to be experienced by nurses throughout their career. In the following sections, some specific forms of psychological stress and their potential impacts on nurses are described: emotional labour, compassion fatigue, burnout and exposure to trauma.

EMOTIONAL LABOUR

The concept of emotional labour was initially developed in relation to flight attendants (Hochschild 1983) and essentially refers to managing emotion to meet the expectations of the work environment. It is the requirement of a worker to supress or create feelings to present an outward appearance that will give another person (e.g. a consumer) a sense of being cared for. Emotions and emotional expression are managed through facial and body language. The emotional expression considered appropriate to a situation is guided by 'feeling rules', which are the personal and professional norms to which we are socialised.

Hochschild (1983) described 'surface acting' and 'deep acting' as strategies for emotional management. Surface acting occurs when workers actively suppress their felt emotion or simulate an emotion that is considered appropriate. The worker does not genuinely experience the emotion but is seen to. Deep acting involves invoking and genuinely feeling emotions appropriate to the situation (Hochschild 1983).

Emotional labour is considered a form of workplace stress for nurses (Theodosius 2008) and has become part of nursing discourse (Delgado et al. 2017; Edward et al. 2017). Theodosius (2008) identified three types of emotional labour in nursing work:

- therapeutic – arising from interactions between nurses and recipients of services
- instrumental – arising from nurses' levels of confidence in their ability to perform clinical work to reduce consumer/carer discomfort
- collegial – arising from interpersonal interactions with colleagues.

Aspects and realities of mental health nursing work that have been identified as emotionally labour-intensive include:

- witnessing human distress and suffering
- feeling and expressing compassion
- managing one's emotions at the same time as managing the emotions (particularly anxiety and distress) of others
- engaging in consumer interactions that are intense and that trigger a range of emotions
- interactions that require a significant degree of effort on the part of the nurse such as working with consumers who are difficult to engage
- interactions where the nurse perceives higher levels of stress and a strong sense of responsibility for consumer outcomes
- managing crisis situations, promoting compliance with treatment and navigating the power structure within the therapeutic relationship
- conflict between professional identity (professionalism) and personal identity (authenticity) of nurses such as in ethical dilemmas or threats that challenge the physical or psychological safety of the nurse
- feeling blamed
- feeling burdened by or unprepared for what is expected
- interpersonal difficulties and conflict with other staff (Delgado et al. 2017; Edward et al. 2017).

Paradoxically, emotional labour in nursing work can also be experienced as a source of satisfaction. The emotional work of nursing has been described as 'emotionful' work and a 'gift' (Bolton 2000). Demonstrating compassion, using oneself as the therapeutic tool and dealing with emotionally charged interpersonal interactions are all sources of both satisfaction and labour (Edward et al. 2017). This view is consistent with the evidence that there is a 'bright side of emotional labour' (Humphrey et al. 2015) in that deep acting as well as the expression of naturally felt emotions have positive impacts on workers. It is surface acting that is associated with negative impacts on worker health and wellbeing (Delgado et al. 2017). The associated emotional discomfort and loss of the 'authentic self' (Humphrey et al. 2015) can result in stress, emotional exhaustion and burnout (Delgado et al. 2017).

To make sense of this, mental health nursing requires emotional work, which is part of its rewards but also its challenges. In my own practice, to be with people during life-changing or life-threatening experiences and to bear witness to their vulnerability and their resilience has been precious and rewarding albeit not easy at times. I recognise that much of the emotional labour of my work was not only deep acting but also genuinely experiencing emotions towards consumers, carers and my work. It is possible that this nourished me and potentially protected me against the negative impacts of surface acting and other workplace stressors.

As nurses we make a choice to be in an occupation that involves emotional labour, and we have a responsibility to undertake activities that help us manage this. Some of these are outlined later in this chapter. However, this responsibility does not rest only with the nurse. The organisation must also contribute to a practice environment that is ethical and healthy that eliminates avoidable harm to staff (Cipriano 2015) and that mitigates against the detrimental impacts of emotional labour on workers. Some of the services you can expect from your workplace are outlined later in the chapter.

COMPASSION FATIGUE

The concept of compassion fatigue entered healthcare discourse in 1992 and was initially seen as a particular form of burnout in caregivers (Joinson 1992). Since then the concept has evolved and is now seen as an individualised, progressive process resulting from the cumulative effects of exposure to others' suffering, distress and pain. This intense exposure threatens one's sense of life integrity (Sabery et al. 2018). Compassion fatigue results in a loss of capacity to care for others (consumers, carers, colleagues and the organisation), and this also flows on to an inability to care for self and family (Sabery et al. 2018). Further to this, if compassion fatigue is not addressed it can lead to disinterest, lack of concern for others' suffering, moral distress and burnout (Cross 2019).

Compassion fatigue and burnout are related concepts that may arise out of different psychological processes. Compassion fatigue is linked with prolonged expression of empathy where the distress of those suffering is absorbed, whereas burnout is more likely to be associated with the cumulative effects of workplace stressors more broadly, particularly the imbalance between expectations and what is achievable (Sabery et al. 2018; Sorenson et al. 2017).

BURNOUT

Burnout research began in the 1970s and those working in caregiving occupations were identified as at risk (Maslach 2017). The phenomenon we now know as burnout initially had no name and it was rarely discussed or acknowledged (Maslach 2017). The literature is now replete with attention to burnout, and it continues to be of concern in the nursing workforce (Laker et al. 2019). Burnout is included in the International Classification of Diseases (World Health Organization 2018) as an occupational phenomenon in the chapter titled 'Factors influencing health status or contact with health services'.

The psychological syndrome of burnout is a response to chronic occupational interpersonal stressors and has three key dimensions:

- feelings of overwhelming physical and emotional **exhaustion** and depletion, lacking the energy to face another day and over-extended by the demands of work without seeing any source of replenishment and recovery
- feelings of cynicism and **detachment**, negative, harsh or disinterested responses, a loss of idealism and doing the bare minimum of work
- a sense of **ineffectiveness** and lack of accomplishment, lowered sense of confidence, competence, self-efficacy and self-regard, regret about career choice and decreased productivity (Maslach & Leiter 2017).

The words 'burnout' and 'stress' are often seen together because stress is seen as a precursor to burnout. However, stress is a feature of life and, when managed properly, does not lead to burnout. Unlike stress, which has some positive features (e.g. it can be a catalyst for effecting positive change such as learning a new skill), burnout has no positive aspects for the person experiencing it or for those around them.

Burnout can lead to significant problems for those experiencing it including poor professional and personal relationships, poor physical health and worsening mental health (Maslach & Leiter 2017) such as depression, substance misuse and suicidal ideation. Fulfilment and identification with the work role are lost. Work becomes a burden without joy or satisfaction, which results in a desire to avoid it to the point of leaving the profession (Maslach & Leiter 2017).

From the perspective of the affected person, there is nothing worse than going to work when feeling unhappy and distressed. Working with colleagues who are irritable, depressed and exhausted adds to everyone's stress. It is not difficult to imagine how distressing it would be for a consumer to be nursed by someone who responded to them and their situation in a cold and unfeeling way rather than with the warmth, caring, empathy and respect we ourselves would wish for if we were sick and needing care.

Burnout comes at significant cost to the employing organisation in terms of poor quality of care provided by that person. This has been demonstrated in decreased consumer satisfaction, increased consumer mortality and increased errors (Maslach & Leiter 2017). It is important to note that burnout is not a personal failing or the sole responsibility of the individual nurse to prevent. Given the high rates of burnout among health professionals, it is more accurate to consider burnout as an organisational and systemic issue that develops as a response of the employee to the workplace (Maslach & Leiter 2017). Therefore, the organisation also has a responsibility for supporting the physical and mental health of employees and to adopt policies and practices that support nurses rather than contribute to stress and burnout. Stress and burnout need to be considered within the organisation as a whole, within teams, and at the individual employee level (Maslach 2017).

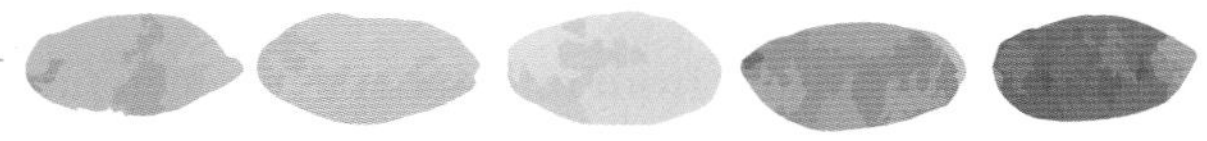

NURSE'S STORY 6.1

James Houghton

Sometimes I find it hard to believe that almost 40 years have passed since I first decided to be a nurse. It's been a challenging and sometimes confronting journey, and I've worked in several different clinical settings as a mental health nurse, including a long period in child and youth services.

When I reflect on resilience and how I've managed to stay passionate about mental health nursing and engaged in this work for so long, I can identify several factors that have been really important. I am part of a team who are kind, supportive, generous with their time and typically very positive in their outlook. We regularly and intentionally celebrate each other's strengths. Over the years I have developed and strengthened my ability to use thought processes such as reframing, depersonalising and not catastrophising situations or events. These skills have enabled me to challenge my thinking so that when I encounter sometimes serious difficulties (which we all do from time to time) I see them as challenges or barriers to be negotiated rather than devastating or insurmountable roadblocks.

Another important factor is my clinical supervision, which has become an essential component of my practice. The people I have had as clinical supervisors have provided me with excellent guidance and support for my practice and encouraged me to become more involved in organisations like the Australian College of Mental Health Nurses and the Australian Clinical Supervision Association. This has contributed positively to my professional identity, which contributes to my self-esteem.

Outside of work I have a caring, supportive partner – one who is willing to listen and sometimes just simply 'be with me' without necessarily having to fully understand things when I need to offload some of my work worries. And I have quite a large group of friends and acquaintances, with a smaller group of really close friends, all of whom are prepared to spend time with me doing the things we all enjoy – be that sport, dancing, live music, movies, theatre or just having dinner and 'hanging out'. Having fun and being able to completely forget about work for a while are really important factors in not burning out.

I'm proud that when anyone asks me what I do for work or I spend time with early career nurses, I can say that I enjoy being a nurse more now than I did when I began my nursing career.

EXPOSURE TO TRAUMA

Mental health nurses are very likely to be exposed to traumatic events within the workplace. Traumatic events are those that are usually unexpected and may involve threats of or actual serious injury, death or sexual violence (Phoenix Australia 2019). While people identify and respond to traumatic events differently, there are common physical, emotional, cognitive, behavioural and social reactions that occur. A sense of shock, disbelief, being overwhelmed and loss of the world as one knew it before the event are common. Most people recover within the first week or two with the help of colleagues, family and friends, but for a few, trauma can have long-term effects. Immediate practical and emotional support goes a long way to alleviating the distress of such events. The Centre for Post-traumatic Mental Health based at the University of Melbourne has resources available to the public on helping yourself and helping others after traumatic events (see the list of useful websites at the end of this chapter).

Mental health nurses are also exposed to trauma through caring for consumers who have had traumatic experiences, which puts them at risk of 'vicarious traumatisation'. Vicarious traumatisation is a change that occurs within a worker that engages with people who have had traumatic experiences, hears their stories and sees the effects of their trauma experiences. The worker may begin to re-experience the trauma stories with hyperarousal and intrusive images and thoughts. They may develop a depressed mood, anxiety and avoid exposure to further traumatic material (Benuto et al. 2018).

Conversely, positive effects and personal growth can occur as a result of exposure to trauma. This growth, which has been called 'post-traumatic growth', is experienced as a greater appreciation for one's own life, improved relationships with others and increased spirituality. Growth following trauma can occur if the trauma is not overwhelming, if there is support available and if the person exposed to trauma has a sense of efficacy to get through it, the ability to reflect, to change core beliefs and to make meaning of the experience (Cosden et al. 2016). The capacity to make meaning from challenging or traumatic experiences is also important when we look at resilience.

While the challenges of stress, emotional labour, compassion fatigue, potential burnout and exposure to trauma exist for nurses, there are many approaches that can successfully mitigate their impact on nurses' health and wellbeing. Mental health nurses can learn and develop skills and strategies that will support their health and wellbeing. In addition, a range of services are available to mental health nurses from within and outside their employing organisation that support them to maintain their health and wellbeing. Some key approaches are described in the next section.

Holistic self-care

Given the challenges and potential stressors in mental health nursing, it is vital that we extend the same care to ourselves that we offer our consumers. As mentioned previously, developing awareness and understanding of what brings us to take up a helping role is important. If we do not do this, we can fall into the trap of compulsive helping, which results in metaphorically 'giving ourselves away' with nothing left for ourselves or anyone else. Self-care is vital for nurses to mitigate against workplace stressors and challenges and to maintain our health and wellbeing. Self-care is also essential to provide compassionate care and should be included as a 'professional expectation inherent to the role of nurses' (Mills et al. 2015, p. 792).

Maintaining a self-care program can be a challenge, especially for shift workers. These challenges include being busy, lack of planning and prioritising self-care, the stigma associated with putting yourself first, a work environment that is not supportive of self-care, inadequate boundaries between work and home, self-criticism and low self-worth (Mills et al. 2018).

These challenges can be addressed by having a commitment to and belief in the need for self-care (Mills et al. 2018). Self-care goes beyond developing skills to cope with and manage the workplace challenges and stressors. Self-care needs to be consciously prioritised, practised deliberately, personalised and ongoing (Mills et al. 2018). Self-care strategies and behaviours need to be in place within and external to the workplace and include work-life balance, adequate sleep, rest and exercise, a healthy diet and general health maintenance.

Work-life balance

Increasingly, the community is recognising the importance of maintaining a balance between our work lives and our personal lives and, for nursing, this has been associated with increased resilience (Brown et al. 2018). As a society we have borne the brunt of focusing on work, money and possessions at the expense of family, community, the environment and what gives meaning to our lives. Many are challenging our society to do something different. Work-life balance is particularly important for nurses and midwives (Schluter et al. 2011) who have the challenge of working unsociable hours through shift work (Leyva-Vela et al. 2018).

> A good work-life balance means you have harmony between different aspects of your life, where benefits gained from each area can support and strengthen the others. Work-life integration is a new concept, where many people are learning to blend their work and personal lives successfully.
>
> (Health Direct 2018)

In a study of nurses and doctors, the participants described that finding harmony between personal and work lives was an effective self-care strategy (Mills et al. 2018). They went on to describe approaches to creating a boundary between work and home was important. The mode of travel to and from work was used as a strategy to ensure not overworking, and the commute itself was an opportunity to unwind from work. Taking a bath at home was described as a way of metaphorically washing away the workplace stressors.

Sleep, rest, exercise and diet

Restful and restorative sleep is an important self-care strategy for both the mind and the body. Sleep is essential to health and vitality and assists us to approach stressful situations more calmly (Chopra 2019). Sleep hygiene is something we teach our consumers, but as nurses we often don't practise it ourselves. Some key principles of sleep hygiene are to obey your body clock, improve your sleeping environment, limit electronic devices (e.g. phones and computers) at bedtime and avoiding drugs/alcohol, stimulants (e.g. coffee), stimulating activity and heavy meals before sleep (Chopra 2019).

Of course, obeying your body clock poses challenges for shiftworkers, especially working overnight and grabbing a meal whenever you can on a busy shift. However, given shiftwork impacts negatively on health, it essential that shiftworkers pay attention to sleep practices, diet and exercise (Wilson & Brooks 2018). Ensuring adequate intake of all food groups, especially fruit and vegetables, avoiding obesity and maintaining enough exercise (especially if the nursing work undertaken involves less activity) are key areas for nurses to pay attention to (Torquati et al. 2018).

Psychological strategies

MEANING MAKING

Making meaning of our work and our lives can also support our energy and passion for our work. It has been postulated that to make meaning out of the experiences of life is central to survival and important in understanding human responses to adversity (Park 2010).

The cognitive process of trying to make sense of stressful events, suffering and death is an important one for nurses. Giving meaning to our work, why we do it and how we evaluate if our input makes a difference are important areas to reflect on. When the meanings made lead to adaptive behaviours (Park 2010) then a cognitive system is developed that supports us in the work we do. The ability to reframe adverse situations into those that are meaningful (Prosser et al. 2017), having the capacity to make sense of challenging situations through placing them in a context or structure and identifying a given situation or action in terms of making a potentially positive contribution (Foster et al. 2019a) are examples of meanings that lead to adaptive behaviours. Meaning making that leads to adaptive behaviours helps us manage our expectations, sit with the suffering of others and maintain the passion of our work, and is also a key part of resilience.

SELF-COMPASSION

As mentioned earlier, having self-compassion is an important part of being self-aware. Self-compassion includes self-kindness, mindfulness and recognising our common humanity and wisdom. Demonstrating self-compassion results in increasing our capacity to self-care, to relate and demonstrate compassion to others, to be autonomous and to develop a sturdier sense of self (Reyes 2012).

SPIRITUAL CARE

For some nurses, holding sustaining belief systems that include cultural and religious dimensions (Marie et al. 2017; Prosser et al. 2017) support practice and form part of self-care. Nurturing our spirit does not solely refer to religious practice but also to 'our life force that gives us the will to live, love and endure' (Lloyd 2019, p. 23). You may have met consumers whose spirit is shattered, but this can also happen to health professionals who overwork or burn out. Ensuring we have work-life balance that includes spiritually nurturing experiences with attention to energising our life force are essential. Mind–body practices and being among nature are effective energisers of our life force (Borradaile 2016). A wise mother once said to me, 'Food nurtures our body, but gardening nurtures our spirit'. While gardening is not everybody's thing, going outside, seeing the light and the sky and the wonders of nature is good for us and can have a revitalising effect.

Mind–body practices

In the workplace, nurses cognitively focus on the issues confronting them at work, continually assessing and considering how to respond and intervene with consumers, carers and colleagues. The body can easily be forgotten and considered a vehicle through which nursing work is delivered. The risk that we treat ourselves as objects is exacerbated by a reductionistic approach to health care. It is a curious thing that the idea that the mind and the body are different entities has dominated Western thinking for centuries. This contrasts with Eastern philosophies that have a long history of understanding the mind and body as an indivisible whole.

A range of practices that bring the mind and body together have been reported by nurses and other health professionals as useful in managing workplace stress and promoting health (Bonamer & Aquino-Russell 2019; Mills et al. 2018; Schueler 2017). Mind–body practices such as mindfulness, yoga, meditation, qi gong and tai chi come from Eastern cultures and are centuries old. These practices involve gentle movements, specific postures and breathing coupled with mental focus that engages the whole person and enhances a sense of wellbeing. A common theme in these practices is they are thought to reduce the physiological and psychological stress response.

> Meditation is a simple yet powerful tool that takes us to a state of profound relaxation that dissolves fatigue and the accumulated stress that accelerates the aging process. During meditation, our breathing slows, our blood pressure and heart rate decrease, and stress hormone levels fall. By its very nature, meditation calms the mind, and when the mind is in a state of restful awareness, the body relaxes too. Research shows that people who meditate regularly develop less hypertension, heart disease, insomnia, anxiety, and other stress-related illnesses.
>
> (Chopra 2019)

Massage is another ancient practice where soft tissue is rubbed or manipulated to enhance relaxation and, sometimes, to relieve pain.

Jon Kabat-Zinn (2019) has been credited for bringing mindfulness from the ancient Eastern practices into medicine and Western society. As a student of Zen Buddhism, he integrated these teachings into mainstream science. There has been a surge of research into mindfulness that has found physical and mental health benefits (Malinowski 2013). You can incorporate mindfulness into your daily work through mindful handwashing (see Box 6.1).

Box 6.1 Mindful handwashing

Handwashing is an essential part of health care and must be done for long enough to be effective. McNamara (2016) suggests:

> ...if you're going to do hand hygiene dozens of times a day anyway, don't just do it for your patients: do it for your**self** too. We're not cold callous reptilian clinicians, we're educated warm-blooded mammals who do emotional labour. We need to nurture ourselves if we are to safely continue to nurture others.

So why not wash mindfully and clear the grime out of your head as well as off your hands? Here are some tips:

1. Step towards the sink with intent and remind yourself you are taking a break.
2. Let the water flow.
3. Feel the water flowing over both hands. Notice the temperature of the water and savour the feeling.
4. Add soap. Notice the frictionless feelings it adds.
5. Start with cleaning. Think about washing stuff away. Let the stuff you need to get rid of flow down the drain. Let it flow away.
6. Move on to restoration, healing. Rub in resilience and health. Let the stuff that sustains you seep into your skin.
7. Check in on the breathing. The slower and deeper the better. If the breathing or the brain are running too fast, slow down and repeat the last two steps.
8. There's no rush. Slowly scan the surroundings. With any luck someone from infection control is watching.
9. Smile.
10. Breathe slowly, thinking: *It is time to rinse both hands.*
11. Then, again breathing slowly, think: 'It is time to thoroughly dry both hands together'.
12. Throw the towel in the bin.
13. Take another slow breath: It is time to get back to work.

Clean hands save lives. Clear heads save lives too!

Adapted from McNamara 2016

Resilience

As has been discussed in this chapter, working in health care is very rewarding but it can be challenging. Resilience is a process of positively adapting to adversity and regaining a sense of wellbeing after stressful situations or difficult events. The presence of resilience has been associated with nurses' improved wellbeing by mitigating against the potentially harmful aspects of nursing work (Craigie et al. 2016; Delgado et al. 2017; Foster et al. 2018b; Mealer et al. 2014). Like burnout, resilience can be constructed as an interaction between an individual and their environment. This view of resilience recognises not only the capacity of the individual to find the resources in their environment to sustain their wellbeing but also the capacity of the environment (family, community and workplace) to provide the resources in a culturally meaningful way (Ungar 2008). Considering resilience in this way provides balance in that the individual nurse has some responsibility, but so too does the employer.

Resilience involves our own resources and skills – that is, managing our thoughts, emotions and responses to challenging situations. Emotional intelligence supports mental health nurses to do this and has been conceptualised as an aspect of personal resilience (Foster et al. 2018a). Emotional intelligence is the ability to recognise the emotions of others, experience and recognise our own emotions, link thought and emotions to assist in our thinking, and manage our emotions (Mayer et al. 2004). The capacity to reflect on and regulate emotions is not only central to emotional intelligence but also an important aspect of being a resilient and well-functioning mental health nurse. Understanding and managing emotions are essential for mental health nurses to be able to effectively work with consumers and carers who are often distressed. The skills of reflection, self-awareness, emotional regulation, social awareness and skilled relationship management (Parsa-Yekta & Abdolrahimi 2016) support the therapeutic use of self. Self-awareness and a strong sense of self as described earlier in this chapter supports mental health nurses to develop resilience in dealing with the difficulties and complexities of human communication and experiences.

However, resilience also involves using the emotional and practical support we get from others and from our workplace. Universities are paying attention to developing emotional intelligence in students (Erkayiran & Demirkiran 2018) and employers are beginning to offer programs aimed at building staff resilience (Foster et al. 2018a). It is argued that resilience can be developed through strengthening skills to manage adversity and stress (Foster et al. 2019a). See Nurses' Story 6.2 for examples of how one nurse has maintained their resilience during their career.

Mental health nursing–specific 'promoting adult resilience programs' are having a promising impact on the health and wellbeing of mental health nurses (Foster et al. 2018a; 2018b). These programs harness the strengths of the participants, integrating cognitive, emotional, behavioural and interpersonal concepts with the aim of promoting 'self and affect/emotion regulation in the face of stress' (Foster et al. 2018b, p. 1,472). A nurse in this study described resilience as:

> ... where you grow and you learn and excel through hardship. That doesn't mean that you can't be affected by something, but that in time you use that positively, or to improve yourself, or improve your practice in some way as you go on.
> (Foster et al. 2018a, p. 342)

General health care

As noted earlier in this chapter, nurses can neglect their own health needs (Christie et al. 2017; Larter 2014; Perry et al. 2018; Ross et al. 2019). Maintaining a healthy diet, getting adequate sleep, rest and relaxation, moderating alcohol intake and maintaining exercise and fitness (Mills et al. 2018) are all important aspects of health care. Engaging in health screening programs as appropriate such as pap smears, and breast and prostate checks as well as having a regular general practitioner are part of maintaining our health. Many organisations offer health programs such as staff clinics and immunisation programs that are easily accessible to employees.

Asking for help with mental health issues can be particularly challenging for nurses (Galbraith et al. 2014). Organisations often offer psychological services to staff services to support the emotional, mental and general psychological wellbeing of its employees and their immediate family members. Services may include educative services on self-care generally or specific programs such as resilience or mindfulness training. They also offer critical incident stress debriefing to help staff regain equilibrium after disturbing experiences or traumatic events.

The profession offers services to nurses through programs such as the Nursing Health and Midwifery Program and Nurse and Midwife Support (see useful websites at the end of this chapter). Whether you make use of the services offered by your organisation or utilise community services, attending to your own health is essential to keeping yourself in the best shape to engage in your professional practice.

Lifelong learning and professional development

In addition to self-care, mental health nurses need to engage in lifelong learning through professional development and further academic pursuits to maintain and develop practice throughout their careers. As you know, health care is an ever-changing world. The developments in technology and treatments, in understanding and preventing the causes of illness, are growing rapidly. To do our job competently as health professionals we need to be willing to continually learn and develop our knowledge and skills; to grow as clinicians.

A growth mindset

An important predictor of achievement is when learners have a 'growth mindset'. This is holding a belief that intelligence can be developed; that it is not fixed (Claro et al. 2016). Carol Dweck (2015) coined the term and says that people who believe their talents and abilities can be developed (i.e. that they can get smarter) through hard work, good strategies and input from others, have a growth mindset. Her research has demonstrated that people with a growth mindset achieve more than those with a fixed mindset (i.e. people who believe their talents are innate). She says this is because people with a growth mindset worry less about looking smart and put more of their energy into learning. Having a growth mindset is not just about putting effort into learning but having a range of approaches to learning and skill development. For example, if you become stuck in the learning process, try out new strategies or seek out others to assist. Instead of looking for praise in your efforts and remaining stuck, ask for help, discuss what you have tried and what you can try next (Claro et al. 2016; Dweck 2015; Masters 2013). In your graduate year you will have access to a range of supports that will help you maintain a passion for learning.

Early graduate programs

Early graduate programs support nurses in the transition from academic learning into professional nursing practice, generally over the first year of employment. These programs aim to assist new graduates to consolidate skills and knowledge and develop independence in practice. Programs typically include:

- orientation days
- designated staff (i.e. coordinators, clinical educators and support staff)
- an average of 6–10 study days
- two to three clinical rotations
- supernumerary days at the start of the program (usually the first week) and at the start of each new rotation (usually 1–2 days)
- a handbook
- progress and performance reviews (usually held quarterly)
- a staged introduction to shiftwork (Healy & Howe 2012).

Graduate programs have a positive impact on work satisfaction and intention to stay in the profession (Kenny et al. 2016). There are mixed views about the value of clinical rotations; there is some evidence it reinforces the idea that graduates are still in need of placements (like students) and other evidence suggesting rotations gives graduates a wider range of clinical exposure (Healy & Howe 2012). Strategies that can maximise your experiences in a graduate program include the following:

- Make the most of your orientation.
- Work at becoming part of the team (Mi 2016).
- Identify and use your team supports and clinical supervision (Hussein et al. 2016).
- Engage with your work (Walker & Campbell 2013).
- Build a professional support network (Jackson et al. 2007).

Professional development

In addition to graduate programs, during your career you will have opportunities to use a range of professional development resources.

POINT-OF-CARE LEARNING

You have already experienced point-of-care learning (Health Education and Training Institute 2013) when on clinical placements in your undergraduate program. These professional development supports form part of graduate programs but may also be available to you throughout your career, especially when joining a new team or transitioning into a new role or specialty area.

Clinical teaching is when a more experienced nurse shares professional knowledge with a less experienced nurse in the workplace.

Clinical facilitation is part of the practice development approach and has a strong focus on collaborating with teams and individuals to influence positive cultural change within a workplace. Practice development mental health nurses may be available in your workplace and, if so, these nurses can be a valuable resource to help you develop specific skills and knowledge.

Buddying is often used for students but also for staff starting in a new work environment. The buddy is usually a skilled and effective team member and resource who can support and engage the new team member into the workplace.

Preceptorship is a formalised relationship with an allocated preceptor who is usually a nurse with considerable experience in a specific clinical environment and who has completed a specialised preceptor training program. The aim of preceptorship is to support the orientation and integration of the nurse into the new roles and responsibilities.

STRUCTURED REFLECTIVE PRACTICE RELATIONSHIPS

Once you graduate, there are other formal relationships where you engage with a colleague or group of colleagues to reflect on your practice and role. As has been already discussed, managing the often intense emotional work of caring for people facing life-threatening or life-changing health problems within the complex health system pose unique and often perplexing challenges for nurses. The importance of reflection in developing self-awareness has been described earlier. Participating in forums that are designed to support reflection on practice contribute to the mental health nurse making meaning of these unique and perplexing challenges.

Through reflecting *on* practice, the supervisee becomes more skilled at reflecting *in* practice and *before* practice. This increases the supervisee's ability to make choices of how to respond to others (be they consumers, carers or staff) in the moment. This decreases reactivity and the risk of impulsive reactions, which results in the increased possibility of helpful communications, less emotional drain on the nurse and the ability for the nurse to practise with increased awareness (Freshwater 2008).

Clinical supervision is a professional development opportunity and an effective forum to reflect on practice after the event as opposed to point-of-care learning, which is in the clinical area and very likely to occur at the time of a practice event.

> Clinical Supervision is a formally structured professional arrangement between a supervisor and one or more supervisees. It is a purposely constructed regular meeting that provides for critical reflection on the work issues brought to that space by the supervisee(s). It is a confidential relationship within the ethical and legal parameters of practice. Clinical Supervision facilitates development of reflective practice and the professional skills of the supervisee(s) through increased awareness and understanding of the complex human and ethical issues within their workplace.
>
> (Australian College of Midwives et al. 2019, p. 2)

The material discussed in clinical supervision relates to the work of the supervisee. This includes clinical care, therapeutic relationships and interactions between the nurse and consumers. Clinical supervision can also provide an opportunity for nurses to reflect on the subjective experience of their work. To develop the nurse's capacity for empathy, acceptance, nurturing and honest reflection, the clinical supervisor needs to be able to model these capacities in their relationship with the supervisee. Clinical supervision can occur in one-to-one sessions or in groups. In both settings establishing a safe, confidential, non-blaming environment in which nurses feel able to share their clinical experiences is paramount (Australian College of Midwives et al. 2019; Buus et al. 2013).

Historical anecdote 6.1: Origins of clinical supervision

The origins of clinical supervision for nurses can be traced back to Florence Nightingale, who had her own experience of depression as a young woman that she related to the intense boredom she experienced as a consequence of her privileged upbringing. After developing an interest in caring for others as a way out of her depression, Nightingale trained as a nurse at a Lutheran community in Kaiserwerth, Germany before returning to England and gaining experience through managing a hospital for upper-class women. In 1854 the British Secretary of War, Sidney Herbert, whom she had met as part of her wealthy social circles, recruited Nightingale as chief nurse for the armed forces during the Crimean War (1853–1856). During the war Nightingale achieved fame for influential work on sanitation, introduced the concept of senior nurses guiding junior nurses in their clinical practice, and organised frequent group meetings for all grades of nursing staff in which, through democratic process, ideas could be pooled for the general welfare of patients and staff.

Read more about it: *Russell L 1990 Clinical supervision: history 23. Nightingale to now: nurse education in Australia. Churchill Livingstone, Sydney*

More information about clinical supervision can be found in the joint position statement for Australian nurses and midwives (Australian Colleges of Midwives et al. 2019) and the suite of documents developed for the New Zealand mental health and addiction workforce (Te Pou o te Whakaaro Nui 2017a; 2017b; 2017c). While the New Zealand documents use the term 'practice supervision', it is one and the same as clinical supervision. These documents outline what your role is as a supervisee, what to expect from a clinical supervisor and what your organisation should provide. The Australian Clinical Supervision Association is also a great resource and, in particular, it offers guidance on how to choose your clinical supervisor.

Mentoring is a relationship where an experienced and knowledgeable professional (mentor) is chosen by a less experienced professional (mentee) to nurture professional growth. Mentors are usually chosen because of their personal qualities and achievements. An effective mentor invests time, effort, knowledge and expertise to nurture the professional expertise of the mentee. Mentoring is particularly useful when transitioning into a more advanced role – for example, from a registered nurse to nurse practitioner (Fedele 2019). Mentors can be short term or lifelong, formal or informal and are not mediated through employment in a particular ward or unit.

Coaching is a professional relationship that can be used for specific knowledge and skill development (Health Education and Training Institute 2013), particularly for advanced practice (Waldrop & Derouin 2019). Coaching relationships are usually over a shorter timeframe than clinical supervision or mentorship and involve a collaborative teaching, training or development process (Health Education and Training Institute 2013).

Peer review is more commonplace in medicine but can also be utilised by nurses. It involves monitoring and improving practice and by purposefully observing, evaluating and discussing our own work with peers, usually within a group (Health Education and Training Institute 2013).

NURSE'S STORY 6.2

Nicola

Nicola is working in an acute inpatient unit. She has two years' experience. She arrives at clinical supervision saying she feels angry with one of her consumers, a young woman with a diagnosis of depression who self-harms. Nicola had spent considerable time with the consumer in the preceding days and felt that she had developed a good relationship with her. Last night, after she had gone home, the consumer cut her arms with a razor blade, and today she is belligerent, appearing to take delight in having 'fooled' the nurses. Nicola says that the other staff have reinforced her belief that she was 'sucked in' and she is now confused about how to proceed with this consumer.

The supervisor asks Nicola to tell in detail the story of what happened. She then asks Nicola to outline her feelings about, and knowledge of, the consumer before and after the incident. The supervisor listens attentively and empathically, encouraging further exploration of the incident and Nicola's feelings about it. Nicola admits to feeling guilty and is concerned that she may have said or done something to provoke the incident. Together they consider how the consumer might have been feeling and what possible triggers to self-harm might have existed. They then consider what Nicola saw as important in developing the relationship with the consumer. The supervisor suggests some reading that Nicola can undertake to increase her understanding of self-harm-related behaviours. Together they identify what might be the goals of nursing interventions with this consumer. Nicola resolves to talk to the consumer about how the consumer was feeling the previous night and what provoked the self-harm incident.

ONGOING EDUCATION AND TRAINING

There are numerous education and training opportunities within and external to your organisation. In addition to mandatory training (e.g. management of clinical aggression, hand washing and emergency procedures), you will be exposed to a range of knowledge and skill development opportunities so make the most of these. Also, remain open to the idea of engaging in post-graduate education. Explore options for support from within your organisation and to external scholarship providers to assist you in your endeavours.

Professional supports and organisations

As has been highlighted throughout this chapter, building positive and nurturing professional relationships has been linked to work satisfaction and resilience (Jackson et al. 2007). Joining professional groups is a very effective way to do this. Te Ao Māramatanga New Zealand College of Mental Health Nursing is the professional body for practising mental health nurses in New Zealand. The Australian College of Mental Health Nurses is the peak professional mental health nursing organisation and the recognised credentialling body for mental health nurses in Australia. Such organisations offer conferences, professional development activities and networking opportunities. In addition to the professional knowledge that can be gained through professional organisations, many nurses have made lifelong colleagues and personal friendships through participating in their professional body throughout their career.

Maintaining a satisfying career

There are many factors that contribute to work satisfaction during our careers, and some have already been described. We spend a large part of our day at work, so it is important we enjoy it. In addition, work satisfaction has been linked to increased resilience (Foster et al. 2019a) and mitigates against burnout (Maslach 2017). It is important to make choices about where to work and who to work with. Carefully consider who you want as your role models, mentors and clinical supervisors. Watch how others work and ask them questions about their practice. Make choices about your professional standards and work environments. You will have many transitions throughout your career, so make sure you support yourself during these times.

Career transitions

Life is full of transitions and stages where we move into new roles. You may remember the mixed feelings you had when finishing secondary school, moving to university or transitioning from the student role into the graduate nurse role. Role transition can be exciting in that it precipitates many opportunities. Simultaneously there may be feelings of vulnerability and uncertainty (Bridges & Bridges 2017). Taking up a new role is a process of change from 'what was' to 'what is' (Duchscher 2009). There are losses and gains in that we need to let go old ways and develop new ways; we need to adapt old skills and learn new ones (Bridges & Bridges 2017) and we need to build new role identities and self-images. The discomfort that comes with role transition is inevitable and necessary for growth to occur (Bridges & Bridges 2017).

Graduation and moving onto the role of a registered nurse can be accompanied by feelings of anxiety, depression and stress (Chernomas & Shapiro 2013) with feelings of doubt, inadequacy and insecurity, a phenomenon that has been called 'transition shock' (Duchscher 2009).

Graduates have reported believing that they will be expected to know everything and doubt their capacities to fulfil meet the responsibilities of a registered nurse (Mooney 2007). This sense of doubt has been termed 'imposter syndrome', where there is a sense of inadequacy, anxiety, lack of self-confidence, frustration and depression. It is accompanied by a tendency to question our sense of belonging to the profession and being up to the task (Christensen et al. 2016).

Thankfully transition shock and imposter syndrome are transient and, as mentioned previously, discomfort during stages of transition are a necessary part of growth and development (Bridges 2004). If you ask most registered nurses, they will be able to recount many tales of challenging transitions, recalling the discomfort and sometimes the hilarity of what it feels like to be so unsure and excited at the same time. The beauty of nursing as a career is that there can be many of these transitions because we have so many choices about where we work and who we work with.

Work environments

The importance of safe and healthy workplaces is being increasingly recognised and promoted (Safe Work Australia 2012). Workplaces with a positive culture are more likely to have satisfied staff, consumers and carers. The key characteristics of safe and healthy workplaces (Hart 2017) are:

- open, effective, respectful and democratic communication where there are opportunities for 'speaking up' and 'speaking out'
- support of the wellbeing of staff where there is access to resources, professional development and staff support programs
- strong leadership where values and professional standards are embedded
- commitment to quality care with clinical review, practice audits, open disclosure and a 'no blame' culture.

MANAGEMENT PROCESSES

It is important for organisations to have clear and effective management processes. These processes are organisationally driven and aim to ensure the goals, standards, procedures and guidelines of the organisation are being maintained and that the service outcomes are being achieved. They include managerial supervision, disciplinary processes, performance review, professional development planning and operational team meetings. Organisations with positive cultures engage in these processes consistently and respectfully.

Managerial supervision is usually undertaken by the nurse's line manager, who reviews both the quality and quantity of the work and can include instruction, direction and evaluation. More senior staff may tend to have individual meetings with their line manager where teams tend to meet in operational team meetings. These meetings should be regular and are a forum for reviewing team functioning and addressing team issues.

Performance review is part of managerial supervision and is where the nurse's work performance is evaluated, and goals are set for the following period. Having access to open and respectful performance reviews can be invaluable in skill and career development.

In addition, use your educators, buddies, preceptors, mentors and clinical supervisors to gather feedback on your performance. Interact with them to explore your successes and failures in an honest and curious way. Not all colleagues will be able to engage in this way, so find those who can. Clarify feedback from others if it is vague or general, ask for specific examples where improvements can be made, and use what you have learned from your successes to help approach the things you find more challenging.

CLINICAL MANAGEMENT PROCESSES

Robust clinical management processes also support nurses and are characteristic of positive work cultures. Processes such as handovers, case reviews, case presentations and grand rounds are examples of clinical management processes that provide clinicians with a place to review clinical work and to gather direct and indirect feedback on their practice.

JOB–PERSON FIT

A key finding from research into burnout is the misfit or misalignment between the worker and the work environment (Maslach 2017). This chapter has offered a range of strategies nurses can use to reduce the risk of burnout. Maslach (2017) also highlighted the importance of getting the right 'job–person fit' in reducing the risk of burnout. She identifies the following areas as important when considering how well a job is right for you:

- **Workload**: is it manageable and sustainable?
- **Control**: Do you feel heard and understood when you discuss your work issues? Do you feel you can influence decision making that relates to your work?
- **Reward**: Do you feel valued and recognised for the contribution you make?
- **Community**: Are the relationships within the workplace supportive and safe? Are conflicts addressed?
- **Fairness**: Are the approaches taken to decision making fair and equitable?
- **Values**: Do the values of the workplace match your professional and personal values?

Maslach (2017, p. 150) describes the 'areas-of-work-life model', which has 'six positive "fits" that promote engagement and well-being can be defined as (a) a sustainable workload; (b) choice and control; (c) recognition and reward; (d) a supportive work community; (e) fairness, respect, and social justice; and (f) clear values and meaningful work'.

Clinical practice settings

In addition to consciously considering the quality of your work environment, exercise choice about the practice settings that suit you. As has been described in other chapters in this book, mental health nurses work in a wide range of settings and practise with a variety of consumers of all ages using different models of service delivery. Gaining experience in a range of practice settings adds a depth and breadth to your practice (see Table 6.1). There are also multiple options for mental health nurses further afield. An observant father once said to me, 'As a nurse you can get a job anywhere in the world'. Nurses can travel the world and work in the most amazing places in developed and developing nations. The experiences and insights gained enhance your career and your life.

Expertise development

The seminal work of Patricia Benner (1984) offered the profession an understanding of the development of nursing expertise. Her book provides numerous exemplars of nursing development through the stages of novice, advanced beginner, competent, proficient and expert practice. She shows how nurses with little or no experience draw on sets of steps and rules to practice and as experience is

TABLE 6.1 Practice settings

SETTING	DESCRIPTION
Inpatient mental health units	• Part of the nursing team that provides around-the-clock care to consumers • Work closely with consumers and as a multidisciplinary team • Has opportunities for increased support and professional development
Generalist inpatient settings and emergency departments	• Work directly with consumers and carers • Work alongside hospital staff • Work with staff to increase their capacity to recognise and attend to the mental health needs of consumers in their care • Work with organisations on mental health-related projects, education, policy development and research
Residential community care	• Focus on the day-to-day functioning of consumers, supporting them to develop skills for recovery
Community	• A range of options available in community services including care coordination, crisis and intensive or early intervention • Can be clinic-based where consumers attend • Can be outreach where the consumers are met in their own environments
Primary health care	• Opportunities for early intervention • Work alongside general practitioners and community health services • Work with staff to increase their capacity to recognise and attend to the mental health needs of the community • Provide assessment and counselling to consumers
Maternal and child health	• Work closely with pregnant women, new mothers and their families • Working alongside midwives and other health professionals • Can be inpatient such as mother-baby units or community-based maternal and child health services
Alcohol and other drugs services	• Can be inpatient and community settings along a continuum of care from detoxification to rehabilitation services
Forensic mental health	• Range of settings including custody centres, courts, custodial diversion services, prisons and specialised forensic mental health services
Schools and tertiary education	• Work with public or private and secondary or tertiary education settings • Provide assessment and counselling services • Address health and wellbeing of students and the school community • Work with teachers and other staff
Asylum seekers and refugees	• Work with refugees and asylum seekers • A range of settings including onshore and offshore immigration detention centres and post-release/re-settlement support and trauma services
e-mental health	• Opportunity to develop web-based education and treatment programs • Provide assessment and counselling over the internet

gathered and reflected on, expertise in nursing practice becomes more imbedded and flexible (Benner 1984).

Expert mental health nursing practice was demonstrated in a study that explored the nature and impact of mental health nursing (Santangelo et al. 2018a; 2018b). The expert mental health nurses in this study drew on a range of experiences to develop meaningful recovery-orientated relationships with consumers and demonstrated the ability and willingness to be with consumers in the here-and-now, in both the extreme and the mundane moments of the consumer's existence. This placed the mental health nurse in a position where they could be alert to disruptions in health and from those observations being able to gauge what needed to be done and when it needed to be done.

ADVANCED PRACTICE

As discussed earlier, career transitions are necessarily uncomfortable. Often when we become proficient in one area of practice, we move to another and can feel like a novice again. Stepping into an advanced practice role for the first time is another of those transitions.

The concept of advanced practice recognises that nurses seeking career progression may wish to retain their clinical focus while incorporating aspects of research, education and leadership into their roles. Advanced practice nursing is 'firmly grounded in the unique body of knowledge that is nursing' (New Zealand Nurses Organisation 2011, p. 1). Advanced practice nurses are expected to be prepared to master's level and are able to draw on nursing and other relevant theories, critically analyse current research and provide a solid understanding and rationale for nursing interventions. Their clinical reasoning, problem-solving skills, judgement and decision making are well developed (New Zealand Nurses Organisation 2011; Nursing and Midwifery Board of Australia 2016). It is important to note that:

> Advanced nursing practice is a level of practice and not a role. It is acknowledged that advanced nursing practice is specific to the individual within their context of practice.
> (Nursing and Midwifery Board of Australia 2016, p. 1)

In the past two decades, nurses in Australia and New Zealand have developed advanced practice roles that reflect contemporary clinical practice within each country. In some cases, advanced practitioners extend their practice to become a nurse practitioner, which is a protected title in New Zealand and Australia that requires licensing by a nursing regulatory body. The growth of advanced practice roles is part of a global development in nursing recognising the contribution that experienced clinicians make to consumer outcomes and are aimed at maximising the nursing contribution to health care and improving health outcomes (Drew 2014).

Advanced practice mental health nurses can choose to go into private practice, providing counselling and psychotherapy to individuals, families and/or groups and, if a nurse practitioner, use their expanded scope of practice to cease, initiate and monitor treatments. Mental health nurses also work as mental health nurse consultants, clinical supervisors and educators in private practice. Nurses choosing to take this path need to identify the client groups that are appropriate to their scope of practice and consider their practice location, fees charged, indemnity insurance and leave coverage.

Management

Progressing along a managerial career path is a popular option for mental health nurses. Nurse unit managers are critical to establishing and maintaining the culture and emotional climate of the unit (Smith et al. 2009) and the quality of consumer care (Siren & Gehrs 2018). Not only has the nurse unit manager role evolved in diversity and complexity, there are many more opportunities for management roles in health organisations. Managers have opportunities to collaborate with a range of staff and groups within and external to the organisation. As managers of clinical services, it is important to demonstrate clinical (Ennis et al. 2016) and managerial (Johnson & Smith 2018) leadership. There are opportunities for ongoing formal education in management through professional development programs and tertiary institutions. In addition, mentoring, coaching and clinical supervision are invaluable supports if you choose this career path.

Education

Moving into education is another potential career path. If you are interested in educating others, look for opportunities to buddy and precept nurses coming into your practice setting. Learn how to be a good preceptor through the many programs that are available. Keep your skills up to date and develop your clinical leadership abilities (Ennis et al. 2015). Within health organisations there will be opportunities for formal education positions in the clinical area and/or in professional development programs. Make use of mentors and clinical supervisors as you endeavour to understand education work and develop skills.

Consider opportunities within the academic sector including with universities and training providers. Take up opportunities that might arise when students are on placement and liaise with the academic staff that are involved with the students. It is not uncommon that mental health nurses working clinically can take up clinical education roles with the students and have input in the classroom.

Research

Undertaking research is often seen as the domain of academics but it is possible to be involved in research and maintain a clinical role. If opportunities arise in your practice setting, consider becoming involved to find out if it is an area you are interested in. A great way to start is to take up the role of participant when researchers are requesting a nursing perspective. You not only learn about research by also add to the professional body of knowledge. Mental health nurses can also be part of research teams as co-investigators or as research assistants or research leads. Mental health nurses can conduct research through postgraduate study on issues of clinical significance through a research master's (commonly referred to as a Master of Philosophy or MPhil) or a PhD (Doctor of Philosophy). Mental health nurses in New Zealand and Australia continue to make a significant contribution to research on the international stage. It is a terrific buzz when you receive feedback from colleagues that your research work has made a difference.

Chapter summary

This chapter has described self-awareness and self-care as essential strategies to maintain wellbeing, to be able to provide compassionate care to consumers and carers, to maintain productive working relationships with colleagues, to manage the demands of mental health nursing practice and to sustain a rewarding career. Mental health nursing is a rich and rewarding career with its own challenges and workplace stressors. This chapter has provided information on these challenges and introduced concepts such as emotional labour, vicarious trauma and, as the process of positive adaptation to stressors, resilience. Individual nurses, organisations and the mental health nursing profession all have a part to play in supporting nurses' professional self-care and development. Understanding the impact of nursing work and developing strategies for addressing workforce health and stress management is an encouraging and developing body of knowledge. Systems of support for mental health nursing are emerging all the time. A nursing career provides an opportunity to work in a range of environments with diverse people and communities. It is also a career of lifelong learning and ongoing professional development. Reflecting on the information in this chapter will assist you to establish healthy self-care and professional development practices early in your career, which will serve you well as you progress through your work in nursing.

NURSE'S STORY 6.3

Julie Sharrock

I have been a nurse for a long time, at least 4 decades in fact. And like most older people, I say things like: 'It feels like yesterday that I was a young woman starting out as a nurse'. I have always been interested in working with people and I also wanted to travel; nursing gave me both.

Nursing gave me the opportunity to understand the dimensions of the human condition. I witnessed the polarities of resilience and vulnerability co-existing in the people I cared for. I was exposed to the absolute mystery of suffering and death. To be with people at the extreme times of their existence has been a privilege, but it has not been without its challenges. In my early years as an intensive care nurse I was close to burnout. Thankfully I had access to staff counselling, which helped me avoid completely imploding. I realised that I was using a lot of energy being angry at the health system and its shortcomings. I also learned that I had choices about what causes to fight for and which jobs to take. These have proved to be important lessons and have helped me to stay in the public health system for most of my working life.

I knew I wanted to be a mental health nurse when I had my first mental health placement. This was after a classmate and I overcame our overwhelming feelings when confronted by a locked women's ward in an old psychiatric institution. By lunchtime on my first day I knew one day I would do my psychiatric nurse training. When I did, I knew I had found my niche and I really found my passion when I became a consultation-liaison nurse in a general hospital. I particularly loved the combination of clinical and education work as well as contributing to quality improvement and becoming involved in research.

The challenges of working with people (consumers, relatives and staff) are ever-present. I have often been asked how I do the work I do and, without doubt, a key component of my survival in health care is good clinical supervision. I continue to enjoy travel and I have had the opportunity to combine travel with my work through conference attendances. In addition, I have maintained my interests outside of work including the surf and the snow, the arts, creative pursuits and of course family and friends. I used my cycling commute (incorporating mindful practices) to bookend my working day. I have engaged in lifelong learning through academic and professional development programs as well as personal growth. Professional associations have always formed part of my support system, and spending time with like-minded colleagues is always energising. I have loved the opportunity to write this chapter and share with you some ideas about how to get the most out of your nursing career. I want you to love nursing as much as I have.

EXERCISE FOR CLASS ENGAGEMENT

An effective way of developing self-awareness is to use questioning. To raise your awareness of some important issues, ask yourself the following questions, and then discuss your responses with other members of your group or class.

1. What kinds of values do I hold important as a framework for living? Where do these values come from? How do they inform my understanding of what it is to be a person in this world?
2. How has my family of origin influenced how I view the world? What values did my family hold as important? What do I see as important in family life?
3. What do I know about why I chose to be a nurse? Does this still hold true or have my ideas changed over time?
4. What are the pervading social attitudes towards people in mental distress or with mental illness? What are my beliefs about people in mental distress or with mental illness?
5. What experiences have I had that influence how I feel about people with mental illness?

Critical thinking challenge 6.1

Reflect on your personality style and unique characteristics:

- How can these characteristics support you in your work?
- How might these characteristics increase your vulnerability in your work?

Reflect on your supports within and outside of work:

- What energises you?
- What calms you?
- Who or what would you turn to if you did not feel you were coping?

How can you use these insights to support yourself during your nursing career?

Acknowledgement

This chapter includes some information adapted from chapters in previous editions of this book by Debra Jackson and Louise O'Brien.

Useful websites

Australian Clinical Supervision Association: http://clinicalsupervision.org.au/.
Australian College of Mental Health Nurses: http://www.anzcmhn.org/.
Centre for Post-traumatic Mental Health: https://www.phoenixaustralia.org/recovery/fact-sheets-and-booklets/.
Health Direct: https://www.healthdirect.gov.au/.
New Zealand Ministry of Health: https://www.health.govt.nz/.
Nurse and Midwife Support Program: https://www.nmsupport.org.au/.
Nursing Health and Midwifery Program: http://www.nmhp.org.au/.
Te Ao Māramatanga New Zealand College of Mental Health Nursing: https://www.nzcmhn.org.nz/.
Te Pou o te Whakaaro Nui: https://www.tepou.co.nz/.

References

Australian College of Midwives, Australian College of Nursing & Australian College of Mental Health Nurses, 2019. Position statement: Clinical supervision for nurses and midwives [Online]. Available: http://www.acmhn.org/publications/position-statements. (Accessed 16 May 2019).
Benner, P., 1984. From Novice to Expert. Addison-Wesley Publishing Company, Menlo Park.
Benuto, L., Singer, J., Cummings, C., et al., 2018. The Vicarious Trauma Scale: confirmatory factor analysis and psychometric properties with a sample of victim advocates. Health Soc. Care Community 26, 564–571.
Bolton, S.C., 2000. Who cares? Offering emotion work as a 'gift' in the nursing labour process. J. Adv. Nurs. 32, 580–586.
Bonamer, J., Aquino-Russell, C., 2019. Self-care strategies for professional development: transcendental meditation reduces compassion fatigue and improves resilience for nurses. J. Nurses Prof. Dev. 35, 93–97.
Borradaile, K., 2016. Self care guide [Online]. Available: http://www.nmhp.org.au/documents/Self-Care-Guide.pdf. (Accessed 26 May 2019).
Bridges, W., 2004. Transitions: Making Sense of Life's Changes. Hachette, London.
Bridges, W., Bridges, S., 2017. Managing Transitions: Making the Most of Change, fourth ed. Nicholas Brearly Publishing, London & Boston.
Brown, S., Whichello, R., Price, S., 2018. The impact of resiliency on nurse burnout: an integrative literature review. Medsurg Nurs. 27 (6), 349–378.
Bulman, C., Lathlean, J., Gobbi, M., 2014. The process of teaching and learning about reflection: research insights from professional nurse education. Stud. Higher Educ. 39, 1219–1236.
Buus, N., Cassedy, P., Gonge, H., 2013. Developing a manual for strengthening mental health nurses' clinical supervision. Issues Ment. Health Nurs. 34, 344–349.
Caldwell, L., Grobbel, C.C., 2013. The importance of reflective practice in nursing. Int. J. Caring Sci. 6, 319–326.
Chernomas, W.M., Shapiro, C., 2013. Stress, depression, and anxiety among undergraduate nursing students. Int. J. Nurs. Educ. Scholarsh. 10, 255–266.

Chiang, Y.M., Chang, Y., 2012. Stress, depression, and intention to leave among nurses in different medical units: implications for healthcare management/nursing practice. Health Policy (New York) 108, 149–157.
Chopra, D., 2019. 7 mind-body practices to transform your relationship with stress [Online]. Available: https://chopra.com/articles/7-mind-body-practices-to-transform-your-relationship-with-stress. (Accessed 25 May 2019).
Christensen, M., Aubeeluck, A., Fergusson, D., et al., 2016. Do student nurses experience Imposter Phenomenon? An international comparison of Final Year Undergraduate Nursing Students readiness for registration. J. Adv. Nurs. 72, 2784–2793.
Christie, C., Bidwell, S., Copeland, A., et al., 2017. Self-care of Canterbury general practitioners, nurse practitioners, practice nurses and community pharmacists. J. Prim. Health Care 9, 286–291.
Cipriano, P.F., 2015. Mitigating the risks of emotional labor. Am Nurse 47 (3), 3.
Claro, S., Paunesku, D., Dweck, C.S., 2016. Growth mindset tempers the effects of poverty on academic achievement. Proc. Natl. Acad. Sci. U.S.A. 113, 8664–8668.
Cosden, M., Sanford, A., Koch, L.M., et al., 2016. Vicarious trauma and vicarious posttraumatic growth among substance abuse treatment providers. Subst. Abus. 37, 619–624.
Craigie, M., Slatyer, S., Hegney, D., et al., 2016. A pilot evaluation of a mindful self-care and resiliency (MSCR) intervention for nurses. Mindfulness 7, 764–774.
Cross, L.A., 2019. Compassion fatigue in palliative care nursing: a concept analysis. J. Hosp. Palliat. Nurs. 21, 21–28.
Delgado, C., Upton, D., Ranse, K., et al., 2017. Nurses' resilience and the emotional labour of nursing work: an integrative review of empirical literature. Int. J. Nurs. Stud. 70, 71–88.
Drew, B.L., 2014. The evolution of the role of the psychiatric mental health advanced practice registered nurse in the United States. Arch. Psychiatr. Nurs. 28, 298–300.
Duchscher, J.E.B., 2009. Transition shock: the initial stage of role adaptation for newly graduated registered nurses. J. Adv. Nurs. 65, 1103–1113.
Dweck, C., 2015. Carol Dweck revisits the growth mindset. Education Week 35, 20–24.
Edward, K.L., Hercelinskyj, G., Giandinoto, J.A., 2017. Emotional labour in mental health nursing: an integrative systematic review. Int. J. Ment. Health Nurs. 26, 215–225.
Ennis, G., Happell, B., Reid-Searl, K., 2015. Enabling professional development in mental health nursing: the role of clinical leadership. J. Psychiatr. Ment. Health Nurs. 22, 616–622.
Ennis, G., Happell, B., Reid-Searl, K., 2016. Intentional modelling: a process for clinical leadership development in mental health nursing. Issues Ment. Health Nurs. 37, 353–359.
Erkayiran, O., Demirkiran, F., 2018. The impact of improving emotional intelligence skills training on nursing students' interpersonal relationship styles: a quasi-experimental study. Int. J. Caring Sci. 11, 1901–1912.
Fedele, R., 2019. Mentoring matters. Aust. Nurs. Midwifery J. 26, 11–12.
Foster, K., Cuzzillo, C., Furness, T., 2018a. Strengthening mental health nurses' resilience through a workplace resilience programme: a qualitative inquiry. J. Psychiatr. Ment. Health Nurs. 25, 338–348.
Foster, K., Roche, M., Delgado, C., et al., 2019a. Resilience and mental health nursing: an integrative review of international literature. Int. J. Ment. Health Nurs. 28, 71–85.
Foster, K., Roche, M., Giandinoto, J.A., et al., 2019b. Workplace stressors, psychological well-being, resilience, and caring behaviours of mental health nurses: a descriptive correlational study. Int. J. Ment. Health Nurs. 29 (1), 56–68.
Foster, K., Shochet, I., Wurfl, A., et al., 2018b. On PAR: a feasibility study of the Promoting Adult Resilience programme with mental health nurses. Int. J. Ment. Health Nurs. 27, 1470–1480.
Freshwater, D., 2008. Reflective practice: the state of the art. In: Freshwater, D., Taylor, B., Sherwood, G. (Eds.), International Textbook of Reflective Practice in Nursing. Wiley-Blackwell, Oxford, UK.
Galbraith, N.D., Brown, K.E., Clifton, E., 2014. A survey of student nurses' attitudes toward help seeking for stress. Nurs. Forum 171–181.
Gardner, A., McCutcheon, H., 2015. A constructivist grounded theory study of mental health clinicians' boundary maintenance. Aust. Nurs. Midwifery J. 23, 30–33.
Gunasekara, I., Pentland, T., Rodgers, T., et al., 2014. What makes an excellent mental health nurse? A pragmatic inquiry initiated and conducted by people with lived experience of service use. Int. J. Ment. Health Nurs. 23, 101–109.
Hart, B., 2017. Identify barriers to best practice. Lamp 74, 18–19.
Hawkins, P., Shohet, R., 2012. Supervision in the Helping Professions. Open University Press, Maidenhead, UK.
Health Direct, 2018. Work-life balance [Online]. Health Direct. Available: https://www.healthdirect.gov.au/work-life-balance. (Accessed 25 May 2019).
Health Education and Training Institute, 2013. The Superguide: A Supervision Continuum for Nurses and Midwives. Health Education and Training Institute, Sydney.
Healy, M., Howe, V., 2012. Study of Victorian Early Graduate Programs for Nurses and Midwives: Final Research Report. TNS Social Research, Hawthorn.
Hochschild, A.R., 1983. The Managed Heart: Commercialization of Human Feeling. University of California Press, Berkeley.
Humphrey, R.H., Ashforth, B.E., Diefendorff, J.M., 2015. The bright side of emotional labor. J. Organ. Behav. 36, 749–769.
Hunsaker, S., Chen, H.C., Maughan, D., et al., 2015. Factors that influence the development of compassion fatigue,

burnout, and compassion satisfaction in emergency department nurses. J. Nurs. Scholarsh. 47, 186–194.
Hussein, R., Everett, B., Hu, W., et al., 2016. Predictors of new graduate nurses' satisfaction with their transitional support programme. J. Nurs. Manag. 24, 319–326.
Jackson, D., Firtko, A., Edenborough, M., 2007. Personal resilience as a strategy for surviving and thriving in the face of workplace adversity: a literature review. J. Adv. Nurs. 60, 1–9.
Johnson, C.S., Smith, C.M., 2018. Preparing nursing professional development practitioners in their leadership role: management and leadership skills. J. Nurses Prof. Dev. 34, 99–100.
Johnson, J., Hall, L.H., Berzins, K., et al., 2018. Mental healthcare staff well-being and burnout: a narrative review of trends, causes, implications, and recommendations for future interventions. Int. J. Ment. Health Nurs. 27, 20–32.
Joinson, C., 1992. Coping with compassion fatigue. Nursing 22, 116–121.
Kabat-Zinn, J., 2019. Guided mindfulness meditation practices with Jon Kabat-Zinn [Online]. Available: https://www.mindfulnesscds.com/. (Accessed 26 May 2019).
Kelly, E.L., Fenwick, K., Brekke, J.S., et al., 2016. Well-being and safety among inpatient psychiatric staff: the impact of conflict, assault, and stress reactivity. Adm. Policy. Ment. Health 43, 703–716.
Kenny, P., Reeve, R., Hall, J., 2016. Satisfaction with nursing education, job satisfaction, and work intentions of new graduate nurses. Nurse Educ. Today 36, 230–235.
La Trobe University, 2019. Nurses and lawyers' heavy drinking study [Online]. Available: https://www.latrobe.edu.au/news/articles/2019/release/nurses-and-lawyers-heavy-drinking-study. (Accessed 12 July 2019).
Laker, C., Cella, M., Callard, F., et al., 2019. Why is change a challenge in acute mental health wards? A cross-sectional investigation of the relationships between burnout, occupational status and nurses' perceptions of barriers to change. Int. J. Ment. Health Nurs. 28, 190–198.
Larter, A., 2014. Nurses need healing. Nurs. Rev. 3, 4.
Leary, M.R., Price Tangney, J. (Eds.), 2012. Handbook of Self and Identity. Guilford Press, New York.
Leyva-Vela, B., Henarejos-Alarcón, S., Llorente-Cantarero, F.J., et al., 2018. Psychosocial and physiological risks of shift work in nurses: a cross-sectional study. Cent. Eur. J. Public Health 26, 183–189.
Lim, J., Bogossian, F., Ahern, K., 2010. Stress and coping in Australian nurses: a systematic review. Int. Nurs. Rev. 57, 22–31.
Lloyd, J., 2019. A hospital is the place to heal a ravaged body, but what about a wounded spirit? Aust. Nurs. Midwifery J. 26, 23.
Malinowski, P., 2013. Flourishing through meditation and mindfulness. In: David, S.A., Boniwell, I., Conley Ayers, A. (Eds.), Oxford Library of Psychology. The Oxford Handbook of Happiness. Oxford University Press, New York.
Marie, M., Hannigan, B., Jones, A., 2017. Resilience of nurses who work in community mental health workplaces in Palestine. Int. J. Ment. Health Nurs. 26, 344–354.
Maslach, C., 2017. Finding solutions to the problem of burnout. Consult. Psychol. J. Pract. Res. 69, 143–152.
Maslach, C., Leiter, M.P., 2017. New insights into burnout and health care: strategies for improving civility and alleviating burnout. Med. Teach. 39, 160–163.
Masters, G.N., 2013. Towards a Growth Mindset in Assessment. ACER (Australian Council for Educational Research) Occasional Essays, pp. 1–5.
Mayer, J.D., Salovey, P., Caruso, D.R., 2004. Emotional intelligence: theory, findings, and implications. Psychol. Inq. 15, 197–215.
McCann, C., Beddoe, L., McCormick, K., et al., 2013. Resilience in the health professions: a review of recent literature. Int. J. Wellbeing 3 (1).
McNamara, P., 2016. Hand hygiene and mindful moments [Online]. Available: https://meta4rn.com/2016/11/26/hygiene/. (Accessed 25 May 2019).
Mealer, M., Conrad, D., Evans, J., et al., 2014. Feasibility and acceptability of a resilience training program for intensive care unit nurses. Am. J. Crit. Care 23, e97–e105.
Mi, Y., 2016. Factors affecting turnover intention for new graduate nurses in three transition periods for job and work environment satisfaction. J. Contin. Educ. Nurs. 47, 120–131.
Mills, J., 2018. Examining self-care, self-compassion and compassion for others: a cross-sectional survey of palliative care nurses and doctors. Int. J. Palliat. Nurs. 24, 4–11.
Mills, J., Wand, T., Fraser, J.A., 2015. On self-compassion and self-care in nursing: selfish or essential for compassionate care? Int. J. Nurs. Stud. 52, 791–793.
Mills, J., Wand, T., Fraser, J.A., 2018. Exploring the meaning and practice of self-care among palliative care nurses and doctors: a qualitative study. BMC Palliat. Care 17, 1–12.
Milner, A.J., Maheen, H., Bismark, M.M., et al., 2016. Suicide by health professionals: a retrospective mortality study in Australia 2001–2012. Med. J. Aust. 205, 260–265.
Monroe, T., Kenaga, H., 2011. Don't ask don't tell: substance abuse and addiction among nurses. J. Clin. Nurs. 20, 504–509.
Mooney, M., 2007. Facing registration: the expectations and the unexpected. Nurse Educ. Today 27, 840–847.
Muir-Cochrane, E., O'Kane, D., Oster, C., 2018. Fear and blame in mental health nurses' accounts of restrictive practices: implications for the elimination of seclusion and restraint. Int. J. Ment. Health Nurs. 27, 1511–1521.
New Zealand Nurses Organisation, 2011. NZNO practice position statement advanced nursing practice. Available: https://www.nzno.org.nz/.
Nursing and Midwifery Board of Australia, 2016. Fact sheet: Advanced nursing practice and specialty areas within nursing.

Park, C.L., 2010. Making sense of the meaning literature: an integrative review of meaning making and its effects on adjustment to stressful life events. Psychol. Bull. 136, 257.

Parsa-Yekta, Z., Abdolrahimi, M., 2016. Concept analysis of emotional intelligence in nursing. Nurs. Pract. Today 3, 158–163.

Perry, L., Xu, X., Gallagher, R., et al., 2018. Lifestyle health behaviors of nurses and midwives: the 'fit for the future' study. Int. J. Environ. Res. Public Health 15, 945.

Phoenix Australia, 2019. What is trauma? [Online]. Centre for Posttraumatic Mental Health, University of Melbourne. Available: http://phoenixaustralia.org/recovery/fact-sheets-and-booklets/. (Accessed 7 July 2019).

Pinel, E., Bosson, J., 2013. Turning our attention to stigma: an objective self-awareness analysis of stigma and its consequences. Basic Appl. Soc. Psych. 35, 55–63.

Prosser, S.J., Metzger, M., Gulbransen, K., 2017. Don't just survive, thrive: understanding how acute psychiatric nurses develop resilience. Arch. Psychiatr. Nurs. 31, 171–176.

Reyes, D., 2012. Self-compassion: a concept analysis. J. Holist. Nurs. 30, 81–89.

Ross, A., Yang, L., Wehrlen, L., et al., 2019. Nurses and health-promoting self-care: do we practice what we preach? J. Nurs. Manag. 27, 599–608.

Russell, L., 1990. Clinical Supervision: History 23. Nightingale to Now: Nurse Education in Australia. Churchill Livingstone, Sydney.

Sabery, M., Tafreshi, M.Z., Hosseini, M., et al., 2018. Compassion fatigue in clinical nurses: an evolutionary concept analysis. J. Nurs. Midwifery 27, 7–14.

Safe Work Australia, 2018. Australian Work Health and Safety Strategy 2012–2022: Healthy, Safe and Productive Working Lives. Safe Work Australia, Canberra.

Safe Work Australia, 2012. Australian Work Health and Safety Strategy 2012–2022. Australian Government, Canberra.

Salzmann-Erikson, M., 2018. Moral mindfulness: the ethical concerns of healthcare professionals working in a psychiatric intensive care unit. Int. J. Ment. Health Nurs. 27 (6), 1851–1860.

Santangelo, P., Procter, N., Fassett, D., 2018a. Mental health nursing: daring to be different, special and leading recovery-focused care? Int. J. Ment. Health Nurs. 27, 258–266.

Santangelo, P., Procter, N., Fassett, D., 2018b. Seeking and defining the 'special' in specialist mental health nursing: a theoretical construct. Int. J. Ment. Health Nurs. 27, 267–275.

Schluter, P., Turner, C., Huntington, A., et al., 2011. Work/life balance and health: the nurses and midwives e-cohort study. Int. Nurs. Rev. 58, 28–36.

Schueler, S.K., 2017. Nurses tending to spiritual self-care through medical therapeutic yoga. Beginnings 37, 22–23.

Siren, A., Gehrs, M., 2018. Engaging nurses in future management careers: perspectives on leadership and management competency development through an internship initiative. Nurs. Leadersh. 31, 36–49.

Smith, P., Pearson, P.H., Ross, F., 2009. Emotions at work: what is the link to patient and staff safety? Implications for nurse managers in the NHS. J. Nurs. Manag. 17, 230–237.

Sorenson, C., Bolick, B., Wright, K., et al., 2017. An evolutionary concept analysis of compassion fatigue. J. Nurs. Scholarsh. 49, 557–563.

Sweet, L., Bass, J., Sidebotham, M., et al., 2019. Developing reflective capacities in midwifery students: enhancing learning through reflective writing. Women Birth 32, 119–126.

Te Pou O Te Whakaaro Nui, 2017a. Te Tirohanga a te Manu 'A Bird's Perspective': Professional Supervision Guide for Nursing Leaders and Managers. Te Pou o te Whakaaro Nui, Auckland.

Te Pou O Te Whakaaro Nui, 2017b. Te Tirohanga a te Manu 'A Bird's Perspective': Professional Supervision Guide for Nursing Supervisees. Te Pou o te Whakaaro Nui, Auckland.

Te Pou O Te Whakaaro Nui, 2017c. Te Tirohanga a te Manu 'A Bird's Perspective': Professional Supervision Guide for Supervisors. Te Pou o te Whakaaro Nui, Auckland.

Theodosius, C., 2008. Emotional Labour in Health Care: The Unmanaged Heart of Nursing. Routledge, London & New York.

Torquati, L., Kolbe-Alexander, T., Pavey, T., et al., 2018. Changing diet and physical activity in nurses: a pilot study and process evaluation highlighting challenges in workplace health promotion. J. Nutr. Educ. Behav. 50, 1015–1025.

Ungar, M., 2008. Resilience across cultures. Br. J. Soc. Work 38, 218–235.

Waldrop, J., Derouin, A., 2019. The coaching experience of advanced practice nurses in a national leadership program. J. Contin. Educ. Nurs. 50, 170–175.

Walker, A., Campbell, K., 2013. Work readiness of graduate nurses and the impact on job satisfaction, work engagement and intention to remain. Nurse Educ. Today 33, 1490–1495.

Wiklund Gustin, L., Wagner, L., 2013. The butterfly effect of caring: clinical nursing teachers' understanding of self-compassion as a source to compassionate care. Scand. J. Caring Sci. 27, 175–183.

Wilson, D.R., Brooks, E.J., 2018. Sleep and immune function: nurse self-care and teaching sleep hygiene. Beginnings 38, 6–23.

World Health Organization, 2018. International Classification of Diseases – revision for mortality and morbidity statistics (11th revision). Available https://www.who.int/classifications/icd/en/. (Accessed 17 January 2020).

Zhang, Y.Y., Han, W.L., Qin, W., et al., 2018. Extent of compassion satisfaction, compassion fatigue and burnout in nursing: a meta-analysis. J. Nurs. Manag. 26, 810–819.

Zugai, J.S., Stein-Parbury, J., Roche, M., 2018. The nature of the therapeutic alliance between nurses and consumers with anorexia nervosa in the inpatient setting: a mixed-methods study. J. Clin. Nurs. 27 (1–2), 416–426.

PART 2

Knowledge for Practice

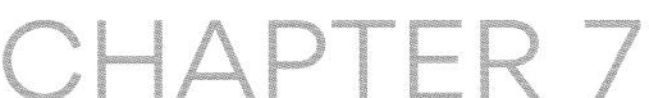

CHAPTER 7

Mental health assessment

Anthony J O'Brien and Mandy Allman

KEY POINTS

- Assessment is the first step in the nursing process and is ongoing throughout each episode of care.
- The purpose of mental health nursing assessment is to understand the mental health problems the person is experiencing and what nurses can do to help.
- Comprehensive assessment involves gathering information about multiple domains of the person's life including their physical and mental health.
- Mental health nursing assessment can involve both conversational and structured interviews, in addition to nursing observation and information from third parties.
- Clinical formulation is the process of developing, with the consumer, a summary of the various influences on the consumer's current problems, and how the consumer and clinician can work towards resolving those problems.

KEY TERMS

- Assessment
- Case formulation
- Cultural assessment
- Diagnosis
- Differential diagnosis
- Documentation
- DSM-5
- ICD-11
- Interviewing
- Mental state assessment
- Narrative
- Physical assessment
- Risk assessment
- Screening
- Spiritual assessment
- Standardised assessment
- Strengths assessment
- Triage

LEARNING OUTCOMES

The material in this chapter will assist you to:

- understand the purpose and process of mental health nursing assessment
- utilise a model of comprehensive mental health nursing assessment in clinical practice
- discuss the place of physical health assessment within comprehensive mental health nursing assessment
- conduct and document a mental state assessment
- discuss the relationship between assessment and clinical decision making.

Introduction

Assessment is one of the most important and fundamental skills of the mental health nurse. Through assessment, we develop an understanding of consumers, formulate a plan of care and contribute to the decision making of multidisciplinary teams. Assessment also tells us about the effectiveness and acceptability of mental health nursing care. A comprehensive assessment encompasses multiple aspects of consumers' lives, including current and past mental health problems, family and social history, use of alcohol and other drugs, physical health, and cultural and spiritual influences on mental health. Assessment focuses on problems in the consumer's life, as well as the strengths and capabilities available to the consumer to respond to those problems. As the consumer's recovery progresses, assessment will reflect the developing understanding between the nurse and the consumer, new issues in response to treatment and the consumer's development of new coping skills and strategies.

This chapter outlines the process of mental health nursing assessment. Assessment is explained as both a structured process in which the nurse seeks to gather important information about the consumer's history and functioning, and as an exploratory process in which the nurse and the consumer review their understandings of the nature of the consumer's problems, and the care and treatment the consumer is receiving. The aim is always one of clarifying the shared understanding that provides the basis of nursing care. The chapter also introduces current models of assessment and the various skills of mental health nursing assessment such as taking a history, assessing mental state, using standardised assessment instruments, clinical formulation and diagnosis. As much as possible the chapter is organised to follow the standard process of psychiatric assessment, from recording the presenting problem through to formulating a plan of care

Critical thinking challenge 7.1

Why is assessment considered fundamental to nursing practice? Why is it important to develop skills in assessment as a basis for any nursing intervention?

Assessment

Assessment is the first step in the nursing process (DeWit & O'Neill 2014) and is ongoing over the time a consumer is engaged with mental health care. Initial assessment occurs when the consumer first accesses mental health care and has the aim of developing a shared understanding of what problems the person seeks help with, their strengths and resources, and what the mental health service can do to assist with those problems. As the nurse and the consumer develop their relationship, and as initial problems are resolved, the shared understanding of the goals of care will change. Ongoing assessment helps review goals, redefine problems and strengths, and develop new strategies to assist in the consumer's recovery.

Assessment is fundamental to mental health nursing and provides the platform on which nursing care is delivered (Coombs et al. 2011; Wand et al. 2019). Nurses are the single largest group of professionals in mental health care and are well positioned throughout the continuum of care to make significant contributions to care delivery. Nursing assessment is carried out in a variety of settings, throughout each episode of care and at key transition points such as discharge and admission. Assessment makes a significant contribution to diagnosis and treatment planning. Mental health nursing assessment adds to the decisions about the care provided by nurses and other members of the multidisciplinary team. As such, nursing assessment is both an independent activity and interdependent with the treating team.

Despite the potential strengths of mental health nursing assessment, there is a lack of clarity over what this entails in practice (Coombs et al. 2013a). The published research literature does little to help here. There is evidence that nurses often gather assessment information in the course of other 'simple social activities' such as making a cup of tea (Coombs et al. 2013b). However, nurses also have difficulty in articulating a model of mental health nursing assessment, and current models do not always reflect nursing's commitment to person-focused care (Wand et al. 2019). Nurses rely on the eclectic nature of nursing, their own intuition and a 'tacit, experiential model of assessment' (MacNeela et al. 2010, p. 1,298) when assessing consumers. The lack of a clear description and demonstration of what constitutes a nursing mental health assessment has contributed to this essential activity being viewed as less than substantial and less reliable than assessment by other team members (MacNeela et al. 2010). This chapter provides a clear way through this maze and offers both a framework for mental health nursing assessment and a description of the key tasks of assessment.

To do a comprehensive assessment well, it is important that a recognised nursing assessment framework is used to identify presenting problems, strengths, health history and risks, and to formulate goals for care. The completion of a robust comprehensive assessment requires the interplay of complex skills and ultimately leads to a sound diagnosis and care planning. Box 7.1 outlines the threads of mental health nursing assessment, threads that must be woven together by each clinical practitioner (see also Fig. 7.1). A suggestion for new graduates is to focus on developing competency in each thread of assessment. While the threads are interdependent, each also has its own skills. Focusing on individual threads will provide a transparent pathway for skill acquisition.

Nurse's Story 7.1 looks at how assessment works in community mental health nursing.

Box 7.1 The threads of mental health nursing assessment

Assessment comprises several main threads woven together:

- process: *the way* information is gathered, including the therapeutic relationship, observation, rating instruments and informal/formal methods
- content: *what* information is gathered such as defining the presenting problem, mental health history, mental state, physical health review and substance use
- interpretation: the *meaning* ascribed to the above content that is jointly understood by the consumer, the nurse and the treating team and informs treatment planning (nursing and other theories help the nurse in the process of interpretation)
- communication: the *articulation* of the assessment – formulation, sharing of assessment information, presentation of assessment at handover, multidisciplinary team meetings and clinical review, and documentation (the written record of assessment findings).

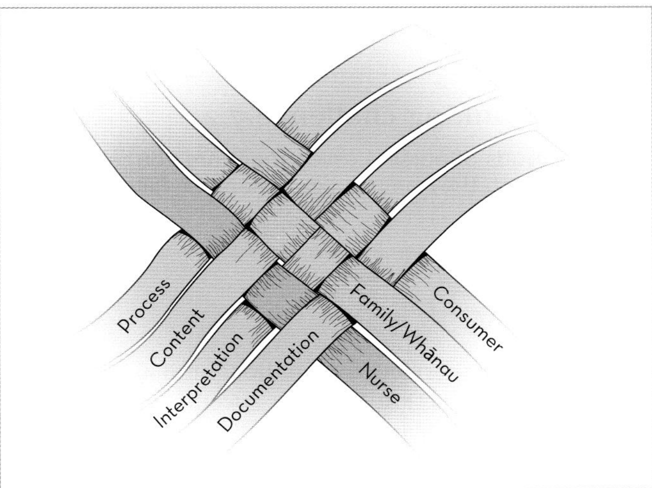

Figure 7.1
The threads of mental health nursing assessment
Adapted from the Ministry of Education New Zealand, CC BY 3.0 NZ.

NURSE'S STORY 7.1
Tania Smith

As a new graduate on the New Entry to Specialty Practice (Mental Health and Addiction) (NESP) program, assessment and diagnosis are utilised daily within my role as a community mental health nurse case manager. This is an autonomous role where I am required to be proactive within a variety of settings from multidisciplinary meetings to liaising with non-government organisations to seek guidance and support regarding my assigned caseload. First and foremost, both professional and therapeutic relationships need to be established to ensure that my assessment and nursing diagnosis is at a consistent level of professionalism to be an advocate and support person for service users on my assigned caseload. I have an affinity with Dr Mason Durie's *Te Whare Tapa Wha*[1] framework and with the utilisation of biopsychosocial comprehensive assessment and relapse prevention plan documentation. I am able to obtain an all-encompassing view of not only the service user's mental and physical health but also a comprehensive history and their understanding of their situation. I utilise this information to assist service users' journeys to wellness, along with being able to monitor their individual progress.

On completion of my 'supernumerary' 6-week period with my preceptor I was effectively 'let loose'. Not surprisingly, around this time the enormity of 'I was now it!' struck, and I found myself doubting my ability to work within the community on my own. After in-depth discussions with my colleagues and other NESP graduates, I found I was not alone in feeling this way and this was considered a normal reaction. Personal acknowledgement and processing of the huge leap across a seemingly endless chasm from a third-year nursing student to registered nurse, responsible for my own caseload, was a lot to decipher.

There are several factors that need to be taken into account when working within the community environment and developing the skill to identify the nuances of when service users are experiencing increased problems. I incorporate a mental state assessment within my notes, which assists in identifying specific issues in a service user's presentation. No one expects me to be an expert as a new grad, but I am expected to build on my core assessment skills and, as time goes on, my individual practice and professional development reflect my learning and growth. Initially, the hardest questions I found to ask were along the lines of: 'Have you cut yourself since I saw you last?', 'Do you want to harm others?', 'Are you having thoughts of suicide?' When the answer is yes to any or all of the above, then your questioning for your assessment teases out the risk component. As my own practice continually develops, it is apparent that a core understanding of not only the nursing process but also a holistic health model assists to form a 'whole picture' of service users, along with input from identified key support people and agencies. Working within a supportive environment is invaluable, and this has assisted my learning and growth immensely. This is reflected in my personal growth and confidence as a community mental health nurse case manager.

[1] *Te Whare Tapa Wha* is a Māori model of health assessment (see Pitama et al. 2014).

Professional standards and mental health nursing assessment

In addition to being a set of clinical skills, assessment is also an obligation of mental health nurses. All nurses are expected to be able to conduct a comprehensive assessment, and this core skill is reflected in nursing standards of practice. Standard 5 of the Nursing and Midwifery Board of Australia (NMBA) competency standards states that nurses can 'conduct a comprehensive and systematic assessment' (NMBA 2013), while Competency 2.2 of the Nursing Council of New Zealand (NCNZ) competencies for registered nurses states that the registered nurse 'undertakes a comprehensive and accurate assessment of health consumers in a variety of settings' (NCNZ 2007). Comprehensive nursing assessment involves considering all aspects of the consumer, including their mental, physical, spiritual, emotional, social and cultural needs (Australian College of Mental Health Nurses 2010). The New Zealand College of Mental Health Nurses standards expect mental health nurses to have knowledge of 'contemporary models of assessment and clinical decision making' (Te Ao Maramatanga New Zealand College of Mental Health Nurses 2012). Professional standards, together with the skills to articulate the findings to others, contribute to sound mental health nursing assessment.

Narrative and descriptive approaches to mental health nursing assessment

Mental health nursing assessment uses formal and semi-formal tools, as well as a range of interpersonal processes. It can sometimes seem that the tools of nursing assessment, such as the assessment templates provided by clinical services, dominate the assessment process due to their requirement to collect a large amount of detailed information. In addition, services usually require clinicians, often nurses, to complete risk assessment forms in which assessment information is used to establish levels of risk. Standardised assessment tools such as mood rating scales, risk scales, symptom scales and measures of cognitive functioning may appear to reduce assessment to eliciting answers to a 'tick box' rather than exploring with consumers the meaning of their experiences.

Mental health nursing assessment can be thought of as comprising two key tasks: collecting and interpreting assessment information (which can be assessed using standard tools and templates); and developing an understanding of each consumer and their perspectives of their current situation. The tasks of assessment should not determine the process of assessment, which can include a variety of methods from conversational interviewing, with its focus on the individual narrative (Barker 2004), to completing consumer- or clinician-rated assessment instruments. Skilled mental health nurses combine the tasks in any assessment and can move between the more descriptive approach of seeking specific information and the exploratory approach of narrative enquiry. Both approaches have an important place in comprehensive assessment, and together they yield a fuller understanding of each consumer and contribute to developing a therapeutic relationship.

Methods of mental health nursing assessment

Mental health nursing assessment uses a range of methods including structured and conversational interviews, standardised assessment instruments, diaries, direct observation and information from third parties including friends and family and clinical records. All these methods have a common purpose: to enhance our understanding of the person seeking mental health care and to help with the problems that led them to seek mental health care. In this section we describe the assessment methods of interviews, mnemonics, standardised assessment tools, diaries, direct observation and information from third parties.

Critical thinking challenge 7.2

What methods of nursing assessment are you familiar with? How can they be used in a mental health clinical setting?

Interviews

An assessment interview can be thought of as a relatively structured conversation that has specific goals: to elicit information about the consumer, to help the nurse understand the consumer's problems and to develop a plan of care. While it is possible to describe a structured assessment interview as a logical series of topics – such as the presenting problem, history of mental health problems and social history – in practice assessment interviews rarely follow a prescribed course. Interviewing is a core skill of mental health nursing and requires a range of nursing skills. Interviews may be brief or lengthy, depending on the demands of the situation and on the needs of the consumer. Interviews may also be formal or informal, and in practice a combination of formal and informal approaches may be necessary. Nurses need to be flexible in their approach to interviews and be ready to change their planned approach as the interview progresses. In particular, at times it may be necessary to stop an interview – for example, if it proves too distressing for the consumer, or if the consumer is not able to concentrate on the interview process. In developing their interview skills, nurses should take opportunities to work with different colleagues from the multidisciplinary team and to observe how colleagues conduct interviews, manage the complex issues that arise and engage with consumers around difficult and sensitive issues such as experiences of trauma, identity, thoughts of self-harm and risk to self and others.

Historical anecdote 7.1: Assessment is ancient

One of the earliest known methods of mental health assessment was invented by the Roman politician and lawyer Cicero (circa 63 BC). He invented an interview schedule that sought to collect the following information: (1) nomen (clan/tribe, region); (2) natura (sex, nationality, family status, age, physique); (3) victus (education, habits/lifestyle); (4) fortuna (rich/poor, free/slave, social class); (5) habitus (appearance); (6) affectio (passions, emotions, temperament); (7) studium (interests); (8) consilium (motivation); (9) factum (working history); (10) casus (significant life events); and (11) orationes (form and content of discourse). Use of similar interview schedules for mental health assessment spread throughout the Roman Empire.

Read more about it: *King H (Ed.) 2004 Health in antiquity. Routledge, New York*

Interviews and therapeutic communication

Interviews should be seen as a form of nursing intervention, thus requiring the interpersonal skills of attending, empathy, listening, reflection, paraphrasing and responding that are inherent in mental health nursing practice. In an interview the nurse is inviting the consumer to share sensitive and personal information, so it is essential that the nurse approaches the interview with an attitude of respect and with a genuine interest in what the consumer has to say. The nurse needs to be available to the consumer, which means not being distracted by other commitments or obligations, and responding to the concerns the consumer expresses. As in any therapeutic relationship, rapport is essential to conducting an interview. The nurse needs to spend the initial part of the interview developing rapport and then maintain that rapport as the interview progresses. Any issues of cultural or language differences need to be acknowledged as they would in any therapeutic interaction. In considering the development of interview skills, it is helpful to review the principles of therapeutic communication outlined in Chapter 3. Some questions and responses that can be used in interviews are listed in Table 7.1.

Interview settings

Interviews take place in a range of locations, and nurses need to be able to adapt their interview skills to the setting. These settings include primary care offices, community clinics, consumers' homes, emergency departments,

TABLE 7.1 Questions and responses for assessment interviews

CONSUMER'S STATEMENT	NURSE'S RESPONSE	COMMENT
I don't know where to start.	Perhaps if we begin by talking about what brought you into the (clinic/hospital/service) today?	At the beginning of the interview the consumer may feel overwhelmed by the issues they are facing. A concrete question or statement can help in initiating dialogue.
I've been seeing my GP for depression, but it's not getting better.	Can you tell me more about the depression? How bad has it been?	By using the term 'depression' the nurse communicates that they are listening and are aware of the significance of the problem.
The voices are there all the time. They never leave me alone.	That sounds very difficult for you. Tell me more about the voices. What sorts of things do they say?	The nurse's responses are designed to validate the consumer's experience and to encourage dialogue about the voices.
I feel so hopeless; I can't seem to do anything right.	It can feel really bad when nothing is going right for you.	This response focuses on the consumer's emotional state and need to have their distress recognised.
I sometimes wish it was all over.	Are you saying that you don't want to be alive any longer?	Consumers may talk indirectly about suicidal thoughts. A direct question can help the consumer to acknowledge suicidal thoughts and can be followed up with further exploration of these thoughts, including intent, available means, etc.

inpatient wards, general hospital wards, courts, prisons and police stations. In planning an interview, the nurse needs to consider the safety of the consumer and themselves, privacy, adequate seating (especially if multiple family members are to be involved) and the availability of the interview room. Some settings, such as general hospital wards or consumers' homes, may present difficulties in ensuring privacy and, whenever possible, an area separate from the consumer's bed space should be sought. The ideal setting is a separate room that is close to other work areas and that provides adequate space and privacy.

SAFETY IN CONDUCTING INTERVIEWS

In arranging an interview, the nurse needs to be mindful of the consumer's safety and their own. An interview can be a challenging experience for a consumer, who may feel vulnerable in the presence of health professionals. Gender, ethnicity and age differences may also contribute to a consumer's feeling of vulnerability. Family members or friends may be present at the interview, although the support they provide needs to be balanced against their potentially inhibiting effect on the interview process. The consumer also needs to consent to the family member or friend being present and should be asked about this confidentially, so they are able to express their preference free of any sense of obligation or coercion.

Another safety consideration is the mental state of the consumer. Before the interview begins the nurse will have some indication of the consumer's level of distress, ability to tolerate the nurse's questions and willingness to participate in the interview. It is often advisable for a second clinician to be present, both as a means of supporting the first clinician and to respond to any difficulties that may arise. In conducting the interview, the nurse needs to continuously assess the consumer's mental state and take steps if the consumer becomes too distressed. If the nurse feels threatened by the consumer's attitude or behaviour (e.g. the emergence of paranoid ideas or anger directed at the nurse), consider abandoning the interview. The nurse should always advise other team members where they will be conducting an interview and how long they expect to take. This allows colleagues to be aware of the consumer and nurse's whereabouts and to be available if additional support is needed.

MANAGING THE INTERVIEW PROCESS

Interviews are more manageable if the nurse and the consumer have a clear idea of the purpose and goals of the interview, the time available and the possible outcomes of the interview. Because the outcomes of an interview depend on the problems identified, their severity and the support available, outcomes should initially be stated in general terms, such as clarifying current problems and planning future care rather than, for example, deciding whether hospital admission is necessary. Although the nurse should always have a plan for an interview, and should be clear about its purpose, the interview should begin informally. The nurse should briefly explain the purpose of the interview and provide an opportunity for the consumer to make opening comments about their current concerns. This may include discussing any concerns the consumer has about the interview such as privacy or confidentiality, what will happen to the information collected and possible outcomes of the interview. From there, the interview can either focus on the concerns expressed by the consumer or begin with background discussion that will provide a wider context for understanding the presenting issues.

It is not possible to prescribe the exact order of an interview – that will very much depend on the needs of the consumer at the time. The interview should begin with general questions and proceed to more specific questions as rapport develops and the consumer's concerns become clearer. In this way the more sensitive areas of assessment can be included naturally in the interview and will seem less intrusive. Some consumers will freely discuss their concerns and may need to be provided with structure to manage issues one at a time. Others may be withdrawn or less forthcoming and may need more prompting with specific questions. The flow of the interview can be determined by the consumer's responses, although the nurse does need to be aware of the need to achieve the aims of the interview. An unstructured interview that simply follows its own course, unguided by a sense of purpose, is of little use to the consumer. It will not help to clarify problems or to decide an appropriate plan of care.

As the interview progresses the nurse should be attentive to the verbal and non-verbal responses of the consumer and to any changes in those responses as the areas of discussion change. A consumer who begins with good eye contact and an open body posture may close up when discussing distressing events, giving valuable clues to the intensity of the feelings involved. The nurse carries responsibility for keeping the interview 'on track' and avoiding digressions that do not help the assessment process. It may be necessary at some points to comment when an interview is losing focus and to gently redirect the focus to the main issues. If friends or family members are present the nurse will need to manage their participation, sometimes by encouraging comment and at other times asking that comments are limited until a more appropriate point in the interview. Interviews are designed to elicit sensitive issues from clients, and it is critical that the nurse acknowledges these issues and validates the consumer's experience. A skilled interviewer will provide opportunities to discuss important issues but will also move the interview on so all important aspects can be covered.

MANAGING POTENTIAL PROBLEMS IN THE INTERVIEW PROCESS

With the best possible plan, and the best attempt to develop rapport, it is still possible that an interview may become 'bogged down' with limited dialogue. There may be interpersonal tension between the nurse and the consumer, or the consumer may have difficulty answering questions or be reluctant to discuss certain topics. There can be many reasons for problems in the interview process, and the nurse should not assume that the source of the problems is the consumer. Problems may arise from cultural, age or ethnicity differences, the nurse's attitude or non-verbal behaviours, as well as factors to do with the interview setting such as noise, limited time and an uncongenial environment. As in any therapeutic interaction, difficulties in the interview process should be acknowledged and discussed as part of the process. Methods to help an interview progress include deferring topics until later, asking questions in different ways, exploring reasons for a consumer's discomfort with specific topics and acknowledging that some issues are hard to discuss. It may be necessary to defer some areas of assessment to a later time. Sensitive areas such as sexuality may be difficult for both the nurse and the consumer and may need to be deferred until a stronger relationship has developed. This can be acknowledged at the time of the interview so the consumer is not left feeling that these issues cannot be addressed. Finally, if the consumer becomes too distressed to continue with the interview, this can be acknowledged and the interview terminated with a plan for further assessment later.

SUMMARISING AND CONCLUDING

As the interview concludes the nurse should begin to move the discussion towards a shared understanding of what has been achieved, clarification of presenting problems and discussion of possible interventions and further care. This can involve the nurse offering a summary or asking the consumer to provide a summary. This phase of the interview is an opportunity to engage the consumer in a plan of care that recognises unresolved problems and draws on the consumer's strengths and supports. The nurse should indicate when the allotted time for the interview is almost up so the consumer is able to introduce any issues not previously discussed. Friends or family members can also be invited to ask final questions at this stage. It can be helpful for the nurse to ask if there are any questions the consumer wishes to raise about the assessment information, further care and so on. Summarising can provide an opportunity to further validate the consumer's concerns. If the nurse feels unsure about the best course of action following an interview, they should openly discuss this with a co-interviewer and include the consumer in that discussion. Acknowledging uncertainty does not need to undermine confidence in the nurse or the clinical service but can be an opportunity for the nurse to share different perspectives on the assessment and future plan. It is important at the end of an interview to establish what has been agreed, as well as where there may be differences between the nurse and the consumer. The interview should terminate with discussing the next step in terms of further care and confirmation of contact details. While an assessment interview is designed to establish a broad understanding of a consumer and the problems they seek help with, it is not the only assessment tool available to nurses. Even the best interviews provide only a limited range of information, and the interview needs to be supplemented with other sources of information.

Mnemonics

Mnemonics (or acronyms) are aids to memory that prompt the nurse to ask specific questions or consider specific areas of assessment. Mnemonics are non-standardised structured assessment tools that provide a convenient reminder when undertaking an assessment.

For example:

- OLDCART can be used for assessing pain, where the letters stand for Onset, Location, Duration, Characteristics, Aggravating factors, Radiation and Timing (Chase 2015).
- The HEADSS assessment is used in youth services, where the letters stand for Home, Education, Activities, Drug and alcohol use, Sexuality and Suicide (Eade & Henning 2013). There are many variations of the HEADSS assessment format, and HEADSS can be adapted for your own practice.
- The SAD PERSONS mnemonic (Sex, Age, Depression, Prior suicidality, Ethanol (alcohol) abuse, Rational thinking, Support systems, Organised support system, No significant other, Sickness) can be used to assess suicidality (Patterson et al. 1983). This mnemonic should be used only as a prompt to memory, not as a rating instrument, as the scoring system of SAD PERSONS has no validity in predicting future self-harm (Warden et al. 2014).

Mnemonics remind clinicians of important areas of enquiry but do not result in a numerical score. Because they are not standardised, mnemonics may be used differently by different clinicians. You can create your own assessment mnemonics by making a list of areas of assessment you have found to be useful, assigning a name to each area and arranging the names so that the first letters form an easily remembered term. Important assessment findings resulting from use of mnemonics identify areas for further assessment.

Standardised assessment tools

In some areas of mental health nursing assessment, standardised instruments are used to gain a quantified measure of some aspect of psychological or social functioning – for example, mood, cognitive functioning, risk or alcohol problems. Wood and Gupta (2017) provide an overview of some useful rating scales. Of the many instruments available, nurses will use only a small number, but it is helpful to be aware of the range of instruments available and their application to clinical practice. A list of commonly used standardised assessments that nurses can incorporate into their practice is shown in Table 7.2. All the instruments listed in the table can be used by nurses in their clinical practice, although in each case training is required to ensure reliable administration of the instrument. Training can occur in formal staff development sessions or as part of supervised clinical practice. Some instruments are subject to licensing, so before using any instrument check whether your service holds the necessary licence.

Critical thinking challenge 7.3

Read the list of standardised assessment instruments included in Table 7.2 and consider the areas of psychological and social functioning they address. How could one of these instruments help you in performing a comprehensive nursing assessment?

TABLE 7.2 Standardised assessment instruments

TEST	PURPOSE	DESCRIPTION
Cognitive functioning		
MMSE (Mini-Mental State Examination) (Folstein et al. 1975)	Measure cognitive impairment	An 11-item test that provides a cut-off score indicating significant cognitive impairment
ACE-R (Addenbrooke's Cognitive Examination—Revised) (So et al. 2018).	Measure cognitive impairment	A 26-item test that provides cut-off scores for severity of cognitive impairment; ACE-R incorporates the 11 items of the MMSE
CAM (Confusion Assessment Method) (Inouye et al. 1990)	Screen for delirium	An 11-item instrument to detect delirium; CAM measures four different areas of cognitive functioning
Substance use		
AUDIT (Alcohol Use Disorder Inventory Test) (Babor et al. 2001)	Detect the presence of alcohol problems	A 10-item test available in clinician- or consumer-rated formats; AUDIT provides cut-off scores for four levels of clinical intervention
Mood		
BDI (Beck Depression Inventory) (McPherson & Martin 2010)	Screen for clinically significant depression	A 21-item self-report of experiences of low mood, with cut-off scores for levels of depression severity; subscales can be used to assess suicidality
GDS (Geriatric Depression Scale short form) (Burke et al. 1991)	Screen for clinically significant depression in older adults	A 15-item clinician-administered instrument with three cut-off scores representing different levels of depression severity
Medication side effects		
LUNSERS (Liverpool University Neuroleptic Side Effect Rating Scale) (Day et al. 1995)	Identify the presence of side effects of antipsychotic medication	A 51-item clinician- or consumer-administered instrument that rates areas of medication side effects on a five-point Likert scale; provides scores for seven different areas of medication side effects
Risk of violence		
HCR-20 (Historical Clinical Risk Management Scale) (Jaber & Mahmoud 2015)	Assess risk of violence	A 20-item clinician-rated instrument that combines historical, current clinical and future risk factors
Non-specific mental health problems		
GHQ 12 (General Health Questionnaire) (Tseliou et al. 2018)	Detect risk of developing mental illness in primary care populations	A 12-item clinician-rated instrument that provides a single cut-off score indicating possible mental illness

Standardisation refers to the statistical evaluation of instruments aimed at ensuring their reliability and validity. Standardised instruments can be regarded as screening tools that alert clinicians to a problematic area of mental health and signal the need for further assessment. An important consideration in using standardised instruments is that they should not be regarded as complete assessments: they do not replace comprehensive assessment. Instead, they augment clinical assessment by providing a uniform means of measuring one aspect of functioning. Most instruments have cut-off scores; that is, scores that indicate levels of severity, need for treatment or need for further assessment. Standardised instruments contribute to assessment in several ways. They provide a benchmark – for example, of mood or cognitive functioning – and a basis for comparing the same area of functioning at some future time. Comparing scores over time allows the clinician to determine any improvement or deterioration in the area measured. This can be very helpful in assessing the response to medication or other interventions, or to determine whether the consumer's problems are escalating, indicating a need for a review of the treatment plan. Standardised measures also allow clinicians to communicate about the extent of a problem, knowing that each is using the same criteria to estimate the level of severity. Another advantage is that they remind clinicians of questions they should ask in assessment. For example, the Alcohol Use Disorder Inventory Test (AUDIT) asks 10 specific questions about alcohol use; without this tool, clinicians may not remember all 10 questions in the course of an interview.

Instruments can be either clinician- or consumer-rated. Self-rated instruments enable consumers to report various experiences to the nurse that they might find hard to express in words. For example, someone who is very depressed might find it difficult to verbalise their low mood but might be able to indicate low mood on a rating form that requires only a tick. If you are using a standardised instrument, take the opportunity to discuss the instrument with the consumer and use the findings to develop collaborative means of addressing significant problems. As clinical problems improve, the changes measured on a standardised instrument can provide the consumer with reassurance of their improvement. On a cautionary note, it is important to consider the conditions under which a standardised instrument is used. We all feel anxious if we feel we are being assessed, and consumers may feel that the findings of an instrument will be used to show there is something wrong with them. Anxiety about completing a rating instrument will adversely affect the results, so it is important that the nurse creates optimal conditions for using the instrument and takes account of factors such as age, literacy level, sensory deficits, pain and discomfort and the explanation provided for using the test.

Diaries

Diaries are records of important experiences that are kept by consumers for their personal use, or in collaboration with clinicians. A diary might record feelings, thoughts, activity level, interpersonal interactions, food intake or other self-observations. If you are going to use a diary as part of an assessment you need to explain the purpose to the consumer, clarify what is to be recorded and discuss how the diary will contribute to care. Diaries can be helpful in developing your understanding of consumers because they contain information that might not be accurately remembered. They also help by actively engaging the person in their care. In addition to contributing to assessment, diaries are a therapeutic intervention because they help increase the consumer's self-awareness of important areas of functioning. Mood diaries have been developed as applications for smartphones (Aguilera et al. 2015), with the additional advantage that information can be shared with a therapist or clinician (see www.anxiety.org.nz).

Direct observation

Of all the professionals involved in mental health care, nurses have the most direct contact with consumers. In inpatient settings this can include contact in the context of activities of living such as care of the bed area, meals and social activities. Other forms of contact are in providing medication, running therapeutic activities such as groups or teaching sessions and discussing issues such as leave requests. In community settings nurses may have contact with consumers in their homes, in community clinics or at a consumer's workplace. Any contact with a consumer is an opportunity to make direct observations of mental state, physical health, socialisation patterns, side effects of medication and other areas. Direct observations can be 'triangulated' with the consumer's self-reports, the observations of other nurses or clinicians and observations of third parties such as friends or family members. Nurses can gain a great deal of information from other clinicians and from clinical notes, but there is no substitute for seeing, talking to and interacting with the consumer. They may seem very different from the picture suggested from other sources, or from your past understanding.

Information from third parties

In addition to information obtained directly from the consumer, nurses use additional information from friends and family members, other clinical services and clinical records. In obtaining information from family members you need to be mindful of confidentiality and potential conflicts between family members. Some consumers welcome the involvement of their family; others prefer not to have family involved (Tambuyzer & Van Audenhove 2013). Using a collaborative approach, nurses can explore the potential contribution of family members to care and the important role played by families in supporting their loved one. Families have a unique perspective on the care of their loved one and often remind mental health clinicians that it is they who know the consumer best. From the above description of the methods of mental health nursing assessment, note that information contributing to an understanding of the consumer as a person comes from a variety of sources. These include consumers, nurses' subjective and objective observations, interviews, information from rating scales and information from a range of other people and clinical records. No one source of information is enough on its own, and some of the information from various sources may appear to conflict. The skill of mental health nursing assessment is to use the range of information available to build a picture of the consumer as a person, to develop a shared understanding of what problems the consumer is seeking help with and a plan of how the nurse and other members of the multidisciplinary team can help with the identified problems. Nurse's story 7.2 illustrates how the scope and purpose of nursing assessment can be expanded.

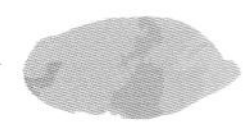   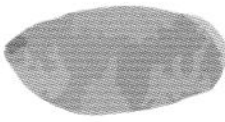 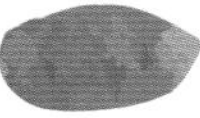

NURSE'S STORY 7.2

Antony Abbey

Reflecting on my early exposure to assessment as a student mental health nurse in 1981, I observed it initially as a linear and two-dimensional procedure. It appeared at the time to sit definitively within the context of gathering information. Clients were on the receiving end of this activity. They (or others who knew of them) would provide information in accordance with a set of questions and observations. Nursing care, although linked to the assessment, was a discrete and subsequent step within an overall process.

I discovered along the way that assessment becomes buoyant and three-dimensional when it allows the client to explore the less familiar and sometimes unknown corridors of his psyche. When this occurs, there is an opportunity for discovery, catharsis and positive change. In this sense, assessment becomes a therapy in its own right. Good questions are enabling, as are the variety of standardised assessment tools that are available. It is also useful to approach the assessment with a comprehensive framework in mind. But we should not be restricted and contained by these tools. We should stop, open up and listen to the client's story, picking up on cues and gently guiding, much like the style that is eloquently described by Brown (1995) in her conversational approach to the assessment interview.

Take the example of Mr C, a man in his 40s who was admitted to the general hospital with severe headache, left-sided weakness and paraesthesia. After medical causes were ruled out, I was asked, within the context of my psychiatric liaison nurse role, if I could help to unravel the mystery of this presentation. Mr C's personal story was one of hard work, stoicism and battling along in the face of any adversity. Emotional expression was not a language that he knew. His narrative was also one of significant recent stressors. It was a story of loss, redundancy and housing and financial struggles. Within the safety of a confidential and non-judgemental setting, and enabled by a conversational approach, Mr C discovered a dialectic side to his story. He discovered that he had been caged in by his emotional illiteracy and 'stiff upper lip' rule. He realised that it didn't have to be that way. Supported with a further three or four sessions, with a focus on learning the language of emotion, Mr C was freed from his rule. He was supported also with developing new tools to help him accept and deal with emotional distress so that he could perhaps be liberated from his somatic manifestation.

Mr C is now free of his neurological symptoms and is working successfully through many of the stressors that he struggled with. So, for this clinician, assessment and intervention work together in partnership but also have interchangeable properties. Assessment as a therapy is one of the most satisfying interventions that a psychiatric nurse can deliver.

Comprehensive assessment process

This section explains the steps of the comprehensive assessment process. Most services will have a template for initial assessment and may have an additional template for risk assessment. The content of these templates will vary between services, so you will need to be familiar with the models used in your own service, as well as with more general assessment issues. A comprehensive mental health assessment involves collecting a wide range of information from the consumer and from other sources.

Identifying information

This is the first part of the comprehensive assessment and includes key demographic information about the consumer including their name, age, gender, employment, ethnicity, main support persons, living situation, address and contact details. Although some of these details will previously have been recorded the nurse needs to ensure they are accurate.

Presenting problem

The presenting problem is the issue that causes the person to present for mental health care. The presenting problem should always be expressed from the consumer's perspective, not from the perspective of the health professional. For example, a consumer may seem to be very depressed when first seen, but their reason for presenting might be expressed as 'I'm desperate. I can't go on.' In the case of a consumer who does not agree that they need mental health care, their presenting problem might be: 'They forced me to come here. I don't need to see anyone.'

HISTORY OF PRESENTING PROBLEM

The history of the presenting problem is concerned with the events leading up to the assessment: the onset, duration, course and severity. Once again, it is important to try to get an understanding of the history as the consumer has experienced it and not only as the health professional sees it. Factors that have led to the presentation will be varied and may be positive (e.g. winning the lottery) or negative (e.g. losing a job) because both positive and negative events can trigger mental health presentations. It is also important to focus on recent precipitants as triggers; for example, the context of a presenting problem may be long-standing relationship discord, but the cause for presentation may be that the spouse has left recently. In documenting the history of the presenting problem, pay attention to the chronological order of events. Consumers may relate events in order of their significance, rather than in chronological order, and while the meaning and significance of events are very important, the order of events is also important in understanding how the presenting problem has developed. Exploring the history of the presenting problem should include a review of symptoms of the most common mental illnesses such as mood disorder, anxiety, psychosis or disorders of cognition. Some symptoms will be obvious, but others might need to be elicited by asking probing questions. As much as possible these questions should be incorporated into an interview; however, you might also need to make a direct enquiry about some symptoms such as unusual perceptions. Factors of significance will not be limited to clinical factors (mood, thoughts, perceptions) but will also include personal factors such as changes in relationships, interests and activities. The nurse should consider the consumer's self-help and support strategies, and how effective these have been. Consumers may have used previously learned methods of stress management and distress tolerance and may have sought support from friends and family members. Other responses can include increased use of prescribed medication, use of non-prescribed medication and use of alcohol or other drugs.

Mental health history

Information gathered for the mental health history is concerned with the consumer's previous mental health concerns. It is important to ask about past attempts the consumer has made to receive help for their mental health. This information should be documented chronologically. Most people will have sought help from various sources at some point in their life; it is important to be aware of this because it helps to better comprehend the nature, longevity and understanding that the person has given their concerns. People may ask a chemist or health-food shop for assistance with symptoms relating to mental health. Some may have been to a naturopath, chiropractor or massage therapist, others to their GP, church minister or school or university counsellor. For some people the main source of help will be family, extended family or their own cultural advisors. All this information is valid and adds to our understanding. It is important to ask what treatment the consumer has tried and what the results were. If the consumer has had psychological therapy or has been prescribed medication such as antidepressants, this should be recorded along with the response. A helpful way to explore past treatment is to enquire whether the consumer found it helpful, how long they had the treatment for and (if relevant) their reasons for discontinuing. Hospital admissions and contacts with community mental health services should also be documented in this part of the assessment. If the consumer has had previous admissions or periods of community care, their legal status should be recorded. Areas of risk should be explored, including history of self-harm or suicidality, history of violence towards others and any history of victimisation such as exposure to domestic violence or assault from others.

Substance use history

Taking a comprehensive substance use history is essential because all substances influence mental health. Some issues of substance use may have been discussed in relation to past mental health experiences and these areas should be explored in more detail (see Chapter 11). Rates of coexisting mental illness and substance use are very high (Gilbert et al. 2014), and substance use will complicate recovery from a mental illness. In some cases, substance use may have precipitated mental illness, or may be a factor in perpetuating mental illness. In taking a substance use history you will need to name the specific substances the consumer has used. Consumers may be concerned that information about use of illegal substances will be passed onto the police, so the assessment should include reassurance that the information is sought for the purposes of health care and will remain confidential. In exploring substance use, consumers should be asked for specific information about the level of use; for example, the statement, 'I don't drink much' could have different meanings for different people. Ask clarifying questions to establish the level and pattern of alcohol or other drug consumption. There are many useful screening tools for assisting with this assessment. Consumers can be asked to complete a brief questionnaire such as the AUDIT (Babor et al. 2001). Assessing substance use provides an opportunity to explore readiness to change using a model such as motivational interviewing (DiClemente et al. 2017) and to discuss whether referral to a substance use agency might be helpful.

Critical thinking challenge 7.4

Mental health assessment involves asking consumers about areas of their lives usually considered private and personal such as questions about sexuality, use of drugs and experiences of trauma. How comfortable do you feel about exploring these areas with consumers? Why is it important that nurses can overcome discomfort about asking very personal questions? What are some of the risks of asking very personal questions and how can those risks be managed?

Family history

It is important to ask about the mental health history of the family, particularly close relatives such as parents, grandparents, siblings, aunts, uncles and cousins. We are interested in knowing this for two reasons. First, some of the major mental health conditions are known to have familial patterns (e.g. schizophrenia, bipolar disorder and depression). These conditions are more common in people with close relatives with the disorder (Rasic et al. 2013). Second, we know that the environment that a person grows up and lives in affects their health generally and their mental health specifically. As we grow, we all role-model our ways of living, behaving and coping on significant others around us. For example, a child raised in a family with a depressed parent who took to their bed for prolonged periods may replicate this behaviour as their way of coping with the world, and this may lead to a mental health presentation. Enquiring about family history can begin with a question such as, 'Has anyone else in your family had problems like these?' The consumer's answers can be explored to gain more detailed information and to gain an understanding of the consumer's past and current relationships with family members.

Developmental and social history

This area of assessment considers the stages of the consumer's life and their possible influence on personality, coping style and the current problem. Understanding experiences at various life stages is an important component of comprehensive assessment. The developmental history can take a chronological approach, although some social stressors may relate to early life experiences and so may have been discussed at other stages of the comprehensive assessment process. Areas of assessment include infancy and early childhood, early family experiences, past relationships with siblings, developmental milestones, peer relationships and friendships, experiences of schooling, academic achievements and relationships with parents and caregivers. Following the life course will lead to discussions about employment, university or other study, intimate relationships and sexuality. Adult relationships are important, especially any pattern of difficulty in maintaining long-term relationships, and relationships with children. For older adults the nurse should discuss later life milestones such as retirement, socialisation patterns, relationships and illnesses, especially those that limit mobility or social functioning or that cause sensory deficits.

Trauma

Trauma is a major contributor to developing mental illness and is a common experience among people with mental illness (Duhig et al. 2015). Experiences of trauma may emerge in any clinical interaction. In many cases you will not need to make a specific enquiry about trauma, but you do need to be prepared to respond empathically to disclosures about trauma and to offer any further intervention or referral if necessary. Consumers commonly feel their experience of trauma is discounted in healthcare services, so any disclosure should be validated, together

Historical anecdote 7.2: Freud and psychoanalysis

One of the most influential paradigms of the 20th century was psychoanalysis, developed by the Austrian neurologist Sigmund Freud (1856–1939). Psychoanalysis was one of the first attempts to assess mental health from a developmental perspective. Although Freud noticed that several of his clients had experienced trauma, he rejected the idea that trauma might be a source of distress and mental ill health. Instead Freud proposed that a person's mental health is heavily influenced by unconscious motivating forces. This premise suggests that all behaviour has meaning and may therefore be understood. According to psychoanalysis, human personality can be understood as comprising three parts: the id, the ego and the superego. These components are thought to develop within the personality by the age of 5 years and often includes inner turmoil, giving rise to anxiety. In response, psychological defence mechanisms are unconsciously created by the personality to deal with such anxiety, which can lead to episodes of mental ill health.

Read more about it: *Westen D 1998 The scientific legacy of Sigmund Freud: toward a psychodynamically informed psychological science. Psychological Bulletin 124(3): 333*

with the opportunity for further exploration. Trauma can take many forms including bullying, physical violence, sexual assault, intimate partner violence, neglect, exposure to traumatic events such as war or military conflict, torture or refugee experiences. Trauma should be approached with tact and sensitivity. Clinicians need to be alert for indications that the consumer does not currently feel safe to discuss experiences of trauma and in such cases should leave exploration of trauma until a more appropriate time. This decision needs to be communicated to the consumer, together with an explanation of how the consumer can seek further help.

Cultural issues

Cultural issues can have a major impact on the expression of mental distress and illness and on consumers' engagement with mental health care (O'Brien et al. 2016). The populations of Australia and New Zealand have increasingly culturally diverse populations, comprising indigenous peoples, descendants of early immigrants and significant populations of new immigrants. Assessment should identify consumers' cultural experiences and seek to understand how these issues might impact on the expression of distress and on care and treatment. Cultural difference between clinicians and consumers can be a barrier to assessment, and clinicians should consider whether the presence of a translator or cultural support person will help facilitate assessment. Clinicians should be cautious in identifying consumers' cultural needs and should check these with each consumer and seek advice if unsure.

Critical thinking challenge 7.5

Consider your own cultural beliefs and practices. How comfortable would you feel discussing these beliefs with a mental health professional? How can you help consumers to feel comfortable discussing these areas as part of their mental health care?

Spirituality

As with culture, spirituality is an important aspect of mental health and should be considered in every comprehensive assessment (Barber 2018). Spirituality can include membership or identification with organised religions or faith communities, or non-religious spiritual beliefs. Spiritual beliefs are important in helping consumers give meaning to their experiences of mental distress and illness. Faith communities are also significant sources of informal support. Consideration of spirituality in assessment can include the consumer's developmental experience of religion, current engagement with religious practices and personal belief systems. Some consumers may say they do not have spiritual beliefs, and this expression should be respected and recorded.

Forensic history

It is not unusual for people with mental illness to have had contact with the police or the legal system and possibly contact with forensic mental health services. These aspects of the personal history may emerge spontaneously or may need to be the subject of specific assessment questions. In the context of an assessment interview, it may become clear from responses to more general questions that the consumer has no history of police involvement, in which case no specific enquiry is needed. In addition to noting specific events, such as any arrests, convictions and sentencing, it is important to know the consumer's current perceptions of events involving legal issues and whether there are any outstanding charges. Forensic history can help in documenting any events involving interpersonal violence and form part of risk assessment. See Chapter 26 for further discussion of forensic mental health issues.

General health history

It is important to gather the consumer's medical history to check for health problems and medical comorbidities that might be affecting their mental health. This is a good chance to ask about medication use that might have been missed earlier in the assessment. The health history should include childhood illnesses, any current or chronic illnesses, history of head injury or loss of consciousness, and known allergies. Having a systematic approach to the medical history will help avoid missing important findings. Thorough questioning may uncover health problems that you might not have considered; for example, pain is an often-overlooked problem that unless specifically asked about can go undetected and may impact greatly on a person's wellbeing. Taking a health history is also an opportunity for discussion about physical issues that might not directly affect the person's mental health but may require attention. It is particularly important to ask about head injuries and any loss of consciousness, including general anaesthetics. Uncovering this information will add to your clinical picture and help the team to decide if seeking historical medical information is pertinent to treatment planning. It may also indicate the need for diagnostic tests such as computed tomography (CT) imaging of the head or psychometric assessments. People with serious mental illness have high rates of physical disorders (Scott et al. 2016), so this part of the comprehensive assessment is an opportunity to reinforce important health messages such as undertaking regular exercise, smoking cessation, cardiovascular screening and sexual health screening. Discussion of physical health issues can also help in checking whether the consumer is enrolled in a primary care practice and is receiving regular primary health care. Chapter 18 provides an extensive discussion of physical health issues experienced by people with mental illness.

Physical health assessment

Like other areas of assessment described in this chapter, physical health assessment is a core skill of mental health nurses. In some research studies mental health nurses have reported that they do not feel well prepared or confident to assess physical health (Gray & Brown 2017; Wand et al. 2018); however, there has been increasing interest among mental health nurses in responding to this need (Dickens et al. 2019). Mental health consumers experience high rates of physical disorders (Bhugra & Ventriglio 2017) and reduced life expectancy (Cunningham et al. 2014). In addition, mental health consumers are frequently prescribed second-generation antipsychotic agents that are associated with higher risk of metabolic syndrome (Wand 2019). Other medications such as clozapine, lithium and sodium valproate require skills of physical health assessment to ensure safe monitoring (see Chapter 18). Sound physical health assessment skills also provide the basis for health promotion interventions in areas such as smoking cessation, exercise regimens, weight management and diet. Physical health assessment should include a health history (see above), both of the consumer's health and that of their immediate family, with special attention to factors that might place the consumer at risk of health problems common in mental health consumers such as cardiovascular disease and metabolic syndrome. Physical health assessment should include a systems review to ensure no areas of health problems are missed. You can use the top-to-toe assessment that you have been introduced to for physical health screening to frame your thinking and questions (see Box 7.3).

Laboratory investigations

Laboratory investigations are part of any comprehensive assessment and have several purposes including to: understand the role of physical illness in the current presentation; establish adherence to prescribed medication; assess organ functioning and how it might be impacted by prescribed medication (e.g. the effect of liver functioning on the half-life of benzodiazepines); identify potentially toxic blood levels of prescribed medication (e.g. lithium carbonate); and identify any use of non-prescribed drugs. Laboratory tests are used in initial assessment and to monitor the impact of prescribed medication (e.g. the development of markers of metabolic syndrome). Nurses should be familiar with the most used laboratory tests and be able to interpret the results of tests using knowledge of the consumer's general health status and the accepted range of values for the particular test. Most results are reported along with the normal range. Full lists of reference ranges are available at www.labtests.co.nz and at www.mps.com.au.

Other investigations

In addition to laboratory tests, there are a range of investigations that may be considered as part of a comprehensive assessment. For example, every consumer should have an electrocardiogram (ECG), both to assess their baseline cardiac functioning and to identify any vulnerability to the effects of prescribed medication. Other tests that might be considered are a CT scan to exclude space-occupying lesions or other pathology, magnetic resonance imaging (MRI) for more detailed imaging of organs, and an electroencephalogram (EEG) to assess possible abnormalities of brain function. A range of other tests may be considered based on the consumer's presenting symptoms.

Historical anecdote 7.3: Assessment and the clinical gaze

In the 18th century clinical work involved doctors listening to patients' stories of symptoms and illness. Diagnoses were made based on indirect evidence rather than direct observation of pathological changes. The advent of new technologies and the proliferation of hospitals as the major site of medical practice meant that assessment shifted in focus from the patient to the disease. Historian Michel Foucault has referred to the new focus on pathology as the 'clinical gaze'. The clinical gaze made the patient's story less important because the 'truth' of their illness was seen to lie inside the patient's body, in diseased organs and tissues, not in their experience of symptoms. Psychiatry has long struggled with this notion of the clinical gaze. While there have been many attempts to provide biological understandings of mental illness, clinical practice in assessment still relies on listening to the patient's story and understanding symptoms in the context of the patient's life and culture. Comment is frequently made that psychiatry is unlike other branches of medicine because there are no objective phenomena (blood tests, laboratory studies) that can be observed to support a diagnosis. In nursing we focus first on the patient as a person. Disease, even where it is present, is not the primary focus of nursing. The clinical gaze of the 18th century helps us to understand diseases, but it is not the basis of nursing assessment.

Read more about it: *Foucault M 1994 The birth of the clinic: an archaeology of medical perception. Vintage Books, New York*

Mental state assessment

In this chapter the term 'mental state assessment' is used in preference to 'mental state examination', as the latter implies an objectified evaluation of the consumer's mental state, whereas we wish to promote an understanding based on an engaged relationship. Mental state assessment is part of every comprehensive assessment and provides a statement of the consumer's emotional and cognitive functioning at a single point in time (Huline-Dickens 2013; Soltan & Girguis 2017). The importance of focusing the mental state assessment on a single point in time is that it can provide a point of comparison for future assessments. Other elements of the consumer's presentation are excluded from the mental state assessment, such as social functioning, history and risk. Many elements of a mental state assessment can be integrated into routine nursing interactions such as the initial assessment interview, reviewing a plan of care or discussing recovery goals. During these interactions the nurse will be able to observe the consumer's behaviour, appearance and mood, and will gain a good understanding of thought content. However, some elements of mental state assessment require specific enquiry on the part of the nurse. For example, the nurse may need to ask direct questions to test their impression that a consumer is disoriented or has problems with memory.

Mental state assessment requires both objective observation and empathic communication. Appearance and behaviour can be objectively observed, while to assess the consumer's mood the nurse will need to establish rapport and enter the consumer's emotional world. Many situational variables affect mental state (e.g. an unfamiliar environment, anxiety or pain), and these can be considered when the findings of the mental state assessment are interpreted.

The structured format used for recording a mental state assessment does not mean that the mental state assessment requires a question-and-answer interview. In fact, the opposite is true: a supportive therapeutic conversation will probably provide most of the information required for a mental state assessment. Additional information can be elicited, if necessary, by direct questions, but these should flow naturally from the interaction with the consumer. A standardised measure of cognitive functioning can be used to augment a mental state assessment (refer back to Table 7.2 for standardised assessments of cognitive functioning).

There is no set format for recording a mental state assessment, but we suggest the BATOMI mnemonic as a useful means of organising the findings (Behaviour and appearance; Affect and mood; Thought and speech; Orientation, cognition and sensorium; Memory; Insight and judgement). An example of a documented mental state assessment using this mnemonic is provided in Box 7.2. The following sections outline the types of observations that can contribute to a mental state assessment.

Box 7.2 Documentation of mental state assessment

The following assessment records the mental state of a woman assessed following an overdose of prescribed medication and medical treatment in an emergency department.

BEHAVIOUR AND APPEARANCE

54-year-old European woman who is attentive to interview, although a little sleepy from lingering effects of overdose. Looks older than her chronological age. Dressed in jeans and T-shirt. Is well groomed and appears well cared for. No unusual movements or mannerisms. Maintains good eye contact. Tearful at times.

AFFECT AND MOOD

Affect sad. Intermittently brighter in response to interview. Mood is objectively depressed. She describes her mood as low, rates it at 4 on a 1–10 scale where 1 is the lowest it has been. Not irritable.

THOUGHT AND SPEECH

Thoughts focus on recent events, and her perception that she is not well supported by family members. Returns to the theme of past long-term relationship that ended 12 months ago. Ruminates about abandonment. Limited ability to focus on problem solving in relation to current stressors. Depressive themes: Loneliness, undeserving of help, lack of confidence in future. Slow rate of thought and talk. No delusional ideas expressed. No unusual perceptions. Has occasional thoughts of suicide but stresses she would not act on these. Has no specific plan. Gives involvement with grandchildren as a protective factor.

ORIENTATION, COGNITION AND SENSORIUM

Alert and oriented to time, place and person. Knows her whereabouts, and the date and time of day. Accurately identifies staff by role or name. Able to perform 'serial sevens' (subtracting in sevens starting from 100).

MEMORY

Both short- and long-term memory are intact. She remembers events of the past few days, and more distant. Able to recall three objects after 5 minutes.

INSIGHT AND JUDGEMENT

Identifies that her mood is currently low and has been low for several weeks. Is aware that alcohol has a disinhibiting role when her mood is low and increases suicidal thoughts. Accepts referral to mental health service and need to review current antidepressant medication. Judgement is unimpaired when not intoxicated.

Behaviour and appearance

Behaviour and appearance refer to the consumer's general appearance and activity. Begin with the most obvious aspects of behaviour such as clothing, grooming and hygiene, evidence of self-care or neglect and distinguishing marks such as tattoos, piercings and notable physical features such as scars. This section also includes observations of motor activity and behaviour such as posture, eye contact, restlessness, tearfulness, nervous mannerisms (e.g. tremors and shaking) and behaviour indicating level of interest in the interaction. The consumer's attitude towards the assessment process can be seen in their appearance, responses, body language and facial expressions. Consider not only what you are observing but how appropriate it is, considering the setting of the assessment. For example, in an assessment in an emergency department you might expect someone to look dishevelled and perhaps sleepy (at least initially). Anxiety about the assessment process will also influence behaviour.

Affect and mood

Affect and mood have various definitions that sometimes conflict. Both refer to emotional state, with mood referring to sustained emotional state (especially because it is experienced by the individual) and affect referring to expressed emotion – something that the clinician can observe. A skilled clinician can often gauge a consumer's mood, especially if a good rapport has been developed and the consumer feels safe to communicate their emotional state. However, it is important that consumers are given the opportunity to describe their mood. Because this may be difficult for people who are depressed, consumers can be asked to rate their mood on a scale of 1 to 10, where 1 is the lowest it has ever been and 10 is the highest. Emotional state can be appropriate or inappropriate to the assessment context – for example, a consumer who is elated and buoyant despite an objectively formal context such as a clinical review. Terms sometimes used to describe affect and mood are dysphoric, flat, elevated, depressed, anxious, labile (fluctuating without obvious reason) and restricted. The term 'euthymic' is often used if the consumer's mood is neither happy nor sad. In assessing mood, you are using your own emotional state as a means of understanding the emotional state of the consumer. Nurses who have established an empathic understanding of a consumer will be best able to assess that consumer's emotional state.

Thought and speech

Thought and speech are usually described together (sometimes called 'thought and talk') and focus on the rate, form and content of thought and the nature of the consumer's verbal communications. It is not possible to assess thoughts directly, so thought is assessed through the indirect medium of speech. Speech is more easily observed because it is the major medium of communication. Aspects of speech are rate (speed of speech), volume, amount of speech, tone and content. Speech that is rapid or slowed, very quiet or loud, hesitant or limited may be significant in assessing mental state and should be recorded. For example, rapid or pressured speech might indicate mania or anxiety; quiet or hesitant speech might indicate low mood or anxiety; and loud speech might indicate anger or suspicion. It is important to note whether speech is goal-directed or circumstantial and tangential. This part of the mental state assessment (sometimes called 'perception') also records any delusional ideas such as ideas of being influenced by others, paranoid ideas, thoughts that radio or television news is referring to the individual and other forms of disordered thinking. Auditory or other hallucinations are noted in this section of the assessment. It is helpful to describe the nature of voices, whether the consumer feels threatened by them or whether they perform an important function for the consumer, such as providing company.

Orientation, cognition and sensorium

Orientation is easily assessed and may not need direct questioning. Orientation refers to understanding of time, place and person and can be assessed by asking questions about time of day and place. Because these might seem odd questions to some consumers it is important to explain that these are part of routine assessment. Cognition refers to the ability to recognise and manipulate information and to perform tasks of reasoning. General interview questions will give some evidence of cognitive functioning. Cognition can also be tested by asking the consumer to perform individual tasks from standardised assessments such as 'serial sevens' or naming different common objects (e.g. pen, book, watch). Disturbances in sensorium are likely to be evident in many interactions, especially in structured interviews. Sensorium can be assessed by observing the consumer's attentiveness and ability to stay focused on tasks. Consumers with an altered level of consciousness may show limited ability to attend and fluctuation in attention and awareness.

Memory

Memory involves the capacity to recall information and extends from initial registration of information to recall of information that is years old. Registration can be assessed by asking the consumer to repeat back to the nurse the names of three unrelated common objects (e.g. pen, clock, tree). Short-term memory can by assessed by asking for recall of the same three objects after 5 minutes, during which time other discussion takes place. Finally, long-term (or remote) memory involves recall of years-old information such as events from childhood or adolescence.

Insight and judgement

Insight can be a controversial area of assessment because it is sometimes interpreted as a test of whether the consumer agrees with the clinician's opinion about what is happening, in particular whether or not the consumer is mentally ill (Diesfeld & McKenna 2007; Lysaker et al. 2018). Insight is best understood as a consumer's perception of their current situation. It is not always helpful to simply record 'lacks insight' because this does not tell us what the consumer believes about their problems. Judgement refers to the person's ability to act safely and with understanding of the possible consequences of their actions. A confused person may have markedly impaired judgement and hence be unsafe unless in a situation where they can be observed.

Clinical formulation

Once all assessment information has been gathered you will have both a subjective impression of the consumer as a person and a set of objective data about the consumer. You will also understand the consumer's perceptions of their current problems and how those problems relate to the consumer's life history. Clinical formulation is the process of bringing this information together to develop an individualised explanatory account of the consumer. Different models of psychological therapy often have their own model of formulation – for example, the cognitive formulation used in cognitive therapy (Johnstone 2018). In this section we discuss a more general model of formulation, but one that can incorporate psychological understandings of the person.

Clinical formulation is a potentially complex process, but fortunately there are several models available to assist nurses in writing clinical formulations and developing skills in this aspect of assessment. Biological, psychological and social theories help explain the relationships between the various aspects of the consumer's history and presentation. Clinical formulation is not undertaken by the clinician alone, although in some literature (e.g. Selzer & Ellen 2014) this is how formulation is described. However, as Crowe et al. (2008) explain, clinical formulation is an opportunity for the nurse and the consumer to discuss their different perspectives and negotiate both common understandings and differences in understandings. If the assessment has been a collaborative process throughout, there will be a strong enough relationship between the nurse and the consumer to allow this negotiation to occur.

A useful model for developing clinical formulation is the 4 P's model described by Selzer and Ellen (2010; 2014) and shown in Table 7.3. In this model the 4 P's (predisposing, precipitating, perpetuating and protective) are used to describe factors that contributed to the current problems, factors that contribute to the persistence of the problem and those that protect the person from the effects of the problem. In addition to the 4 P's, this model allows for consideration of biological, psychological and social factors. Theoretical and philosophical understandings, such as learning theory, adaptation theory and recovery philosophy, can be used to interpret the contribution of the various factors. Using this model, the clinician can focus on factors in any cell of the matrix, depending on what the significant factors are for the individual consumer. With some consumers there will be a greater emphasis on social factors, while with others psychological or biological factors will be more important.

Clinical formulation is written in narrative form. The clinician and the consumer work together to reach agreement regarding how different aspects of the consumer's history affect the current presentation. It may not always be possible to reach agreement. In such cases, the formulation is written to reflect the different perspectives of the clinician and the consumer (Crowe et al. 2008). The written formulation concludes with a statement about the possible future for the consumer and focuses on how strengths and protective factors can be enhanced by support from clinical services. Writing clear, clinical formulations takes practice. A typical difficulty encountered by clinicians is attempting to include too much information. Remember, the clinical history contains all the relevant information about the consumer. The formulation is a selective summary: only the most pertinent information should be included, and the emphasis is on how the various factors interact.

Diagnosis

A diagnosis is a definition of a problem once all available information has been considered (Zanotti & Chiffi 2015). A diagnosis is, first, identifying diseases via signs and symptoms and by other investigations, and second, developing an opinion or conclusion based on those investigations. The current model of psychiatric diagnosis most employed in Australia and New Zealand is the *Diagnostic and Statistical Manual of Mental Disorders* (DSM), now in its fifth edition (American Psychiatric Association 2013). In most clinical practice settings, psychiatric diagnoses are assigned by medical practitioners, not always by psychiatrists, especially in primary care. Nurses need to be familiar with the diagnostic criteria of the more common mental illnesses and of the diagnostic reasoning process applied to making these diagnoses. A full list of DSM-5 diagnoses and criteria is available on the American Psychiatric Association website (www.psychiatry.org).

Critical thinking challenge 7.6

Psychiatric diagnosis is a process of assigning a category to a consumer's unique subjective experiences and problems in living. How can you work with consumers to help them understand the process of diagnosis and to consider whether their diagnosis accurately reflects their experiences?

TABLE 7.3 Clinical formulation

FACTOR	BIOLOGICAL	PSYCHOLOGICAL	SOCIAL
Predisposing	Genetic Birth trauma Brain injury Illness – psychiatric, physical Medication Drugs/alcohol	Pain Personality Modelling defences (unconscious) Coping strategies Self-esteem Body image Cognition Trauma	Socioeconomic status Culture/spirituality
Precipitating	Medication Drugs/alcohol Trauma Acute illness	Pain Stage of life Grief Loss Treatment Stressors	Work Finances Connections Relationships
Perpetuating	Any of the above factors that are continuing	Any of the above factors that are continuing	Any of the above factors that are continuing
Protective	Physical health	Engagement Insight Adherence Coping strategies Intelligence	Group belonging and affiliations Family and social relationships

Adapted from Selzer & Ellen 2010

Triage

Triage refers to the assessment that takes place when a consumer first contacts a health service. A consumer may present with self-harm, hearing voices, self-neglect or suicidal thoughts. Presentations may involve use of alcohol or other substances. Triage assessments may occur in the emergency department, at community mental health clinics, at ambulance callouts, in primary care settings or in private homes. Triage may also be conducted by telephone. The aims of triage are to establish how urgent the problem is, any immediate safety issues and the immediate priorities for health service response.

In an emergency department setting, clinicians may use an instrument such as the Australasian Triage Scale (see www.acem.org.au), which has five categories of increasing urgency of response, with a response time associated with each category. However, the Australasian Triage Scale has been found to have relatively low reliability with mental health consumers (Broadbent et al. 2010) and an instrument more sensitive to the needs of these consumers, the Victorian Emergency Department Mental Health Triage Tool, has since been developed (Sands et al. 2014). Questions to be addressed in mental health triage are outlined in Box 7.3. Triage is usually followed by comprehensive assessment, once immediate issues of safety have been addressed.

Box 7.3 Important questions for mental health triage

- Does the consumer feel safe in their current situation?
- Is the consumer at imminent risk of self-harm?
- Is the consumer at risk of harming others?
- If there are risks of harm to self or others, does the consumer have the means in their possession to carry out that harm?
- Is the consumer likely to stay where they are or are they likely to leave?
- How soon does the consumer need to be seen?
- Are there physical health problems that may be contributing to the presentation?

Risk assessment

Risk assessment is a requirement of most mental health service providers and it is therefore important that nurses understand the language and limitations of risk assessment. However, there is controversy about the value of risk assessment (Wand 2015) and about the ability of clinicians to accurately identify consumers at high risk and to predict the likelihood of adverse events. The most commonly identified areas of risk are risk to self through self-harm or neglect, risk of violence to others and risk of victimisation. In inpatient settings nurses also need to assess risk of absconding. Risk assessment is not a separate form of assessment: it is a process that selectively draws on information obtained in the comprehensive assessment to identify the existence of risk, the level of risk and a plan to manage risk.

A very good summary of risk assessment and management, including the limitations of risk assessment, is provided by Flewett (2010). Flewett makes the important point that risk assessment and management are not about eliminating risk or about predicting the occurrence of adverse events. Rather, they are about understanding the factors that contribute to risk and working with consumers to manage that risk. Nurses also need to balance awareness of risk with the positive value of risk in the lives of consumers and of the value of learning from the consequences of decisions (Morgan & Andrews 2016). Risk assessment is further discussed in Chapter 4.

Assessing strengths

Assessment of strengths considers the personal resources consumers can access to manage their mental health concerns (Rapp & Goscha 2012). Many consumers have had years of experience of adversity and self-management and have developed individual and interpersonal strategies for preventing and responding to their issues. Consumers who are newly presenting to mental health services will also have developed life skills that will be valuable to them in coping with their mental health challenges. As in all areas of mental health nursing assessment, developing a therapeutic relationship is essential for understanding the strengths a consumer may have. At times of crisis, consumers may feel they have no available strategies, so it is important initially to respond to the consumer's current concerns and distress before exploring strengths. Assessing strengths involves inviting the consumer to identify their individual strategies and how they have responded to life challenges in the past. Rather than being the expert, the nurse needs to ask what they can learn from the consumer. Examples of individual strengths that consumers may identify include pleasurable activities that provide distraction and reduce stress, the availability of family members and friends, spiritual beliefs, and skills learned in stress management and problem solving.

CONSUMER'S STORY 7.1
Gareth Edwards

I'd never been in a police cell before. Without a comparison, or a Lonely Planet guide to incarceration, I assumed it was your bog-standard police cell. Concrete block walls painted institutional grey with hint of drab, a formidable steel door and a thin bench and/or bed next to a half-wall discreetly housing a metal toilet. So at least I got en suite. It was very much like a room at an airport hotel, though with possibly a little more charm. Not exactly what most people would think of as an ideal environment for a 'health assessment'. But then assessment is different in mental health than physical health. There's no blood tests, MRI scans or even an old man in a leather-elbowed jacket tapping your knee with a fairy hammer. Sometimes you might get a questionnaire, like those Facebook games that tell you if you are 'an extrovert who likes to stay home' or 'an introvert who likes to go out'. But mostly my assessment involved a psychiatrist looking at the way I talked and behaved and deciding if I was fit for society.

In the cell, the assessment took less than a minute. Though all it actually did was buy the system some time by sectioning me for 28 days for further assessment. Assessment then became a 24/7 activity. It's hard enough being paranoid without knowing that your every moment is under close scrutiny by people who are writing secret notes about you.

Then every week there was 'the day' when you were formally assessed. My most vivid memory was sitting in the ward lounge with over a dozen strangers with clipboards and being asked, 'How are you today?'. 'Er … intimidated and overwhelmed' would have been an accurate answer. However, assessment in mental health once you are sectioned is less about 'How are you?' and more about 'Will this end up in the headlines if you are discharged?' So, when asked 'How are you?' the right answer is 'Not a threat to myself or others'. Once you have found a way to say and demonstrate that, you are rewarded with your freedom. And then you can really start answering the question 'How am I?'

'Health assessment' in mental health is mostly 'risk assessment'. The small 'health' portion is more like those shape-matching toys toddlers have. If it looks enough like depression, you go through the antidepressants-shaped hole. If it looks enough like mania or psychosis, you go through the antipsychotics-shaped hole. And if you don't fit the holes neatly, you are called 'complex' and pushed through anyway, like a frustrated child pushing a star-shaped block through a square-shaped hole. And if all this sounds pretty bleak, it is. But the worst part is no-one ever does a 'final assessment' to say you are no longer ill. Like a puppy bought at Christmastime, assessment is for life.

For more insights, see Gareth's website: www.positivethinking.co.nz.

Classification in psychiatry

There have been many attempts at developing systems of psychiatric classification. One notable early example is that of psychiatrist Emil Kraepelin in the late 19th century. Kraepelin's system, which included just 13 diagnoses, assumed that each mental illness is distinct rather than comprising clusters of symptoms with a significant degree of overlap. The most common system of psychiatric diagnosis in current use, the DSM-5, is also based on the assumption of distinct illnesses, although such categorical systems do not reflect the human experience of distress and illness. For a full analysis of these issues, see Zachar et al. (2014). There are two manuals of diagnoses in psychiatry: the *International Classification of Diseases and Health Related Problems* (ICD) (World Health Organization 1989) and the DSM. Since their initial establishment, both manuals have undergone numerous revisions. The most current versions are the ICD-11 and the DSM-5. The ICD-11 is a comprehensive manual of all known diseases, with its fifth chapter being devoted to mental and behavioural disorders, while the DSM-5 exclusively catalogues mental illnesses. The two systems are broadly similar and have become more so in their most recent editions. In Australia and New Zealand, the ICD AM (Australasian Modification) is more commonly used for collecting administrative health information, while the DSM is more commonly used in clinical practice.

Psychiatric diagnosis is not formally part of the practice of most mental health nurses, but it is important for nurses to understand the diagnostic process and the criteria for the most used diagnostic categories. Consumers may have questions about their diagnoses, and nurses need to be able to respond knowledgeably to these questions. Nurses may at times question the diagnosis assigned to a consumer in their care, and it is important that such questioning is well informed. Understanding diagnoses does not mean that nurses are practising within a biomedical model. Diagnostic models are only one of many frameworks for practice, but they are important because they form part of the common language of mental health care. The purpose of diagnosis is to accurately group people whose clinical symptoms are sufficiently similar, with the aim of optimising treatment and clinical outcomes for each group. Accurate diagnosis is essential to identifying optimal treatment. To assist clinicians in making diagnoses the DSM-5 provides lists of criteria and decision rules about applying those criteria in individual cases.

Despite the statement of explicit criteria and rules in the DSM-5, a diagnosis may not be clear, especially for consumers new to a mental health service or with complex histories. For those reasons, clinicians may defer diagnosis, assign a provisional diagnosis or make a list of differential diagnoses. A differential diagnosis is a list of possible diagnoses, any of which may eventually prove to be the final diagnosis (Baid 2006). Diagnosis should always be regarded as open to revision as clinicians' understanding of the consumer develops. Clinicians should also discuss the diagnosis with the consumer and should be prepared to share their uncertainty about the diagnosis and the role of diagnosis in clinical care.

Chapter summary

Assessment is one of the foundational skills of mental health nursing. Assessment begins with the person's first contact with a health service and continues throughout the episode of care. The aim of assessment is to develop an understanding of the person and the problems that have led them to seek mental health care. Assessment is based on developing a therapeutic relationship. It is both a structured process in which the nurse seeks information about many aspects of the life of the consumer and a process of exploration in which consumers are encouraged and supported to share their experiences with the nurse. Assessment methods include structured and conversational interviews, standardised assessment instruments and diaries recording aspects of functioning such as thoughts, feelings, activities and social interactions. A range of tools are available to assist in the process, including standard assessment templates and standardised assessment instruments. In conducting assessments nurses need to use the standard tools available as well as engage in dialogue in which consumers feel safe to share significant aspects of their lives. The tools of mental health nursing assessment provide the structure for the assessment to occur, while the process of assessment allows the nurse to integrate philosophical and theoretical frameworks into the assessment.

EXERCISES FOR CLASS ENGAGEMENT

You are a newly registered nurse working in a community mental health clinic. One of your roles in the service is to take phone calls from health practitioners and members of the public who are considering whether someone they know has a mental illness and would benefit from assessment and treatment. You receive a call from Donna, who describes her 19-year-old son (Matthew) as moody and irritable for the past 6 months after losing his job as a shop assistant. Soon after the loss of his job Matthew ended a 12-month relationship with his girlfriend. During the past 6 months he has been drinking excessively but will not discuss his problems with anyone in the family.

1. In mental health telephone triage, it is quite common to have limited information, and rapport with the caller may be tenuous. Refer to the 'Triage' section of this chapter where mental health triage is discussed. Discuss the triage nurse's phone call with Donna with members of your class and make a list of six questions you would want to ask at some point during the telephone interview. List the questions in order of priority. What interview skills would you use to ensure you have the opportunity to ask these questions?
2. Donna tells you that Matthew does not know that she is calling as he is currently out of the house. During the telephone interview, how would you work with Donna to help her in discussing her concerns with Matthew and supporting him to accept a face to-face assessment?

3. Two days later Matthew presents at the mental health clinic for a face-to-face assessment. Reflecting on the narrative and descriptive approaches to mental health assessment, how could you use each approach in your assessment of Matthew?
4. The face-to-face assessment involves Matthew, his mother and several members of the multidisciplinary team. The assessment interview takes an hour and the team works with Matthew to develop a collaborative understanding of what is happening for him and what the service can do to help. A plan is agreed that you will visit Matthew at home in a week's time. After Matthew has left, the team discusses psychiatric diagnosis. Most agree that Matthew is experiencing an adjustment disorder with depressed mood. In small groups, discuss the place of diagnosis in Matthew's care. The groups should consider:
   a Is a diagnosis necessary for Matthew to receive appropriate care?
   b What problems could a diagnosis of adjustment disorder with depressed mood cause for Matthew?
   c On your visit next week, how you will discuss Matthew's diagnosis with him? What questions might he have and how you will respond to those questions?

Useful websites

Clinical guideline for mental state assessment: https://www.rch.org.au/clinicalguide/guideline_index/Mental_state_examination/
Diagnostic and Statistical Manual of Mental Disorders, 5th edn (DSM-5): www.dsm5.org
HEADSS assessment: https://headspace.org.au/health-professionals/clinical-toolkit/psychosocial-assessment/
Head-to-toe assessment: https://nurse.org/articles/how-to-conduct-head-to-toe-assessment/
International Classification of Diseases (ICD): https://icd.who.int/en
Laboratory values: www.labtests.co.nz (New Zealand); https://www.mps.com.au/ (Australia)
Mental health assessment: https://www.integration.samhsa.gov/clinical-practice/screening-tools
Risk assessment (information about the HCR-20 instrument): http://hcr-20.com
Strengths-based assessment: https://www.iriss.org.uk/resources/strengths%c2%adbased%c2%adapproaches%c2%adworking%c2%adindividuals
Suicide risk assessment: http://www.psychiatryadvisor.com/home/topics/suicide-and-self-harm/is-this-patient-suicidal-tips-for-effective-assessment/

References

Aguilera, A., Schueller, S.M., Leykin, Y., 2015. Daily mood ratings via text message as a proxy for clinic-based depression assessment. J. Affect. Disord. 175, 471–474.
American Psychiatric Association (APA), 2013. Diagnostic and Statistical Manual of Mental Disorders, fifth ed. APA, Washington.
Australian College of Mental Health Nurses, 2010. Standards of Practice for Australian Mental Health Nurses. Australian College of Mental Health Nurses, Canberra.
Babor, T.F., Higgins-Biddle, J.C., Saunders, J.B., et al., 2001. AUDIT: The Alcohol Use Disorders Identification Test Guidelines for Use in Primary Care. World Health Organization, Geneva.
Baid, H., 2006. Differential diagnosis in advanced nursing practice. Br. J. Nurs. 15 (18), 1007–1011.
Barber, C.F., 2018. Mental health and spirituality. BJMHN 7 (3), 124–128.
Barker, P.J., 2004. Assessment in Psychiatric and Mental Health Nursing: In Search of the Whole Person. Nelson Thornes, Cheltenham, UK.
Bhugra, D., Ventriglio, A., 2017. Mind and body: physical health needs of individuals with mental illness in the 21st century. World Psychiatry 16 (1), 47.
Broadbent, M., Creaton, A., Moxham, L., et al., 2010. Review of triage reform: the case for national consensus on a single triage scale for clients with a mental illness in Australian emergency departments. J. Clin. Nurs. 19 (5–6), 712–715.
Brown, S.J., 1995. An interviewing style for nursing assessment. J. Adv. Nurs. 21, 340–343.
Burke, W.J., Roccaforte, W.H., Wengel, S.P., 1991. The short form of the Geriatric Depression Scale: a comparison with the 30-item form. J. Geriatr. Psychiatry Neurol. 4 (3), 173–178.
Chase, S.K., 2015. The art of diagnosis and treatment. In: Dunphy, L.M., Winland-Brown, J., Porter, B., et al. (Eds.), Primary Care: The Art and Science of Advanced Practice, fourth ed. FA Davis, Philadelphia.
Coombs, T., Crookes, P., Curtis, J., 2013a. A comprehensive mental health nursing assessment: variability of content in practice. J. Psychiatr. Ment. Health Nurs. 20 (2), 150–155.
Coombs, T., Curtis, J., Crookes, P., 2013b. What is the process of a comprehensive mental health nursing assessment? Results from a qualitative study. Int. Nurs. Rev. 60 (1), 96–102.
Coombs, T., Curtis, J., Crookes, P., 2011. What is a comprehensive mental health nursing assessment? A review of the literature. Int. J. Ment. Health Nurs. 20 (5), 364–370.
Crowe, M., Carlyle, D., Farmar, R., 2008. Clinical formulation for mental health nursing practice. J. Psychiatr. Ment. Health Nurs. 15 (10), 800–807.
Cunningham, R., Sarfati, D., Peterson, D., et al., 2014. Premature mortality in adults using New Zealand psychiatric services. N. Z. Med. J. 127 (1394), 31–41.
Day, J.C., Wood, G., Dewey, M., et al., 1995. A self-rating scale for measuring neuroleptic side-effects. Validation

in a group of schizophrenic patients. Br. J. Psychiatry 166 (5), 650–653.
DeWit, S.C., O'Neill, P.A., 2014. Fundamental Concepts and Skills for Nursing, fourth ed. Elsevier, St Louis.
Dickens, G.L., Ion, R., Waters, C., et al., 2019. Mental health nurses' attitudes, experience, and knowledge regarding routine physical healthcare: systematic, integrative review of studies involving 7,549 nurses working in mental health settings. BMC Nurs. 18 (1), 16.
DiClemente, C.C., Corno, C.M., Graydon, M.M., et al., 2017. Motivational interviewing, enhancement, and brief interventions over the last decade: a review of reviews of efficacy and effectiveness. Psychol. Addict. Behav. 31 (8), 862.
Diesfeld, K., McKenna, B., 2007. The unintended impact of the therapeutic intentions of the New Zealand mental health review tribunal. Therapeutic jurisprudence perspectives. J. Law Med. 14 (4), 552–566.
Duhig, M., Patterson, S., Connell, M., et al., 2015. The prevalence and correlates of childhood trauma in patients with early psychosis. Aust. N. Z. J. Psychiatry 49 (7), 651–659.
Eade, D.M., Henning, D., 2013. Chlamydia screening in young people as an outcome of a HEADSS; Home, Education, Activities, Drug and alcohol use, Sexuality and Suicide youth psychosocial assessment tool. J. Clin. Nurs. 22 (23–24), 3280–3288.
Flewett, T., 2010. Clinical Risk Management: An Introductory Text for Mental Health Clinicians. Elsevier, Sydney.
Folstein, M.F., Folstein, S.E., McHugh, P.R., 1975. 'Mini-Mental State': a practical method for grading the cognitive state of patients for the clinician. J. Psychiatr. Res. 12 (3), 189–198.
Foucault, M., 1994. The Birth of the Clinic: An Archaeology of Medical Perception. Vintage Books, New York.
Gray, R., Brown, E., 2017. What does mental health nursing contribute to improving the physical health of service users with severe mental illness? A thematic analysis. Int. J. Ment. Health Nurs. 26 (1), 32–40.
Huline-Dickens, S., 2013. The mental State examination. Adv. Psychiatr. Treat. 19 (2), 97–98.
Inouye, S.K., van Dyck, C.H., Alessi, C.A., et al., 1990. Clarifying confusion: the Confusion Assessment Method. A new method for detection of delirium. Ann. Intern. Med. 113, 941–948.
Jaber, F.S., Mahmoud, K.F., 2015. Risk tools for the prediction of violence: 'VRAG, HCR–20, PCL–R'. J. Psychiatr. Ment. Health Nurs. 22 (2), 133–141.
Johnstone, L., 2018. Psychological formulation as an alternative to psychiatric diagnosis. J. Humanist. Psychol. 58 (1), 30–46.
King, H. (Ed.), 2004. Health in Antiquity. Routledge, New York.
Lysaker, P.H., Pattison, M.L., Leonhardt, B.L., et al., 2018. Insight in schizophrenia spectrum disorders: relationship with behavior, mood and perceived quality of life, underlying causes and emerging treatments. World Psychiatry 17 (1), 12–23.
MacNeela, P., Scott, A., Treacy, P., et al., 2010. In the know: cognitive and social factors in mental health nursing assessment. J. Clin. Nurs. 19 (9–10), 1298–1306.
McPherson, A., Martin, C.R., 2010. A narrative review of the Beck Depression Inventory (BDI) and implications for its use in an alcohol–dependent population. J. Psychiatr. Ment. Health Nurs. 17 (1), 19–30.
Morgan, S., Andrews, N., 2016. Positive risk-taking: from rhetoric to reality. J. Ment. Health Train. Educ. Pract. 11 (2), 122–132.
Nursing and Midwifery Board of Australia (NMBA), 2013. National Competency Standards for the Registered Nurse. Nursing and Midwifery Board of Australia, Melbourne.
Nursing Council of New Zealand (NCNZ), 2007. Competencies for Registered Nurses. Nursing NCNZ, Wellington.
O'Brien, A.J., De Souza, R., Baker, M., 2016. Cultural safety. In: Barker, P. (Ed.), Psychiatric and Mental Health Nursing: The Craft of Caring, third ed. Hodder Arnold, London.
Patterson, W.M., Dohn, H.H., Bird, J., et al., 1983. Evaluation of suicidal patients: the SAD PERSONS scale. Psychosomatics 24 (4), 343–349.
Pitama, S., Huria, T., Lacey, C., 2014. Improving Māori health through clinical assessment: Waikare o te Waka o Meihana. N. Z. Med. J. (Online) 127 (1393).
Rapp, C.A., Goscha, R.J., 2012. The Strengths Model. A Recovery-Oriented Approach to Mental Health Services, third ed. Oxford University Press, New York.
Rasic, D., Hajek, T., Alda, M., et al., 2013. Risk of mental illness in offspring of parents with schizophrenia, bipolar disorder, and major depressive disorder: a meta-analysis of family high-risk studies. Schizophr. Bull. 40 (1), 28–38.
Reilly, J., McDermott, B., & Dillon, J. (2019). Standardized drug and alcohol questions at admission to an acute adult mental health unit: Clarifying the burden of dual diagnoses across a five-year period. Australasian Psychiatry 27 (3), 270–274.
Sands, N., Elsom, S., Berk, M., et al., 2014. Investigating the predictive validity of an emergency department mental health triage tool. Nurs. Health Sci. 16 (1), 11–18.
Scott, K.M., Lim, C., Al-Hamzawi, A., et al., 2016. Association of mental disorders with subsequent chronic physical conditions: world mental health surveys from 17 countries. JAMA Psychiatry 73 (2), 150–158.
Selzer, R., Ellen, S., 2014. Formulation for beginners. Australas. Psychiatry 22 (4), 397–401.
Selzer, R., Ellen, S., 2010. Psych-Lite: Psychiatry That's Easy to Read. McGraw-Hill, Sydney.
So, M., Foxe, D., Kumfor, F., et al., 2018. Addenbrooke's cognitive examination III: psychometric characteristics and relations to functional ability in dementia. J. Int. Neuropsychol. Soc. 24 (8), 854–863.
Soltan, M., Girguis, J., 2017. How to approach the mental state examination. BMJ 357, j1821.
Tambuyzer, E., Van Audenhove, C., 2013. Service user and family carer involvement in mental health care: divergent views. Community Ment. Health J. 49 (6), 675–685.
Te Ao Maramatanga New Zealand College of Mental Health Nurses, 2012. Standards of Practice for Mental

Health Nursing in Aotearoa New Zealand, third ed. Te Ao Maramatanga New Zealand College of Mental Health Nurses, Auckland.
Tseliou, F., Donnelly, M., O'Reilly, D., 2018. Screening for psychiatric morbidity in the population-a comparison of the GHQ-12 and self-reported medication use. Int. J. Popul. Data Sci. 3 (1), 5. https://doi.org/10.23889/ijpds.v3i1.414.
Wand, T., 2019. Is it time to end our complicity with pharmacocentricity? Int. J. Ment. Health Nurs. 28 (1), 3–6.
Wand, T., 2015. Recovery is about a focus on resilience and wellness, not a fixation with risk and illness. Aust. N. Z. J. Psychiatry 49 (12), 1083–1084.
Wand, T., Buchanan-Hagen, S., Derrick, K., et al., 2019. Are current mental health assessment formats consistent with contemporary thinking and practice? Int. J. Ment. Health Nurs. doi:10.1111/inm.12656.
Wand, T., Wynaden, D., Heslop, K., 2018. Who is responsible for metabolic screening for mental health clients taking antipsychotic medications? Int. J. Ment. Health Nurs. 27 (1), 196–203.
Warden, S., Spiwak, R., Sareen, J., et al., 2014. The SAD PERSONS scale for suicide risk assessment: a systematic review. Arch. Suicide Res. 18 (4), 313–326.
Westen, D., 1998. The scientific legacy of Sigmund Freud: toward a psychodynamically informed psychological science. Psychol. Bull. 124 (3), 333.
Wood, J.M., Gupta, S., 2017. Using rating scales in a clinical setting: a guide for psychiatrists. Curr. Psychiatr. 16 (2), 21–25.
World Health Organization (WHO), 1989. ICD-10: International Statistical Classification of Diseases and Related Health Problems, 10th Revision. WHO, Geneva.
Zachar, P., Stoyanov, D.S., Aragona, M., et al. (Eds.), 2014. Alternative Perspectives on Psychiatric Validation: DSM, IDC, RDoC, and Beyond. Oxford University Press, Oxford.
Zanotti, R., Chiffi, D., 2015. Diagnostic frameworks and nursing diagnoses: a normative stance. Nurs. Philos. 16 (1), 64–73.

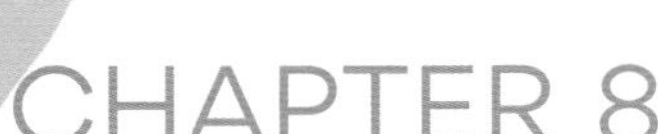

CHAPTER 8

Legal and ethical issues

Anthony J O'Brien and Scott Trueman

KEY POINTS

- Mental health care involves reflecting on ethical issues and applying principles of ethical reasoning.
- Codes of ethics guide members of the professions as to the nature of proper conduct and their obligations to the public.
- Ethical principles provide nurses with guidelines for ethical practice.
- A sound knowledge of legal issues is critical to contemporary mental health nursing.
- Mental health legislation is the legal framework that informs the involuntary treatment of individuals, defines their rights and ensures appropriate treatment.
- Australia and New Zealand have high rates of use of community treatment orders, raising questions about coercion and human rights.

KEY TERMS

- Autonomy
- Beneficence
- Code of ethics
- Community treatment orders
- Confidentiality
- Consent
- Duty of care
- Ethics
- Human rights
- Involuntary treatment
- Justice
- Least restrictive alternative
- Mental health legislation
- Non-maleficence

LEARNING OUTCOMES

The material in this chapter will assist you to:

- identify common ethical issues in mental health nursing
- apply ethical principles to the analysis of ethical issues in mental health nursing
- understand the importance of health legislation in mental health care
- identify issues related to privacy and confidentiality
- discuss the issue of informed consent in relation to compulsory mental health care
- understand the significance of the United Nations *Convention on the Rights of Persons with Disabilities*
- identify how the concept of duty of care applies in the mental health setting.

Introduction

Mental health nursing is practised within an ethical and legal context and within a framework of ethical principles. This chapter outlines the ethical and legal context of mental health nursing and provides guidance to assist nurses in maintaining professional practice that meets professional, legal and ethical standards. Mental health nurses are legally mandated to practise nursing in accordance with professional competencies and societal expectations. As professionals, mental health nurses must be aware of legislation specific to the domain of mental health. Ethical principles and theories assist nurses to make decisions on issues of conflict and to maintain clear and safe boundaries around their practice. In addition to the ethical issues inherent in every practice setting, the mental health context presents unique issues of coercion and treatment without consent.

The mental health context presents unique challenges for nurses because the use of compulsory treatment under mental health legislation involves significant departures from normally accepted human and healthcare rights. The United Nations *Convention on the Rights of Persons with Disabilities* is an international instrument aimed at protecting the rights of people with mental illness. In recent years countries have been challenged under the Convention to rethink how they protect the rights of mental health consumers. In particular, the basis for compulsory treatment under mental health legislation has been challenged. Mental health legislation provides a legal framework for treatment without consent and specific guidelines for procedures such as electroconvulsive therapy (ECT), psychosurgery and seclusion. Rates of compulsory treatment in Australia and New Zealand are high by international standards.

This chapter explores the ethical and legal context of practice. It outlines the principles of ethical conduct and discusses some ethical issues commonly encountered in mental health nursing. It also outlines use of mental health legislation and the rights issues raised by compulsory treatment. Capacity-based legislation, advance directives and supported decision making are explored as responses to the challenges of the *Convention on the Rights of Persons with Disabilities*.

Historical anecdote 8.1: A fairer society can improve mental health

The French Revolution (1789–1799) heavily influenced understanding of how to manage mental disorders, emphasising principles such as individual rights and equality. As a consequence of the revolution, people in France who experienced mental illness began to be considered victims of a poorly ordered society. This attitude shifted the focus of blame for mental ill health away from the individual concerned and onto the ills of society. It also supported the idea that mental health care should take a social form and prompted hope for recovery if their environment could be more supportive. The ideals of the revolution emboldened French psychiatrist Phillippe Pinel and asylum superintendent Jean Baptise Pussin, who led development of a kinder, more humane approach to mental health care, which came to be referred to as 'moral therapy'.

Read more about it: *Pinel P 1806 A treatise on insanity. Messers Cadell & Davies, Strand*

Ethics and professional practice

A profession is a collective with a clear definition of its roles and responsibilities to ensure the quality of work and knowledge produced by its members. The right to call itself a profession arises through the credibility and trust that are built with the people to whom the group provides a service. For nursing to assert itself as a profession, ethics and identity are inseparable. This is because the identity of nursing and the self-regulatory processes that ensure continued trust within the community are inextricably interwoven. In other words, nursing and nursing practice are guided by the law, ethical principles and the public trust in the nurse as an ethical practitioner. Nurses must practise within the law and adhere to a code of ethical conduct.

Internationally, professional nursing organisations have identified the need for codes of ethics to guide practice. The first international code of ethics for nurses was developed by the International Council of Nurses in 1953, with the most recent revision published in 2012 (International Council of Nurses 2012). As early as 1993 a code of ethics was developed for Australian nurses (Australian Nursing and Midwifery Council 2008), and a New Zealand code of ethics was developed in 1995 (New Zealand Nurses Organisation 1995). Codes of ethics are informed by conventionalised ethical principles. The four most commonly adopted principles (Beauchamp & Childress 2019) – autonomy, beneficence, non-maleficence and justice – are explained in Box 8.1.

Ethical frameworks

A code of ethics provides a formalised set of rules or expectations that reflects the ideals and values of a group. Codes of ethics are informed by ethical theories and value statements. Such codes are not a 'means to an end' in and of themselves; they are a guide to ethical conduct and decision making. A nurse remains a moral agent in every situation. The following section outlines the three major ethical theories that inform professional practice.

Box 8.1 Seven areas that need to be considered when thinking about clinical scenarios and applying ethical reasoning

1. **Rights:** Rights form the basis of most professional codes and legal judgments and consider ideas such as self-determination rights, rights and cultural relativism, the right to health care and rights to privacy and confidentiality.
2. **Autonomy:** Autonomy involves the right of self-determination, independence and freedom. Autonomy promotes the right of an individual to make their own decisions and implies that the person will also take responsibility for decisions made. Respect for autonomy means that nurses recognise the individual's uniqueness, right to lead a life they want and right to set personal goals. Nurses who follow the principle of autonomy respect a client's right to make choices even if they are not always the best options in the opinion of the nurse.
3. **Beneficence and non-maleficence:** Beneficence means 'doing good'. Nurses should work towards actions that support and benefit clients and their family members. However, in an increasingly technological healthcare system, doing the best by a person can also do harm by potentially putting that person at risk (e.g. intensive therapy programs). Non-maleficence means the duty to do no harm. Harm can be caused deliberately, or it may involve actions that put the person at risk of harm, even if this was unintentional. In nursing, intentional harm is always unacceptable. The risk for potential to cause harm is not always clear. For example, a nursing intervention that is implemented to be helpful may cause harm (e.g. medication administration).
4. **Justice:** Justice can also be considered as fairness. Nurses frequently face decisions in which a sense of justice should prevail. For example, a person may be detained under mental health legislation, but justice requires this to be the case only while that person is at risk to themselves or other people and unable to self-assess and manage their own risk.
5. **Fidelity:** Fidelity means to be faithful to agreements and responsibilities one has undertaken. Nurses have responsibilities to clients, employers, government, society, the profession and themselves. Circumstances often affect which responsibilities take precedence at a particular time.
6. **Veracity:** Veracity means telling the truth. Consumers expect nurses to be truthful in matters such as planned treatment and any limits on autonomy. Veracity also applies to information about medication where the nurse has the obligation to be truthful about risks and side effects as well as the benefits of medication.
7. **Trust and reciprocity:** We trust that colleagues will act in ways that are mutually supportive and do no harm to each other. The principle of reciprocity is essential for nurses to build trust in working relationships between professionals as well as their clients. Consumers also rely on trust and the principle of reciprocity to ensure health practitioners do their best to do no harm and promote recovery.

UTILITARIANISM

Utilitarian theory is a subset of consequentialism, which is informed by teleology (from the Greek word *telos* meaning 'end'). The theory of utilitarianism requires that an action is right if it produces the best or most desirable consequences compared with other action(s). Actions are right if they *maximise* happiness/pleasure/interests/preferences and simultaneously minimise unhappiness/pain/harm (measured against utility). This requires one to do the 'greatest good for the greatest number'.

DEONTOLOGY

Deontological theory guides the *duty* to perform acts that are *intrinsically good* or *inherently good*. We have a duty to refrain from acts that are *intrinsically bad* or *intrinsically wrong*. Ethical concepts guide us in our everyday work as health professionals. The seven areas shown in Box 8.1 need to be considered when thinking about clinical scenarios and applying ethical reasoning.

VIRTUE ETHICS

In contrast to the emphasis of utilitarianism on action based on its consequences and the emphasis of deontology on the right action with reference to one's duty to fulfil moral obligation(s), virtue ethics emphasise the moral character of the agent. Some consider virtue ethics to be especially pertinent to nursing because of nursing's concern with the moral character of the nurse (Sellman 2017).

Critical thinking challenge 8.1

Consider the current diagnostic label of 'borderline personality disorder' (BPD) and the clinical signs and symptoms of BPD (see Chapter 14). People with BPD often present in states of high arousal with varying degrees of self-harm, and clinicians can find these presentations stressful and difficult. They provide major challenges to the healthcare service, and the label 'BPD' often invokes feelings of helplessness in clinicians, who may respond by attempting to dissuade the person from accessing the health service. If we were to take into account the fact that many people labelled with BPD have been invalidated in their lives, often as a result of sexual or physical abuse, and if this consideration persuaded us to view BPD as post-traumatic stress disorder, would this change our attitudes to working with people who are given this diagnostic label?

Ethical principles

Ethical principles (sometimes referred to as 'ethical principlism') represent the view that ethical decision making requires adhering to reasoned/reliable ethical standards, sometimes described as 'imperatives'. The four principles below, identified by Beauchamp and Childress (2019) and universally adopted, specify actions or conduct that is either prohibited, permitted or required in the circumstances.

AUTONOMY

This term derives from the Greek *autos* (meaning 'self') and *nomos* (meaning 'rule' or 'governance) and means that people are free to choose, make decisions and act on their own preferences, so long as they do not impinge on the moral interests of others. Hence, consumers' decisions are to be respected concerning what is 'in their best interests'. Accordingly, in providing care and treatment a consumer's *consent* is usually required. Some exceptions to this requirement are outlined later in this chapter.

BENEFICENCE

This term derives from the Latin *beneficus*, in turn from *bene* (meaning 'well' or 'good'), and *facere* (meaning to 'do good') – 'above all, do good'. It mandates a positive obligation on nurses to act for the benefit of others. Beneficence embraces such virtuous acts as compassion, empathy, kindness, altruism, care, charity, friendship and mercy in providing care. An important qualification is that a nurse is not obliged to so act if it would impinge on or compromise their own moral interests.

NON-MALFEASANCE

This term derives from the Latin word *male* (meaning 'ill' or 'wicked') and prescribes 'above all, do no harm'. Accordingly, in providing care it obliges nurses to refrain from acts that unnecessarily cause injury, harm or suffering. 'Harm' includes violating a consumer's wellbeing or interests. Importantly, if there is a conflict between beneficence and non-malfeasance concerning a nurse's proposed action the latter is usually more stringently applied.

JUSTICE

In the context of providing health care, 'justice' usually means facilitating what is due and owed to a consumer. With the limited resources available, this often means making decisions about rationing to ensure an equal distribution of benefits and harms – distributive justice. To make such a decision requires impartiality and objectivity on the part of the nurse to ensure fairness for all consumers.

Critical thinking challenge 8.2

Using the four most commonly cited principles of ethical conduct (autonomy, beneficence, non-maleficence and justice), consider when and if it is appropriate to administer an intramuscular injection of medication against a consumer's will.

Ethical issues in mental health practice

People experiencing mental illness can be marginalised by their illness and this can cause them to be politically powerless through a lack of ability to plan and speak for themselves. They can therefore be a group that is vulnerable to human rights abuse and stigmatisation. Manifestations of mental illness often include low self-esteem, withdrawal, self-doubt and distortions in thinking. Consequently, people with mental illness may have difficulty in making autonomous decisions at various times in their life and may find it difficult to advocate for themselves. Because of this vulnerability, mental health nurses frequently encounter complex issues, requiring ethical decision making. This section considers some critical areas of mental health nursing practice requiring the need for ethical reasoning.

PSYCHIATRIC DIAGNOSIS

Psychiatric diagnosis is a fundamental aspect of ethical reflection in mental health care. Personal consequences of a diagnosis may include loss of personal freedom, imposed treatment regimens and the possibility of being 'labelled' as mentally ill for life. Diagnostic labelling and hospitalisation of people with mental illnesses often marginalise them from their community and thus jeopardise their chances of achieving or regaining social integration and recovery.

Diagnosis can be a powerful tool, with the capacity to label behaviour that is seen as odd or objectionable. Diagnosis has been used to explain behaviour that is unlawful, such as acts of theft or violence, in terms of a medical issue rather than applying the usual social sanctions. In the latter case, the law recognises that mental illness compromises a person's free will and can classify the person as not legally responsible for their actions. Therefore, a diagnosis of mental illness can, in some cases, 'benefit' a person through exculpation for their actions by transforming their criminal act into a symptomatic one. However, the process of psychiatric diagnosis has been reported as being of poor or questionable reliability (Zachar et al. 2014). In mental health, objective signs of mental distress are not always evident, so diagnosis may be a difficult procedure. Consumers may not always have enough trust in professionals to tell their story, and some aspects of their history may be too painful to recount in full. Also, people are influenced by processes such as denial and fantasy in describing their lives. Diagnosis plays a powerful role in some people's lives, but it has its limits. People can be left with a lifelong label, and care must be taken not to label culturally determined experiences as signs of mental illness. It can be helpful to think of making a diagnosis as a social act of assessing behaviour against accepted social norms, rather than simply as a matter of applying diagnostic criteria.

A diagnosis of mental illness may label the consumer as deviant from the normal population and result in predetermined clinical and social behaviours, in both the person diagnosed and the health professionals caring for them. Illich (2001) first suggested in his classic 1977 text that while some people are transformed into consumers, others are transformed into clinicians by enculturation that attributes to them the power to diagnose and heal. If a consumer is described to you as 'Mr Brown, the man who has been hearing voices and is afraid that others are talking about him', you will have certain expectations based on this description. However, if Mr Brown is described as 'the schizophrenic in room 4', how might your initial perceptions differ? In this case the ethical concern is one of non-maleficence. Consumers should not be harmed by the actions of health professionals, including the practice of diagnosis. There are strong messages in the words we use, especially when they become labels.

Some of the questions that need to be considered are: Who has the right to decide which types of behaviour are mental illness rather than moral deviance? How do we classify people who become verbally abusive when drunk, who are addicted to psychoactive substances, are antisocial, have sexual preferences different from our own, hold unusual religious beliefs or gamble excessively? We do have systems of classification that differentiate normal from abnormal behaviour – for example, the *Diagnostic and Statistical Manual of Mental Disorders* (DSM) (American Psychiatric Association 2013). But criticism has been aimed at the DSM for creating ever-expanding criteria for mental illness, resulting in more people being labelled with mental illness. Flaskeraud (2010) suggests that the DSM turns general problems or traits of personality into psychiatric disorders that are then treated with pharmaceuticals. Further, future behaviours and actions will be referable to the assigned label and hence become proof of the original diagnosis. The label becomes self-confirming. The cultural sensitivity of these diagnostic criteria and the disempowerment that the consumer feels from the confusing terminology used have also been questioned.

PSYCHIATRIC TREATMENT

Mental health clients are critical of the use of coercive practices (e.g. overuse of pharmaceuticals, restraint and seclusion and treatment orders) and perceive their use by nurses as punishment (Mayers et al. 2010). Worldwide, lengths of stay in hospital have decreased, while admission rates have increased, resulting in changes to the overall milieu of inpatient units where acute interventions and containment are the predominant care provided and less attention is paid to rehabilitation and comprehensive discharge planning.

Community treatment orders (CTOs) raise several ethical issues that need to be considered concerning consent (lack of), autonomy (breach), coercion (enforced), paternalism (forced) and beneficence (weighing against non-maleficence). There is concern that CTOs can be non-inclusive and coercive by requiring the client to comply with treatment plans. This raises issues concerning the human rights of a person diagnosed with a mental illness compared with members of the general public. CTOs are legally enforceable documents that can have an enormously negative impact on the patient's privacy and autonomy (Light et al. 2012b). Further discussion of CTOs is provided later in this chapter.

PSYCHOPHARMACOLOGY

The drugs prescribed for mental illness are potent agents, often causing major side effects and problems with toxicity and, in the case of major tranquillisers such as clozapine, producing cardiac complications and metabolic disorders (Moncrieff 2013). Psychotropic medications can also interact with other therapeutic agents and so need to be monitored closely. Side effects such as metabolic syndrome and dependence raise ethical issues of non-maleficence, while administration of medication without consent, as frequently occurs in mental health nursing, compromises the consumer's autonomy. People who have been taking psychotropic medication may find it difficult to stop their medication due to discontinuation syndrome (Massabki & Abi-Jaoude 2020; Salomon & Hamilton 2014), which carries further ethical implications. As with other psychiatric treatments, nurses may argue that their practice in this area is motivated by beneficence, but issues of non-maleficence and compromised autonomy also need to be considered.

With respect to drug treatment, a question that needs to be considered is: What are a person's rights when placed on psychopharmacological agents? These rights include access to effective non-pharmacological treatment and information concerning the drug prescribed (desired effects, side effects, contraindications, complications) and the freedom to accept or refuse treatment. These rights may be limited if the person is an involuntary patient under mental health legislation. However, all consumers should have some voice in drug selection. If the side effects of a particular drug are difficult to live with, the person should be able to ask for a review and change of treatment, including a non-pharmacological alternative. Considerations of psychopharmacology invoke the legal dictum – *primum non nocere* – the principle of least harm; the benefits of the medication must outweigh the hazards (Stein & van Niekerk 2015). Psychopharmacology is further discussed in Chapter 19.

ELECTROCONVULSIVE THERAPY

ECT is used mainly for major depression (Griffiths & O'Neill-Kerr 2019). A significant ethical problem occurs when a psychiatrist prescribes ECT in order to reduce a consumer's risk of self-harm or harm through neglect but where the individual does not give consent for the therapy. The thought of having ECT can be traumatic to consumers and families due to the negative perceptions about this form of treatment and the potential for memory loss (Smith et al. 2009). Cleary and Horsfall (2014) outline issues of choice and effectiveness of ECT and urge nurses to carefully consider their views on ECT. As with all treatments, ECT needs to be carefully negotiated with consumers to prevent occurrences of medical paternalism. For depressed people, their lowered mood and pessimistic outlook may mean they are unable to see any solution to their depression. In the case of refusal to consent, doctors in New Zealand and in some Australian states have the power under mental health legislation to administer ECT without the consumer's consent but require a second psychiatric opinion to do so. Treatment without consent involves a significant limitation on the consumer's autonomy and so needs sound ethical justification. Nurses need to ensure consumers and their families are informed of the nature of the procedure and why substituted consent has been provided by treating psychiatrists. ECT is also discussed in Chapter 10.

NURSE'S STORY 8.1

Simon

I have worked in many areas of nursing but found my way into mental health about 15 years ago. All clinical areas have their challenges, and the challenges are often about the legal requirements as well as ethical issues about practice and treatment options for consumers. Nurses make a big difference in consumer advocacy and are often the person who checks the legal requirements and thinks about ethical decision making. It is an essential part of reflective practice for a nurse. Thinking how the benefits of treatment outweigh the harm of treatment is often difficult in mental health. We have mental health legislation that governs our practice. That gives us a lot of power, but it also places a greater amount of responsibility and decision making on the nurse working in mental health with people who are detained and prescribed treatment without their consent. We work in partnership when we can with consumers and their carers, but often when a person is severely depressed or psychotic it is difficult to engage. That doesn't mean you don't try.

One of my main roles is ECT nurse coordinator. This means I work with the medical staff, the psychiatrist and the anaesthetist to administer ECT. I'm responsible for the consumer's care once they come to the ECT suite and during the procedure, and I manage and support the nurses who are escorting people and providing after treatment care in the recovery suite. We also have a lot of students come through as it is a teaching hospital.

ECT is a controversial topic. I have care-coordinated ECT for years and seen good outcomes, but there is a lot of stigma and misunderstanding about ECT as a treatment. The Mental Health Act provides direction for the procedure and that the person needs to have given voluntary consent. If they are unable to do this, then there are provisions to provide the prescribed ECT treatment against the consumer's wishes. So, this may be legal to do but it reduces the person's autonomy in decision making, and you have to ensure the benefits outweigh the potential harms. ECT is a safe treatment and it is conducted within guidelines and standards directed by the Chief Psychiatrist's Office.

Consumers are often quite frightened by the thought of having ECT, and this has been influenced by the media. Consumers can also be passive in their treatment, especially if the psychiatrists have prescribed and consented for them. What we try to do here is bring the person down to the ECT suite and take them through. I think this really helps them to be more at ease and also to have a better recovery. The idea to do an orientation came from the number of events we had with people becoming distressed and disoriented in recovery. So, we take them to a room and say this is where you will come and wait for the treatment, explain the procedure and that they need to fast and encourage questions. Then they go into the suite and we say this is where you will lie down and be given a short-acting anaesthetic and how they will be hooked up to some monitors. We then show them the recovery area and say you will wake up here and once you are ready you can go back to the ward area and have breakfast. I try to include student nurses in this orientation as well and always ask the consumer if it would be OK to have students in the room during the procedure. It is very rare that they have a problem with students.

I like to have student nurses. They don't just observe, they can have supervised but hands-on experience with the care of the consumer, placing on the monitoring equipment, turning them, taking vital signs and recovering them. They also get to see the Mental Health Act in practice and how we check the consent and that it is the correct consumer and the prescription is correct and current. The whole team takes an interest in students and we encourage them to ask questions and speak to the consumer after the treatment once they are recovered.

SECLUSION AND RESTRAINT

Seclusion is the involuntary supervised isolation of a person in a locked, non-stimulating room. This room may be spartan, containing only a mattress with a blanket and a bed pan. Limited furnishment is aimed at preventing consumers from hurting themselves or others (Bowers et al. 2010). Australian courts have interpreted mental health legislation to determine that seclusion is deemed to be treatment and not a management action; however, advice to clinicians is that seclusion should not be regarded as a therapeutic intervention (Ministry of Health 2010). In recent years both Australia and New Zealand have followed policies of reducing or eliminating seclusion (Australian College of Mental Health Nurses 2016; Te Pou o te Whakaaro Nui 2015).

Seclusion is generally deemed lawful when it is necessary to protect the mental health consumer's health and welfare or to protect another person from imminent risk to their health or safety. While the wording and procedures of the various mental health Acts might differ, there are common themes in relation to consumer safeguards.

The use of a restraint and seclusion in a designated mental health service must be authorised by either:

- an authorised psychiatrist or delegate, or
- if an authorised psychiatrist or delegate is not immediately available, a registered medical practitioner or the senior registered nurse on duty.

An authorised psychiatrist must then be notified as soon as practicable. They then must examine the consumer as soon as practicable to decide whether continued use of the restrictive intervention is necessary. A registered nurse may only approve urgent physical restraint if:

- it is necessary and urgent to prevent imminent and serious harm to the consumer or another person
- an authorised psychiatrist, registered medical practitioner or senior on duty registered nurse is not immediately available for authorisation.

Urgent physical restraint without authorisation must be for the minimum time necessary and after all reasonable and less restrictive options have been tried or are considered unsuitable.

A consumer being bodily restrained (including urgent physical restraint) must be under continuous observation by a registered nurse or registered medical practitioner. Further, a registered nurse or registered medical practitioner must clinically review the use of bodily restraint (including urgent physical restraint) on a consumer as often as is appropriate but not less frequently than every 15 minutes. An authorised psychiatrist must examine a consumer in seclusion or being bodily restrained as frequently as is appropriate but not less than every 4 hours.

Consumers and some clinicians and researchers have been influential in raising awareness about the negative impact of seclusion for consumers. Consumers have expressed dissatisfaction with seclusion, finding the experience negative, frightening, cold, drab and untherapeutic and increasing their feelings of distress or agitation (Askew et al. 2019; Larue et al. 2013). While the World Health Organization (2019) has suggested that authorities should pursue the elimination of isolation rooms and prohibit the provision of new ones, such recommendations have not yet been fully implemented in Australia or New Zealand.

NURSE'S STORY 8.2

Rachael

I was educated to believe that we should have shared male/female wards. The end of the 1970s was when they had segregated wards and that was before my time. After that, wards only had beds, and nurses would care for consumers, be they male or female. We always tried to allocate a female with a female nurse and a male with a male nurse when personal care was required, but largely we based the ward bed allocation not on gender but on consumers' need for safety. And when I went into the community you had to go to people's homes and give injections, be they either gender.

On reflection this has caused a lot of concern for consumers coming into the ward environment and I am glad to say it has been identified as a major need by the Department of Health. Our ward has had funding to develop a female-only area. This provides a space for meeting and also a separate corridor for female-only beds and bathrooms. It was controversial at first, but it is part of everyday practice now.

Women feel more comfortable having a separate space to go to and an area where they can rest and shower without the fear of males coming in. Doors on bathrooms don't lock in mental health facilities, and that can make many women feel uncomfortable and unsafe. No matter how hard we try to make this a welcoming and home-like environment it is still a public space. We don't want women coming into mental health facilities and feeling uncomfortable when there is no need for them to feel this way.

Management obtained the funding and a committee of clinicians and the carer and consumer consultant guided the development of policy as well as the spending to redesign the ward. A great outcome! It was also an example of how you can work with consumers, listen to them and develop ways to provide the least restrictive environment possible as per the Mental Health Act. So, in this case an environment where women can move freely and attend to their ablutions in a safe-feeling environment. Where we aim to care but do no harm.

We did also plan for transgender consumers. There is a room with an en-suite bathroom so anyone who identifies as transgender can have the option to stay here if their risk assessment upon admission allows for this plan of care. If they need closer monitoring, then we consider this as part of their care plan.

It is important to think about the restrictive environments we work in within mental health. There has been a lot of work done on reducing the use of seclusion, but we often find that this means the person is within a high dependency area that has secure doors and a quite rigid routine. Nurses need to ensure that consumers feel comfortable in this environment and monitor this. Once needing less observation and care, we transfer people to the open ward as soon as we can. But sometimes the doors to these units are locked as well, as there are many people on the ward who are a danger to themselves. The locked ward resolves a lot of the problems that you would experience with consumers in a general ward where you don't have this facility, but it poses human rights and ethical issues. Legally the wards can be locked if even one consumer at the time poses a danger to themselves or to others. For example, if they were actively wanting to harm themselves. But the guidelines of the Mental Health Act do not take away from the ethical decision making we must do to always place the consumer in the least restrictive environment, promote their self-advocacy and choice. We must ensure that the benefits of a locked ward area are clear and that the need for this is conveyed to the consumer and their family. We must also make provision for others to have leave from the ward to go about their business without restriction. This can be time consuming to do, but it is very much part of the day-to-day work of a mental health nurse to ensure we provide the best care we can.

SUICIDAL BEHAVIOUR

Caring for suicidal people is one of the most challenging clinical situations that mental health professionals face. The topic of suicide is well documented, but few realise that the number of unsuccessful attempts at suicide (parasuicide) is eight to ten times the figure for actual suicide (Ministry of Health 2019). The high incidence of suicide and suicidal behaviour makes this a significant issue for mental health nurses. The prospect of members of our community considering whether they wish to live at all challenges the image of life as cherished and worthwhile. The ethical debate about suicide largely centres on the justification (paternalism) for intervening in a person's choice to live or die. Healthcare workers have a duty to intervene by preventing the intentional act of suicide, but this brings about a conflict with respecting a person's autonomy. Compounding this ethical dilemma is that a suicidal person may not be suffering from a mental illness and may have decision-making capacity. In clinical settings nurses have a duty of care to prevent suicide but must weigh up what the limits of that duty are, and when a consumer should retain autonomy to make and take responsibility for their own decisions.

Historical anecdote 8.2: Australian mental health care began in a jail

In the early days of New Zealand and Australia the colonial governments of both countries were unable to afford the cost of establishing standalone mental health facilities, which meant people who became mentally ill were kept in jails alongside criminals. Australia's first 'lunatic asylum' was opened in 1811 when Governor Macquarie and his wife, Elizabeth, inspected Parramatta jail and were so moved with compassion for people in the jail who were experiencing mental ill health that he gave orders to open Australia's first asylum at Castle Hill. Macquarie's empathy was linked to his older brother Donald's experience of mental illness following return form the Napoleonic wars. New Zealand's first asylum was opened some years later in 1844 for remarkably similar reasons when Wellington jail became overcrowded.

Read more about it: *Raeburn T, Liston C, Hickmott J, Cleary M 2018 Life of Martha Entwistle: Australia's first convict mental health nurse. International Journal of Mental Health Nursing, 27(1): 455–63*

INVOLUNTARY TREATMENT

Guidelines for ethical conduct are particularly relevant to mental health nurses because involuntary status under mental health legislation places restrictions on the therapeutic nurse–consumer relationship. Consumers who feel they have few rights and are restricted by legislation may be less likely to engage in a working relationship with a mental health nurse. In this situation, where the consumer is subject to mental health legislation, the nurse exercises social control over the consumer. If the consumer is involuntarily hospitalised, the nurse can lawfully initiate medication compliance and restrain and seclude the consumer. No consent is required. However, mental health is not an area where the nurse can always refer the consumer to doctors for the answers because the nurse is often the person delivering care and it is frequently the nurse's actions that the consumer is questioning.

When a person is committed to a mental health facility, the major ethical debate centres on the tension between the state's legal responsibilities (parens patriae – the state's duty to act as a parent) versus individual moral rights (liberty, autonomy). When should a person be admitted involuntarily under mental health legislation? The answer is usually about when the person is a danger to themselves or others *and* suffering from a mental illness. However, consider whether you would feel comfortable committing a person to a mental health facility if the person was a member of your family or a close friend.

A consumer voluntarily seeking treatment for a mental illness should be treated as fully competent and retains the right to give or withhold consent to treatment, unless assessed otherwise. Conversely an involuntary consumer admitted to hospital under mental health legislation is deemed to have limited legal capacity to refuse or consent to treatment (Mandarelli et al. 2018). As nurses we should advocate for such disempowered consumers, but we must ensure we advocate in collaboration or else we risk being paternalistic. Paternalism is when nurses believe that they know what is best for the consumer (i.e. in their best interests) and that they are most qualified to speak on the consumer's behalf. Although the intention is good, consumer autonomy is at risk. All consumers should be treated with the same degree of respect that you would require for yourself and, whenever practicable, their autonomy should be maintained (e.g. benefit paternalism). This ensures consumers maintain their integrity and do not feel so vulnerable and powerless.

Critical thinking challenge 8.3

Beth is 23 years old and is admitted to an acute mental health inpatient unit as an involuntary patient. She has been diagnosed with a drug-induced relapse of psychosis and it is expected that she will have a short admission. Beth remembers a past admission where a male consumer came into her room at night and rummaged through her things. Because of that experience, she is having problems sleeping on the ward this time. Should Beth be prescribed prn (*pro re nata*) sedatives? Considering contemporary beliefs concerning gender equality and mixed-sex wards, is allocating beds on a needs basis always appropriate? What gender issues arise from having integrated ward environments with involuntary consumers, and what can we do about them?

INTERPERSONAL THERAPY

Consumers place trust in their therapist, expecting that the therapist will not exploit it. The relationship between therapist and consumer is therapy's strength and weakness. The therapist gains recognition as a health professional, but also power within the relationship. The ethical issue is how to use this power. Does the power remain egalitarian or become authoritarian? And to what extent does transference within the relationship hinder the therapeutic process? The therapist may become the most important person in the consumer's life and runs the risk of assuming priority over all others.

In general, the ethical guidelines for one-on-one therapy and group work are threefold: (1) to protect the consumer from exploitation, incompetence and pressure to coercion; (2) to uphold the right of the consumer to be provided with information and make informed decisions concerning their life; and (3) to foster personal growth and wellness (Holmes & Adshead 2009). The first two goals protect and promote the consumer's rights, while the third outlines the true goal of therapy. It is often taken for granted that therapy is beneficial for the consumer. After all, looking at oneself or sharing beliefs during group or individual therapy should help consumers to grow and understand why their lives have evolved as they have. This aim is compromised when the therapy is focused on the needs of the therapist or institution, rather than on those of the consumer. In extreme cases this can lead to unprofessional conduct, including sexual exploitation of the consumer.

PROFESSIONAL BOUNDARIES

The therapeutic relationship is a privileged relationship for both the consumer and the clinician. Courts often refer to the relationship as a 'fiduciary relationship' – one where the clinician upholds and respects the ethical principle of *fidelity*. However, responsibility for maintaining the required professional boundaries rests with the clinician, who needs to have safeguards in place that will enable issues involving professional boundaries to be identified and appropriately managed (Griffith & Tengnah 2013). Without adequate professional standards there is a risk that the consumer may suffer emotional harm, which would be a breach of the ethical principle of non-maleficence. Safeguards include reflective practice, especially use of a colleague or supervisor to discuss consumer care confidentially. You may notice at times when you are working closely with a consumer that you have feelings of friendship, wanting to save the consumer from reckless behaviour, boredom with their lack of progress or a sense of knowing better than the consumer what their needs are. These are all signs of potential countertransference.

You should be aware of the boundaries needed to keep nursing care therapeutic and consumer-centred. When a nurse moves outside the therapeutic relationship and establishes a friendship or social relationship with a consumer, the professional boundaries between the nurse and the consumer become confused. When professional boundaries are blurred, the relationship can become non-therapeutic and potentially harmful to both the consumer and the nurse. Utilising ethical decision-making principles is especially important to ensure that professional boundaries are not transgressed.

Critical thinking challenge 8.4

Kirsty has been employed in an inpatient ward for 3 months and has been working with her clinical supervisor on developing interpersonal skills and maintaining professional boundaries. One of the consumers Kirsty is caring for is Marissa, a young woman close to Kirsty's age. In talking with Marissa, Kirsty becomes aware that they share certain life issues. These are to do with trust, forming intimate relationships and a fear of being abandoned if they let anyone get too close to them. Because they have so much in common Kirsty feels able to help Marissa more than the other nurses on the ward. Kirsty's friends are having a party next weekend and she decides to invite Marissa so that Marissa can meet some new people and perhaps form some friendships. Kirsty decides to discuss this with her supervisor after the party, when she will be able to report on how the intervention has worked. Do you think Kirsty is at risk of breaking professional boundaries? What suggestions can you make that would help Kirsty to develop safe and positive interpersonal relationships?

CONFIDENTIALITY

Consumers often reveal personal information to nurses and ask that we keep that information secret. Confidentiality is a primary principle of the therapeutic relationship and is based on the ethical principle of autonomy. For nurses to engage in professional practice, consumers need to be able to trust that their personal information will not be disclosed to others. However, there are some limitations to confidentiality. In some cases, ethical principles of non-maleficence and justice might dictate that confidential information should be disclosed to a third party. For example, if a consumer reveals information about an intention to harm others, that information must be shared with the rest of the team. In this case the principle of justice might override that of autonomy. There might also be occasions where it is necessary to share a consumer's health information with another practitioner, such as a general practitioner, to ensure that harm does not result from the general practitioner being unaware of prescribed treatments. Most health services have policies for these situations, which guide professional practice within the law and within codes of ethics. Nurses should seek guidance in cases where they are unsure. Consumers sometimes ask nurses to keep secrets. Secrets are appropriate within a friendship but never within a therapeutic relationship. It is paramount that the consumer is made aware that information will be shared with the team and that this information will remain within the team. Hence, confidentiality in such circumstances is a *prima facie moral principle* and not an *absolute principle*. This is reflected in the common law and also in nursing codes of conduct and professional practice.

Law and mental health

Like other areas of nursing, mental health nursing occurs within a framework of legislation and the common law. Every jurisdiction has legislation that governs professional practice, such as privacy, guardianship and health care rights. In addition to these various legal frameworks, mental health care is unique compared with other areas of nursing because mental health is the only specialty in which a significant proportion of services can be provided under a framework of legal compulsion and without consent. This section outlines the major areas of law that impact on the care of mental health consumers and the practice of mental health nurses.

Professional regulation

In Australia, nursing and other health practitioners, including students, are registered with and regulated by, the Australian Health Practitioner Regulation Authority (Ahpra) and through boards such as the Nursing and Midwifery Board of Australia (NMBA). Ahpra and the NMBA operate under what is known as statutory law – that is, an Act of Parliament. In Australia there is uniform regulation of nurses through the *Health Practitioner Regulation National Law Act*, also known as the National Law, passed by all Australian states and territories parliaments. This mandates registration of health practitioners annually, certification and reporting of any adverse relevant events (e.g. a charge or finding of guilt relating to serious criminal offences).

New Zealand nurses' practice is governed by Te Kaunihera Tapuhi o Aotearoa/The Nursing Council of New Zealand (NCNZ). This is a statutory body authorised under the *Health Practitioners Competence Assurance Act 2003*. Both the New Zealand and Australian Acts are primarily concerned with protecting the safety of the public. The nursing regulatory boards are therefore authorised to make judgements about individual nurse's eligibility for registered and fitness to practice. Decisions made by regulatory boards are subject to court rulings on appeal.

The National Law (Australia) defines professional misconduct, unprofessional conduct and notifiable conduct (ss. 5, 140), and the relevant board (e.g. the NMBA) may investigate nurses whose practice or conduct is or may be unsatisfactory. For example, the board may assess a nurse's knowledge, skill, judgement or care, and evaluate this in relation to the standard reasonably expected of a nurse of an equivalent level of training or experience. Additionally, the Act authorises boards to intervene if nurses or students have an impairment (e.g. a physical or mental health impairment) that affects patients' safety. Furthermore, there is a mandatory requirement for nurses, employers and (in the case of students) educators to report such an impairment (ss. 140, 143); that is, impairment is one ground for 'notifiable conduct'. The other grounds for notifiable conduct (and hence mandatory reporting) are when a nurse:

- provides care while affected by alcohol or drugs
- engages in sexual misconduct in connection with practice
- places consumers at risk of harm by significantly departing from professional standards (s. 140).

The NMBA has adopted codes and competency standards to articulate minimum standards – including compliance with relevant law (NMBA 2008; 2016) – and the values that should inform practice. Similarly, the NCNZ (2012) refers to Acts that impose legal obligations on New Zealand nurses, as well as the council's expectations about the values nurses are expected to demonstrate. Failure by nurses to practise according to the standards of conduct and values could lead to disciplinary proceedings, with the form of investigation, hearing and outcome outlined in the regulatory legislation regimes.

Privacy legislation

Privacy is important to health consumers in any setting, and especially in mental health where consumers may be subject to stigma or discrimination if their mental health history is known. In clinical practice nurses have many therapeutic encounters with consumers in which sensitive, deeply personal information is discussed. There may also be conflict within families that accentuate the need for privacy in consumers' relationships with mental health professionals. Legislation has been introduced to address these issues, although privacy also remains an ethical obligation on the part of nurses.

At common law, medical and nursing notes, whether in paper, electronic or other form, belong to the health service, although the information is owned by the consumer. For clarity, the Commonwealth created a legislative scheme in relation to the issues of privacy and confidentiality including health records and data. The Commonwealth Australian Information Commissioner is responsible for administering the *Privacy Act 1988*. The 13 Australian Privacy Principles (APPs), which are contained in Schedule 1 of the Privacy Act, outline how most Australian Government agencies (e.g. Medicare, health services and hospitals) and all private health service providers must handle, use and manage personal information.

The APPs are not prescriptive; each agency needs to consider how the principles apply to its own situation. The principles cover:

- the open and transparent management of personal information including having a privacy policy
- rules for collecting solicited personal information and receiving unsolicited personal information including giving notice about collection
- how personal information can be used and disclosed (including overseas)
- maintaining the quality of personal information
- keeping personal information secure
- the right for individuals to access and correct their personal information.

APP 12 requires agencies that hold personal information about an individual (e.g. a consumer) to give the individual access to that information on request, although there are limits. APP 12.3 lists 10 grounds on which an organisation can refuse to give access to personal information including:

- the organisation reasonably believes that giving access would pose a serious threat to the life, health or safety of any individual (consumer), or to public health or public safety (APP 12.3(a))
- giving access would have an unreasonable impact on the privacy of other individuals (APP 12.3(b))
- the request for access is frivolous or vexatious (APP 12.3(c)).

Some mental health legislation contains laws about confidentiality and when information can be disclosed. For example, where the consumer does not consent, information may be disclosed to carers under s. 120A(3)(ca) of the *Mental Health Act 1986* (Vic) if the information is reasonably required for the ongoing care of the person and the carer will be involved in providing that care. Conversely, where a consumer does not consent to the disclosure of information to a carer, this must be respected (see, for example, s. 288 (2)(a) of the *Mental Health Act 2016* (Qld)). However, there is some tension between carers' requests to be lawfully provided with more information and consumers' concern about protecting their rights to privacy and confidentiality (National Mental Health Consumer and Carer Forum 2011).

The New Zealand Privacy Commissioner's website (www.privacy.org.nz) provides information about the New Zealand *Privacy Act 1993*, which applies to all health agencies. A Health Information Privacy Code sets out specific rules for agencies in the health sector and covers health information collected, used, held and disclosed by health agencies. The code requires that health information is kept confidential but also allows information to be passed on to third parties under certain circumstances, such as where other legislation requires it. Within the health sector, health information can only be disclosed if the reason for the disclosure is the same reason the information was collected (i.e. for providing health care). Other legislation with implications for consumers' privacy includes the *Mental Health (Compulsory Assessment and Treatment) Act 1992* and the *Health and Disability Commissioner Act 1996*.

Finally, codes of conduct and ethics for nurses require nurses to respect the privacy of consumers. The NMBA *Code of Conduct for Nurses in Australia* and *Code of Ethics for Nurses in Australia* outline the requirement for nurses to observe confidentiality in the course of their practice. Privacy is one of the principles of the NCNZ's *Code of Conduct for Nurses*.

Guardianship legislation

Issues of guardianship arise when an adult lacks legal capacity or competency and therefore is deemed to be unable to provide a valid consent (Chesterman 2018). Each jurisdiction has guardianship legislation that facilitates consent for treatment on behalf of incompetent adults. In Australian jurisdictions (except the Australian Capital Territory and the Northern Territory), the consent of a relative or carer may be lawful where no other legal guardian has precedence. For example, the Victorian *Guardianship and Administration Act 1986* includes a hierarchy whereby a person appointed by the Victorian Civil and Administrative Tribunal, under a guardianship order, and by the consumer as an enduring guardian, all precede the consumer's spouse or domestic partner and primary carer, and all the former precede the further hierarchy of nearest relative (ss. 3, 37).

Depending on the circumstances of the consumer for whom an order is made, a guardian's authority may be full or limited (e.g. in decision-making scope or period of authorisation). Typically, the legislation refers to the guardian acting in the consumer's best interests or the consumer's health and wellbeing, along with acting according to the consumer's wishes if these are known. Mental health (or sometimes guardianship) legislation may limit the capacity of guardians to consent to or refuse some psychiatric treatments (e.g. ECT and psychosurgery); it may be necessary to obtain authorisation from a guardianship authority or mental health tribunal. This highlights the need for nurses to become familiar with both the relevant mental health and guardianship legislation in their jurisdiction.

In New Zealand, guardianship for adults is provided for in the *Protection of Personal and Property Rights Act 1988*. Under that legislation a person can assign an enduring power of attorney (EPOA) to a trusted individual, as long as they are competent to do so. The Act provides two forms of guardianship – one for personal affairs (financial affairs, personal business, etc.) and another for welfare (including decisions about health care). If an EPOA has been assigned it must be 'activated' to become effective. Activation requires a health professional to determine that the individual now lacks decision-making capacity. Once activated the power of attorney allows the nominated person to make decisions on behalf of the incompetent individual. Most mental health consumers, including compulsory patients under the Mental Health (Compulsory Assessment and Treatment) Act, retain the legal capacity to make decisions, including about health care, apart from those directly related to their mental health. If the individual has not named an EPOA, this role can be assigned by the Family Court.

Mental health legislation

Compulsory treatment under mental health legislation carries significant human right implications for consumers and presents unique clinical, ethical and professional issues for mental health nurses. This section on law and mental health provides an outline of the rationale for mental health legislation, the process of enacting civil commitment, discussion of the rights of people subject to compulsory treatment, ethical issues for mental health nurses, and human rights issues related to mental health legislation. Several Australian states have passed new legislation in recent years, and a full list of current legislation is provided in Table 8.1. The mental health legislation of New Zealand is described, and some aspects of the legislation of the state of Victoria are outlined as an example of Australian legislation. A detailed comparison of Australian and New Zealand mental health legislation has been provided by the Royal Australian and New Zealand College of Psychiatrists (see the list of useful websites at the end of this chapter). Discussion of mental health legislation is followed by a section discussing the human rights implications of mental health legislation, with special reference to the *Convention on the Rights of Persons with Disabilities*. Many jurisdictions provide separate legislation for the compulsory treatment of alcohol and other addictions. That legislation is not covered in this chapter, and readers are referred to more specialised resources and the websites of each jurisdiction. A list of key concepts related to mental health legislation is provided in Box 8.2.

RATIONALE FOR MENTAL HEALTH LEGISLATION

Legal powers to protect individuals from the consequences of their behaviour resulting from mental illness, or to protect others from such behaviour, has a long tradition in Western societies (Scull 2015). In Australia and New Zealand these provisions are contained in mental health legislation by a process known as 'committal' or 'civil commitment'. These two terms are used interchangeably in the discussion that follows. The term 'civil commitment' indicates that the legal procedure is a civil rather than a criminal process. Civil commitment provides states with two powers to restrain an individual and hence breach their autonomy. The first is the 'parens patriae' (Latin; 'parent of the state'), a doctrine that grants courts and the government inherent powers and authority to protect individuals who are unable to act on their own behalf and in their best interests. The second is the public policy powers of the state to empower certain persons or services (e.g. police, ambulance officers, medical and authorised mental health practitioners) to breach the autonomy of individuals if their behaviour is considered a significant risk to themselves or others. An example of this power would be the case of an individual who might harm another person because of a false belief that that person means to harm them.

Two consequences of civil commitment are that the individual is either physically restrained by being forcibly hospitalised or has conditions placed on their freedoms as a member of society. Conditions typically include accepting mental health care (e.g. medication) or may include living at a particular location (usually the consumer's home). From an ethical perspective civil commitment is usually based on an ethical justification of paternalism, which means that the harm of breaching a consumer's autonomy

TABLE 8.1 Mental health legislation and related guidelines in Australia and New Zealand

JURISDICTION	LEGISLATION	GUIDELINES
Australian Capital Territory	*Mental Health Act 2015*	Information about the Act www.health.act.gov.au
New South Wales	*Mental Health Act 2007*	Mental Health Act 2007: guide book www.health.nsw.gov.au
Northern Territory	*Mental Health and Related Services Act 1998*	Mental health information for health professionals https://health.nt.gov.au/professionals/mental-health-information-for-health-professional
Queensland	*Mental Health Act 2016*	Mental Health Act 2016: Chief Psychiatrist policies and guidelines www.health.qld.gov.au
South Australia	*Mental Health Act 2009*	Clinicians' guide and code of practice www.sahealth.sa.gov.au
Tasmania	*Mental Health Act 2013*	Mental Health Act 2013: a guide for clinicians www.dhhs.tas.gov.au
Victoria	*Mental Health Act 2014*	Mental Health Act 2014: handbook www.health.vic.gov.au
Western Australia	*Mental Health Act 2014*	Clinicians' practice guide to the Mental Health Act 2014 www.mentalhealth.wa.gov.au
New Zealand	*Mental Health (Compulsory Assessment and Treatment) Act 1992*	Guideline to the Mental Health (Compulsory Assessment and Treatment) Act 1992 www.health.govt.nz

is justified by being in the best interests of the person restrained. Justification is vexed, but according to prima-facie paternalism is part of the state's obligations to individuals. Mental health legislation provides clinicians with a legal framework within which to provide involuntary treatment for people who meet the criteria of that legislation. It will be apparent that civil commitment involves significant departures from the normally accepted rights of citizens and health consumers, especially the right to personal freedom and the right to consent to treatment.

THE PROCESS OF CIVIL COMMITMENT

The exact process of civil commitment varies from one jurisdiction to another, and the section below is intended as an overview of the main steps of the process. In most Australian and New Zealand jurisdictions legislation requires that the individual concerned has a mental illness (sometimes termed 'mental disorder') *and* that a degree of risk is present. It is not enough that the person has a mental illness and in the opinion of professionals would benefit from treatment that they refuse. Mental illness must also coexist with a significant degree of risk. An example would be a person who hears voices commanding them to harm others, where it seems likely that the person will act on those voices if not prevented from doing so. Note that this example includes features of mental illness (hearing voices) *and* risk (risk of harm to others). It is important to note that hearing voices is not always associated with mental illness and that most people with mental illness are not at risk of harming others. Mental health legislation therefore only applies to a small minority of people with mental illness, and only when their symptoms are assessed as sufficiently severe. Exceptions to the assessment of the degree of mental illness and risk are the states of Tasmania and Victoria, which have introduced a capacity standard for civil commitment (Callaghan & Ryan 2012). Capacity is also referenced in the assessment criteria of the legislation in Queensland, South Australia and Western Australia. Under an assessment of capacity, the focus is on the consumer's capacity for decision making, not on mental illness and risk. 'Capacity' is a legal concept requiring an individual to demonstrate the cognitive ability to understand, consider and make rational choices.

If a person becomes acutely mentally unwell, a clinician or family member may feel that they represent a significant risk to themselves or others and begin the process of civil commitment. Civil commitment may be initiated in a variety of settings including consumers' homes, primary care, court hearings, police custody, emergency departments and community or inpatient mental health services. The initial step is usually an application whereby a concerned person requests that the individual with signs of a mental illness be assessed with a view to civil commitment. Applications may be completed by family

Box 8.2 Key concepts related to mental health legislation and compulsory mental health care

Advance directive: A legal document in which a person specifies what actions should be taken for their health if they are no longer able to make decisions for themselves because of illness.

Assessment: For the purposes of mental health legislation, assessment is a clinical assessment with the specific purpose of determining whether the consumer meets the criteria of the legislation for civil commitment.

Capacity: The cognitive ability of a consumer to make informed healthcare decisions.

Case law: Rulings (judgments) of courts that create precedents about how legislation is interpreted and the law is to be applied.

Civil commitment or committal: The process being made subject to mental health legislation.

Committed: The legal status of a person under mental health legislation.

Coercion: Care or treatment in which a consumer's autonomous decision making is limited. Coercion may be formal or informal and is not limited to consumers subject to mental health legislation.

Community treatment order (CTO): A determination for compulsory treatment applying to consumers living in the community.

Compulsory treatment or involuntary treatment: Treatment provided under mental health legislation that does not involve informed consent.

Convention on the Rights of Persons with Disabilities: A United Nations Convention that outlines the rights of people with disabilities, including people with mental illness.

Dangerousness: The assessed degree of risk concerning the level (amount) and likelihood of self-harm, self-neglect or harm to others occurring as a result of mental illness.

Duty of care: The legal obligation owed by nurses to consumers to take all reasonable actions (both positive and negative) to provide the standard of care necessary to avoid foreseeable harm or injury to a consumer. Failure to meet the standard of care can result in a case of negligence.

Forced treatment: Compulsory treatment (usually medication and hospitalisation) provided when a consumer is not consenting and usually when physically restrained.

Informed consent: The process of making healthcare choices based on full information about alternatives and free from coercion or undue influence. Informed consent is an ethical and legal obligation on health practitioners.

Inpatient order: A form of compulsory treatment provision applying to consumers admitted to hospital.

Judicial review: A review by a judge of a consumer's legal status under mental health legislation.

Least restrictive alternative: The legal and general principle that requires clinicians to use the least possible restrictive measures in providing care and treatment.

Mental health legislation: Legislation (Acts of parliament) that are specific to mental health that govern the provision of mental health services and treatment whether with or without consent.

Parens patriae power: Power invested in the state to protect individuals who are mentally unwell and who are considered to be at risk as a result of mental illness. Use of parens patriae power may involve a restraint on individual autonomy.

Police power: Power invested by the state in the police to restrain or breach the autonomy of individuals who are mentally unwell and considered to represent a risk to themselves or others.

Review tribunal (Mental Health Review Tribunal): A quasi-judicially empowered panel established under mental health legislation to review the legal status of consumers and/or appeals brought by consumers seeking judicial review.

Statutory officials Nurses, doctors, lawyers and others (e.g. ambulance officers) who are assigned specific roles and powers under mental health legislation.

Supported decision making: A tool that allows people with disabilities to retain their decision-making capacity by choosing supporters to help them make choices.

Voluntary treatment: Treatment that involves informed consent and is provided voluntarily and freely – for example, without inducement, threat or sanction.

members, general practitioners or other authorised health professionals (e.g. mental health nurses). There may be a need for a supporting certificate written by a nurse as part of the application. Next, the individual will be formally assessed by a health practitioner, who will decide about whether there is a need for the person to be committed. If this assessment demonstrates there is a need, a 'committal order' will be made. This normally occurs in an inpatient setting, although in some regions involuntary treatment can be provided out of hospital. The initial period of involuntary treatment is from 1 day or up to 2 weeks, depending on the jurisdiction, usually with a proviso that if the consumer 's mental state improves, the period of compulsory treatment can cease. Once a consumer is subject to committal, the period of compulsory treatment can be extended. In some jurisdictions the extension may be indefinite.

Although the initial process of committal is undertaken by clinicians, including nurses, committal is a legal procedure and so is subject to appeal and review by a mental health tribunal or a judge in a court of law. The judge will ultimately determine whether the clinician's actions are consistent with the requirements of legislation and/or whether the consumer continues to require involuntary treatment. Mental health legislation includes various support and appeal processes that allow the consumer to question decisions and to have legal representation in the decision-making process. If an application for civil commitment has been made, the consumer will need to be informed of their rights, and about the possible decision to make an order for compulsory treatment. Other processes include the right to have a family member or a nominated support person involved in care and decision making, the right to consult a lawyer, the right to seek review by a judge and the right to have their legal status considered by a review tribunal.

ASSESSMENT UNDER MENTAL HEALTH LEGISLATION

An assessment under mental health legislation involves a clinical assessment that follows the standard process of a comprehensive assessment (see Chapter 7) but with a focus on whether the consumer meets the legislative criteria for committal. Assessments under mental health legislation are usually conducted by psychiatrists and include careful consideration of current and historical risk issues. Nurses may also be involved and, in some cases, may have initiated the process by raising concerns about the consumer and their safety. Although the psychiatrist will complete and sign the assessment document, nurses often contribute important observations and information to the assessment. Nurses may also be able to advocate for alternatives to committal – for example, by exploring additional community and home support, utilising respite care and negotiating the consumer's voluntary engagement with the mental health team. These considerations are important to ensure the care provided involves the least restrictions for the consumer. Care should be voluntary whenever possible and compulsory only if options for voluntary care cannot be safely employed. It is important to understand that in most cases assessment under mental health legislation is not an assessment of the consumer's capacity for informed decision making, although as noted above Tasmania and Victoria have adopted a capacity standard for civil commitment. Rather, assessment is one of mental state in the context of the person's social and clinical history, thoughts, behaviours and level of risk. The issue of assessing capacity is addressed in a separate section below.

COMPULSORY TREATMENT

Once subject to civil commitment a consumer can be treated without their consent, although as discussed below there is still a continuing obligation on clinicians to seek consent. People made subject to civil commitment have very often refused to consent to voluntary treatment – that is one of the reasons for seeking an order for compulsory treatment. The plan of compulsory treatment will include ensuring safety by providing a secure environment, ongoing clinical assessment, medication aimed at reducing acute symptoms, personal care for those consumers unable to care for themselves (hygiene, hydration, nutrition) and supportive psychological care (being with the person, psychotherapeutic support, safe socialisation, visits or contact with friends or family members).

Although the power to treat without consent is provided by legislation, nurses should always attempt to obtain consent rather than simply exercising the legal right to treat without it. Compulsory treatment does not override nurses' ethical and professional obligation to work collaboratively with consumers. For example, a consumer may have medication prescribed but might refuse to accept that medication when it is first offered. The nurse should then work with the consumer to negotiate obtaining consent by explaining the intended benefits of the medication, validating any concerns the consumer has about the medication and providing the consumer with choices about how the medication is administered. An option might be to provide as much explanation as possible and give the consumer time to reconsider their refusal. In these situations, nurses should always be honest in disclosing whether administering the medication by force is a possibility. In cases where medication does need to be administered by force, safety of the consumer and the nurse is paramount. This includes psychological and physical safety. Every service has policies and procedures relating to the use of force and these should be followed carefully. In addition, these policies will outline the explanations to provide to consumers, how to offer reassurance to consumers about the nurse's actions and use of the least possible force necessary in the situation. Remember that the law only permits reasonable and proportionate force in the circumstances. Consumers should be provided with subsequent opportunities to review their experience of forced medication, and nurses should have an opportunity to debrief with colleagues.

PROTECTIVE MECHANISMS IN MENTAL HEALTH LEGISLATION

Because mental health legislation involves significant limitations on normally accepted health care and human rights, mental health Acts include a range of measures aimed at counterbalancing the legislative power to detain consumers and impose compulsory treatment. Protective mechanisms include the right to advocacy (legal or otherwise), processes of appeal and review by tribunals and courts, appointment of statutory officials (e.g. district inspectors) to oversee the operation of legislation and complaints procedures. Readers should consult the legislation for their own jurisdiction, as well as the guidelines for applying mental health legislation listed in Table 8.1.

As with other legislation, actions taken under mental health laws may be subject to challenge in the courts, where clinical decisions can be tested and may be legally overturned. Decisions arising from legal challenges create a body of case law that instructs and provides guidance concerning legal actions, decision making and procedures implemented by clinicians pursuant to mental health legislation. Case law precedents can affect clinical practice because clinicians are obliged to work within the precedents. One set of cases in New Zealand involved mental health nurses acting as duly authorised officers under the legislation. This role includes arranging assessments under mental health legislation, which in New Zealand requires a person subject to an assessment to be advised of the assessment in the presence of a member of their family, a caregiver or a person concerned with their welfare. Three cases were heard where the consumers, through their lawyer, argued that an appropriate third party was not present. As a result of these cases, nurses acting in the duly authorised officer role must now be vigilant that the third party is an appropriate person. A full discussion of these cases is provided by Thom et al. (2009).

WORKING WITH COERCION AND COMPULSION: THE ROLE OF PROCEDURAL JUSTICE

The legal concept of the doctrine of procedural fairness and due process (procedural justice) provides a template for working with consumers whose autonomy is restricted by their legal status or by any imposed limiting conditions. Procedural justice is a branch of natural justice and can be defined as fairness in which decisions are made. Fairness relates to both decision-making processes and their outcome for the consumer. Procedural justice includes nursing skills such as listening, treating consumers with respect, offering choices, being open and transparent and availing the consumer time to consider their position and how to respond when their autonomy is limited. Because these skills are inherent in therapeutic relationships, nurses do not need to develop a new set of skills. It is therefore especially important for nurses to be aware of any coercive actions and how they affect consumers. When interactions are legally coercive the principles of procedural justice demand limitations on the use and impact of those interactions such as undue influence and duress.

An example of procedural justice is provided by Maguire et al. (2014), who studied the coercive practice of limit setting in a mental health inpatient setting. Limit setting can be important to the safety of inpatient setting and can help consumers by providing clear boundaries for their behaviour. At the same time, limit setting can constrain a consumer's autonomy. In Maguire et al.'s (2014) study nurses and consumers were interviewed about their experience of limit setting and reported that empathic engagement helped in maintaining therapeutic relationships. The researchers also found that treating consumers in a fair, respectful, consistent and knowledgeable way enhanced positive outcomes compared with interactive styles that were controlling and indifferent. This example from an inpatient setting has application in many situations when nurses are working with consumers who are subject to the restraints of mental health legislation or other forms of coercion. In community settings, where nurses are working with consumers under compulsory community treatment, researchers have reported that procedural justice is associated with a reduced experience of coercion (Galon & Wineman 2011). Procedural justice is not a substitute for ensuring that consumers' rights are respected and upheld, but it does help to guide interactions towards being less coercive.

NEW ZEALAND MENTAL HEALTH LEGISLATION

New Zealand's Mental Health (Compulsory Assessment and Treatment) Act was introduced towards the end of the period of deinstitutionalisation and reflected a shift from a therapeutic (need for treatment) standard to a legal standard based on dangerousness in decisions about involuntary treatment. This shift has influenced mental health legislation in many Western countries (Brown 2016). Consumers have access to legal counsel, appeal processes and reviews of their status under legislation by courts of law (Dawson & Gledhill 2013). In addition to establishing criteria for civil commitment, the Act contains provisions for ECT, psychosurgery and seclusion. For nurses, the Act introduced changes in their responsibilities by creating a range of new roles, from providing advice to the public to the exercise of temporary holding powers (McKenna & O'Brien 2013).

A decision to place a person under involuntary status does not mean the person needs to be admitted to hospital. Treatment can occur in a hospital or in any other place deemed suitable by the treating clinician. The intent and wording of the Act allow clinicians to explore less-restrictive alternatives such as care in a community respite facility or care at home. Criteria for invoking mental health legislation involve two components: 'abnormal state of mind' and 'serious danger to self or others' (Dawson &

Gledhill 2013). Section 2 of the Act defines mental disorder as:

> an abnormal state of mind (whether of a continuous or intermittent nature), characterised by delusions, or by disorders of mood or perception or volition or cognition, of such a degree that it:
> (a) Poses a serious danger to the health or safety of that person or of others; or
> (b) Seriously diminishes the capacity of that person to take care of himself or herself.

There are certain exclusions to the application of the New Zealand legislation. Section 4 of the Act specifies that the Act cannot be invoked solely by reason of the person's:

- political, religious or personal beliefs
- sexual preferences
- criminal or delinquent behaviour
- substance abuse, or
- intellectual disability.

In keeping with recognition of the Treaty of Waitangi, s. 5 of the Act requires that powers be exercised under the Act with respect for the cultural identity of consumers.

For an individual to be placed under mental health legislation, there first needs to be an application by a person over 18 years of age and an accompanying certificate of assessment. Following an initial assessment examination, the person may be required to undergo further periods of assessment and treatment, coordinated by a 'responsible clinician' appointed under the Act. During this time the individual can apply under s. 16 of the Act for a review of their condition by a judge. At the conclusion of the assessment, if the individual is thought to meet the criteria for compulsory treatment, the responsible clinician applies to the court for a compulsory treatment order. Compulsory treatment orders can be either inpatient orders or CTOs, and are for an initial period of six months. Other provisions of the Act apply to consumers following the issue of a CTO. These include the right to seek a review by a judge, regular clinical review, access to a review tribunal and specific rights under the Act. A detailed outline of the process of compulsory assessment and treatment, including definitions of key concepts, is provided by the Ministry of Health (2020).

Nurses are involved, through several statutory roles, in facilitating assessment and treatment under the Mental Health Act. The role of duly authorised officers involves aiding members of the public who may be concerned that a person is mentally disordered and in need of treatment under the Act. Although the legislation does not specify the professional background of individuals acting as duly authorised officers, in most cases this role has been assumed by nurses.

As discussed above, consumers with involuntary status may, under s. 16 of the Act, seek a review of their condition by a District Court judge. In most s. 16 reviews, the second health professional providing an opinion to the court is a nurse. Acting as second health professional can cause a sense of conflict between a custodial and a therapeutic role (O'Brien & Kar 2006), but with specific training nurses have demonstrated an increased sense of confidence and competence in the role (McKenna et al. 2011).

AUSTRALIAN MENTAL HEALTH LEGISLATION

Each Australian state and territory has mental health legislation (mental health Acts) designed to: protect individuals with mental illness from inappropriate treatment; direct the provision of mental health care and the facilities in which it is provided; and instruct mental health professionals' practice in providing treatment and care. For example, mental health Acts detail physical treatments involving 'prescribed' actions such as ECT, psychosurgery and some invasive medical interventions such as seclusion practices. While the Acts vary regarding the requirements of psychiatrists and mental health nurses, core issues such as a definition of mental illness and basic criteria for the admission and detention of voluntary and involuntary consumers deliberately reflect United Nations' human rights principles and are purposively present in all Acts.

Like New Zealand legislation, several Australian mental health Acts identify behaviours and personal characteristics that are *not* indicative of mental illness. For example, the Victorian Mental Health Act stipulates:

- particular political views or activities
- particular religious views or activities
- particular philosophies
- particular sexual preferences or sexual orientation
- particular illegal conduct or use of drugs and/or alcohol
- an antisocial personality
- having an intellectual disability.

This is expressly included to ensure that mental health Acts are not used perniciously and unconscionably against the individual as a form of social control.

Australian mental health Acts provide for the care and treatment of both voluntary and involuntary consumers. In amendments made to the Acts in recent years, caution has been taken to prescribe the consumers' perspective such as providing an appropriate and timely response to complaints about care during treatment (in the hospital and the community). As part of this consumer movement, detained consumers are more likely than ever before to receive care in the community, and the Acts facilitate this via CTOs. Remember that in cases where consumers are prescribed depot medication, they may be forcibly removed to hospital for treatment.

Australian mental health Acts have a stronger treatment focus than in other Commonwealth countries such as Canada. An involuntary admission will only occur if a person requires treatment and all other alternatives have been considered. For example, a person will be admitted if they are assessed to be a danger to themselves or others and there is no other less restrictive alternative available to manage that risk and provide treatment. Conversely, where the consumer is voluntary (i.e. with informed consent), two criteria common to Australian mental health Acts are that: (1) the severity of the mental illness requires treatment in an 'approved mental health facility' (Act defines such a facility); and (2) the individual is suffering from an acute episode of a mental illness. Mental health Acts generally include statements about the need to involve consumers in all appropriate aspects of their care and treatment regardless of their status (voluntary or detained). Consumer advocates and advance directives are examples of this. Again, this reflects the consumer movement. Circumstances may occur where a consumer is admitted voluntarily and then asks to leave but is deemed too unwell and is therefore detained against their will. For a consumer to be detained in such circumstances, they must be mentally ill and in need of immediate treatment that can only be provided in an approved mental health facility. In such circumstances the detention is lawful.

Australian mental health Acts vary in the time for which they specify that consumers can be detained involuntarily when first admitted to a mental health unit. Generally, a person may be detained against their will for an initial period of 24 hours by a medical practitioner but then must be reviewed by a psychiatrist as soon as is practicable. The consumer may be further detained for 21 days, or the detention may be revoked, and the consumer will assume voluntary status. Under a continuing detention order, consumers have a right of appeal, which is heard through a sitting of the state or territory mental health tribunal. For consumers, there is an uneasy tension between self-determination and the determinations made by mental health authorities 'in their best interests'.

Although all Australian mental health Acts have adopted the tenets of least-restrictive and consumer-focused practice in relation to the law, an issue facing Australian consumers and mental health nurses is the variation in language and provisions contained in the various state and territory Acts. In different jurisdictions, various terms are used for 'compulsory detention' (e.g. 'section' is used in one state; 'schedule' or 'order' in another), the length of time for which a person may be detained varies, and there are contrasting conditions surrounding the use of seclusion and restraint. In addition, the protective provisions of the various mental health Acts are different across regions, and there are different processes for obtaining legal advocacy.

Critical thinking challenge 8.5

1. How would you feel if a friend or a member of your family was admitted to hospital under mental health legislation?
2. What rights should consumers have to have their involuntary status reviewed?
3. How can you support consumers who express dissatisfaction at being treated under mental health legislation?
4. What long-term effects might compulsory admission to hospital have on a consumer?

COMMUNITY TREATMENT ORDERS IN AUSTRALIA AND NEW ZEALAND

For the past three decades compulsory mental health care in the community has been implemented through CTOs. CTOs are recommended as an alternative to hospitalisation (Rugkåsa et al. 2014) and as a means of providing care in the least restrictive environment. There are, however, concerns that CTOs represent part of an increasing preoccupation with minimising 'risk' (McMillan et al. 2019) and contribute to stigmatisation of consumers by reinforcing a perception of dangerousness.

CTOs vary in their conditions but generally require consumers to attend and consent to treatment or be sanctioned with the possibility of rehospitalisation. Hence, CTOs are legally enforceable against a consumer's consent but are subject to judicial review on appeal by consumers. Justifications for CTOs are that they reduce rates of hospitalisation, improve access to services, reduce relapse rates and improve the consumer's social functioning by assisting them to remain in the community.

A consumer subject to a CTO will live in their own home, whether a private residence, boarding house or some form of supported community accommodation. A CTO's conditions may specify the residential address where they must live and that they must refrain from using alcohol and other recreational drugs. Consumers under CTOs will usually receive follow-up care from a community-based mental health service, which will provide coordination of wraparound care such as social support, psychological treatment, medication and support to navigate the health and social services. Services are delivered in the consumer's home or at a community mental health centre, or some combination of both, often by community mental health nurses. Another frequent CTO condition stipulates compliance with prescribed medications, usually an antipsychotic in depot (long-acting) form. Part of the community mental health nurse's role will also be to monitor the consumer's physical health and ensure they receive primary health care. This last function is important to address the health disparities experienced by people with severe mental illness, particularly those who have been prescribed second-generation antipsychotic medication for long periods of time (see Chapter 18 for further discussion of physical health).

CTO rates are high in Australia and New Zealand. Light et al. (2012a; 2012b) surveyed Australian mental health tribunals and health district providers concerning the frequency of CTOs and the number of consumers subject to them. The lowest rate was in Tasmania, with 30.2 per 100,000 population, and the highest was Victoria, with 98.8 per 100,000. These rates are high by world standards. New Zealand's rate of 84 per 100,000 is also high by world standards (O'Brien 2014).

Although CTOs are now an established and frequent treatment option facilitated by mental health legislation in Australasia, debate about their human rights implications and effectiveness continues (O'Brien 2014). Critics have argued that the CTO represents an unnecessary extension of coercion into community settings and that this coercion and compulsory care/treatment is likely to lead to consumer resistance by disengaging from services. As a nurse you need to be aware of your legal obligations for consumers subject to CTOs and of their potential to negatively affect your therapeutic relationships.

Critical thinking challenge 8.6

1. How would you feel if a friend or a member of your family was discharged from hospital under a CTO?
2. What rights should apply to consumers subject to CTOs?
3. Why is it important that countries commit to international treaties such as the United Nations *Convention on the Rights of Persons with Disabilities*?
4. What domestic legislation is aimed at protecting the rights of mental health consumers?

HUMAN RIGHTS AND MENTAL HEALTH LEGISLATION

People with mental illness have historically been subject to specific discriminatory laws and, systemic denial of rights has been enshrined in mental health legislation (e.g. insanity commitment orders and lunatic Acts) Much of this denial of rights stemmed from medical ignorance, few treatment options and stigma. With greater awareness various international instruments have been drafted and ratified to help protect the rights of individuals with mental illness. Until 2008 human rights protections under mental health legislation were protected mainly by three instruments: the 1966 *International Covenant on Civil and Political Rights*; the 1966 *International Covenant on Economic, Social and Cultural Rights*; and the 1991 United Nations *Principles for the Protection of Persons with Mental Illness and the Improvement of Mental Health Care*. Australia and New Zealand are signatories to all three instruments. However, because international conventions are not binding or mandatory on Australian and New Zealand domestic laws, people with mental illness continued to experience discrimination, often reflected in and perpetrated by mental health legislation.

The *Convention on the Rights of Persons with Disabilities* was adopted in 2006 and entered into force in May 2008. The Convention has been ratified by both Australia and New Zealand and is now considered to be the most internationally authoritative document articulating the rights of people with mental illness. The Convention does not create new rights for people with disabilities but clarifies existing rights under other instruments such as those mentioned above. Unlike some other rights instruments, the Convention does not focus solely on one issue, in this case mental illness. Instead, it focuses on the concept of disability and provides a wide definition that includes mental illness alongside other disabilities. A foundation principle of the Convention is equality; that is, not only should people with disabilities enjoy the rights to be free from prejudice and discrimination but also barriers to social inclusion should be removed so that people with disabilities are able to enjoy the full range of opportunities available to other members of society. The 50 Articles of the Convention make this a wide-ranging instrument, covering issues such as equal access to justice, gender issues, housing, rights of children and older people, and mobility. The full text of the Convention can be downloaded from www.un.org/disabilities.

One of the major implications of the Convention is the Article 12 requirement for equality before the law. Internationally, this requirement has been interpreted to mean that any legislation that limits rights based on an individual's membership of a 'status group' (e.g. people with disabilities) is considered discriminatory (Dawson 2015). As noted in the discussion of mental health legislation above, most Australian and New Zealand mental health legislation exclusively limits the rights of people with mental illness and is therefore considered discriminatory under the terms of Article 12 (Szmukler et al. 2014). The argument is that this legislation is discriminatory because it only applies to people with mental illness.

Recent reforms in mental health legislation have attempted to give effect to concerns raised under the Convention. Tasmania and Victoria amended their mental health legislation to respond to the Convention and have adopted a capacity-based standard for treatment without consent (Callaghan & Ryan 2012). An argument has been made for adopting the same standard in New Zealand (Gordon & O'Brien 2014), and legislative reform is now planned for New Zealand. In light of the Convention, understandings of the rights of people with mental illness and how legislation should address the issue of treatment without consent continue to evolve (Dawson 2015).

Substituted and supported decision making

When consumers are subject to mental health legislation, traditional approaches to decision making have seen health professionals, usually doctors, replacing the individual's usual autonomous decision making with a decision made by the health professional. This is known as substitute decision making and is frequently used when adults are considered to lack capacity (White et al. 2018), sometimes with some form of legal guardianship. Substitute decision making has been challenged under Article 12 the *Convention on the Rights of Persons with Disabilities*, which has been interpreted to require that health consumers should always make their own decisions, even when they lack capacity. The argument is that with adequate support the individual will be able to articulate their preferences and make the decision they would have made if they had capacity. This is an argument for supported decision making: providing consumers with the support they need to make their own decisions, rather than have another person make that decision for them (Gooding 2013). Supported decision making helps professionals meet their ethical obligations to respect consumers' autonomy and is also likely to promote consumers' recovery (Kokanović et al. 2018). Barriers to supported decision making include clinicians' lack of skills in this area and the lack of legal requirements for it. Although supported decision making does not need to be legally mandated, changing legislation to require supported rather than substitute decision making would help to promote this practice and would likely address some of the coercion experienced by people on CTOs (Brophy et al. 2019). Some arguments have been made that rejection of any form of substitute decision making is likely to have adverse effects on consumers and instead efforts should be made to improve the quality of substitute decision making – for example, by promoting the use of advance directives (Scholten & Gather 2018). Within the current framework of mental health legislation nurses can work with consumers to assist them to make their own decisions rather than impose decisions under the guise of paternalism (Davidson et al. 2016).

Duty of care and decision-making capacity

In this section, we discuss emergency situations arising in general health settings. In emergency situations of a threat to life or a serious threat to health and injury, restraint, hospitalisation and treatment without consent is a common-law protected duty of clinicians. Emergency situations might arise in mental health settings or general health settings, including community settings, mental health inpatient units, emergency departments and general hospital wards. In emergency departments, individuals may temporarily lose capacity because of the toxic effects of recreational drugs or the high emotional arousal associated with self-harm. A common example of impaired decision-making capacity in a general health setting is where an individual has developed delirium and become acutely confused. There are many causes of delirium, which is characterised by a rapid deterioration in mental state that can fluctuate rapidly. This may be secondary to medical illness, anaesthesia, high temperature or other causes. In some cases, the precise cause of delirium is not known, and the diagnosis is based on the clinical history. However, in delirium there is often severe impairment of cognitive functioning, with loss of decision-making capacity.

In people displaying acute confusional states such as delirium, clinicians commonly apply a test of capacity. Capacity refers to the mental or cognitive ability to understand the nature and effects of one's actions. Note that legally an individual is presumed to have capacity unless otherwise demonstrated. Although it is not a standardised test, the applied test contains four criteria:

- **Comprehension:** Does the person understand the information provided by a health professional?
- **Expressing a choice:** Is the person capable of weighing alternatives and stating their preferences?
- **Appreciation:** Does the person appreciate their situation and its consequences?
- **Reasoning:** Is the person able to think rationally about the situation?

In most situations it is necessary for the person to meet all four criteria in order to have decision-making capacity. Additional assessment may involve using standardised assessment instruments that can be repeated to detect improvement or deterioration in mental state (Cheung et al. 2015), as capacity can change over time.

Assessment of capacity is dependent on the seriousness of the situation the person faces. For example, deciding to leave hospital while confused is clearly more serious than making a decision about whether or not to have a shower. Each situation must be assessed individually, and clinicians should consult with colleagues if they are unsure. Family members should also be consulted to establish what the person's normal preferences would be. Factors such as cultural and language differences, sensory impairment, pain and an unfamiliar environment need to be considered to contextualise a capacity assessment. If an individual's decision-making capacity is thought to be permanently impaired (e.g. in dementia), clinicians should consider provisions for legal guardianship. This normally involves a court process, to appoint a 'substitute decision-maker'. This can be a family member, lawyer or the Guardianship Board, who will make decisions on the individual's behalf and in their best interests. Again, if the person regains capacity the guardianship order on application may be discharged.

Advance directives

Mental health advance directives are statements of preferences for mental health care if a mental health crisis leaves the person unable to express their preferences. The aim is to increase consumer autonomy in mental health crises. Many mental health consumers experience crisis events when they may be too distressed or cognitively impaired to state their preferences. In such cases, a statement of preferences, prepared in advance at a time when the consumer is well, can act as a guide to clinicians as to what the consumer's preferences are.

Various models of advance instructions have been developed, including psychiatric advance directives, joint crisis plans, wellness recovery action plans, advance statements and mental health advance preference statements (Henderson et al. 2008; Lenagh-Glue et al. 2018). An advance directive can include treatment preferences such as which medication to use or avoid, preferences about use of seclusion and restraint, involvement of particular clinicians, treatment setting and methods of calming and de-escalation (Thom et al. 2019). They can also include preferences for personal affairs such as care of the consumer's house or flat, care of pets, who to contact in the event of a crisis, and who the consumer would prefer not to have involved. Research has shown that consumers value the opportunity to make an advance directive, although in practice many are not given that opportunity (Shields et al. 2014). Mental health advance directives help to meet obligations under the *Convention on the Rights of Persons with Disabilities* (Szmukler 2019), and several Australian states have recognised advance directives in their mental health legislation (Ouliaris & Kealy-Bateman 2017). Advance directives have been proposed for inclusion in revised legislation in New Zealand (Lenagh-Glue et al. 2020).

A mental health advance directive does not override mental health legislation, although even for consumers subject to mental health legislation clinicians have an ethical and legal obligation to attempt to work with consumers' competently expressed preferences. A mental health advance directive can only be effective if clinicians take the trouble to access it from the consumer's clinical records and then work with the consumer towards meeting the preferences expressed. This presents a key advocacy role to mental health nurses within multidisciplinary teams in helping ensure the advance directive is used to negotiate care and treatment with consumers.

Chapter summary

This chapter has explored ethical and legal issues associated with mental health nursing practice in Australia and New Zealand. Mental health nursing is fraught with ethical issues arising from the classification of mental illness, diagnoses, treatment and working within the constraints of mental health legislation and guidance provided by professional codes of ethics. The mental health setting poses unique challenges to nurses in the form of treatment without consent under mental health legislation. In addition, nurses must practise within legislation governing consumer rights, privacy and guardianship. The United Nations *Convention on the Rights of Persons with Disabilities* provides challenges to current legislation and practice. Capacity-based legislation, advance directives and supported decision making provide some responses to these challenges.

EXERCISES FOR CLASS ENGAGEMENT

Read the four scenarios below and consider appropriate responses to the questions that follow. You can either split into discussion groups or work individually.

SCENARIO 1

A 33-year-old woman under a CTO is refusing to have her regular antipsychotic medication, although she does agree that her symptoms were lessened when taking the medication. She is concerned about her increase in weight as a result of taking the medication and tells you that you do not understand what it is like taking medication with such side effects.

SCENARIO 2

A 59-year-old male widower, who has been diagnosed with liver and bowel cancer, presents with considerable pain and distress. He tells you he has always believed in euthanasia and has decided that his time is now up. He does not want to be a burden on his daughter and wishes to die with dignity. He is open about his wish to die and has planned his suicide. All his affairs are in order. He believes that he will carry this out sooner rather than later, as the pain is now too great, and he just wants it to end.

SCENARIO 3

A 15-year-old girl presented at an emergency department after ingesting 24 paracetamol tablets. She had been struggling with anorexia nervosa since she was 11 and felt that her life was heading nowhere. She was transferred as an involuntary consumer to the local mental health hospital and prescribed nasogastric tube feeding, which was given without her consent. Three weeks later she remains suicidal and is still being tube fed. She wants to be left alone as she cannot face the pain of life anymore.

SCENARIO 4

An 84-year-old well-known actor has refused food and fluid for 6 days as she does not want to live anymore. She has right-sided paralysis following a cerebrovascular accident. She wants to be remembered as young and beautiful. She feels that her life has been full and now wants it to end, as she feels that her prospects are hopeless.

QUESTIONS

1. Considering the above four scenarios:
   - Who is making a rational choice to die?
   - What are our responsibilities in each case as health professionals?
   - Do health professionals have the right to stop people when they wish to die?
2. Discuss contemporary developments in mental health services globally and in Australia and New Zealand, and their impact on how people with mental illness are cared for in the community.
3. Think about some recent clinical experiences you have had with consumers with a mental health problem or illness and discuss your responses to the following questions with your group or class members.

- Identify some controlling interventions you have been involved with or have observed. If you were involved, how did you feel about being involved?
- Were there alternatives that could have been less restrictive?
- What are your own beliefs about how and where people with mental illness should be cared for?
- Should legislation have the power to contain or control people with a mental illness to protect them from themselves and/or other people?

Useful websites

Australian Commission on Quality and Safety in Health Care: https://www.safetyandquality.gov.au/.

Australian Health Practitioner Regulatory Agency: https://www.ahpra.gov.au/.

Australian Human Rights Commission: https://www.humanrights.gov.au/.

Australian Nursing and Midwifery Accreditation Council: https://www.anmac.org.au/.

Community Law (New Zealand): http://communitylaw.org.nz.

End Seclusion Now (Facebook group): https://www.facebook.com/End-Seclusion-Now-653392888041998/.

Involuntary commitment and treatment (ICT) criteria in Australian and New Zealand Mental Health Acts: https://www.ranzcp.org/files/resources/college_statements/mental-health-legislation-tables/mental-health-acts-comparative-tables-all.aspx.

Mental Health Coordinating Council (New South Wales) – online Manual of legal and human rights related to the mental health system: http://mhrm.mhcc.org.au/home.

MindFreedom – ethics and mental health page: https://mindfreedom.org/.

Nursing and Midwifery Board of Australia: https://www.nursingmidwiferyboard.gov.au/.

Nursing Council of New Zealand: https://www.nursingcouncil.org.nz/.

Office of the Health and Disability Commissioner: https://www.hdc.org.nz/.

Office of Disability Issues (New Zealand): https://www.odi.govt.nz/.

Office of the Public Advocate (South Australia) (click on 'Mental health treatment and your rights'): http://www.opa.sa.gov.au/.

United Nations *Convention on the Rights of Persons with Disabilities*: https://www.un.org/development/desa/disabilities/.

Universal Human Rights Instruments: https://www.ohchr.org/EN/ProfessionalInterest/Pages/UniversalHumanRightsInstruments.aspx.

References

American Psychiatric Association (APA), 2013. Diagnostic and Procedural Manual of Mental Disorders, fifth ed., text rev. APA, Washington.

Askew, L., Fisher, P., Beazley, P., 2019. What are adult psychiatric inpatients' experience of seclusion: a systematic review of qualitative studies. J. Psychiatr. Ment. Health Nurs. 26 (7–8), 274–285.

Australian College of Mental Health Nurses, 2016. Seclusion and restraint position statement. http://www.acmhn.org/images/stories/FINAL_Seclusion_and_Restraint_Position_Statement_-_August_2016.pdf.

Australian Nursing and Midwifery Council, 2008. Code of Ethics for Nurses in Australia. ANMC, Canberra.

Beauchamp, T.L., Childress, J.F., 2019. Principles of Biomedical Ethics, eighth ed. Oxford University Press, New York.

Bowers, L., Van Der Merwe, M., Nijman, H., et al., 2010. The practice of seclusion and time-out on English acute psychiatric wards: the City-128 Study. Arch. Psychiatr. Nurs. 24 (4), 275–286.

Brophy, L.M., Kokanović, R., Flore, J., et al., 2019. Community treatment orders and supported decision making. Front. Psychiatry 10, 414.

Brown, J., 2016. The changing purpose of mental health law: from medicalism to legalism to new legalism. Int. J. Law Psychiatry 47, 1–9.

Callaghan, S., Ryan, C.J., 2012. Rising to the human rights challenge in compulsory treatment: new approaches to mental health law in Australia. Aust. N. Z. J. Psychiatry 46 (7), 611–620.

Chesterman, J., 2018. Adult guardianship and its alternatives in Australia. In: Spivakovsky, C., Seear, K., Carter, A. (Eds.), Critical Perspectives on Coercive Interventions: Law, Medicine and Society. Routledge, New York, p. 180.

Cheung, G., Clugston, A., Croucher, M., et al., 2015. Performance of three cognitive screening tools in a sample of older New Zealanders. Int. Psychogeriatr. 27 (06), 981–989.

Cleary, M., Horsfall, J., 2014. Electroconvulsive therapy: issues for mental health nurses to consider. Issues Ment. Health Nurs. 35 (1), 73–76.

Davidson, G., Brophy, L., Campbell, J., et al., 2016. An international comparison of legal frameworks for supported and substitute decision-making in mental health services. Int. J. Law Psychiatry 44, 30–40.

Dawson, J., 2015. A realistic approach to assessing mental health laws' compliance with the UNCRPD. Int. J. Law Psychiatry 40, 70–79.

Dawson, J., Gledhill, K., 2013. The complex meaning of 'mental disorder'. In: Dawson, J., Gledhill, K. (Eds.), New Zealand's Mental Health Act in Practice. Victoria University Press, Wellington, pp. 29–45.

Flaskeraud, J., 2010. DSM proposed changes, part I. Criticisms and influences on changes. Issues Ment. Health Nurs. 31 (10), 686–688.

Galon, P., Wineman, N.M., 2011. Quasi-experimental comparison of coercive interventions on client outcomes in individuals with severe and persistent mental illness. Arch. Psychiatr. Nurs. 25 (6), 404–418.

Gooding, P., 2013. Supported decision-making: a rights-based disability concept and its implications for mental health law. Psychiatr. Psychol. Law 20 (3), 431–451.

Gordon, S., O'Brien, A., 2014. New Zealand's mental health legislation needs reform to avoid discrimination. N. Z. Med. J. 127 (1403), 55.

Griffith, R., Tengnah, C., 2013. Maintaining professional boundaries: keep your distance. Br. J. Community Nurs. 18 (1), 43–46.

Griffiths, C., O'Neill-Kerr, A., 2019. Patients', carers' and the public's perspectives on electroconvulsive therapy. Front. Psychiatry 10, 304.

Henderson, C., Swanson, J.W., Szmukler, G., et al., 2008. A typology of advance statements in mental health care. Psychiatr. Serv. 59 (1), 63–71.

Holmes, J., Adshead, G., 2009. Ethical aspects of the psychotherapies. In: Bloch, S., Green, S. (Eds.), Psychiatric Ethics, fourth ed. Oxford University Press, Oxford, pp. 367–384.

Illich, I., 2001. Limits to Medicine. Medical Nemesis: The Expropriation of Health. Marian Boyers, London.

International Council of Nurses (ICN), 2012. The ICN Code of Ethics for Nurses. ICN, Geneva.

Kokanović, R., Brophy, L., McSherry, B., et al., 2018. Supported decision-making from the perspectives of mental health service users, family members supporting them and mental health practitioners. Aust. N. Z. J. Psychiatry 52 (9), 826–833.

Larue, C., Dumais, A., Boyer, R., et al., 2013. The experience of seclusion and restraint in psychiatric settings: perspectives of patients. Issues Ment. Health Nurs. 34 (5), 317–324.

Lenagh-Glue, J., O'Brien, A., Dawson, J., et al., 2018. A MAP to mental health: the process of creating a collaborative advance preferences instrument. N. Z. Med. J. 131 (1486), 18–26.

Lenagh-Glue, J., Potiki, J., O'Brien, A.J., et al., 2020. The content of mental health advance preference statements (MAPS): a qualitative assessment of completed advance directives in the Southern District Health Board. Int. J. Law Psychiatry doi.org/10.1016/j.ijlp.2019.101537.

Light, E., Kerridge, I., Ryan, C., et al., 2012a. Community treatment orders in Australia: rates and patterns of use. Australas. Psychiatry 20 (6), 478–482.

Light, E., Kerrige, I., Ryan, C., et al., 2012b. Out of sight, out of mind: making involuntary community treatment visible in the mental health system. Med. J. Aust. 196 (9), 591–593.

Maguire, T., Daffern, M., Martin, T., 2014. Exploring nurses' and patients' perspectives of limit setting in a forensic mental health setting. Int. J. Ment. Health Nurs. 23 (2), 153–160.

Mandarelli, G., Carabellese, F., Parmigiani, G., et al., 2018. Treatment decision-making capacity in non-consensual psychiatric treatment: a multicentre study. Epidemiol. Psychiatr. Sci. 27 (5), 492–499.

Massabki, I., Abi-Jaoude, E., 2020. Selective serotonin reuptake inhibitor 'discontinuation syndrome' or withdrawal. Br. J. Psychiatry 1–4.

Mayers, P., Keet, N., Winker, G., et al., 2010. Mental health service users' perceptions and experiences of sedation, seclusion and restraint. Int. J. Soc. Psychiatry 56 (1), 60–73.

McKenna, B.G., O'Brien, A.J., 2013. Mental health nursing and the Mental Health Act. In: Dawson, J., Gledhill, K. (Eds.), New Zealand's Mental Health Act in Practice. Victoria University Press, Wellington, pp. 198–212.

McKenna, B.G., O'Brien, A.J., O'Shea, M., 2011. Improving the ability of mental health nurses to give second opinion in judicial reviews: an evaluation study. J. Psychiatr. Ment. Health Nurs. 18 (6), 550–557.

McMillan, J., Lawn, S., Delany-Crowe, T., 2019. Trust and community treatment orders. Front. Psychiatry 10, 349.

Ministry of Health, 2020. Guideline to the Mental Health (Compulsory Assessment and Treatment) Act (1992). Ministry of Health, Wellington.

Ministry of Health, 2010. Seclusion Under the Mental Health (Compulsory Assessment and Treatment) Act 1992. Ministry of Health, Wellington.

Ministry of Health, 2019. Every Life Matters – He Tapu te Oranga o ia Tangata: Suicide Prevention Strategy 2019–2029 and Suicide Prevention Action Plan 2019–2024 for Aotearoa New Zealand. Ministry of Health, Wellington.

Moncrieff, J., 2013. The Bitterest Pills: The Troubling Story of Antipsychotic Drugs. Palgrave Macmillan, Basingstoke.

National Mental Health Consumer and Carer Forum 2011. Privacy, confidentiality and information sharing – consumers, carers and clinicians. National Mental Health Consumer and Carer Forum. West Deakin, ACT. Retrieved from: nmhccf.org.au/sites/default/files/docs/nmhccf_pc_ps_brochure.pdf.

New Zealand Nurses Organisation (NZNO), 1995. Code of Ethics. NZNO, Auckland.

Nursing and Midwifery Board of Australia, 2016. Registered Nurse Standards for Practice for Nurses in Australia. NMBA, Canberra.

Nursing and Midwifery Board of Australia, 2008. Code of Ethics for Nurses in Australia. NMBA, Canberra.

Nursing Council of New Zealand, 2012. Code of Conduct for Nurses. NCNZ, Wellington.

O'Brien, A., 2014. Community treatment orders in New Zealand: regional variability and international comparisons. Australas. Psychiatry 22 (4), 352–356.

O'Brien, A., Kar, A., 2006. The role of second health professionals under New Zealand mental health legislation. J. Psychiatr. Ment. Health Nurs. 13 (3), 356–363.

Ouliaris, C., Kealy-Bateman, W., 2017. Psychiatric advance directives in Australian mental-health legislation. Australas. Psychiatry 25 (6), 574–577.

Pinel, P., 1806. A Treatise on Insanity. Strand, Messers Cadell & Davies.

Raeburn, T., Liston, C., Hickmott, J., et al., 2018. Life of Martha Entwistle: Australia's first convict mental health nurse. Int. J. Ment. Health Nurs. 27 (1), 455–463.

Rugkåsa, J., Dawson, J., Burns, T., 2014. CTOs: what is the state of the evidence? Soc. Psychiatry Psychiatr. Epidemiol. 49 (12), 1861–1871.

Salomon, C., Hamilton, B., 2014. Antipsychotic discontinuation syndromes: a narrative review of the evidence and its integration into Australian mental health nursing textbooks. Int. J. Ment. Health Nurs. 23 (1), 69–78.

Scholten, M., Gather, J., 2018. Adverse consequences of article 12 of the UN Convention on the Rights of Persons with Disabilities for persons with mental disabilities and an alternative way forward. J. Med. Ethics 44 (4), 226–233.

Scull, A., 2015. Madness in Civilization. A Cultural History of Insanity From the Bible to Freud, From the Madhouse to Modern Medicine. Princeton University Press, New Jersey.

Sellman, D., 2017. Virtue ethics and nursing practice. In: Scott, A.P. (Ed.), Key Concepts and Issues in Nursing Ethics. Springer, Cham, pp. 43–54.

Shields, L.S., Pathare, S., Van Der Ham, A.J., et al., 2014. A review of barriers to using psychiatric advance directives in clinical practice. Adm. Policy Ment. Health 41 (6), 753–766.

Smith, M., Vogler, J., Zarrouf, F., et al., 2009. Electroconvulsive therapy: the struggles in the decision-making process and the aftermath of treatment. Issues Ment. Health Nurs. 30 (9), 554–559.

Stein, D.J., van Niekerk, A.A., 2015. Ethics of psychopharmacology. In: Sadler, J.Z., Van Staden, W.C.W., Fulford, K.W.M. (Eds.), International Perspectives in Philosophy and Psychiatry. The Oxford Handbook of Psychiatric Ethics. Oxford University Press, Oxford, pp. 1175–1190.

Szmukler, G., 2019. 'Capacity','best interests','will and preferences' and the UN Convention on the Rights of Persons with Disabilities. World Psychiatry 18 (1), 34–41.

Szmukler, G., Daw, R., Callard, F., 2014. Mental health law and the UN Convention on the Rights of Persons with Disabilities. Int. J. Law Psychiatry 37 (3), 245–252.

Te Pou o te Whakaaro Nui, 2015. Towards Restraint-Free Mental Health Practice. Supporting the Reduction and Prevention of Personal Restraint in Mental Health Inpatient Settings. Te Pou o te Whakaaro Nui, Auckland.

Thom, K., Lenagh-Glue, J., O'Brien, A.J., et al., 2019. Service user, whānau and peer support workers' perceptions of advance directives for mental health. Int. J. Ment. Health Nurs. 28 (6), 1296–1305.

Thom, K.A., O'Brien, A.J., McKenna, B.G., et al., 2009. Judging nursing practice: implications of habeas corpus rulings for mental health nurses in New Zealand. Psychiatr. Psychol. Law 15 (1), 31–39.

White, B., Then, S.N., Willmott, L., 2018. Adults Who Lack Capacity: Substitute Decision-Making. Health Law in Australia, third ed. Thomson Reuters, Pyrmont, New South Wales, pp. 207–270.

World Health Organization, 2019. Strategies to End Seclusion and Restraint: WHO Quality Rights Specialized Training: Course Slides. World Health Organization, Geneva. https://apps.who.int/iris/handle/10665/329747.

Zachar, P., Stoyanov, D.S., Aragona, M., et al. (Eds.), 2014. Alternative Perspectives on Psychiatric Validation: DSM, IDC, RDoC and Beyond. Oxford University Press, Oxford.

CHAPTER 9

Anxiety

Anna Elders

KEY POINTS

- Anxiety is a necessary, protective emotion that functions to elicit several adaptive responses in the face of a stressor or threat. Anxiety can become problematic for some people, leading to significant impacts on functioning and quality of life.
- Most people presenting with anxiety disorders receive treatment and support within primary care settings; however, anxiety disorders have a high level of comorbidity with substance use, depressive disorders and suicidality.
- Therapies such as cognitive behaviour therapy and acceptance and commitment therapy are evidence-based treatments for anxiety, trauma and stress-related disorders. Combined psychological and pharmacological treatment may be warranted in more severe and complex presentations.
- Nurses are in a good position to develop collaborative, therapeutic relationships, undertaking assessment and offering psychoeducation, socioeconomic support and psychological interventions for people with anxiety, trauma and stress-related disorders.

KEY TERMS

- Avoidance behaviours
- Chronic stress
- Cognitions
- Hyperarousal
- Hypervigilance
- Hypothalamus–pituitary–adrenal (HPA) axis
- Intrusive anxious thoughts
- Post-traumatic stress disorder
- Psychological interventions
- Rumination
- Stress response
- Stressor
- Trauma-informed care

LEARNING OUTCOMES

The material in this chapter will assist you to:

- understand anxiety from evolutionary, adaptive and functional perspectives
- consider the aetiology of stress and anxiety and their mechanisms of action
- be aware of the demarcation between anxiety as a normal stress response and anxiety disorders
- be aware of the diagnostic symptoms and characteristics of specific anxiety disorders
- understand the considerations in assessing a person presenting with anxiety and identify suitable interventions for alleviating the distress and symptoms of anxiety disorders.

Introduction

To clinically define and understand what an anxiety disorder is, we must first consider anxiety as it naturally occurs within the human experience. Anxiety is as an evolutionary survival trait that allows for the identification and development of necessary responses to potentially dangerous stimuli (Malan-Müller et al. 2013). Anxiety can be defined as a future-oriented mood state associated with cognitive, physiological and behavioural reactions designed to reduce the level of perceived danger within a stimulating situation (Craske et al. 2009). Commonly known as the fight/flight/freeze response, such stress-based reactions are essential in the face of the numerous dangerous situations human beings can experience over a lifetime.

Anxiety can move from a response that ensures survival to one that creates ongoing levels of distress and impairment within a person's life. Considering anxiety and fear responses on a continuum and within a functional framework assists us to normalise anxiety and to work alongside consumers to make better assessments as to whether an anxiety disorder may be present.

This chapter examines the complex interactions that occur during an anxiety response and looks at the different anxiety, trauma and stress-related disorders, their common symptoms and the current evidence-based treatments available. A concise overview of symptoms is provided in Table 9.1 later in the chapter.

The chapter also explores some of the internal triggers and reinforcing elements of anxiety shaped by past experiences and significant events that may include trauma and childhood adversity (Craske et al. 2009). Being able to view anxiety through a trauma-informed lens can help nurses to better consider the origins and function of anxiety, enabling us to provide much more supportive and effective care.

Aetiology of stress, fear and anxiety

Stress, fear and anxiety are normal internal experiences that occur in response to a stressor. A stressor can be defined as any internal or external stimulus that promotes a stress response within a person. Historically, humans have been exposed to numerous life-threatening situations on a regular basis, from tribal warfare to naturally occurring environmental hazards such as famine. When we study the role that stress, fear and anxiety play in human evolution, we begin to see a system containing inbuilt mechanisms that allow for early recognition, physiological priming and behavioural adaptation in the face of danger. For the purposes of survival, the human brain developed the capability to learn and store information to aid timely responses in the face of threats. Human behaviour is shaped by our stress response system, and it is this system that is implicated in developing anxiety disorders and most other mental health disorders.

The physiological response to stress is a complex myriad of feedback mechanisms involving nearly every system of the body. The initial processes of a stress response are contained within the hypothalamus, located within our central nervous system. Incoming sensory information is sent directly to the amygdala for a rapid preparatory response. At the same time, information is processed against stored memories in the hippocampus. This process allows us to ascertain the level of risk and prepare for further physiological and behavioural responses. The sympathetic nervous system is activated, and a cascade of hormonal signalling responses work to stimulate action on the body's systems such as the cardiovascular system to ensure we are ready to respond to potential danger through our fight or flight response. The system responsible for these responses is the hypothalamic–pituitary–adrenal axis, or HPA axis (see Fig. 9.1). The HPA axis plays other important roles such as being part of our immune response in the face of infection and assisting in the regulation of glucose levels during times of stress.

Exposure to high levels of stress, such as those experienced through childhood abuse, is associated with heightened stress responses (Faravelli et al. 2012; Leonard 2005), identifying early trauma as a significant contributor to developing psychopathology.

Chronic stress, such as that experienced during an enduring, traumatic stressor like an abusive relationship, also leads to hypersecretion of cortisol and sustained

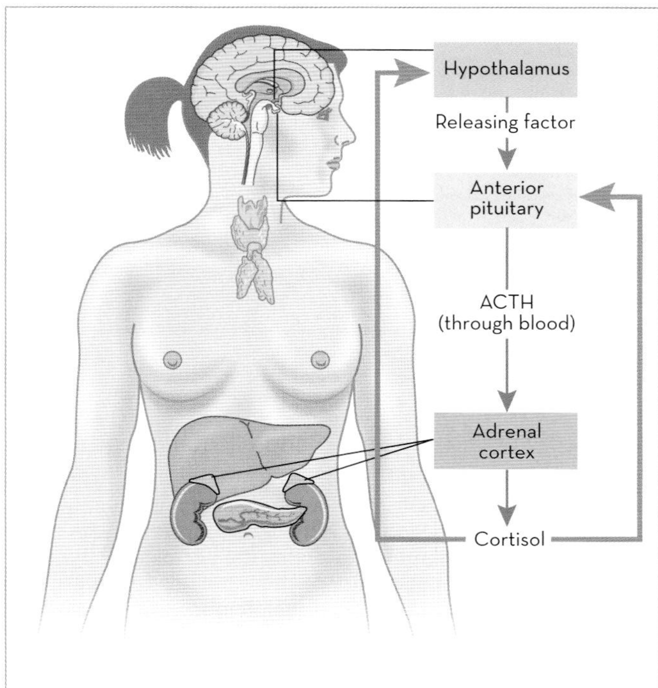

Figure 9.1
The hypothalamic–pituitary–adrenal axis
Adapted from Simon 2015

sympathetic nervous system response (Lowrance et al. 2016). Sustained sympathetic nervous system activity and excessive systemic exposure to cortisol have been shown to result in both physical illness and psychopathology due to the production of an ever-increasing and difficult-to-manage allostatic load (see Fig. 9.2), causing damaging effects on systems such as the central nervous and cardiovascular systems.

Differing responses to stressful life experiences can be understood as a combination of individual genetic (nature) and environmental (nurture) differences. Genetic vulnerability has been shown to greatly contribute to the presence of depression and anxiety symptoms in children up until age seven. However, environmental factors (positive or negative) are known to be important predictors of the presence and stability of symptoms throughout adolescence and adulthood (Nivard et al. 2015).

Chronic stress can thereby be thought of as a direct contributor to developing difficulties in mental health and general wellbeing. Stress is initially activated by real-life crises and adversity; however, it can continue years after the alleviation of these triggering events through the fear generalisation process. The fear generalisation process is thought to support survival through the ability to retain fear information and fear responses in the face of a similar future threat. In chronic stress, however, the limbic system becomes hypersensitive and more reactive, increasing and expanding the experience of risk and threat in a person's environment and thereby creating an unhelpful generalisation of fear.

Over the course of our lives, each of us develops belief systems and associated cognitive or thinking styles based on our early environments and experiences that help us to make sense of ourselves, others, the world and our future. These cognitions help to guide decision making and event processing as we move through life and play an important role in the generation of stress and development of reactive mood states or affects (Riskind et al. 2013). Hammen's (1991) stress generation effect refers to the contribution that our cognitive vulnerabilities (depressive thinking styles, hopelessness and rumination) make towards increasing the likelihood of experiencing negative events with catastrophic perceptions, thereby generating further stress and anxiety. And so develops a potentially vicious cycle of anxious physiological reactions, anxious thinking, anxious feeling and anxious doing, all perpetuating each other and increasing the risk to our mental wellbeing.

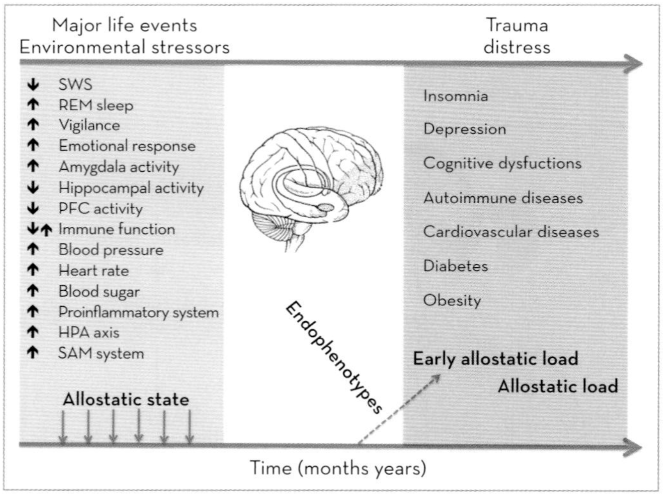

Figure 9.2
The effects of allostatic state and allostatic load on the brain

Major life events and environmental stressors can create an allostatic state (imbalance) within pivotal centres of the brain such as the hypothalamus, the prefrontal cortex and the amygdala due to increased adaptive responses to stress (indicated in the blue column). If maintained over months or years, this can create an allostatic load (wear and tear), increasing susceptibility to insomnia, mental health disorders, cardiovascular disease, diabetes and so on. SWS: slow wave sleep; HPA axis: hypothalamic–pituitary–adrenal axis; REM: rapid eye movement; SAM system: sympatho–adreno–medullary system.

Source: *Palagini et al. 2013. Copyright © 2012 Elsevier Ltd.*

Anxiety disorders

Anxiety symptoms are commonly experienced as high levels of fear with thoughts of imminent danger and perception of risk, safety behaviours and notable physiological arousal on presentation of an anxiety trigger. In a clinical sense, the term 'anxiety disorder' is applied following a diagnostic reasoning process in which symptoms of anxiety and related distress causing significant impairment in functioning and quality of life are recognised.

Most people experiencing anxiety disorders receive treatment within the primary care setting. Symptoms of anxiety disorders can be missed in people with commonly presenting major depressive symptoms, which have much higher rates of detection and gain a larger focus for treatment (NICE 2014). This presents a challenge for those living with symptoms of anxiety as well as for healthcare systems, as anxiety disorders are associated with high service usage due to the chronically disabling nature of the symptoms that can arise (Johnson & Coles 2013).

People with anxiety disorders often delay seeking treatment, thought to be partly due to avoidant behavioural coping styles. This delay can result in ongoing distress, impairment in functioning and considerable reduction in quality of life.

Anxiety disorders contribute significantly to the risk of self-harm and suicide, partly due to the way in which symptoms impair coping in the face of presenting psychosocial stressors (Hawton et al. 2013). Anxiety as an emotion can distort perceptions, leading to the person feeling overwhelmed, fearful and hopeless.

Although there are no fail-safe treatments for anxiety disorders, there are many options available that provide hope and relief of symptoms. Screening and assessment for anxiety disorders and other mental health conditions should be a necessary part of all nursing assessments.

The demarcation between 'normal' anxiety and that which may be considered 'disordered' can be difficult to make if we do not obtain all the information to make an informed assessment. Collaboration and a good therapeutic rapport are therefore imperative to ensure all necessary information, including trauma histories, are collected. The context or environment in which a consumer is experiencing anxiety provides a basis on which to formulate possible precipitating and perpetuating factors that we must consider during assessment and treatment. Anxiety disorders can lead to misinterpretations of presenting triggers; for example, a person's catastrophic response to noticing a change in their heart rate may lead them to believe that they are going to die of a heart attack. On the other hand, symptoms of anxiety disorders can appear in response to dangerous external stimuli, such as generalised anxiety in relation to emotional or physical abuse from a violent partner.

Salkovskis (1996) provides a helpful illustration for understanding the role that perception of danger plays in the development and intensity of anxiety (see Fig. 9.3). Our interpretation of the world, others and ourselves dictates our emotional, physiological, cognitive and behavioural responses. Many symptoms of anxiety can be understood in relation to the level of threat perceived by the individual. Any potential threat is processed through an estimation of the likelihood that such an event will occur and, if so, how catastrophic it would be for the person. Internal coping resources are considered alongside any external support/rescue that may be available. When the likelihood of catastrophic danger seems high without a sense of protection from self and others, we experience high levels of anxiety and fear, resulting in a cascade of survival-focused responses until a sense of safety returns.

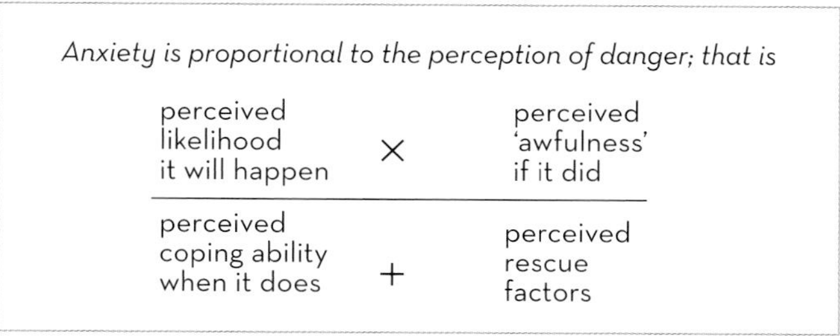

Figure 9.3
Anxiety and perceptions of danger
Source: Salkovskis 1996

Salkovskis' model (1996) provides a way of understanding how previous trauma and the associated impact on our cognitions affects our processes of threat assessment. Trauma can negatively change our perception and responses to future situations. If we no longer feel capable of protecting ourselves and we do not trust others to come to our aid, we feel less in control and therefore more vulnerable. These factors are often at play in the experiences of those living with high levels of anxiety. They can wreak havoc on a person's functioning, reducing their behaviours to those that appear to reduce the sense of immediate risk and avoid further anxiety-triggering situations rather than behaviours that provide engagement meaningful, valued activities. These safety behaviours then reinforce anxiety as the person begins to act as if there is significant threat in the present and/or future, thereby continuing an internal physiological stress response and reinforcing the perceptions the person may currently be living with. It is these physiological, behavioural, emotional and cognitive experiences that form the basis for the diagnostic symptoms of anxiety and other mental health disorders (Schmidt 2012) and leave them vulnerable to developing depression.

Historical anecdote 9.1: Early descriptions

One of the earliest written descriptions of anxiety disorder was a condition known as 'irritable heart' described by Dr Jacob Da Costa during the American civil war (1861–1865). He described soldiers exhibiting symptoms such as sweaty hands, palpitations, dizziness, tunnel vision, diarrhoea and chest pain, which resolved when soldiers were moved to lighter duties. An early description for anxiety disorder that is still used today is 'agoraphobia'. It was first written about by neurologist Moritz Benedikt (1835–1920) in an article in 1870 where he described a condition in which people are 'well so long as they remain indoors or in narrow streets; yet as soon as they enter a boulevard, or especially a public square are seized by dizziness so that they fear falling down or are seized by such anxiety that they do not dare to cross the space'.

Read more about it: *Klein DF 2002 Historical aspects of anxiety. Dialogues in Clinical Neuroscience, 4(3): 295*

Epidemiology of anxiety disorders

Data describing the prevalence of anxiety disorders was last collected in Australia by the Australian Bureau of Statistics in 2007 and in New Zealand between 2003 and 2004 (Wells 2006). The Australian survey highlighted a population prevalence of lifetime mental health disorders at 45%, with 20% of the sample experiencing symptoms in the 12 months prior to data collection (Australian Bureau of Statistics 2007). Anxiety disorders were found to be the most prevalent of all disorders, with 14.4% of survey participants reporting symptoms in the preceding 12 months. The most commonly experienced anxiety disorder was post-traumatic stress disorder (PTSD) (6.4%), followed by social anxiety disorder (SAD) (4.7%), with reasonably comparable prevalence rates in other anxiety disorders (agoraphobia 2.8%; generalised anxiety disorder [GAD] 2.7%; panic disorder 2.6%; obsessive-compulsive disorder [OCD] 1.9%). Data regarding adjustment disorder or specific phobia was not collected within the survey and separate data on Indigenous Australians was not reported.

New Zealand survey results indicated a 46.6% lifetime prevalence rate of mental health disorders in the general population, with 20.7% of respondents indicating prevalence in the 12 months prior to data collection (Wells 2006). At the time of the study, prevalence estimates indicated that 24.9% of the population would experience an anxiety disorder over their lifetime. Specific phobia (7.3%) and SAD (5.1%) were the most commonly experienced of the anxiety disorders, while other disorders were found at lower rates: PTSD, 3%; GAD, 2%; panic disorder, 1.7%; agoraphobia, 0.6%; and OCD, 0.6%. The survey found higher lifetime prevalence of mental health disorders for Māori (50.7%, with a 29.5% 12-month prevalence). Anxiety disorders for Māori were found to be most prevalent at 19.4% in the 12 months prior to the study, with an estimated lifetime prevalence of 31.3%. Māori not only experience higher rates of mental health disorders compared with non-Māori but also experience greater levels of severity (Wells 2006), highlighting the importance of current national health strategies within New Zealand to address these inequalities.

Pacific peoples living in New Zealand were shown to have slightly higher 12-month prevalence rates (23.9%) than non-Pacific peoples (not including Māori) but lower rates of service utilisation for severe mental health disorders. An interesting finding to consider was an increased vulnerability to mental health disorders for Pacific peoples who were born in New Zealand versus those born in Pacific Island countries (Wells 2006).

Collective Australasian survey findings show that anxiety disorders are the most commonly occurring mental health problems within our populations. Females experience higher rates of anxiety disorders than males, and younger people (16–24 and 25–44) generally experience higher rates than older groups within the surveys (Australian Bureau of Statistics 2007; Wells 2006). Lifetime prevalence rates of mental health disorders and anxiety disorders appear very similar throughout Australasia and compare with other first-world populations such as Britain (Baldwin et al. 2014).

Mental health statistics for Māori and Pacific peoples highlight the importance of considering the impact that loss of culture and connection to their land through acculturation and colonisation can have on a person's mental wellbeing and sense of self. Although there were no formal statistics collected in the 2007 Australian survey on the mental health of Aboriginal and Torres Strait Islander peoples, it is well known that colonisation has created a significant loss of land and culture and associated impact on the wellbeing of these people. These issues are also discussed in Chapter 1.

Critical thinking challenge 9.1

How do you currently deal with stress and anxiety in your own life? What thoughts do you notice you experience regularly during these times and what behaviours do you engage in? What things do you do that provide the most effective support for yourself? Do you have any responses that are not so helpful? What would be the most helpful way to think and act towards stress and anxiety when it shows up? How could you use this learning in your practice?

Comorbidity

Comorbidity in anxiety disorders is so prevalent that it is often considered the rule, rather than the exception. Lifetime prevalence rates of comorbidity within anxiety disorders have been shown to be as high as 80%, with a strong correlation with depressive disorders (Katzman et al. 2014); however, anxiety-anxiety comorbidity (presentation of more than one anxiety disorder) is very common and has been shown to be associated with earlier age of onset and greater chronicity of symptoms (Hofmeijer-Sevink et al. 2012).

It is important to consider the heightened anxiety identified within many mental health disorders. Studies have shown that people diagnosed with schizophrenia show clinically significant anxiety symptoms at rates between 16% and 85% (Hartley et al. 2013). Comorbid anxiety disorders have been shown to be related to positive symptoms of schizophrenia; for example, suspiciousness and paranoia appear correlated with social anxiety and panic (Hartley et al. 2013). Anxiety has also been shown to be related to an increase in the number of hospitalisations among people with schizophrenia (Cosoff & Hafner 1998). These findings support the need for therapeutic interventions for anxiety in those with a primary diagnosis of schizophrenia and other mental health disorders.

Diagnoses such as SAD, panic disorder and GAD may occur with substance abuse disorders (APA 2013), where in some cases substance use acts as a way of self-medicating to manage anxiety symptoms. Anxiety disorders are also known to occur with other severe mental disorders such as bipolar disorder and have been commonly associated with personality disorders (APA 2013). Box 9.1 provides recommendations for increasing awareness of anxiety disorders.

Box 9.1 Recommendations for increased awareness of anxiety disorders

- Become familiar with the main features of anxiety disorders, PTSD and OCD and the main symptoms that distinguish them from each other.
- Develop systematic questions to ask about the nature, severity, duration, distress and associated impairment in people presenting with anxiety symptoms to decide whether an anxiety disorder, PTSD or OCD is present.
- Become familiar with the fluctuating nature of symptoms in patients with anxiety disorders, and with the tendency for symptoms to change in nature over time

Source: Baldwin et al. 2014.

Assessment and diagnosis

Engaging with services can initially heighten people's anxiety due to uncertainty regarding outcomes, experience of self-stigma and feared judgement from others as well as exposure to fear-inducing stimuli through the initial assessment and treatment processes. Becoming adept with the skills of engagement and conveying a sense of unconditional positive regard supports consumers to begin to have a sense of safety and trust (for further discussion of assessment, see Chapter 7), allowing consumers to begin to open up about their current and historical experiences. It is through gaining an understanding of these experiences that we begin to build a picture of predisposing aspects and precipitating and perpetuating factors that impact on a person's anxiety.

Due to the high prevalence of trauma and childhood adversity, trauma screening should be incorporated into assessment to help identify the level of contribution to presenting symptoms. This is particularly pertinent for refugee communities that experience extremely high rates of trauma. Trauma screening does not assess exactly what happened to the person but gathers enough information to ascertain that trauma has occurred. When trauma is disclosed, assessment should focus on whether there is any present risk of harm to the person and screening should be conducted for symptoms of PTSD following on from the trauma (see later information on PTSD within this chapter).

In Nurse's story 9.1 Karen Jones describes her use of assessment skills to develop an understanding of a consumer's anxiety and to plan effective intervention.

Conducting a thorough nursing assessment includes reviewing relevant psychosocial information, enabling exploration of current stressors that may be producing an understandable anxiety response such as financial threat, physical danger or significant losses (employment, relationships, health status, acculturative stress).

NURSE'S STORY 9.1

Karen Jones

I recall working with a man in his 40s who was so anxious he wasn't sleeping or eating at all and couldn't sit still. He described walking around with earmuffs on his head to try to block noise, which he felt was worsening his anxiety. The man took a year off work and felt unable to drive or participate in his usual daily life, including caring for his two young children due to his hyper-anxious state and lack of concentration. This took a real toll on his family, as his wife was required to take over running the household. His children did not understand what had happened but noticed their father had completely withdrawn into himself. Through thorough assessment and ongoing support from his GP, practice nurses and primary mental health services it was established that certain changes occurring within his workplace were the cause of his anxiety. A combination of medication and cognitive behaviour therapy assisted him in identifying coping strategies, enabling him to recover and regain the ability to get back into his life. A variety of further resources were also accessed to support the patient and his family, including help from a social worker, financial support and guidance in accessing educational and self-help websites.

Karen Jones is a designated nurse prescriber and practice nurse working in a marae-based health clinic.

Box 9.2 General screening questions

During the past 2 weeks, how much have you been bothered by the following problems:

- Feeling nervous, anxious, frightened, worried or on edge?
- Feeling panicked or being frightened?
- Avoiding situations that make you anxious?

Source: APA 2013

General screening questions have been recommended to support consumers to disclose any aspects of anxiety that are becoming problematic (see Box 9.2). Questioning relating to anxiety needs to be simple, time-specific and inclusive of both an experience of heightened anxiety and behavioural changes such as avoidance.

Exploring the impact of anxiety symptoms on quality of life and functioning helps to consider whether a clinically significant level of anxiety is being experienced.

New migrants and refugees often experience major stress adapting to a new country, and culture and language barriers may affect engagement. There may also be misunderstandings about what services can and cannot provide if the person has little experience of healthcare systems. Integrating care with other social and healthcare service providers can provide huge benefits to assistance with essential needs such as housing, which can then support the person to better focus on other issues.

Pervasiveness of anxiety across roles and life domains should be assessed to help identify generalised anxiety over that which may be experienced in reaction to a particular stress-inducing trigger (such as flying). Scaling questions (0–10) can assist with identifying the intensity of anxiety. Questions assessing the presence of physiological arousal (e.g. tachycardia, sweating, hyperventilation) and behavioural responses (avoidance of triggers or other described behaviours to reduce anxiety and promote sense of safety) assist in determining functional and physical levels of impact of anxiety.

Assessing other presenting issues or difficulties – such as depressive mood states, alcohol and drug abuse, psychotic symptoms or mood lability – helps ascertain the presence of possible comorbid disorders. Equally, anxiety should be assessed if one of these presents as the primary disorder due to the high levels of comorbidity with anxiety disorders.

Assessment should include special consideration of the consumer's health history, particularly conditions known to cause anxiety (e.g. Graves' disease) and those that are negatively affected by anxiety (e.g. hypertension).

It is important to be aware of the different cultural presentations and beliefs about anxiety that people may present with. In some cultures, symptoms may present more somatically, such as physical symptoms experienced throughout the body (e.g. pain), or intrusive thoughts may be perceived as being caused by spiritual or supernatural experiences (Hinton 2012). It is important to gain the consumer's perspective and attempt to understand the cultural context from which they come to support a shared understanding and approach to treatment. Cultural advisors can be extremely helpful in bridging the cultural–clinical gap and ensuring that care remains acceptable, culturally inclusive and safe for the consumer. Assessment should also consider the specific cultural aspects of wellbeing of indigenous peoples to identify pathways to support them to regain their health. See Chapter 1 for further discussion of cultural safety in mental health nursing.

Finally, the prevalence of self-harm and suicidal ideation and behaviours in anxiety disorders has been previously discussed: it is imperative that nurses become comfortable asking about these issues in order to assess any risk of harm that may be present.

In the following section symptoms of the different anxiety disorders are outlined. A summary of key features is provided in Table 9.1.

Assessment tools

There are several assessment tools available for general use by nurses that can assist in screening for anxiety disorders. Below are a few examples, many of which are self-administered and available for free use and download via the internet. Most of the tools mentioned can be used within any health setting and are sensitive for detecting mild to severe presentations, although in themselves they do not determine the diagnosis. Outcomes from such assessments need to be viewed together with historical and current information to ensure a thorough diagnostic reasoning process. Experienced nurses, particularly those in autonomous roles such as clinical nurse specialists and nurse practitioners, can diagnose anxiety disorders. Other nurses can provide essential support in gathering information that may help clarify any eventual diagnoses made.

GAD-7

The GAD-7 (Spitzer et al. 2006) is a seven-question self-report assessment tool designed to screen and measure the severity of any presenting symptoms of excessive worry and generalised anxiety. Scores of 5, 10 and 15 are considered cut-off points for mild, moderate and severe anxiety, respectively. Scores above 10 indicate that further assessment is required to enable exploration as to whether a diagnosis of GAD may be present.

Yale-Brown Obsessive-Compulsive Scale (Y-BOCS)

The Y-BOCS (Goodman et al. 1989) is a lengthy, comprehensive measure of the severity, impact and type of symptoms of OCD. The Y-BOCS requires a reasonable degree of experience to administer because it is carried out as a semi-structured interview.

Impact of event scale – revised (IES-R)

The IES-R (Weiss & Marmar 1996) is a 22-item short self-report tool designed to measure symptoms following exposure to a trauma that may indicate the presence of PTSD. Questions aim to measure the presence of the major cluster of symptoms of PTSD: intrusive re-experiencing, hyperarousal and persistent avoidance (see later information on PTSD within this chapter).

Anxiety disorders

Generalised anxiety disorder

GAD is a debilitating condition characterised by constant, excessive and consuming worry about numerous everyday situations. Worry is often difficult to control and highly disrupting to day-to-day functioning due to the intrusive nature of the thoughts and physical symptoms of anxiety

TABLE 9.1 Key features of specific anxiety, trauma- and stress-related disorders

DISORDER	KEY FEATURES
Panic disorder (PD)	• Recurrent unexpected panic attacks, in the absence of triggers • Persistent concern about additional panic attacks and/or maladaptive change in behaviour related to the attacks
Agoraphobia	• Marked, unreasonable fear or anxiety about a situation • Active avoidance of feared situation due to thinking that escape might be difficult or help unavailable if panic-like symptoms occur
Specific phobia	• Marked, unreasonable fear or anxiety about a specific object or situation, which is actively avoided (e.g. flying, heights, animals, receiving an injection, seeing blood)
Social anxiety disorder (SAD)	• Marked, excessive or unrealistic fear or anxiety about social situations in which there is possible exposure to scrutiny by others • Active avoidance of feared situation
Generalised anxiety disorder (GAD)	• Excessive, difficult-to-control anxiety and worry (apprehensive expectation) about multiple events or activities (e.g. school/work difficulties) • Accompanied by symptoms such as restlessness / feeling on edge or muscle tension
Obsessive-compulsive disorder (OCD)	• Obsessions: recurrent and persistent thoughts, urges or images that are experienced as intrusive and unwanted and that cause marked anxiety or distress • Compulsions: repetitive behaviours (e.g. handwashing) or mental acts (e.g. counting) that the individual feels driven to perform to reduce the anxiety generated by the obsessions
Adjustment disorder (AD)	• Development of emotional or behavioural symptoms occurring within 3 months of the onset of a stressor (not including normal bereavement) • Distress is noted to be out of proportion to the severity or intensity of the stressor
Post-traumatic stress disorder (PTSD) and acute stress disorder (ASD)	• Exposure to actual or threatened death, serious injury or sexual violation • Intrusion symptoms (e.g. distressing memories or dreams, flashbacks, intense distress) and avoidance of stimuli associated with the event • Negative alterations in cognitions and mood (e.g. negative beliefs and emotions, detachment), as well as marked alterations in arousal and reactivity (e.g. irritable behaviour, hypervigilance)

experienced. GAD can be considered a persistent, chronic disorder accompanied by somatic complaints, restlessness, irritability, insomnia, fatigue and hyperarousal arising out of a constant state of anxiety-induced alertness (APA 2013).

GAD is considered a chronic condition, often exacerbated by stressors (Andrews et al. 2018) and is thought to cause the most interference with life compared with other anxiety disorders, with almost half (48%) of responders in one study stating that it impacted considerably in at least four domains of their life (McEvoy et al. 2011). GAD is often not well recognised in primary care because people may present with more complaints about their physical health and mood rather than anxiety symptoms (Baldwin et al. 2014).

Lifetime prevalence of GAD in Australasia of is around 6% of the general population (Andrews et al. 2018) and mean age of onset is around 33 years of age (McEvoy et al. 2011; Wells 2006). Having an anxious temperament is considered a vulnerability factor, with people often reporting that they have always been a worrier (APA 2013). There are noted inherent genetic risks (APA 2013), increasing the prevalence of comorbidity with other anxiety and depressive disorders sharing similar predisposing risk factors. Major depressive disorder commonly occurs alongside GAD (Baldwin et al. 2014), which can cause a more chronic and debilitating range of symptoms.

It is important to note that differences in expression of anxiety symptoms have been identified within certain cultures, with some people presenting with more somatic complaints while others experience more cognitive symptoms (APA 2013).

Recent guidelines developed by the Royal Australian and New Zealand College of Psychiatrists identify psychoeducation and active monitoring as an important first-step, with delivery of either face-to-face cognitive behaviour therapy (CBT) or supported e-CBT as a second-step and consideration of a pharmacological treatment such as a selective serotonin reuptake inhibitor (SSRI), specifically sertraline in combination with psychological intervention as a third step (Andrews et al. 2018). Consumer's story 9.1 provides an account of how one consumer developed strategies to help manage an anxiety disorder.

CONSUMER'S STORY 9.1

Thomas

Quite often I don't know when anxiety is going to hit as it can creep up or come on suddenly; however, I know the warning signs: feeling more tense and on edge, getting irritable with my family, feeling something just isn't right and having a sense of urgency to everything. I notice my thoughts begin to race and it is harder to enjoy things or be as present in the moment because I'm either thinking about something I have to do or worrying about something I've done and whether it was right or not.

My anxiety comes partly from my temperament (I've always been a worrier), partly from my lifestyle (I don't always get a good balance between work and life) and from experiences in my childhood. I grew up with a parent who worried a lot. The older I get, the more I can see my parent's worries in the way that I see the world when anxiety descends.

Learning about how anxiety works and what goes on in my body, how to identify anxious thinking and focus on slowing down and looking after myself have been the most helpful approaches to anxiety. Quite often, stopping and paying attention to my distress, being willing to feel it and not fight with it, and being kinder to myself really helps. The next step is making lifestyle changes to ensure I protect my sleep, keep a balance in diet and activity and do things I enjoy with people I love. I know it is important to keep these important wellbeing behaviours in my everyday life to maintain balance.

Obsessive-compulsive disorder

OCD involves a recurring experience of anxiety-creating intrusive cognitions (thoughts, impulses or images) that become obsessive in nature, risking dominating a person's internal world over time. Obsessive cognitions often involve themes of risk of harm to self or others, such as developing a life-threatening disease or harm coming to family members. These cognitions are experienced with significant accompanying physiological symptoms of anxiety, giving the person a sense of danger (APA 2013; Wells 2006). In response to the obsessive cognitions and anxious bodily sensations, compulsive behaviours develop that serve the purpose of reducing the perception of harm and creating a sense of safety. Compulsive behaviours may be directly related to the obsessions, such as washing hands to prevent acquisition or transmission of disease, or totally unrelated, such as tapping surfaces a particular number of times to reduce the risk of an unwanted outcome. The relief provided and sense the compulsive behaviours have successfully averted catastrophe 'fuse' the compulsive behaviours to the obsessions. Thus, the more the obsessions are experienced, the more the compulsions are carried out.

Despite attempts to reduce anxiety by carrying out the compulsions or attempting to suppress intrusions, both reoccur. This leads into a very disruptive and often distressing reinforcing cycle as the compulsions take up more time and the obsessive thinking disrupts usual day-to-day cognitive processes.

OCD is not a particularly common anxiety disorder. Twelve-month prevalence rates in New Zealand were last recorded at about 0.6% and lifetime rates at 1.2%; however, Māori rates were higher, with 12-month prevalence at 1% and lifetime rates at 2.6% (Wells 2006). The Australian survey noted higher 12-month prevalence at 1.9%, with the lifetime rate at 2.8% (Australian Bureau of Statistics 2007).

Despite lower rates of OCD, symptoms are often more severe compared with other anxiety disorders, with higher rates of suicidal ideation, plans and suicide attempts (Wells 2006) indicating necessity to ensure treatment and close monitoring of risk.

Treatment involves a combination of medication and concurrent talking therapies due to the severity of symptoms. Exposure and response prevention, a specific type of CBT, appears to be the most successful talking therapy for OCD, with long-term improvement in symptoms reported in 75% of individuals engaging in therapy (Neziroglu & Mancusi 2014). Pharmacotherapy options include SSRIs at higher doses than prescribed for depression as a first-line treatment (Seibell et al. 2015).

Historical anecdote 9.2: Socratic questioning

In modern times CBT has become well known as a first-line treatment for several types of anxiety disorder. CBT has historical links to the stoic philosophy of ancient Greece, which observed that because life perpetually changes, people need to strive to maintain clear thinking. In particular a key tenant of CBT is the ancient technique skill known as 'Socratic questioning'. This refers to a method of learning named after the ancient Greek philosopher Socrates (470–399 BC). He believed that rather than teaching people information laid out as facts people learnt more when they were taught how to ask thoughtful questions to examine ideas and determine their validity.

Read more about it: *Brickhouse TC, Smith ND 2009 Socratic teaching and Socratic method. In: Siegel H (ed). The Oxford handbook of philosophy of education. Oxford University Press, New York, pp. 177–94*

Panic disorder

PD is characterised by unpredictable experiences of intense, episodic surges of anxiety that occur in the form of panic attacks. Intense physiological anxiety symptoms are experienced (tachycardia, sweating, shaking, dyspnoea, chest pain, dizziness, nausea, tingling), along with a sense of depersonalisation (feeling detached from oneself). Panic attacks can occur outside of PD in relation to other presentations of anxiety; however, the higher frequency, non-selective triggering environments and anticipatory anxiety helps differentiate PD from other diagnoses.

Panic attacks reach a peak of severity within approximately 10 minutes and can last up to 45 minutes (Baldwin et al. 2014). It is common to experience catastrophic cognitions during panic attacks due to the surge of physiological symptoms. These can include a sense of imminent death ('I'm going to have a heart attack and die'), mental health deterioration ('I'm going to lose my mind') or a negative outcome regarding fear of losing consciousness ('I'll pass out and something will happen to me when I'm unconscious'). As a result, people engage in rapid safety behaviours during panic attacks in order to seek help (e.g. phoning emergency services), escape the attack (e.g. sit down) and further monitor symptoms (e.g. body scanning, taking one's pulse).

As the panic attack begins to abate, the person obtains a false impression that (a) they were on the brink of a catastrophic event and (b) their safety behaviours prevented the imminent catastrophe that was occurring during the attack. This signals a major misinterpretation of anxiety symptoms (e.g. 'I could have a panic attack and die'), leading to scanning for a further attack and greater anticipatory anxiety. A number of preventive safety behaviours develop to avoid future attacks and reduce perceived risk should one occur – becoming dependent on others to go out, body hypervigilance (body scanning for symptoms) and avoiding potential triggering/high-risk situations. These safety behaviours can lead to agoraphobia (see later description) in approximately two-thirds of cases (Baldwin et al. 2014; Royal Australian and New Zealand College of Psychiatrists (RANZCP) 2003) and vicious cycles of panic attacks, anxiety and ever-increasing safety behaviours – see Fig. 9.4, which illustrates Clark's cognitive model of PD.

PD is one of the less common anxiety disorders, with a 12-month prevalence rate of 1.7% in New Zealand and 2.6% in Australia (Australian Bureau of Statistics 2007; Wells 2006). However, PD often presents with high levels of severity, with 44.9% of cases within the New Zealand survey being classified as serious (Wells 2006).

PD has a high comorbidity rate with conditions such as depression (Baldwin et al. 2014) and is strongly correlated with suicidal ideation, planning and completed suicide (Wells 2006). PD is linked to higher rates of help-seeking (Wells 2006) due to both the accompanied fear of medical illness linked attacks causing high rates of presentation to medical services during and after attacks.

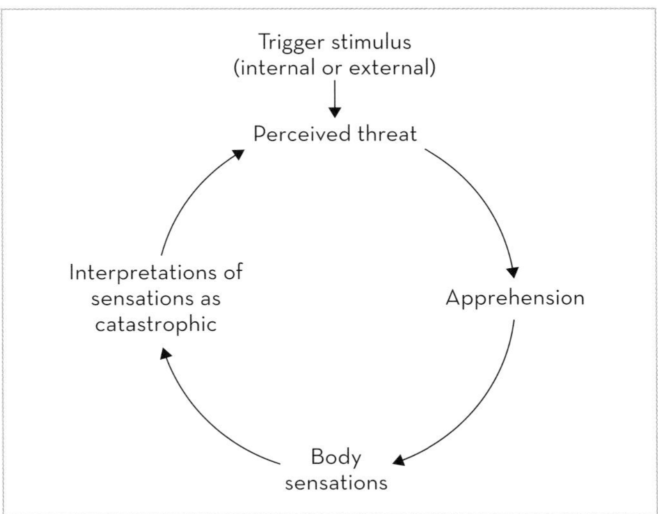

Figure 9.4
Clark's cognitive model of panic disorder
Source: Clark 1986

Treatment for PD largely centres on brief psychological interventions such as CBT, which can be delivered through online CBT courses or in face-to-face sessions (Sawchuk & Veitengruber 2016). There has been conflicting evidence for pharmacological treatment, with SSRIs and benzodiazepines showing only modest efficacy and tricyclic antidepressants often causing side effects that reduce adherence over longer periods (RANZCP 2003).

Agoraphobia

Agoraphobia is characterised by generalised, consistent and significant unrealistic fear responses to exposure or anticipated exposure to public spaces such as shopping centres, crowded areas or open spaces. Common associated anxious cognitions relate to fears help may not be available or escape possible should the person begin to panic or experience considerable symptoms of distress. Avoidance is commonly used as a safety behaviour, thereby causing impairment in day-to-day functioning. Techniques such as distraction and dependency on others to go out are used regularly in order to enter areas or situations that trigger anxiety.

Agoraphobia is highly comorbid with panic disorder and functional impairment can be significant, though panic attacks are not always experienced (Asmundson et al. 2014).

Agoraphobia has been found to occur at 12-month prevalence rates of 2.8% within the Australian population (McEvoy et al. 2011) and 0.6% within the New Zealand population, with the highest age representation being between 25 and 44 years old (Wells 2006). Despite its lower prevalence rate compared with other anxiety disorders, agoraphobia is highly correlated with suicidal ideation, plans and suicide attempts (Wells 2006), highlighting the significance of screening for suicide risk in assessment.

Social anxiety disorder

SAD is poorly recognised in primary health care (Baldwin et al. 2014) and may be misconstrued as shyness and introversion (Sawchuk et al. 2015). People with SAD experience high levels of socially induced distress and impairment in day-to-day functioning due to persistent and objectively unreasonable fear in social situations of embarrassment, humiliation and negative judgement by others. This is particularly true where there may be performance expectations, such as within a classroom or at a party. Negative and inflexible beliefs about self may occur as a result of internalising past or present emotional abuse, with fear others may 'discover' perceived physical or personality flaws or perceived lack of intelligence.

It is the intense focus and over-monitoring of the self in social situations that reinforce and perpetuate the condition. Experienced distorted cognitive appraisals of self lead to social avoidance or high social anxiety in social situations. Developed safety behaviours such as conversation rehearsal, conversation redirection towards others or avoidance of interactions during social events fuel further anxiety as the person acts as if they are socially incompetent and unacceptable to others. Post-event analysis of behaviours is often biased towards perceived negative social interactions and flawed social behaviours, increasing fear and potential avoidance in future situations.

It is common for people with SAD to have considerable fear of losing control of their bodies (incontinence, vomiting, blushing or shaking) in social situations, causing further fear of social humiliation and negative evaluation by others.

SAD can have serious impacts on a person's family and romantic relationships, occupational opportunities and day-to-day functioning as it becomes both harder to make and maintain relationships and present oneself for educational and career development opportunities.

SAD was found to be the second most common anxiety disorder after GAD in terms of lifetime prevalence within New Zealand (Wells 2006). Australian prevalence rates for SAD are comparable to those of New Zealand, with 4.7% and 5.1% of the respective populations presenting with SAD within a 12-month period. However, prevalence rates are higher for Māori (6.2%) and Pacific peoples (5.8%) (McEvoy et al. 2011; Wells 2006). In the most recent mental health survey in New Zealand, youth (16–24 years) had the highest rates of SAD, with a median age of onset of 12 years of age (Wells 2006). However, there is an estimated 28-year delay in treatment from age of onset, with only 4.9% of affected youth seeking help at the start of symptoms (Wells 2006), indicating a lack of screening within primary care youth services and reluctance to engage no doubt due to feared negative appraisals by clinicians. While SAD shows greater comparability of rates between the sexes (males 4.5%, females 5.6%) in youth in contrast with other anxiety disorders (Wells 2006), females have higher rates of SAD in adult populations (Sawchuk et al. 2015).

SAD is strongly correlated with comorbid depression and drug and alcohol abuse. These issues often lead to engagement in services, rather than symptoms of SAD itself (Baldwin et al. 2014).

Treatment for SAD depends on the severity of symptoms and whether comorbid conditions such as depression or another anxiety disorder are present (Sawchuk et al. 2015). A recent meta-analysis of treatment options produced a recommended optimal combination treatment of CBT with administration of either an SSRI or a selective noradrenaline reuptake inhibitor (SNRI), with CBT showing greater enduring effect than pharmacotherapy (Canton et al. 2012). Other medications such as benzodiazepines are not suggested due to the risk of developing dependence. Case study 9.1 describes the experience of social anxiety.

CASE STUDY 9.1
Jenny

Jenny is a 21-year-old woman with a diagnosis of dyslexia and marked anxiety in social situations. Jenny constantly fears the judgement of others and believes that when she speaks to others they can 'hear her dyslexia' and will think she is stupid. Jenny regularly avoids social situations and, when she has to attend, has a number of safety behaviours to protect her from making a fool of herself, such as practising her replies to discussions in her head and deflecting attention by asking other people a lot of questions.

Jenny very much believes that her problem lies in her level of intellect and that her low perceived intelligence will mean that people won't want to know her when they discover this about her. Jenny is unsure how she can make any changes and is beginning to experience low moods as a result of her lack of social contact and constant anxiety.

Specific phobia

It is common to experience transient fears of situations, animals or natural environments. However, a fear that becomes disproportionate to the actual level of risk posed and causes distress and functional impairment can be considered a specific phobia. Specific phobias involve a persistent, irrational (out of proportion), intense fear reaction in the face of triggers that are generally clustered into animal, situational, natural environment or blood-injection-injury subtypes. Blood-injection-injury phobic reactions are often accompanied by a vasovagal fainting/near-fainting response due to a sudden increase then decrease in heart rate and blood pressure (APA 2013).

The major criterion for diagnosis involves a consistently elevated anxiety response for a period of 6 months or more on presentation of the phobic stimulus, considerable avoidance or intense fear being endured throughout exposure, reduction in functioning and increase in distress.

Fear of phobic objects can be experienced through direct contact, distant proximity or anticipation of contact with the stimulus and can produce a continuum of anxious responses, including panic attacks at the more severe end. The degree of anxiety experienced can be reduced/increased by the presence/absence of accompanying contextual elements of safety such as having others around or being exposed to a phobic stimulus with less perceived danger (e.g. for a person with a dog phobia, seeing a smaller dog versus seeing a bigger dog or seeing a dog on a lead across the street versus seeing a dog off the lead on the same side of the road). Longer contact with the phobic stimulus will often draw greater anxiety responses due to an increased perception of risk.

Up to 75% of people with a diagnosis of specific phobia have multiple phobias of certain objects or situations (APA 2013; Baldwin et al. 2014).

The 12-month prevalence rates of specific phobia in New Zealand are around 7.3% within the general population (Wells 2006). Although specific phobias were found to produce the least interference with life in the most recent New Zealand mental health survey (Wells 2006), severity and impact need to be considered on an individual basis. In some instances, phobias can produce life-threatening dangers, such as a person with a serious medical illness refusing treatment via needles because of a blood-injury-injection phobia.

Specific phobias typically develop between 7 and 11 years of age, although situational or natural environment subtypes have a later age of onset (APA 2013). Some phobias spontaneously remit during childhood and adolescence; however, they can persist into adulthood. It is important to assess factors around the development of phobias as they can occur secondary to trauma; for example, fear of the dark may develop following childhood sexual abuse or fear of dogs may develop after witnessing or being attacked by a dog. Other developmental factors may include media coverage of plane crashes or storms, witnessing an incident or experiencing an intense reaction during contact with a stimulus such as having a panic attack on top of a tower.

Avoidance behaviours can have a major influence over time in terms of how people live their lives, dictating choice of home and work locations and routines. It may be a change in circumstances that leads to help-seeking, such as a move that increases the person's direct contact with their phobic stimulus.

Treatment of phobic disorders has been relatively under-researched in comparison with other anxiety disorders (Baldwin et al. 2014). Current treatment indications depend on the level of severity and impairment in functioning. In the case of subclinical or mild symptoms, monitoring and face-to-face or online psychoeducation through CBT tools are recommended to assist in normalising distress and assisting people to begin to identify their triggers for anxiety. Internationally, CBT with graded exposure to phobic stimuli is considered a first-line treatment, with use of benzodiazepines considered only in cases of acute treatment – for example, if someone has a needle phobia and requires medical intervention using needles (Freidl & Zakarin 2016).

Critical thinking challenge 9.2

Many people experience mild symptoms of anxiety disorders throughout life due to the number of significant life stressors that come their way. What are the benefits of making a diagnosis of an anxiety disorder versus using a more normalising approach for mild presentations? When can a diagnosis be helpful and when might it not be?

Trauma- and stressor-related disorders

PTSD, acute stress disorder (ASD) and adjustment disorder (AD) were previously categorised as anxiety disorders. Their separated classification as trauma and stress-related disorders reflects and identification of the significance of trauma both in itself and as a cause of mental health distress and other developmental lifespan challenges.

Exposure to potentially traumatising events is common, with up to 75% of people reporting at least one traumatic event over their lifetime (Australian Centre for Posttraumatic Mental Health (ACPMH) 2013). A variety of distress responses are both common and normal following trauma, from insomnia to fear and anxiety, but some people may go on to develop ASD, PTSD or other anxiety or affective disorders.

Post-traumatic stress disorder

PTSD can develop following direct exposure to a traumatic event or multiple traumas, either by first-hand experience or by vicarious traumatisation (witnessing a trauma, hearing about a loved one's trauma or extreme/repeated exposure to details of trauma via interviews with people who have experienced trauma). The types of trauma considered for the purposes of diagnosis include threatened or actual physical or sexual harm, personal violence, war, serious accidents, natural disasters and sudden, catastrophic medical events.

PTSD is characterised by symptoms located within four distinct symptom clusters (APA 2013): intrusive re-experiencing (nightmares, dissociative flashbacks, recurrent memories), hyperarousal (heightened startle response, intense physiological response to trauma recall, hypervigilance), persistent avoidance of trauma stimuli (avoiding external reminders and internal trauma-related experiences such as memories) and mood and cognitive alterations (emotional numbing, anhedonia, fear, low mood, impartial trauma memory recall, poor concentration, generalised thoughts about danger). Behavioural changes occur such as avoidance of associated triggers, sleep disturbance, increased interpersonal irritability, violence, recklessness or self-destructive behaviours such as substance abuse. Individuals may experience more severity of symptoms such as dysphoric mood states, dissociation or arousal (APA 2013).

Symptoms typically develop within 3 months of the trauma; however, it is possible for a delayed expression of symptoms to occur months or years later (APA 2013). A diagnosis of PTSD is not made in the first month after the trauma as approximately 50% of people fully recover within 3 months, although some still experience symptoms years or even decades later (APA 2013).

Associative learning processes aid future survival responses when we experience danger, helping us to recall processed threat triggers and respond accordingly when required. In PTSD, it is thought that a fault occurs during and after the trauma in terms of memory processing, resulting in the development of 'broken trauma memories' that are incomplete, inappropriately stored with associated generalised, catastrophic threat cues that later become identified with non-dangerous stimuli. Inaccurate processing of trauma memories is hypothesised to contribute to an inaccurate sense of placement of the memory in time, leading to a perceived sense (physiologically and cognitively) of current danger and associated and behaviour responses. As a result, traumas are re-experienced rather than simply remembered. Significant avoidance strategies develop due to the emotional load and sense of danger created through continual trauma re-experiencing, leading to functional impairment in day-to-day life. The trauma is thought to also create a heightened fear response within the person, triggered by the traumatic event itself and other predisposing genetic, cognitive and temperamental vulnerabilities (Zoellner et al. 2014). These and other mechanisms are considered integral to perpetuating the vicious cycle of PTSD, leaving the person feeling overwhelmed and struggling to function under the weight of their symptoms while expending considerable effort trying to avoid the memories that haunt them and reduce the likelihood of the trauma recurring.

The 12-month prevalence rates for PTSD in New Zealand and Australia are similar, with 4.4–6.4% of the general population receiving a diagnosis within a year (Cooper et al. 2014; McEvoy et al. 2011; RANZCP 2003; Wells 2006). However, prevalence rates for Māori are significantly higher at 9.7% (Wells 2006). A recent study of PTSD in Aboriginal people living in remote Western Australia showed concerningly high lifetime prevalence rates of 55.2% in the sample of 221 people, while 91% of the sample with PTSD had comorbid alcohol-related disorders (Nadew 2012). The authors cite this as the highest ever recorded PTSD rate found within a sample when compared with other studies around the world. The comorbidity of substance abuse within this sample points to a link between use of substances as a way of self-medicating for symptoms of PTSD. This is supported by findings by Benton et al. (2012), in which one-third of people in treatment for substance abuse met criteria for a diagnosis of PTSD.

Rates of PTSD are shown to be much higher after exposure to specific types of interpersonal trauma; for example, in one study 50% of rape survivors were noted to have PTSD (Cooper et al. 2014).

Many people diagnosed with PTSD report multiple trauma events (Kessler 2000), leading to the concept of complex PTSD. Complex PTSD symptoms relate to the impact of the enduring and/or compounding nature of multiple traumas and can cause ongoing interpersonal difficulties, emotional dysregulation, prolonged dissociative states, somatic distress/symptoms and fixed, distorted belief systems (Resick et al. 2012).

It is important to note that prevalence of PTSD has been found to be much higher for health consumers accessing specialist mental health services, with some studies reporting rates as high as 67.2% (Simpson et al. 2011). A large multi-site American study found that 84% of its sample of 782 reported experience of lifetime interpersonal violence, while 52% of the sample reported lifetime sexual assault. When the sexual assault was reported to occur in childhood, higher rates of further traumas into adulthood were found (Mueser et al. 2004). In addition, 34.8% of the sample met the criteria for PTSD, with high comorbidity of mood disorders and current substance abuse. Those identified with PTSD had higher rates of psychiatric readmission over the past year, poorer physical health and higher rates of hospitalisation for physical health issues in the past 6 months. These findings highlight the potentially widespread and disabling effects of trauma over a lifetime.

An important consideration is the rate at which PTSD is screened for in relation to other diagnoses in clinical settings. One early study identified an alarming rate of under-diagnosis within a multi-site study containing a sample of 275 service users. Of the sample, 98% reported exposure to at least one traumatic event, with 43% (119) meeting criteria for a diagnosis of PTSD. Of these 119 service users, only three had the diagnosis documented in their clinical notes (Mueser et al. 1998). A later study containing 70 participants with schizophrenia (Newman et al. 2010) noted a significant effect on severity of symptoms and increased chronicity of illness when participants had a comorbid diagnosis of PTSD. It was noted that none of the 70 participants had been diagnosed with PTSD before the study (Newman et al. 2010).

PTSD has high rates of comorbidity, particularly with anxiety and affective disorders and substance abuse (ACPMH 2013; APA 2013). Screening for risk of harm to self is essential because trauma is a known risk factor for suicide, particularly when a person has experienced violence or trauma in childhood (APA 2013). Due to the potential for current trauma, assessment should also cover risk of harm from others so that necessary protective measures can be considered.

Current Australasian and international guidelines for treating PTSD advise offering trauma-focused psychological interventions such as eye movement desensitisation reprocessing (EMDR) and trauma-focused CBT (ACPMH 2013; Cooper et al. 2014; Forbes et al. 2007; NICE 2005). These specialist psychological interventions are offered by experienced health professionals (including nurses) who have undertaken training in trauma-focused talking therapies and engage in ongoing supervision. There is little evidence to show benefit from use of pharmacological treatments, although SSRIs can be used if a consumer does not wish to engage in or is not finding benefit from psychological therapies alone and may be supportive if there is a comorbid moderate-to-severe affective or anxiety disorder (ACPMH 2013).

Critical thinking challenge 9.3

How does anxiety operate as part of different mental health diagnoses such as schizophrenia, depression or eating disorders? What challenges does anxiety pose to people experiencing these conditions? Which interventions for anxiety might be helpful within these different presentations?

Acute stress disorder

ASD is clinically very similar to PTSD; however, ASD can be diagnosed within a month of exposure to a traumatic event, whereas PTSD is not diagnosed until after 1 month. It is important to note that people who receive a diagnosis of ASD do not necessarily go on to develop PTSD – thus one is not predictive of the other. Similarly, those who receive a diagnosis of PTSD may not have had symptoms of ASD within the first month of exposure (ACPMH 2013).

The evidence and guidelines for treatment of ASD are similar to those of PTSD, with trauma-focused CBT recommended as a first-line treatment (ACPMH 2007).

Adjustment disorder

AD is characterised by an objectively determined, significant, enduring and atypical stress response to one or more life stressors such as a potential or an actual significant event like a relationship ending, job loss, socioeconomic difficulties, developmental events (retirement) or ongoing illness or disability. Symptoms typically involve emotional or behavioural changes such as low mood, worry, a sense of inability to cope and withdrawal from activities, which often impairs social or occupational functioning (APA 2013). Symptoms develop within 3 months and remit within 6 months of cessation of the stressor. Diagnosis of AD following bereavement is complicated and only considered if grief symptoms occur at a level of intensity and persistence considered outside of expected grief responses (APA 2013).

AD is fairly common (APA 2013), though is relatively under-researched, with few validated diagnostic tools available. Delineation from other disorders such as major depressive disorder is difficult (Patra & Sarkar 2013), therefore recognition of AD in primary care services is relatively low (Casey & Doherty 2012).

There are few epidemiological studies of AD, particularly in Australasia. Worldwide prevalence is thought to be between 5% and 20% in outpatient settings (APA 2013), with rates of 14% identified in people experiencing physical health conditions (Kenardy 2014). An Australian study found AD with features of depressive and anxiety symptoms was the most prevalent mental health condition (13.4%) in a sample of 172 postpartum couples (Wynter et al. 2013). This identifies a need to assess for AD in populations entering significant life transition (parenthood, retirement) due to increased vulnerability and potential significant impact on individual and family functioning.

AD is found across all cultures (Patra & Sarkar 2013); however, cultural responses to life stressors differ. Careful consideration and input from cultural advisors is recommended during assessment.

Treatment works to enhance individual coping mechanisms through cognitive behavioural, mindfulness-based and solution-focused therapies (Kenardy 2014). Despite a lack of evidence to support the use of pharmacological treatments for AD, antidepressant prescribing is high in primary care, possibly due to the misdiagnosis of symptoms as major depressive disorder (Casey & Doherty 2012).

Treatment and nursing interventions

Nurses play a significant role in supporting people with anxiety or a history of trauma. Validation is the first and perhaps most helpful intervention we can provide. Conducting a thorough assessment supports us to assist in making sense of the origins of anxiety and its impacts on a person's life. Nurses can provide numerous helpful interventions to support people to develop greater peace of mind and functioning. For an account of how a consumer made use of interventions for anxiety, see Consumer's story 9.2 on the next page.

Psychoeducation

'Psychoeducation' refers to knowledge that is provided to increase a person's mental health literacy and self-awareness in order to inform future decision making. Poor mental health literacy and self-stigma have been associated with low levels of help-seeking behaviours in people struggling with their mental wellbeing (Taylor-Rodgers & Batterham 2014). Psychoeducation is a powerful therapeutic tool in alleviating the distress caused by anxiety disorders (Tursi et al. 2013) and helps improve consumer engagement, treatment outcomes and psychosocial functioning.

CONSUMER'S STORY 9.2

Amy

I think one thing that is misunderstood about anxiety is its physical nature. It is often uncomfortable but can become quite painful at times. At my worst, my physical anxiety was at or near a panic attack level for most of the day and night for the final 2 months of my last pregnancy. My thought processes were rational, but I was unable to shut down the adrenaline and cortisol pumping through my body by trying to use calming, rational thoughts. From the moment I woke, I was acutely aware of my body and how it was feeling. It was in overdrive and hyped up to such a level of discomfort that focusing on anything else was difficult. Medication helped me sleep for 4 hours at a time, but the only time I could find peace during the day was if I was deeply engaged in an activity. Even then these moments were fleeting. My psychiatrist described me as being minute to minute and there were many times throughout this that I was not sure I would survive until the next minute.

Several things helped me through. I had to be busy, constantly and without question. I asked for tasks and my family kindly made jobs up if they needed to. Looking back, the tasks needed to be both physical and productive for them to distract my mind and allow some moments of peace. Puzzles were a failure as my panic easily broke through the level of distraction they provided, but actively playing with my son worked for a few minutes at a time. On one of my worst days, my psychologist told me to drive to a park on my way home and walk barefoot in the grass while focusing on nature and the feeling of the grass underneath me. I thought he was the crazy one, but I also knew I had to do it. It worked. I survived that day and all the other days using medication, therapy, mindfulness techniques, active distraction and family support. Three years later and after EMDR (eye movement desensitisation reprocessing) therapy, I use only one medication instead of the six I needed at delivery, I run and practise Pilates, and try every day to look at one thing in nature very closely. I try to analyse it in detail and remind myself that the moment I am in is actually all there is.

Psychoeducation involves teaching people about the function and purpose of anxiety so it can be viewed as a normal, necessary and shared human experience that does not necessarily have to be avoided or feared. Heightened anxiety responses can be explored by talking through real-life scenarios to help raise insight and reflection regarding mechanisms in which anxiety is perpetuated.

Psychoeducation should always be provided free from unnecessary jargon and delivered in a well-paced, collaborative manner, allowing time for processing of information and questions. Self-directed learning through websites, handouts and self-help books provide flexibility and choice for learning, therefore it is invaluable to identify and carry helpful resources for use in clinical settings.

Social support

Social support has consistently been found to protect individuals against the potential long-term negative effects of trauma and distress (Kazantzis et al. 2012). Social support provides multiple benefits such as companionship, a sense of connection and increased access to resources and opportunities for engaging in activities that provide enjoyment. Identifying and enhancing a person's current level of social support can have powerful impacts on recovery.

Unmet socioeconomic needs (housing, poverty, social isolation, etc.) can be huge barriers and need to be considered alongside other interventions, with referrals made to other agencies as required.

Trauma-informed care and psychological formulations

A trauma-informed approach ensures a strong emphasis on attempting to understand what has happened to the person as opposed to what is wrong with them and seeks first to do no harm by ensuring sensitivity, choice and collaboration in all aspects of service provision. Consideration must be given to any trauma-based experiences that may predispose and perpetuate current heightened states of anxiety such as bullying, any type of abuse, significant loss, disaster or exposure to parental mental health difficulties. See the assessment section of this chapter for more information on trauma screening.

Psychological formulations are essential in the delivery of trauma-informed care and are therapeutic interventions in themselves, providing an opportunity to understand the reasons people may be struggling as they are. In this sense, psychological formulations are very much about making meaning, providing insight to both clinicians and consumers and assisting in the careful process of intervention selection.

Collaborative formulations provide the potential to deepen the therapeutic alliance, align the wider clinical team and assist in empowering consumers through gaining a deeper understanding of themselves.

Psychological formulations have been considered a tool of psychologists yet are being used more and more by nurses.

Psychological interventions

Psychological interventions help to modify feelings, cognitions, attitudes and behaviours using a variety of resources such as experiments, education, psychotherapy, skills training, taught relaxation or written activities.

Psychological interventions are considered efficacious, evidence-based and often preferable treatment options for anxiety and trauma-related disorders (Baldwin et al. 2014; Peters 2007). They can be provided as a one-off session, over a brief to long-term package of therapy (6–20+

sessions), within group treatment settings or through the use of guided online or written self-help packages. Psychological or talking therapies are delivered by suitably trained health professionals, including registered nurses who adhere to evidence-based treatment protocols while engaging in specialist supervision.

Current evidence-based psychological interventions for anxiety disorders include CBT, acceptance and commitment therapy (ACT), applied relaxation and mindfulness-based stress reduction. Research generally shows that psychological therapies have large effects compared with waiting list controls for anxiety symptoms (Cuijpers et al. 2014), and CBT has been evidenced to show lower relapse rates than medication alone (Baldwin et al. 2014).

Nurse's story 9.2 provides an outline of a nurse using psychological interventions in nursing practice.

NURSE'S STORY 9.2

Katie Waite

Jerry fills his chair, his eyes wide open, eager and willing. He has been doing this with others like me, on and off, for 10 years. I quickly notice Jerry is eager to please and open to suggestions. I must tread carefully. Jerry has anxiety. We all have anxiety; with Jerry this very natural experience has been amplified, turning life into a world of fear.

Together we talk about what isn't working in his life. His anxiety is crippling. Finding joy is close to impossible when you're trapped behind your rented curtains, frightened to come out. Joy is in a bag of chips, a bottle of fizzy.

The irrational fears are everywhere. They feel as if they are closing in. A social invitation has become a threat to Jerry: 'My friend invited me round ... I was so angry. How dare he? He knows I can't go!' Any situation where he may come under scrutiny, Jerry fears. He fears he will come up short, like he always has, especially as a little boy trying to impress his unimpressed dad.

His thoughts are twisted: 'I can't go ... I won't cope ...' – from these thoughts, a cascade is launched. Anxious emotions ping through the air. His heart races, pupils dilate, muscles tense, palms sweat. These physical sensations become so severe he could fear for his heart. All of these sensations feed an old belief: 'I must stay here behind my curtain where it's safe ... I'm not feeling good enough to leave.'

In this safe room we put words to his struggles: the thoughts, feelings and fears. Jerry's fears are spoken and heard and explored objectively. The power of the fear begins to fall away. We explore anxiety, its natural rhythm and purpose. As we explore this, he begins trusting himself to manage any negative outcome. He then exposes himself to his fears one by one. Bringing these experiences to our room to discuss, critique and learn from. Now Jerry can challenge his thoughts. He uses mindfulness and relaxation to calm the physical sensations. Emotions are noticed and acknowledged.

Today, Jerry sits with a grin and an air of confidence. He was at work earlier, it wasn't easy, but it was OK. He's been visiting a friend; he'll be off soon to a family gathering and he's thinking of starting up rugby again. Today, Jerry is thoughtful about his life and the scary parts it holds, but he is not afraid.

Katie Waite works as a nurse practitioner intern for a community mental health team. She has previously completed a postgraduate paper in psychological therapies. Jerry is a pseudonym.

Cognitive behaviour therapy

CBT is an effective, evidence-based talking therapy used to treat a multitude of mental health conditions, particularly anxiety disorders (Baldwin et al. 2014; Schmidt 2012). Originally developed by Aaron Beck in the 1960s as a short-term treatment for depression, CBT has been modified and enhanced for a range of mental and physical health disorders, including anxiety and trauma-related disorders. Table 9.2 provides a summary of cognitive behavioural interventions, which are further discussed below.

CBT focuses on the collaborative establishment of a working formulation that attempts to make sense of the consumer's historical experiences, developed belief systems and current-day cognitions, physiological symptoms, emotional experiences and behavioural reactions within the context of their current environment. By identifying how these factors interact with each other to perpetuate distress and difficulty, the therapist and client can identify behavioural change experiments and work to restructure cognitions to allow for greater flexibility and function in life. Changes to long-held belief systems and habitual ways of behaving towards distress and distressing experiences may explain the research findings on CBT's enhanced effectiveness for relapse prevention in comparison with pharmacological treatment for anxiety and depressive disorders (Baldwin et al. 2014).

CBT can be delivered as an online intervention, within a brief package of care (3–6 sessions), over a longer period for more intensive benefits (6–20+ sessions) or pared down as part of brief, one-off psychological intervention in crisis work.

CBT has been adapted into what are considered 'third-wave' approaches such as dialectical behavioural therapy, ACT (see below), schema therapy and behavioural activation.

TABLE 9.2 Components of cognitive behavioural interventions

Exposure	• Encourages patients to face fears • Patients learn corrective information through experience • Extinction of fear occurs through repeated exposure • Successful coping enhances self-efficacy
Safety response inhibition	• Patients restrict their usual anxiety-reducing behaviours (e.g. escape, need for reassurance) • Decreases negative reinforcement • Coping with anxiety without using anxiety-reducing behaviour enhances self-efficacy
Cognitive strategies	• Cognitive restructuring, behavioural experiments and related strategies target patients' exaggerated perception of danger (e.g. fear of negative evaluation in SAD) • Provides corrective information regarding the level of threat • Can also target self-efficacy beliefs
Arousal management	• Relaxation and breathing control skills can help patients control increased anxiety levels
Surrender of safety signals	• Patients relinquish safety signals (e.g. presence of a companion, knowledge of the location of the nearest toilet) • Patients learn adaptive self-efficacy beliefs

Acceptance and commitment therapy

Developed by Steven Hayes, Kirk Stroshal and Kelly Wilson in the late 1980s, ACT takes quite a different approach to working with distress by changing the way we relate to internal representations of it (negative thoughts, distressing emotions, physiological manifestations) as opposed to directly challenging or trying to change the level of distress itself (Hayes et al. 2012). ACT proposes that internal experiences such as negative thoughts, distressing emotions and their accompanying physical symptoms are normal aspects of the human experience and that rather than trying to avoid or battle to attempt to get rid of them, we can choose to accept and work with them using mindfulness and commitment to values-based actions to create greater flexibly in life and a present-moment focus. Treatment involves developing skills to improve psychological flexibility, allowing us to have a more flexible view of ourselves, being able to tolerate distress and difficult thoughts without being governed by them, and being able to be in contact with the present moment.

ACT is well evidenced with more than 60 randomised controlled trials providing a good empirical base in working with anxiety and other mental health conditions (Hayes et al. 2012).

Transdiagnostic treatment approaches

Despite the differences between the anxiety disorders, several shared vulnerabilities have been found, leading to the belief that single treatments targeting these commonalities could be efficacious and more cost-effective than targeting interventions at single disorders. Transdiagnostic treatments are adapted to be more easily implemented across healthcare settings by different clinicians, though are considered to retain the known scientifically evidenced interventions that support their use (Craske 2012).

Sensitivity to the experience of anxiety itself is one of the transdiagnostic vulnerabilities found within all anxiety disorders. Anxiety sensitivity is a fear of the arousal symptoms of anxiety and is particularly problematic in PD and PTSD. ACT is a good example of a transdiagnostic treatment that aims to reduce fear of anxiety itself through promoting acceptance of anxiety as a necessary and important human experience. In this way, if such vulnerability is noted, ACT can be utilised no matter which anxiety disorder may be diagnosed.

Digital mental health resources

We are increasingly identifying the benefits of harnessing technology to deliver psychological interventions due to their ability to be digitalised and disseminated relatively inexpensively across large populations. E-CBT and online resources offer greater flexibility of engagement with often little to no cost to consumers. Most internet-based tools are based on CBT and provide users with the opportunity to: access CBT through regular online lessons with between-lesson activities; assess and monitor their own wellbeing; learn integral psychoeducation about different conditions; and select the time, place and pace of utilisation. Tools can support people seek further support and input in times of high distress through built-in prompts. Tools such as 'Just a Thought' in New Zealand or 'THIS WAY UP' in Australia provide specialised courses to support people experiencing an array of mental health disorders and general wellbeing challenges and can be undertaken independently or with support and monitoring by a health professional. Research shows that concurrent guidance and support provided by a health worker allows for greater adherence and outcomes than non-guided forms of e-CBT (Andrews et al. 2018).

Some websites offer free downloads of self-help treatment manuals, while others such as SPARX (an abbreviation of Smart, Positive, Active, Realistic, X-factor thoughts; Merry et al. 2012) and Quest – Te Whitianga (Christie et al, 2019) incorporate learning and self-help utilising CBT through an interactive gaming program targeted at supporting young people with anxiety and depression.

There is a growing number of studies comparing face-to-face with online CBT showing similar levels of effectiveness (Cuijpers et al. 2014) and generally better than waiting list comparisons (Baldwin et al. 2014). Therapies delivered via the internet can be considered a helpful first step for people with mild to moderate anxiety in line with stepped-care models of treatment (Earl et al. 2014) and are supportive for people waiting for face-to-face therapy.

Cultural support

Our culture is inherently as much a part of who we are as are our mind and body, and connection to our culture is essential for wellbeing. Culture can be difficult to define, but it is commonly thought to comprise a set of collective values, practices, customs and traditions (Gee et al. 2014) and is not necessarily bound solely by ethnic identity. Connection to culture provides a multitude of protective factors and resilience because it gives people a sense of belonging, security and meaning, as well as helping them to find their place within their histories and in the present moment, assisting with a vision of themselves into the future.

Our health systems typically originate from Western models of health, bringing about potential implications and challenges for those from other cultures. The indigenous cultures of New Zealand and Australia – Māori, Aboriginal and Torres Strait Islander – contain their own unique belief systems and health practices, which are known to provide protective factors for their peoples. In order to strive for equitable outcomes for indigenous peoples, we must work to identify connection to culture as an important factor and learn from and utilise current indigenous models of health in care such as Sir Mason Durie's (1982) model, *Te Whare Tapa Wha*. This model diagrammatically depicts the deep connections and essential roles that *taha whānau* (extended family health and wider social systems), *taha hinengaro* (mental wellbeing and the inseparable nature of the mind and body), *taha tinana* (physical health) and *taha wairua* (spiritual health) have for Māori, as well as the importance of their connection with *whenua* (land), their *whakapapa* (genealogy) and *tikanga* Māori, or the Māori way. Cultural issues in mental health care are also discussed in Chapter 1.

Psychopharmacology

Generally, medication is not a first-line approach for anxiety and trauma-related disorders given the risk of side effects, costs involved and inability to target important perpetuating factors that psychological interventions work with. It has also been difficult to prove the efficacy of medication in treating mild anxiety disorders because assessment and monitoring of symptoms alone have often provided high placebo responses, indicating that placebo alone can play a large part in positive outcomes (Baldwin et al. 2014).

The drivers for using pharmacological treatments for anxiety disorders are the intensity, impact on daily functioning and duration of symptoms experienced by consumers. Psychopharmacology should always be utilised through a process of obtaining informed consent once all aspects of the medication, including the side effects and adverse risks, have been discussed.

Short-term use of medication can be supportive for people with more moderate to severe symptoms, assisting them to engage in psychological therapies (Baldwin et al. 2014), and combined use in more severe cases of GAD, for example, has been shown to be more efficacious than either treatment alone (Andrews et al. 2018).

Psychotropic medications used for anxiety (apart from benzodiazepines) often do not produce an immediate response. There can be a short-term worsening of symptoms, which the consumer should be prepared for. Choice of medication is steered by levels of evidence, safety in terms of side effects and any contraindications for the individual, as well as any prior positive responses with past use.

SSRIs are used to treat depression and affective disorders and are commonly prescribed when necessary for the treatment of anxiety disorders due to a comparable evidence base, broad-spectrum efficacy and high levels of tolerability in terms of side effects (Baldwin et al. 2014). SNRIs are less well tolerated, with a higher side effect profile, though have proven efficacy in anxiety disorders, particularly GAD, and the acute treatment and relapse prevention phase of PD (Baldwin et al. 2014). Benzodiazepines such as lorazepam and diazepam have some proven efficacy for short-term treatment of PD, SAD and GAD (Baldwin et al. 2014), though often cause sedation and cognitive impairment and there is risk of dependence in prolonged use.

Chapter 19 contains further discussion of psychopharmacology.

Chapter summary

High levels of anxiety can be responsible for sending anxious intrusive thoughts into our consciousness, filled with myriad dangerous possibilities that can create further anxiety and fear of what might be happening now and into the future. However, as an emotion in itself, anxiety is normal and necessary, playing a protective mechanism in our day-to-day lives.

Anxiety and trauma-related disorders can develop following several significant life events and early experiences and are often perpetuated by the stress of day-to-day life, impairing functioning and connectedness with values and sense of meaning in life. Psychological interventions play a large role and may be complemented with thoughtful pharmacological treatment.

Nurses will be well equipped to work alongside people with anxiety disorders if they can enhance their assessment and formulation skills, as well as identifying and learning psychological interventions that are effective across different diagnoses and problems. The greatest tool we have to work with, however, is the collaborative therapeutic relationship, recognising consumers' own expertise and helping them harness this expertise within their own lives.

EXERCISE FOR CLASS ENGAGEMENT

Separate the class into two groups in order to undertake a debate on the benefits of living life with a lot of anxiety versus living life with no anxiety. Allow time for each group to discuss and devise arguments on its allocated topic and then set up a debate, either inviting an impartial group or devising one from within the class to decide which team wins the debate. Ensure the major points of argument are written down in full view of students for discussion after the debate.

Useful websites

CALM (Computer Assisted Learning for the Mind) – online self-care package: https://www.calm.auckland.ac.nz/

e-Couch – free, self-help modules for depression and anxiety: https://ecouch.anu.edu.au/welcome

GET Self-Help – cognitive behaviour therapy self-help resources: https://www.getselfhelp.co.uk/

Just a Thought – free CBT tool that can be used independently or prescribed by a health worker: https://justathought.co.nz

MindSpot – a free service for Australian adults experiencing anxiety, stress, depression and low mood: https://mindspot.org.au/

National Institute for Health and Care Excellence (NICE) – guidelines for a range of mental health conditions: https://www.nice.org.uk/guidance

Royal Australian and New Zealand College of Psychiatrists (RANZCP): https://www.ranzcp.org/home

SPARX – self-help e-therapy tool for young people: https://www.sparx.org.nz/

This Way Up – low-cost online CBT courses: https://thiswayup.org.au

References

American Psychiatric Association (APA), 2013. Diagnostic and Statistical Manual of Mental Disorders, fifth ed. APA, Washington, DC.

Andrews, G., Bell, C., Boyce, P., et al., 2018. Royal Australian and New Zealand College of Psychiatrists clinical practice guidelines for the treatment of panic disorder, social anxiety disorder and generalised anxiety disorder. Aust. N. Z. J. Psychiatry 52 (12), 1109–1172.

Asmundson, G.J.G., Taylor, S., Smits, J.A.J., 2014. Panic disorder and agoraphobia: an overview and commentary on DSM-5 changes. Depress. Anxiety 31, 480–486.

Australian Bureau of Statistics, 2007. National survey of mental health and wellbeing: summary of results. ABS, Canberra. Available: www.abs.gov.au/ausstats/abs@.nsf/mf/4326.0. (Accessed 1 July 2015).

Australian Centre for Posttraumatic Mental Health (ACPMH), 2013. Australian Guidelines for the Treatment of Acute Stress Disorder and Posttraumatic Stress Disorder. ACPMH, Melbourne. Available: http://phoenixaustralia.org/wp-content/uploads/2015/03/Phoenix-ASD-PTSD-Guidelines.pdf. (Accessed 1 July 2015).

Australian Centre for Posttraumatic Mental Health (ACPMH), 2007. Australian guidelines for the treatment of adults with acute stress disorder and posttraumatic stress disorder. ACPMH, Melbourne, Victoria. Available: www.nhmrc.gov.au/_files_nhmrc/publications/attachments/mh13.pdf. (Accessed 1 July 2015).

Baldwin, D.S., Anderson, I.M., Nutt, D.J., et al., 2014. Evidence-based pharmacological treatment of anxiety disorders, post-traumatic stress disorder and obsessive-compulsive disorder: a revision of the 2005 guidelines from the British Association for Psychopharmacology. J. Psychopharmacol. 28 (5), 403–439.

Benton, D.M., Deering, D.E.A., Adamson, S.J., 2012. Treating co-occurring posttraumatic stress disorder and substance use disorders in an outpatient setting in New Zealand. NZ J. Psychol. 41 (1), 30.

Brickhouse, T.C., Smith, N.D., 2009. Socratic teaching and socratic method. In: Siegel, H. (Ed.), The Oxford Handbook of Philosophy of Education. Oxford University Press, New York, pp. 177–194.

Canton, J., Scott, K.M., Glue, P., 2012. Optimal treatment of social phobia: systematic review and meta-analysis (report). Neuropsychiatr. Dis. Treat. 8, 203–215.

Casey, P., Doherty, A., 2012. Adjustment disorder: implications for ICD-11 and DSM-5. Br. J. Psychiatry 201, 90–92.

Christie, G.I., Shepherd, M., Merry, S.N., et al., 2019. Gamifying CBT to delivery emotional health treatment to young people on smartphones. Internet Interv. 18, 100286.

Clark, D.M., 1986. A cognitive approach to panic. Behav. Res. Ther. 24, 461–470.

Cooper, J., Metcalf, O., Phelps, A., 2014. PTSD: an update for general practitioners [online]. Aust. Fam. Physician 43 (11), 754–757.

Cosoff, S.J., Hafner, R.J., 1998. The prevalence of comorbid anxiety in schizophrenia, schizoaffective disorder and bipolar disorder. Aust. N. Z. J. Psychiatry 32, 67–72.

Craske, M.G., 2012. Transdiagnostic treatment for anxiety and depression. Depress. Anxiety 29, 749–753.

Craske, M.G., Rauch, S.L., Ursano, R., et al., 2009. What is an anxiety disorder? Depress. Anxiety 26, 1066–1085.

Cuijpers, P., Sijbrandij, M., Koole, S., et al., 2014. Psychological treatment of generalised anxiety disorder: a meta-analysis. Clin. Psychol. Rev. 34, 130–140.

Durie, M., 1982. Whaiora: Māorihealth Development. Oxford University Press, Auckland.

Earl, T., Hodgson, E., Bunting, A., et al., 2014. Talking therapies in times of change. J. NZCCP 24, 5–24.

Faravelli, C., Lo Sauro, C., Lelli, L., et al., 2012. The role of life events and HPA axis in anxiety disorders: a review. Curr. Pharm. Des. 18 (35), 5663–5674.

Forbes, D., Creamer, M., Phelps, A., et al., 2007. Australian guidelines for the treatment of adults with acute stress disorder and post-traumatic stress disorder. Aust. N. Z. J. Psychiatry 41 (8), 637–648.

Freidl, E.K., Zakarin, E.B., 2016. Phobias. BMJ Publishing Group, London. Available: http://bestpractice.bmj.com.

Gee, G., Dudgeon, P., Schultz, C., et al., 2014. Aboriginal and Torres Strait Islander social and emotional wellbeing. In: Dudgeon, P., et al. (Eds.), Working Together: Aboriginal and Torres Strait Islander Mental Health and Wellbeing Principles and Practice. Commonwealth of Australia, Canberra.

Goodman, W.K., Price, L.H., Rasmussen, S.A., et al., 1989. The Yale–Brown Obsessive–Compulsive scale. I. Development, use, and reliability. Arch. Gen. Psychiatry 46, 1006–1011.

Hammen, C., 1991. Generation of stress in the course of unipolar depression. J. Abnorm. Psychol. 100, 555–561.

Hartley, S., Barrowclough, C., Haddock, G., 2013. Anxiety and depression in psychosis: a systematic review of associations with positive psychotic symptoms. Acta Psychiatr. Scand. 128 (5), 327–346.

Hawton, K., Saunders, K., Topiwala, A., et al., 2013. Psychiatric disorders in patients presenting to hospitals following self-harm: a systematic review. J. Affect. Disord. 151 (3), 821–830.

Hayes, S.C., Pistorello, J., Levin, M.E., 2012. Acceptance and commitment therapy as a unified model of behaviour change. Couns. Psychol. 40 (7), 976–1002.

Hinton, D.E., 2012. Multicultural challenges in the delivery of anxiety treatment. Depress. Anxiety 29, 1–3.

Hofmeijer-Sevink, M.K., Batelaan, N.M., van Megen, H.J.G.M., et al., 2012. Clinical relevance of comorbidity in anxiety disorders: a report from the Netherlands Study of Depression and Anxiety (NESDA). J. Affect. Disord. 137 (1–3), 106–112.

Johnson, E.M., Coles, M.E., 2013. Failure and delay in treatment-seeking across anxiety disorders. Community Ment. Health J. 49 (6), 668–674.

Katzman, M.A., Bleau, P., Blier, P., et al., 2014. Canadian clinical practice guidelines for the management of anxiety, posttraumatic stress and obsessive-compulsive disorders. BMC Psychiatry 14 (Suppl. 1), S1–S83.

Kazantzis, N., Kennedy-Moffat, J., Flett, R., et al., 2012. Predictors of chronic trauma-related symptoms in a community sample of New Zealand motor vehicle accident survivors. Cult. Med. Psychiatry 36 (3), 442–464.

Kenardy, J., 2014. Treatment guidance for common mental health disorders: Adjustment disorder. InPsych October (online). Available: www.psychology.org.au/Content.aspx?ID=6213. (Accessed 1 July 2015).

Kessler, R.C., 2000. Posttraumatic stress disorder: the burden to the individual and to society. J. Clin. Psychiatry 61 (Suppl. 5), 4–12.

Klein, D.F., 2002. Historical aspects of anxiety. Dialogues Clin. Neurosci. 4 (3), 295.

Leonard, B.E., 2005. The HPA and immune axes in stress: the involvement of the serotonergic system. Eur. Psychiatry 20, S302–S306.

Lowrance, S.A., Ionadi, A., McKay, E., et al., 2016. Sympathetic nervous system contributes to enhanced corticosterone levels following chronic stress. Psychoneuroendocrinology 68, 163–170.

Malan-Müller, S., Hemmings, S.M.J., Seedat, S., 2013. Big effects of small RNAs: a review of microRNAs in Anxiety. Mol. Neurobiol. 47, 726–739.

McEvoy, P.M., Grove, R., Slade, T., 2011. Epidemiology of anxiety disorders in the Australian general population: findings of the 2007 Australian National Survey of Mental Health and Wellbeing. Aust. N. Z. J. Psychiatry 45 (11), 957–967.

Merry, S.N., Stasiak, K., Shepherd, M., et al., 2012. The effectiveness of SPARX, a computerised self-help intervention for adolescents seeking help for depression: randomised controlled non-inferiority trial. BMJ 344, e2598.

Mueser, K.T., Goodman, L.B., Trumbetta, S.L., et al., 1998. Trauma and posttraumatic stress disorder in severe mental illness. J. Consult. Clin. Psychol. 66, 493–499.

Mueser, K.T., Salyers, M.P., Rosenberg, S.D., et al., 2004. Interpersonal trauma and posttraumatic stress disorder in patients with severe mental illness: demographic, clinical, and health correlates. Schizophr. Bull. 30 (1), 45–57.

Nadew, G., 2012. Exposure to traumatic events, prevalence of posttraumatic stress disorder and alcohol abuse in Aboriginal communities. Rural Remote Health 12 (4), 1667. Available: www.rrh.org.au. (Accessed 1 July 2015).

Newman, J.M., Turnbull, A., Berman, B.A., et al., 2010. Impact of traumatic and violent victimization experiences in individuals with schizophrenia and schizoaffective disorder. J. Nerv. Ment. Dis. 198, 798–814.

Neziroglu, F., Mancusi, L., 2014. Treatment resistant OCD: conceptualization and treatment. Curr. Psychiatry Rev. 10 (4), 289–295.

National Institute for Health and Care Excellence (NICE), 2014. Anxiety disorders. In: NICE Quality Standard QS53. NICE, UK.

National Institute for Health and Care Excellence (NICE), 2005. Post-traumatic stress disorder: management. In: NICE Quality Standard CG26. NICE, London.

Nivard, M.G., Dolan, C.V., Kendler, K.S., et al., 2015. Stability in symptoms of anxiety and depression as a function of genotype and environment: a longitudinal twin study from ages 3 to 63 years. Psychol. Med. 45, 1039–1049.

Palagini, L., Baglioni, C., Ciapparelli, A., et al., 2013. REM sleep dysregulation in depression: state of the art. Sleep Med. Rev. 17 (5), 377–390.

Patra, B.N., Sarkar, S., 2013. Adjustment disorder: current diagnostic status. Indian J. Psychol. Med. 35, 4–9.

Peters, J., 2007. We Need to Talk: Talking Therapies – a Snapshot of Issues and Activities Across Mental Health and Addition Services in New Zealand. Te Pou O Te Whakaaro Nui, Auckland.

Riskind, J.H., Kleiman, E.M., Weingarden, H., et al., 2013. Cognitive vulnerability to anxiety in the stress generation process: further investigation of the interaction effect between the looming cognitive style and anxiety sensitivity. J. Behav. Ther. Exp. Psychiatry 44, 381–387.

Royal Australian and New Zealand College of Psychiatrists (RANZCP), 2003. Australian and New Zealand clinical practice guidelines for the treatment of panic disorder and agoraphobia. Aust. N. Z. J. Psychiatry 37, 641–656.

Resick, P.A., Bovin, M.J., Calloway, A.L., et al., 2012. A critical evaluation of the complex PTSD literature: implications for DSM–5. J. Trauma. Stress 25 (3), 241–251.

Salkovskis, P.M. (Ed.), 1996. Frontiers of Cognitive Therapy. Guilford Press, New York.

Schmidt, N.B., 2012. Innovations in the treatment of anxiety psychopathology. Behav. Ther. 43, 465–467.

Sawchuk, C.N., Veitengruber, J.P., 2016. Panic Disorders. BMJ Publishing Group, London. Available: http://bestpractice.bmj.com.

Sawchuk, C.N., Veitengruber, J.P., Olatunji, B.O., et al., 2015. Social Anxiety Disorder. BMJ Publishing Group, London. Available: http://bestpractice.bmj.com.

Seibell, P.J., Pallanti, S., Bernardi, S., et al., 2015. Obsessive-Compulsive Disorder. BMJ Publishing Group, London. Available: http://bestpractice.bmj.com.

Simon, D.P., 2015. The science of stress and addiction: A mini-review of the research, Part 1. Available: https://drsimonsaysscience.org/2015/03/22/the-science-of-stress-and-addiction-a-mini-review-of-the-research-part-1.

Simpson, T.L., Comtois, K.A., Moore, S.A., et al., 2011. Comparing the diagnosis of PTSD when assessing worst versus multiple traumatic events in a chronically mentally ill sample. J. Trauma. Stress 24, 361–364.

Spitzer, R.L., Kroenke, K., Williams, J.B., et al., 2006. A brief measure for assessing generalized anxiety disorder: the GAD-7. Arch. Intern. Med. 166 (10), 1092–1097.

Taylor-Rodgers, E., Batterham, P.J., 2014. Evaluation of an online psychoeducation intervention to promote mental health help seeking attitudes and intentions among young adults: randomised controlled trial. J. Affect. Disord. 168, 65–71.

Tursi, M.F., Baes, C.V., Camacho, F.R., et al., 2013. Effectiveness of psychoeducation for depression: a systematic review. Aust. N. Z. J. Psychiatry 47 (11), 1019–1031.

Weiss, D.S., Marmar, C.R., 1996. The impact of event scale: revised. In: Wilson, J., Keane, T.M. (Eds.), Assessing Psychological Trauma and PTSD. Guilford Press, New York, pp. 399–411.

Wells, J.E., 2006. Twelve-month prevalence. In: Oakley Browne, M.A., Wells, J.E., Scott, K.M. (Eds.), Te Rau Hinengaro: The New Zealand Mental Health Survey. Ministry of Health, Wellington.

Wynter, K., Rowe, H., Fisher, J., 2013. Common mental disorders in women and men in the first six months after the birth of their first infant: a community study in Victoria, Australia. J. Affect. Disord. 151 (3), 980–985.

Zoellner, L.A., Pruitt, L.D., Farach, F.J., et al., 2014. Understanding heterogeneity in PTSD: fear, dysphoria, and distress. Depress. Anxiety 31, 97–106.

CHAPTER 10

Mood disorders

Greg Clark and Sophie Temmhoff

KEY POINTS

- There are key nursing principles and interventions for working with people experiencing a mood disorder.
- As with all mental health disorders, establishing a therapeutic, interpersonal relationship is critical to treatment success.
- Mood disorders respond to a variety of psychological, sociocultural and biological interventions.
- Antidepressants and mood stabilisers are the major classes of medication used to treat mood disorders.
- People with depression and bipolar disorder are more likely to think about suicide, but this is not the case for everyone with depression and bipolar disorder, and we need to assess this on an individual basis

KEY TERMS

- Bipolar disorder
- Depression
- Family history
- Physical health and comorbidity
- Psychology and medicine
- Signs and symptoms
- Spirituality and culture

LEARNING OUTCOMES

The material in this chapter will assist you to:

- describe behaviours associated with mood disorders
- describe cognitive (thinking) changes associated with mood disorders
- understand communication changes associated with mood disorders
- describe mood changes associated with major depressive disorder and bipolar disorder
- describe changes in physical functioning associated with mood disorders
- explain the reasons for nursing interventions and the expected client responses
- outline cognitive, social and biological theories that contribute to the understanding of the aetiology (origin) of mood disorders
- understand the use of antidepressants and mood stabilisers
- examine the nature of medication collaboration
- outline psychotherapies, cognitive behaviour therapy and other therapeutic options
- describe the therapeutic use of self
- recognise some of the personal challenges arising for nurses working with people who are experiencing major depressive disorder and bipolar disorder.

Introduction

This chapter examines the nature of mood disorders. It also explores mental health assessment, interventions, knowledge and attitudes that nurses need to work effectively with people with mood disorders. A holistic view is essential because mood disorders affect all aspects of daily living.

Depression and elevated mood commonly occur in many mental disorders. This chapter considers disorders where the change in mood predominates. When a person has a mood disorder, the changes they experience are more intense and persistent than those that most people experience in their day-to-day lives and may affect functioning both at work and at home. The person experiences a range of disturbances in behaviour, cognition, communication and physical functioning.

This chapter addresses major depressive disorder (major depression), bipolar disorder, postpartum depression and depression associated with ageing. It also makes a distinction between major depressive disorder (major depression) and feeling sad.

The key to working effectively with someone with a mood disorder is a collaborative relationship characterised by openness and respect. This is emphasised throughout the chapter. The collaborative relationship is an essential part of counselling and pharmacotherapeutic interventions. At all times, the nurse must be a partner in the client's recovery.

Historical anecdote 10.1: From melancholia to depression

For most of human history the term 'melancholia' was used to describe people who struggled with low mood. The term 'depression', which stems from the Latin '*de*' and '*premere*', which means 'to press', began to be used by physicians during the 18th century when Scottish neurologist Robert Whytt (1744–1766) used the term 'depression of the mind'. Unfortunately for patients at the time, there were few treatments, and Whytt wrote that 'nothing has such sudden good effects as bleeding' (Whytt 1765). Pioneer of American psychiatry Benjamin Rush was another writer to use the term 'depression'. He observed that 'depression of the mind may be induced by causes that are forgotten' (Rush 1827, p. 44).

Read more about it: *Whytt R 1765 Observations on the nature, causes, and cure of those disorders which have been commonly called nervous, hypochondriac, or hysteric, to which are prefixed some remarks on the sympathy of the nerves. Printed for T Becket and P DuHondt, London, and J Balfour, Edinburgh.*

Types of mood disorders

The *Diagnostic and Statistical Manual of Mental Disorders*, 5th edition (DSM-5) (American Psychiatric Association (APA) 2013) lists several diagnoses relating to mood disorders. These include diagnoses related to depression and bipolar disorder, the two major categories of mood disorder.

Diagnoses relating to depression include disruptive mood dysregulation disorder, major depressive disorder (including major depressive episode), persistent depressive disorder (dysthymia), premenstrual dysphoric disorder, substance/medication-induced depressive disorder, depressive disorder due to another medical condition, other specified depressive disorder and unspecified depressive disorder (APA 2013).

Postpartum or perinatal depression are types of depression that affect women who are pregnant or who have recently given birth. Some women develop depression during their pregnancy, while other women become depressed soon after the birth of their child. This is different from the 'baby blues', a relatively common phenomenon after the birth of a child. Postpartum depression is more severe and enduring than the baby blues. Depression in the postpartum period can have significant consequences for the woman and her baby, and it is important to ensure help is delivered as soon as possible after the problems become evident. Depression can affect the mother's bonding with her baby and her availability as the primary carer. Attachment and early bonding are important for the welfare of the baby, both in the immediate postpartum period and throughout childhood. It is also important for the woman to feel she is doing her best in caring for her baby and providing everything her baby needs to thrive.

Bipolar disorder can also affect both the mother and baby. Many women already have a diagnosis of bipolar disorder when they become pregnant and are already taking pharmacological treatments for this. As with many medications, mood stabilisers can cause problems for the fetus, and managing a pregnant woman with bipolar disorder requires a high level of specialist knowledge. Some medications are specifically contraindicated in pregnant women, such as those in the anticonvulsant class, but lithium carbonate seems to be a safer choice (Rosso et al. 2016). The safest choice is no medication at all, but this is rarely possible with women who have a history of bipolar disorder. Accessing a psychiatrist with specialist knowledge in perinatal and postpartum mental illness is essential. Mental health nurses also work in this specialist field and can provide ongoing support and therapeutic interventions to overcome the problems.

Depression seems to occur more frequently in older people. This may follow on from a previous history of depression, but in many cases the consequences of ageing bring on an episode of depression (Freeman et al. 2016). Common issues are loss of purpose following retirement, the death of a spouse or other close relative or friend, difficulty accepting the limitations produced by an ageing body and the effects of 'ageism'. Older people may feel they are no longer as valued as they were when they could be seen to be contributing members of society. Older people with a pre-existing diagnosis of bipolar disorder may also be seen in mental health services. It is extremely rare for bipolar disorder to appear for the first time in later life. Older people with bipolar disorder may also be experiencing the long-term effects of their medications, and this can affect their physical health. There are some psychiatrists who specialise in older people's mental health, and it is helpful to access this expertise when possible.

Diagnoses relating to bipolar disorder include bipolar 1 disorder, bipolar 2 disorder, cyclothymic disorder, substance/medication-induced bipolar and related disorder, bipolar and related disorder due to another medical condition, other specified bipolar disorder and unspecified bipolar disorder (APA 2013).

Although not usually classified as a mood disorder it is useful to be aware of another condition that has a significant mood component. This is schizoaffective disorder. It is essentially a type of schizophrenia that also has a significant alteration in mood as part of the presentation. The mood can be either depressed or elevated, but the predominant problem is psychotic symptoms.

Diagnoses help to clarify the problems that people are experiencing and indicate the treatment options that could be used for that specific diagnosis. People with mental health problems can also find a diagnosis helpful in making sense of the problems they are experiencing. Knowing that the problems they are experiencing can be identified and named can be reassuring for some people. However, formal diagnosis can be more relevant to medical practitioners and psychiatrists than nurses. Barker (2009) has suggested that mental health nurses do not need to be overly concerned with diagnostic issues because the work of mental health nurses is guided by the person's explanations of their problems, what they call these problems and the type of help that they identify that will be useful to them. He suggests we use three questions developed by American psychiatrist Loren Mosher to guide our work with people:

- Why are you here?
- What has happened in your life that resulted in you coming here (or being brought here) for help?
- What needs to be done to 'fix' the situation, and how can we help you with the 'fixing' process? (Barker 2009, p. 131)

Mental health nurses have the experience and expertise to help people with their problems of daily living, however these problems are labelled.

Historical anecdote 10.2: Virginia Woolf

Mental ill health can affect people from all walks of life. Virginia Woolf (1883–1941) was one of the most famous novelists of the 20th century, but she had a long battle with bipolar disorder. Exceptionally intellectual, Woolf used her writing to cope with her mental health challenges. This particularly related to her relationship with her parents from whom she is thought to have inherited a predisposition to mood disorder. In books such as *The Lighthouse* she included her parents as central characters and was able to experience some therapeutic effect. Some critics have argued Woolf's suicide in 1941 suggested she lacked insight. Another way of understanding this, however, is that in her era there were very few effective treatments for mood disorder and her suicide may well have been considered a rational act given her ongoing struggle with unremitting episodic illness.

Read more about it: *Caramagno TC 1996 The flight of the mind: Virginia Woolf's art and manic-depressive illness. University of California Press, Berkeley.*

Prevalence of mood disorders

Approximately 10% of the Australian population will experience depression at some time in their life (ABS 2018). The population of New Zealand has a similar rate for experiencing depression (Mental Health Branch 2018).

Prevalence rates for bipolar disorder vary between 1% and 4.6% (Bipolar Australia 2019; Black Dog Institute 2018; Best Practice Advocacy Centre New Zealand 2014). In New Zealand the rates for Māori people are higher (4.6%) than for Pacific peoples (3.7%) and people of European and other ethnicities (1.8%) (Best Practice Advocacy Centre New Zealand 2014). This variation in prevalence rates may be related to the controversial nature of the diagnosis, with some suggesting that this diagnosis is overused and does not reflect the prevalence rates for 'true' bipolar disorder (Whitaker 2010). In the past, bipolar disorder was known as manic-depressive psychosis and this was thought to be a rare condition with a prevalence rate of 0.3% to 0.4% of the population in 1973 (Sainsbury 1973). In more recent times, and with a change of name, bipolar disorder has become a more acceptable diagnosis, and it has been suggested that psychiatrists overuse this diagnosis so they can treat problems medically rather than psychologically (Zimmerman 2016). This means that problems that may not be true bipolar disorder become medicalised and are treated with medications, even though this may not be the best or most effective treatment option (Whitaker 2010). Whatever the merits or problems with these issues, the reality is that there are a group of people who are diagnosed with bipolar disorder and treated with mood-stabilising medications. Psychological or talking therapies and psychosocial interventions are also beneficial for people with bipolar disorder, and an integrated approach using medication and other therapies is the optimal approach.

Factors contributing to mood disorders

Depression and bipolar disorder are complex phenomena that have a range of contributing factors. Shea (2018) suggests that we need to consider several factors when considering the origins of mood disorders. These include biological issues, psychological issues, relationship issues, family and societal issues and the worldview and spirituality of the person. Each of these factors may contribute to developing mood disorders in different ways, and not all factors will have an impact on every person, although it is worthwhile exploring all of these areas when assessing a person who presents with a mood disorder (Shea 2018).

McLaren (2007) offers a different view on the origins of depression. He suggests that depression has its origins in uncontrolled, longstanding anxiety. Because of this longstanding anxiety, people gradually give up on various activities and aspects of their lives and this 'giving up' process eventually leads to depression because the person essentially gives up on pleasure and enjoyment.

It is also important to differentiate depression that seems to appear out of the blue, for no specific reason, and depression that has an identifiable cause. People can become depressed following a major loss of some type such as the death of a loved one, loss of employment or following some other calamity in their lives. In the past, this type of depression was known as exogenous depression – that is, depression with an identifiable, external cause. This terminology is no longer used but it remains a helpful way of considering the factors that may lead to depression in some people.

The experience of mood disorders

Mood disorders disrupt people's lives. This applies with both depression and bipolar disorder.

Depression saps people of their energy, ability to think clearly and their feelings of enjoyment and pleasure in life. It can make simple tasks like shopping or cooking extremely difficult. Some people have great difficulty leaving their house or doing the things that keep them functioning at an acceptable level, such as going to work, looking after their personal hygiene or fully participating in the important relationships in their lives.

People often feel guilty, frequently with no real basis for their guilt. They withdraw from those around them because they feel they are a burden or unworthy of other people's love and attention. It can be a very isolating experience, and people often feel hopeless about the possibility of feeling better and getting back to a normal level of functioning.

In the manic phase of bipolar disorder, however, the opposite happens. People may feel very happy and energetic. They may also engage in behaviours that are out of character for them, and this can lead to feelings of guilt and shame when their mood returns to normal levels. People in a manic state may also exhaust themselves physically because they feel they have boundless energy and a reduced need for sleep. Their judgement may be impaired and so they can make poor decisions that can have long-term consequences. This includes issues such as overspending, accruing debt and possibly engaging in indiscrete sexual behaviours that the person would not usually consider. Harm to their reputation is a real possibility for people in the manic phase of bipolar disorder, and this is one of the criteria for involuntary treatment due to the damaging effects of this harm.

Signs and symptoms of mood disorders

The signs and symptoms of depression and bipolar disorder are listed in diagnostic manuals such as the DSM-5 (APA 2013) and the ICD 11 (World Health Organization 2018). In Australia and New Zealand, most doctors and other health professionals in mental health services use the DSM-5 as the main diagnostic classification system. However, health systems tend to rely more on ICD 11 as their main diagnostic system because ICD 11 also includes diagnoses for physical health problems and this makes ICD 11 more useful across all areas of a health system, particularly in the area of data collection.

The main symptoms of depression are depressed mood most of the day, nearly every day as indicated by self-report or observations made by others. The other main symptom is loss of enjoyment and pleasure in life. Either one or both of these symptoms need to occur nearly every day, for most of the day, for at least 2 weeks, before a diagnosis of depression could be considered. Other psychological symptoms include excessive feelings of inappropriate guilt, anxiety, worthlessness and hopelessness. Another symptom of depression is recurrent thoughts of death (not just fear of dying), recurrent suicidal thinking without a specific plan or a suicide attempt or a specific plan for attempting suicide (APA 2013).

There is also decreased energy or increased feelings of fatigue, psychomotor agitation or retardation nearly every day, insomnia or hypersomnia and significant weight loss when not dieting, or weight gain or changes in appetite (APA 2013).

Some people can have psychotic symptoms as part of their depressive illness. The most common psychotic symptoms are delusional beliefs. These delusional beliefs tend to be congruent with the experience of depression and include nihilistic delusions and somatic delusions.

These are delusions where the person believes their internal organs have deteriorated or died or that parts of their body or their self no longer exists. This is a rare but serious type of depression that usually needs hospital treatment in the initial stages.

DSM-5 has two main diagnoses for bipolar disorder: bipolar 1 disorder and bipolar 2 disorder. The main difference between these two diagnoses is the severity of the problems. The signs and symptoms are similar, but bipolar 2 includes the criterion that 'the episode is not severe enough to cause marked impairment in social or occupational function, or to necessitate hospitalisation' (APA 2013, p. 22).

The distinctive feature of bipolar disorder is fluctuations in mood between a depressed mood state and a manic or hypomanic mood state. A person must experience a manic mood state before a diagnosis of bipolar disorder can be made. If a person only ever has a depressive mood state, then they are diagnosed with major depressive disorder. These fluctuations in mood can be rapid in some people, with the mood fluctuating over periods of days to weeks. This is known as rapid-cycling bipolar disorder and is, fortunately, rare. It is more common for the mood fluctuations to occur over periods of months to years.

The main symptoms of a manic episode in bipolar disorder are a distinct period of persistently elevated, expansive or irritable mood and abnormally and persistently increased energy or activity, present for most of the day, nearly every day and lasting at least 1 week (or any duration if hospitalisation is needed). The person also needs to demonstrate three or more of the following symptoms:

- inflated self-esteem or grandiosity
- decreased need for sleep
- more talkative than usual or pressure to keep talking
- flight of ideas or a subjective experience that thoughts are racing
- distractibility, as reported or observed
- increase in goal-directed activity (either socially, at work/school or sexually) (APA 2013).

The mood disturbance is sufficiently severe to cause marked impairment in social or occupational functioning or to necessitate hospitalisation. This last criterion is where the main difference between bipolar 1 and bipolar 2 is noted.

DSM-5 states that in bipolar 2 the episode is associated with an unequivocal change in functioning, but the episode is not severe enough to cause marked impairment in social or occupational functioning or to necessitate hospitalisation (APA 2013, p. 20). Based on this criterion, bipolar 2 is obviously a less severe form of bipolar disorder and is not as disruptive to the person's life as bipolar 1 disorder.

The depressive phase in bipolar disorder is remarkably similar to major depressive disorder. For a diagnosis of bipolar disorder to be made, a hypomanic or manic episode must occur at some point in the course of the illness.

It is important to differentiate between what might be called normal unhappiness or happiness and what might be depression or mania. It is normal for people to experience unhappiness and joy in response to the ups and downs of life. Many people experience fluctuations in their mood and there is nothing pathological in this process. It is a normal response to the vicissitudes and triumphs of life. We need to avoid the tendency to medicalise normal responses. A good understanding of the person's life story can help us determine where a person falls on the spectrum from normal to abnormal and to distinguish between a temporary state and a longer term problem. Unnecessary and inappropriate treatment can be harmful and needs to be avoided.

Physical health and mood disorders

Depression and bipolar disorder both have physical symptoms that can affect a person's physical health and wellbeing. In both disorders sleep problems can manifest. In depression insomnia is one of the symptoms of the illness, whereas in bipolar disorder, people feel they need less sleep because of their heightened energy levels.

Decreased appetite can also cause physical health problems because of decreased nutritional input. As with sleep problems, reduced appetite manifests differently in depression and bipolar disorder. Reduced appetite is a symptom of depression, whereas people with bipolar disorder may be just too busy to eat properly.

Some physical health problems can lead to or exacerbate depression. Issues such as chronic pain or a chronic, disabling illness are examples of this. This is understandable when we think of the problems of living with chronic pain, for example. Pain relief is sometimes minimally effective, and the burden of chronic pain can affect many aspects of a person's life. Even simple tasks like washing and dressing can become difficult. Going out and doing the shopping can also be a pain-laden experience. People with chronic pain restrict their activities to reduce their level of pain and, as their world becomes more restricted, they can become depressed. There are no simple solutions to these complex issues, but some alternative approaches such as mindfulness and meditation can be helpful.

People with other chronic illnesses such as diabetes may neglect their health care when they have depression or mania. Those with insulin-dependent diabetes may not check their blood sugar levels regularly and may neglect their diet, which can lead to deterioration in their physical health.

Assessment areas

Assessing people experiencing depression and bipolar disorder can be complex, with a number of issues that need to be considered and managed throughout the assessment process. These include biological issues, psychological issues, relationship issues, family and societal issues and the worldview and spirituality of the person.

Patience is required when assessing a person with a mood disorder because there are several issues that can make the assessment process more complex. People experiencing depression may have difficulty with their thinking and concentration. Their thinking may be slower than usual and, along with reduced concentration, this can make it difficult for the person to put their thoughts and feelings into words. It is usually necessary to give the person more time to formulate answers and to think through the issues at hand. This also means that more time may need to be allocated when assessing someone with depression.

On the other hand, people experiencing the manic phase of bipolar disorder often speak too much, have racing, disorganised thoughts, and have problems with concentration because their mind is constantly racing. It is usually necessary to use strategies to help the person stay focused. This may require constant redirection to keep the person on task.

An assessment is an opportunity to undertake therapeutic work with a person, even when it is a one-off process. Engaging a person in an assessment process requires good interpersonal skills. Engagement is a skill set that can be developed and refined. One of the most powerful tools for engagement is a respectful, courteous approach on the part of the nurse. Being respectful and courteous conveys acceptance and a preparedness to listen to the person's story and to be helpful. Being fully present and available during an assessment also has a strong therapeutic effect (Younger 1995). If a person feels you are fully focused on them, their story and their needs, they are more likely to engage in the assessment process. Collaboration is also important. This involves promoting a sense of working with a person rather than doing things to them. We increase collaboration with a person through careful listening and encouragement to tell their story, involving them in decision making about the therapeutic options and treating them as a partner in their care rather than us being the 'expert' and provider of care.

The use of good therapeutic relational skills can have a profound impact on the person we are caring for. For many people, a well-conducted mental health assessment can provide a sense that they are being listened to and taken seriously and that help is available to resolve the difficulties they are facing. This can promote hope, an important factor in recovery. Many consumers express the view that hope is an important ingredient in their recovery journey (Denton 2008). We, as mental health nurses, have an important role to play in promoting hope.

Health history

It is important to obtain a complete history of the course of a mood disorder, including the time preceding the onset of the problems. Depression, in particular, rarely appears out of the blue, and it is also the case that the manic phase of bipolar disorder builds up over several weeks or months. It is therefore important to go back as far as necessary to find a time when the person was not experiencing any problems. Finding out more about the times before the person became unwell can give us a good baseline as to how the person functions when they are well. It may also indicate the existence of any precipitating factors that contributed to the person becoming unwell.

We need to know if the person has experienced a disturbance in mood in the past. This helps build a picture of the course of their illness over time and to understand what may have helped them in the past. This information is particularly relevant for medication choices and can take the guesswork out of prescribing if we know what worked for the person in previous episodes of disturbed mood.

It is also helpful to gain knowledge about any other interventions that were helpful in the person's recovery. This may include a range of therapeutic and psychosocial interventions such as cognitive behaviour therapy, other talking therapies and assistance with work, daily activities or developing social networks.

Substance abuse

Alcohol and other substances can have a negative impact on a person's mood, producing either depression or elevated mood. Alcohol is a depressant drug and can induce depression in susceptible people. Likewise, amphetamines and other stimulant drugs can induce mania in susceptible individuals.

Some people use drugs or alcohol to self-medicate in an effort to overcome their difficulties. This is seldom an effective approach and generally leads to more problems as people may then need to deal with and manage addiction. Drugs and alcohol can also lead to physical health problems that further complicate the recovery process.

Alcohol and other drugs can also interfere with pharmacological treatments used in mental health. For these reasons it is important to take a complete history of alcohol and other drug use.

Physical health

Physical health problems can imitate mental health problems or can produce mental health problems as part of their symptomatology. Chronic pain or longstanding, disabling physical health problems can lead to depression. Conditions such as hyper- or hypothyroidism can mimic the manic phase of bipolar disorder or depression. It is, therefore, informative and necessary to take a full physical health history.

The other aspect of physical health that needs to be considered is any treatments the person may be taking for physical health problems. Some of these treatments can cause problems for a person either due to side effects or effects of the medications or other treatments. We also need to consider any potential interactions that may occur with medications used to treat depression or bipolar disorder.

Psychological (cognitive and affective) state

A person's worldview is an important aspect of their approach to life in general and any difficult issues they might be dealing with. It is important for us to understand this worldview and how it shapes the person's perceptions of issues in their life and their responses to these issues. This is a broad description of issues that fit within the psychological realm.

Some aspects of a person's worldview that may assist or hinder their recovery are their level of optimism or pessimism and their feelings of being in control of things in their lives. If a person has a generally pessimistic view of the world and their place within the world, and also has a feeling of limited control over their life circumstances, then it is difficult for them to mobilise their internal resources and work towards recovery.

Included in this category is the person's feeling state. This is generally referred to as 'mood', and assessment of mood relies on what the person tells us about how they are feeling. We can also get some idea of how the person is feeling by how they look, in terms of emotional expression. This latter aspect is known as 'affect'. A person's affect may, in some cases, provide a more accurate picture of their feeling state than what they tell us about how they are feeling. Some people find it difficult to acknowledge that they have a problem such as depression and they may attempt to put on a 'happy face' to convince others that they are okay. They may not be able to sustain their 'happy face' for prolonged periods of time and this is when we may see the 'sad face' that reflects their true feeling state. It is therefore important to closely observe a person's affect during an assessment interview. Any change in affect should be noted and commented on. Gentle questioning can reveal the true emotional state of the person.

Mental health problems can also affect a person's cognitive capacities such as concentration and planning. One of the symptoms of both depression and mania is reduced capacity for concentration. This may be reflected in an inability to read or perform necessary tasks in the workplace.

Social networks

A person's social networks can be either helpful or unhelpful in their efforts to manage a mental illness. It is, therefore, useful to understand the social networks surrounding the person we are assessing.

Do they have strong, supportive family connections or are they in conflict with or unconnected with their families? Do they have friends who are supportive? Do they have interests that help them find purpose in life and that require a commitment of time and effort? Are they part of wider social networks with people with shared interests such as sport or hobbies? Do they work and have positive relationships with their work colleagues or are there difficulties with colleagues in their workplace?

It is useful to know about these issues because people generally do better if they have good family and social networks. These networks not only provide support to the person but can also be instrumental in the person's recovery, providing interests and activities that can help the person re-engage with the world around them. Sometimes, something as simple as going for a walk around the neighbourhood can provide connections with other members of the community, and this can be the start of a positive recovery process, particularly for people experiencing depression.

Spiritual beliefs

Spirituality is a broad-based concept that is not only concerned with religious affiliation. Spirituality can provide a sense of meaning and purpose in a person's life. For example, many Aboriginal and Māori people have strong traditions and beliefs that do not fit within mainstream religious systems of belief, but these traditions and beliefs provide a spiritual foundation for the lives of these people.

For some people, religious affiliations provide the foundations for their understandings of life and their place and purpose in the world. There are a wide range of religions and associated belief systems, and it is important for us to gain an understanding of these issues.

This may be a sensitive issue for some people, and it is important that our enquiries about a person's spiritual beliefs are conducted in a sensitive way. It is vitally important to maintain a respectful approach when discussing a person's spiritual beliefs and to not do or say anything that may come across as critical or negative. There are several current conflicts in the world that have religious connections such as Islamic State and its associations with the Muslim religions. People of Muslim faith have also been subjected to persecution and discrimination, and for these reasons a person of Muslim faith may be reluctant to speak about their religious affiliations. People of other religious faiths may have similar experiences, perhaps dating back in their family for several generations, but their family culture and beliefs may still hold grievances about past treatment so it is vital that we approach the topic of spirituality in a highly sensitive and compassionate way.

Ethnically based spiritual associations may also generate difficulties for people such as the issue of the 'Stolen Generations' in Indigenous Australian populations. This may produce, in some parts of these communities, strong negative feelings that may affect our ability to connect with them. We need to be aware of and sensitive to these types of situations and respond in a caring and supportive way. If we show genuine interest in a person's spirituality and work from a compassionate frame of reference, we are more likely to gain an understanding of each person's spiritual frameworks.

Cultural views

Cultural issues are also a broad concept. This not only refers to a person's ethnic background but can include issues like sexuality and cultural identities imposed by events. An example of this is people who become refugees when they are fleeing from difficult circumstances in their home country. Being a refugee can attract many negative experiences and interactions with others and their refugee status takes over other aspects of the person's cultural background. Refugees are particularly prone to developing feelings of hopelessness, particularly those who are detained in processing centres. Procter et al. (2017) discuss the effects of isolation and trauma on the mental health of refugees as well as the iatrogenic (medically induced) effects of the systems used to manage people seeking refugee status, such as the use of temporary protection visas. These visas create high levels of uncertainty and stress and contribute to the poor mental health of refugees.

There are many different cultural views about what we, in mainstream Australian and New Zealand culture, call mental illness. The white, Anglophile view of mental illness is not universal, and it is important that we gain an understanding of an individual's cultural perspectives on mental illness. Their views may be quite different, and while it is not expected that we can be experts on all cultural views about mental illness we are expected to be experts on discovering these differences. A sensitive, non-judgemental, non-critical enquiry into these issues can provide the perspectives we need to understand the different ways that people from other cultures think about mental illness.

It is also important to be aware of and sensitive to a person's ability and capacity to communicate in English. Australia and New Zealand have significant migrant populations whose first language is not English. Using interpreters can help facilitate good communication, but it requires some skill and experience to work effectively with interpreters. Working with interpreters increases the amount of time required to undertake assessments and clinical work, so we need to factor this into our clinical planning. It also sometimes happens that concepts that can be expressed in the person's native language cannot be easily translated into English. This is where the use of skilful, qualified interpreters is most useful. It is always recommended that qualified interpreters be used in preference to family members. Interpreters are more likely to provide accurate interpretations of what a person is saying, and this can assist us in gaining a clear picture of the issues. One problem that can arise, however, is when working with people who come from a very small language group – for example, the Tibetan language and some African languages. In these cases, the interpreter may know the person socially, and this can influence the interpreting process. When using interpreters from small language groups it is useful to know if this is the case and whether a pre-existing relationship may affect the interpretation process.

Risk assessment

Suicidal thinking can increase, particularly during an episode of depression, but also in the manic phase of bipolar disorder, so it is important to enquire about this. Risk assessment requires high levels of skill and knowledge and sound clinical judgement. These skills can be developed over time with input from experienced mental health nurses. It is important to not overreact when suicidal risk is revealed but rather to develop a clear understanding of the levels of risk and whether the person has the capacity and resources to manage their risk. It is rarely necessary to admit people to hospital due to suicide risk. With the right type and level of support from mental health workers it is possible to maintain people with suicide risk in the community.

We need to enquire about issues such as whether the person has a plan about how they will kill themselves and, if so, whether they have access to the means to carry out this plan. We also need to understand their level of intent. This refers to the likelihood that the person will act on their plans. Intent is one of the more accurate predictors of suicide risk. We also need to gain an understanding about why the person thinks suicide might be an option for resolving their problems. When we understand why a person is thinking about suicide as a solution to their problems, we can then instigate interventions to address these issues. It is easy to feel overwhelmed and helpless when working with people with suicide risk, but a clear-headed, supportive, flexible approach can make all the difference. Most people move beyond suicidal thinking if they have the right levels and types of support, and this is valuable mental health nursing

Historical anecdote 10.3: Suicide has always been with us

Experiences of mental ill health and suicide are as old as time itself. The ancient Greek document *The Histories* contains one of the earliest written descriptions of mental illness and suicide. Author Herodotus (490–425 BC) describes the plight of Cleomenes of Sparta who probably experienced mental illness throughout his life. In the end his state of mind deteriorated so badly that his family had him confined to stocks, bound and guarded. Cleomenes' suicide occurred when he tricked a guard who was a slave into giving him a knife. Herodotus describes how 'as soon as the knife was in his hands, Cleomenes began to mutilate himself, beginning on his shins. He sliced his flesh into strips working upwards to his thighs, and from them to his hips and sides until he reached his belly and while he was cutting it into strips he died'.

Read more about it: *Strassler RB, Purvis AL 2009 The landmark Herodotus: the histories. Anchor Books/Random House, New York*

work. Whenever risk is present, we need to ensure we monitor the level of risk as an ongoing process.

Interventions

Interpersonal interventions

The interpersonal relationship is one of the foundation principles and interventions of mental health nursing. Much has been written about this type of relationship, beginning with the work of Helena Render in 1947 (Render 1947), with further contributions from Hildegarde Peplau in 1952 (Peplau 1952) and Joyce Travelbee in 1966 (Travelbee 1966).

One of the essential elements of the therapeutic relationship is engagement. Engagement arises out of several attitudes and behaviours on the part of the nurse. The aim of engagement is to help the person in care to feel safe and valued as a fellow human being.

Presence is one of the most important aspects of engagement. Presence means being fully present and available to the person in care. It requires being fully conscious of the person and their needs with a minimum of unconscious behaviour (Younger 1995). Other factors that influence engagement are a respectful, non-judgemental approach combined with active listening – that is, looking beneath the surface of what is being said to detect underlying issues and themes. Listening and clarifying are two important aspects of engagement. We do not learn anything when we are speaking, but listening provides a gateway into another person's experiences. If we do not fully understand what a person is telling us, then we need to seek clarification so we are clear about what is being discussed. This can also help the person to clarify their own perceptions and thoughts.

Much has been written about the interpersonal aspects of mental health nursing. It is still, in some ways, a poorly articulated approach to helping people (Clark 2017). It can be helpful to return to the original works on interpersonal nursing such as those by Peplau and Travelbee, mentioned above. These authors articulated the core principles and concepts of interpersonal nursing, and these principles and concepts are as relevant today as they were when they were first discussed (Clark 2017). Interpersonal relationships are a fundamental aspect of life and of being human and, as Travelbee (1966) stated, it is a human-to-human process that requires an educated heart and an educated mind on the part of the nurse to turn this fundamental human process into a therapeutic wonder.

Establishing a good interpersonal relationship provides the foundation for the other interventions we use. If we can establish a positive, supportive relationship with the person in our care it is more likely that they will follow through with the interventions we suggest to them. They are also more likely to let us know when things are not going well, and this provides us with additional opportunities to finetune our interventions.

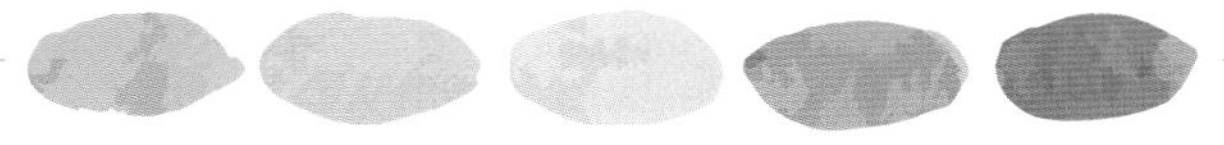

NURSE'S STORY 10.1

Greg Clark

I am a registered nurse who has worked in mental health services for 40 years. Working in mental health has provided me with an enjoyable mix of challenges and rewards. When I reflect on my practice a story that comes to mind is that of Henry. Henry was a man in his 70s who was referred to the mental health service by his general practitioner because of depression. Henry had recently returned from an overseas trip he had taken with his wife. She had inherited money from one of her relatives and embarked on a lifelong dream to travel through Europe. During the trip Henry became increasingly anxious and depressed. This occurred because of the constant changes of location, time zones and accommodation during their journey. He had a long history of diabetes and he became increasingly anxious and rigid around the management of his blood sugar levels and insulin dosing, and the constant changes exacerbated his anxiety. This led to a state of deep depression, partly because he felt guilty about the effect of his behaviour on his wife and her enjoyment of the travel, and partly because he was constantly worried that he would give himself too much insulin and die. He normally had a very strict routine around his mealtimes and blood sugar testing, and this was thrown into disarray because of the travel. Anxiety and depression are frequently found together in a person and they exacerbate each other, as in this story.

When Henry retuned to Australia his general practitioner referred him to the local community mental health service. The psychiatrist started Henry on an antidepressant, venlafaxine. I arranged to see Henry at his home. I worked on helping Henry manage his anxiety and depression through talking about the issues that led to his depression and the current difficulties Henry was experiencing as well as assisting him to develop skills and strategies that would help him get back to his more usual way of being. I also worked with Henry and his wife to work through the feelings of disappointment and anger that arose as a result of the difficulties in their overseas holiday. Henry was seen every week over a period of months, and I encouraged him to gradually take up some of the interests and activities that he had before the emergence of depression. Henry had worked as a motor mechanic all his adult life and, following retirement, he had taken on the job of repairing and maintaining his neighbour's lawn mowers and other motorised garden equipment. Once Henry overcame his reluctance and inertia and repaired his first lawn mower since becoming depressed, he was on the road to recovery. He felt pleased with himself and his confidence returned, but most importantly he again felt useful and competent.

Henry and his wife began planning a cruising holiday around New Zealand, which was a very positive sign of recovery. They chose a cruising holiday because of the stable accommodation aboard the ship and the lack of disruption it would cause in Henry's diabetes routines. It was very gratifying for me to see the effects of my work with Henry and his wife as exemplified in their thinking and planning around future travel plans.

As a nurse it is important to be patient and work with the person at the pace with which they are comfortable. Recovery cannot be rushed, and when working with people with depression it is important to pay attention to and acknowledge the small steps that lead to recovery. Recovery is not usually a dramatic process. It is incremental and takes time. It is a great privilege to work with people like Henry and to see positive outcomes from careful, thoughtful work over sometimes lengthy periods of time.

Pharmacological interventions

The main pharmacological treatments for depression are antidepressants. There are many different types of antidepressant medications available and these will be described in more detail below. The main pharmacological treatments for bipolar disorder are antidepressants for the depressive phase and mood stabilisers for both the manic phase and for maintenance.

Effective antidepressants were first developed in the 1960s. The early medications included tricyclic antidepressants and monoamine oxidase inhibitors (MAOI). Both these groups of medications are still used, although MAOIs require dietary restrictions in their use and are now prescribed less frequently.

During the 1970s and since, there has been a significant growth in the number and types of antidepressants available. These include selective serotonin reuptake inhibitors, serotonin noradrenalin reuptake inhibitors, selective noradrenaline reuptake inhibitors, alpha 2 antagonists and melatonin agonists, plus others. Unfortunately, it is not possible to determine in advance the most effective antidepressant for any particular person, and so a process of trial and error is needed. Given that antidepressants usually take 2–3 weeks before their full effects become evident, this can be a difficult period for people hoping for fast relief. Ongoing support is necessary during this period of waiting, to maintain hope and to help the person manage their symptoms as best they can while waiting for the medications to provide relief (Stahl 2013). This initial few weeks is also when side effects from the medications are most prominent, and this is another area where mental health nurses can help people with strategies to manage their side effects.

One of the dangers of using antidepressants in people with bipolar disorder is that these medications can induce a manic phase, so caution and close monitoring are needed for people receiving antidepressants during the depressive phase of their illness. If a manic phase develops, the antidepressant medication needs to be stopped, following medical advice.

A variety of mood stabilisers are available for people experiencing the manic phase of bipolar disorder. The first mood stabiliser that became available in the 1940s was lithium carbonate. This medication was discovered in 1948 by an Australian psychiatrist, John Cade (1949). Lithium carbonate is a mineral salt, similar to common table salt, but it has a strong therapeutic, stabilising effect on elevated mood. Lithium is used less commonly these days because it requires regular monitoring of blood levels to avoid the risk of toxicity and it has some significant long-term adverse effects on the kidneys and thyroid gland (Cheung 2018). It also causes a hand tremor in many people who take it.

An alternative treatment to lithium carbonate that is now used far more commonly is a group of medications that are designed as anticonvulsants – that is, treatments for epilepsy. These medications include sodium valproate (Epilim), carbamazepine (Tegretol) and lamotrigine (Lamactil). These medications are generally safe and effective, although, as with all medications, they do have side effects.

Some antipsychotic medications also have mood-stabilising effects and these can be quite effective for some people. Antipsychotics that are used as mood stabilisers include quetiapine (Seroquel), olanzapine (Zyprexa) and ziprasidone (Zeldox). These medications can be particularly helpful for women who are pregnant or breastfeeding because the other mood stabilisers cannot be used during pregnancy. Sodium valproate is particularly harmful to a developing fetus and it is recommended that this medication not be used in any woman with child-bearing potential (Austin et al. 2017).

Although not a pharmacological treatment, electroconvulsive therapy (ECT) is included among the medical treatments for mood disorders. It is particularly effective for depression but is also used very infrequently for mania. ECT involves applying electrodes to a person's head. The small electric current that is delivered via the electrodes induces an epileptic-like seizure. A course of treatment usually involves 12 episodes of ECT delivered three times a week. The person receives a general anaesthetic and a muscle relaxant before beginning each treatment, so they have no conscious experience of the treatment. The main side effects from ECT are transient memory loss and the after-effects of the anaesthetic. For people with severe depression who need access to a faster recovery than can be achieved with medications, ECT can be a valuable addition to their treatment armamentarium. ECT is rarely used as a sole treatment option and is usually combined with antidepressant medications.

Digital/web-based interventions

Organisations such as The Black Dog Institute and Beyond Blue provide information about mood disorders on their websites. Information can be a powerful tool in helping people understand what is happening in their lives. See the 'Useful websites' section at the end of this chapter for more details.

Other interventions

There are a range of alternative therapies that people access independently such as chiropractic care, homeopathy, herbal medicine, acupuncture and traditional Chinese medicine. Many of these treatment approaches have a limited evidence base and their use is generally not supported by conventional medical practitioners. Nevertheless, people do use these alternative approaches and may find them helpful.

Whatever your thoughts about these alternative practices, it is important to keep an open mind and develop an understanding of why people find them helpful. It is not up to us to dissuade people from using alternative practices unless they are clearly dangerous. The alternative treatments listed above are not generally considered dangerous. Many consider them useless but harmless.

The role of nursing

Nurses have a range of roles in interventions for people with mood disorders. As previously mentioned, the interpersonal relationship is the foundation of mental health nursing work and has therapeutic outcomes as a result of establishing this relationship. However, and probably more importantly, the therapeutic, interpersonal relationship facilitates a range of other interventions. If people have a sense of trust in their nurse, they are more likely to accept the interventions offered by the nurse (Clark 2017).

Psychosocial issues are one area where nurses can provide helpful interventions. This covers a range of possibilities and it is helpful to think broadly about psychosocial issues. For example, helping a person to re-engage with their community in some way can facilitate recovery from depression. This may involve helping the person re-connect with activities or groups that they were previously involved with. This can also involve connecting a person with services that might help them manage their lives more easily. Accessing home help or personal care services may be very helpful for people with issues like chronic pain and the ensuing depression. Getting help with personal hygiene and shopping can relieve some of the burden of living with depression. An added advantage with services like these is the personal contact with someone from outside the person's usual circumstances.

Walking alongside people during their recovery journey and providing the gift of time is a valuable but underappreciated aspect of mental health nursing work (Jackson & Stevenson 1998). Sometimes, just sitting with people and letting them tell whatever story is important to them at that moment in time can be a valuable intervention for people with mood disorders. Spending unfocused, unprogrammed time with someone can make a difference to their mental health, perhaps through the simple act of spending time with someone who is interested, non-judgemental and available – a rare experience in today's often busy world. Using a non-directive, sensitive approach, allowing people to focus on whatever is important to them at any moment in time is valuable nursing work that can make a positive difference to a person's mental wellbeing.

Helping people access other services such as employment assistance or government services like Centrelink or the Department of Housing can be a useful intervention. Many services are overly bureaucratic and require knowledge and persistence to navigate. Nurses working in community settings can help people access and successfully navigate these bureaucratic processes.

Mental health nurses can also provide a range of formal therapies, following appropriate training. Nurses are engaged in providing cognitive behaviour therapy, psychotherapy and mindfulness practices; however, these therapies are also provided by other suitably qualified and trained health professionals and are not the exclusive remit of mental health nurses. The unique contribution that mental health nurses make is the person-centred, practically focused, holistic care that helps people get on with their lives and have the best quality of life possible. Mental health nurses engage in helping people with the ordinary, small details of life that other disciplines do not have access to. In an inpatient setting, mental health nurses 'inhabit the liminal space between the doctors and the patients, affecting in important ways the fate of both' (Clark 2017, p. 185). We have access to this liminal space 24 hours per day, 7 days a week, and this provides us with a unique opportunity to help people manage the difficulties they are facing. It also provides us with a unique opportunity to gain a more detailed understanding of the issues that are important for each person. This is a great privilege that should never be underestimated. Maddison, Day and Leabetter (1975) discuss the importance of seeking out therapeutic opportunities in a hospital setting every minute of the day and night and that this opportunity for therapeutic work is only available to nurses.

CONSUMER'S STORY 10.1

Sophie Temmhoff

In my early 20s, the deep heavy depression that had come off and on since I was a child was back again, and this time it was not leaving. I had just left an abusive marriage and was rebuilding from nothing. I had lived for six months with family and during that time had experienced constant suicidal thoughts. By the time I had moved into my own small flat, I was a complete mess, drinking heavily and self-harming daily. I didn't know where to start getting help, so I saw my GP. He prescribed me antidepressants, and that was all. They made things worse, and I ended up in the mental health unit at hospital for an extended stay.

Being on the ward was like some strange kind of holiday. I was in a bad state, the most vulnerable I had ever been. I was scared, alone and had everything taken away from me. All of a sudden, my outside responsibilities were gone. All I had to do was eat, sleep, shower and take my meds. I was forced to stop and confront just how bad things had become.

Being on the ward can feel dehumanising. You don't have your usual comfort and freedom, and you suddenly have little contact with the outside world. All of this happens while you are in an incredibly vulnerable space. It meant so much to me for the nurses to treat me in a way that respected my autonomy. A collaborative effort during treatment helped me to still be in control of myself, even though everything else was stripped away. The compassionate care of the nurses was really vital during my stay.

The nurses did their best to spend time with the patients socially, which helped foster some friendships and a sense of comfort. This was really helpful for the times when I needed to speak to a nurse about how I was feeling. For me to be able to speak freely and having a connection with the nurses meant it didn't feel like I was unloading on to a stranger. For a nurse to sit with me for an extended period of time without making me feel rushed or like I was bothering them was really important. It not only helped me but I feel it gave the nurses a wider scope of information that would then help my treatment plan as well as fostering an open dialogue where I felt comfortable expressing myself.

I think it's really important to have information on medications. I am the sort of person who reads as much as possible about a medication before I start taking it. This was tricky on the ward as there was no internet access. It was incredibly helpful when the nurses were able to readily give me information about my medications by giving me print-outs as well as spending time with me discussing side effects and what the medication might do for me. It helped me feel like I was still in control of my treatment. Otherwise it would have felt really dehumanising to just be told. 'Here, take this!', with no information and no say on my part whether I even wanted to try the medication. Being able to collaborate with the nurses and doctors to figure out what I wanted to do with my treatment really helped me come to terms with my diagnosis, as it wasn't just something that was happening to me, I was guiding it.

One of the worst things a nurse could do while on the ward was treat me like a child. Thankfully, this happened rarely, but there were definitely a few nurses who thought just because I was mentally ill and on the ward that I mustn't have known what I needed. This mostly happened with a change of shift. Often the night or weekend nurses wouldn't know the patients very well and would question my requests that previous nurses had no issues with. This felt really infantilising and like my autonomy had been taken. I understand that the nurses would need to question things sometimes and say no to some requests, but to have it done in a very dismissive way, as if I had no idea what I was talking about, was extremely upsetting.

It was hard to know what was going on in the ward at times – when you were going to see the psychiatrist, if you had been written up for leave, when you were going home. It was important that the nurses kept communicating to me what was happening. When you are in the ward you don't have much control over when things were happening, so to be vaguely told you were seeing the psychiatrist and then waiting all day for nothing was really horrible. It helped for the nurses to keep me in the loop with what was going to happen, if they could.

Most nurses spoke in a positive way, where recovery was something attainable for me. They held space and listened to me while supporting me with my discharge plans. The next year or so, I was unable to work and spent most of my time in and out of the mental health unit. The nurses were compassionate every time I reappeared in the ward for another stay; they remembered me and never made me feel as if I had failed by returning. Recovery is never linear, and the open and welcoming support I received each time helped me to feel like even though I was back in hospital, I was still on my way to recovery.

I was referred to the community mental health team and started seeing a clinical psychologist weekly. I did my best to wade through my past and untangle the beliefs I had made about myself while my psychologist held space and facilitated growth and resilience. It was during this time I was diagnosed with bipolar 2, and things started making more sense from a treatment point of view. The next 6 years were spent trying countless medication combinations, in therapy, and with more trips to the mental health unit. At times treatment felt pointless, but my psychiatrist and case manager never seemed to give up trying to find a way to stabilise me. I had built myself a strong support base with family and friends and eventually found myself in an incredibly supportive and healing relationship.

One of the catalysts for my healing was starting to undo my trauma with mindfulness and therapy. Thankfully, I had started a combination of desvenlafaxine and quetiapine and I was finally stable for the first time I could remember in my whole life. The stability from my psych meds allowed me to be in the right space to start understanding and applying the years of therapy, and I am ever thankful for learning how trauma works and how to move it through my body.

I know I am incredibly lucky with the experiences I have had through the public health system. Having continuous compassionate care throughout my journey has been truly priceless, and I am aware that not everyone has this same experience.

Chapter summary

This chapter has provided an overview of mood disorders – their symptoms and presentations, issues that need to be considered in assessment and some of the things that nurses can do that will be helpful for people with mood disorders. We have also discussed some of the treatment options such as medications, ECT and talking therapies. The importance of psychosocial interventions delivered by nurses has also been discussed.

Interpersonal relations, a foundation process in mental health nursing, have been described and the essential elements of this work have been elucidated. Mental health nursing as a person-centred, relational process is a fundamental aspect of working with people with mood disorders and any other type of mental illness or life problem, however labelled. The importance of working with people in a respectful, non-judgemental, compassionate framework is a key concern for mental health nurses. Being fully present and available to those in need of our help is a vitally important aspect of mental health nursing.

Useful websites

Beyond Blue: https://www.beyondblue.org.au/.
Bipolar Australia: http://www.bipolaraustralia.org.au/services-directory/wpbdp_category/support-groups/.
Black Dog Institute: https://www.blackdoginstitute.org.au/clinical-resources/bipolar-disorder/seeking-help.
ReachOut: https://au.reachout.com/articles/support-services-for-bipolar-disorder.

References

American Psychiatric Association (APA), 2013. Diagnostic and Statistical Manual of Mental Disorders, fifth ed. APA, Washington DC.

Austin, M.P., Highet, N., the Expert Working Group, 2017. Mental Health Care in the Perinatal Period: Australian Clinical Practice Guidelines. Centre of Perinatal Excellence, Melbourne.

Australian Bureau of Statistics, 2018. National Health Survey: First Results, 2017–18. Commonwealth of Australia. Released December 2018.

Barker, P. (Ed.), 2009. Psychiatric and Mental Health Nursing: The Craft of Caring, second ed. Hodder Arnold, London.

Best Practice Advocacy Centre New Zealand, 2014. Bipolar disorder: identifying and supporting patients in primary care. Accessed at: http://bpac.org.nz/bpj/2014/july/bipolar.aspx.

Bipolar Australia, 2019. Bipolar information. Accessed at: www.bipolaraustralia.org.au/bipolar-information/.

Black Dog Institute, 2018. Facts and figures about mental health. Accessed at: www.blackdoginstitue.org.au.

Cade, J.F., 1949. Lithium salts in the treatment of psychotic excitement. Med. J. Aust. 2 (10), 349–352.

Caramagno, T.C., 1996. The Flight of the Mind: Virginia Woolf's Art and Manic-Depressive Illness. University of California Press, Berkeley.

Cheung, D.S., 2018. Bipolar patient presenting with lithium-induced hyperparathyroidism following years of lithium-induced hypothyroidism. Proceedings of UCLA Health, 22.

Clark, G.J., 2017. The past is not a foreign country: a history of ideas in psychiatric nursing scholarship – 1885 to 2013. PhD Thesis. University of Newcastle. Newcastle, Australia.

Denton, A., 2008. Enough Rope. Angels and Demons. ABC TV/Zapruder's Other Films, Sydney.

Freeman, A.T., Santini, Z.I., Tyrovolas, S., et al., 2016. Negative perceptions of ageing predict the onset and persistence of depression and anxiety: findings from a prospective analysis of the Irish Longitudinal Study on Ageing (TILDA). J. Affect. Disord. 199, 132–138.

Jackson, S., Stevenson, C., 1998. The gift of time from the friendly professional. Nurs. Stand. 12 (51), 31–33.

Maddison, D., Day, P., Leabetter, B., 1975. Psychiatric Nursing. Churchill Livingstone, Edinburgh.

McLaren, N., 2007. Humanizing Madness: Psychiatry and the Cognitive Neurosciences. Future Psychiatry Press, Ann Arbor.

Mental Health Branch, 2018. NSW Strategic Framework and Workforce Plan for Mental Health 2018–2022 and NSW Mental Health Workforce Plan 2018–2022. NSW Ministry of Health, North Sydney.

Peplau, H., 1952. Interpersonal Relations in Nursing. G.P. Putman's Sons, New York.

Procter, N., Hamer, H.P., McGarry, D., et al., 2017. Mental Health: A Person-Centred Approach, second ed. Cambridge University Press, Cambridge.

Render, H.W., 1947. Nurse–Patient Relationships in Psychiatry. McGraw-Hill Book Company Inc, New York.

Rosso, G., Albert, U., Di Salvo, G., et al., 2016. Lithium prophylaxis during pregnancy and the postpartum period in women with lithium-responsive bipolar I disorder. Arch. Womens Ment. Health 19 (2), 429–432.

Rush, B., 1827. Medical Inquiries and Observations Upon the Diseases of the Mind, third ed. Grigg & Elliott, Philadelphia.

Sainsbury, M.J., 1973. Key to Psychiatry: A Textbook for Students. Australian and New Zealand Book Co. Pty. Ltd, Sydney.

Shea, S.C., 2018. Psychiatric Interviewing: The Art of Understanding. Elsevier, Edinburgh.

Stahl, S.M., 2013. Stahl's Essential Psychopharmacology, fourth ed. Cambridge University Press, Cambridge.

Strassler, R.B., Purvis, A.L., 2009. The Landmark Herodotus: The Histories. Anchor Books/Random House, New York.

Travelbee, J., 1966. Interpersonal Aspects of Nursing, first ed. F.A. Davis Company, Philadelphia.

Whitaker, R., 2010. Anatomy of an Epidemic. Magic Bullets, Psychiatric Drugs and the Astonishing Rise of Mental Illness in America. Crown Publishers, New York.

Whytt, R., 1765. Observations on the nature, causes, and cure of those disorders which have been commonly called nervous, hypochondriac, or hysteric, to which are prefixed some remarks on the sympathy of the nerves. Printed for T Becket and P DuHondt, London, and J Balfour, Edinburgh.

World Health Organization, 2018. The International Classification of Diseases, 11th Revision. WHO, Geneva.

Younger, J., 1995. The alienation of the sufferer. ANS Adv. Nurs. Sci. 17 (4), 53–72.

Zimmerman, M., 2016. Improving the recognition of borderline personality disorder in a bipolar world. J. Personal. Disord. 30 (3), 320–335.

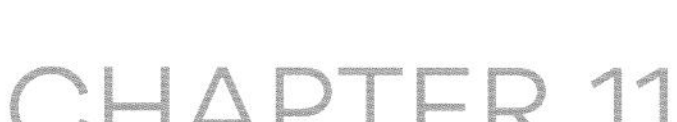

CHAPTER 11

Substance use and co-occurring mental health disorders

Megan McKechnie

KEY POINTS

- Excessive alcohol consumption is the cause of a wide range of health harms including being the major cause of road accidents, domestic violence, public violence, crime, chronic health problems and brain damage. It contributes to family breakdown and broader social dysfunction.
- There is a considerable degree of co-occurrence between substance use disorders and other mental health disorders.
- Psychoactive drugs can cause harm through intoxication or addiction.
- Interventions may include harm reduction, intoxication management, detoxification, management of pharmacotherapy, early interventions, brief interventions and longer term maintenance therapies.
- Treatment may include pharmacological, psychological and psychosocial interventions to assist with reducing the harm associated with substance use.

KEY TERMS

- Co-occurring disorder
- Dependence
- Detoxification
- Harm reduction
- Intoxication
- Novel psychoactive substance
- Psychoactive drug
- Psychosis
- Substance use disorder
- Synthetic cannabinoid
- Tolerance
- Withdrawal

LEARNING OUTCOMES

The material in this chapter will assist you to:

- discuss the incidence and impact of substance-related disorders and co-occurring disorders in Australia and New Zealand
- describe the pharmacokinetics and pharmacodynamics of psychoactive drugs
- identify the importance of undertaking a drug and alcohol assessment for all mental health clients
- describe a range of interventions that can be used for clients with a co-occurring substance use disorder and a mental illness
- describe the different substance withdrawal syndromes
- apply your knowledge of the nursing process to clients who are dependent on alcohol and other drugs
- describe a range of harm minimisation strategies that can be used for clients with substance use disorders
- critically analyse the range of treatment services available for clients with a co-occurring diagnosis.

Introduction

Wherever nurses work they will come across people who have substance use problems. This may involve using legal and illegal substances, as well as working with clients who have accidentally developed an iatrogenic (medically induced) dependence on prescribed medication. We may have experienced our own mental health or substance use problems or that of family and friends and we need to consider the impact of this pre-existing bias on treatment. If we understand the nature of these problems, we can offer the best care possible, in a non-biased and empathetic way.

This chapter explores issues of substance use, substance use disorders and co-occurring disorders (mental health problems and substance use problems) in Australia and New Zealand. It highlights the costs of drug and alcohol use to the person, their family and community. The pharmacology of psychoactive drugs is explored, and various terms are defined. The skills needed to ask targeted questions and to provide a comprehensive drug and alcohol assessment are detailed. Specific interventions such as early interventions, brief interventions and harm reduction strategies are explored. The assessment and treatment of clients who are intoxicated or withdrawing from substances is described.

The final section of the chapter discusses co-occurring substance use and mental health disorders, the significance of co-occurring diagnosis and why people with a mental illness use alcohol and other drugs. You will find additional information and specific nursing interventions for co-occurring presentations in other relevant chapters.

Types of substance use disorders

Substance use exists on a spectrum that ranges from abstinence to occasional use to harmful use to addiction. Occasional use may not cause problems or may even be therapeutic. In general, the more often the substance is used or the greater the amount used, the more severe the health consequences, psychosocial consequences and risk of dependence. Substance use disorders may be defined as disorders that develop due to the use of psychoactive substances that result in mental and behavioural changes over time (World Health Organization (WHO) 2018a). The severity of these disorders will vary significantly between individuals (American Psychiatric Association 2013).

Intoxication

Intoxication refers to a clinically significant yet transient state that develops rapidly after using alcohol or other substances and is characterised by a range of changes to consciousness, cognition, perception, affect, behaviour or coordination (WHO 2018a). Nurses need to manage intoxication effectively because it may complicate assessment and client management and increase the risk of mortality. Intoxication can mask serious illness or injury (e.g. infections, hypoxia, head injury and cerebrovascular accidents). It can also be life threatening by directly altering physical functions (e.g. depressed respiration, temperature dysregulation) or via secondary events associated with altered mental/conscious states (e.g. aspiration when acutely intoxicated on alcohol, motor vehicle accidents).

Dependence

Dependence can be both physical and psychological; specifically, dependence is when withdrawal symptoms occur after abrupt cessation or reduction in use after a sustained period of time. Physiological dependence is the cluster of physiological, behavioural and cognitive symptoms that lead to an individual re-prioritising their substance use over other behaviours that were once important (WHO 2018a). There are two central processes to dependence: the desire to continue taking the substance (despite a clear knowledge of the potential negative consequences of use) and the continued use to avoid symptoms of withdrawal (WHO 2018a).

'Psychological dependence' refers to the process of impaired control of alcohol or other drug use, whereas 'physiological dependence' is associated with developing tolerance and withdrawal (WHO 2018a). Often, physical and psychological dependence are combined, but not always. A person might be psychologically dependent on cannabis (with regular daily consumption and cravings) but demonstrate no significant withdrawal symptoms upon cessation of use.

Tolerance

Physiological tolerance occurs as a result of the brain being repeatedly exposed to a substance over time. Brain neural circuitry involving a range of neurotransmitters (e.g. dopamine and serotonin) adapts to the addition of the drug and reduces the responsiveness of those receptors. This decreased responsiveness leads to tolerance, which reduces the positive effect that the drug may have. Simply put, greater amounts of the drug are required to create the same effect as the first time it was used. This may also occur with behavioural addictions such as problem gambling.

Withdrawal

Withdrawal is the presence of a range of clinically important symptoms and behaviours, of varying intensity and duration, that occur upon cessation or reduction in alcohol or other drug use in those who have developed dependence (WHO 2018a). The different withdrawal syndromes will be discussed in more detail later in the chapter.

Behavioural addictions

There is increasing recognition of disorders that occur as a result of repetitive behaviours. The *International Classification of Diseases, 11th Revision* (ICD-11) and *Diagnostic and Statistical Manual of Mental Disorders, 5th Edition* (DSM-5) both recognise behavioural disorders, in particular, gambling disorders (American Psychiatric Association 2013; WHO 2018a). Behavioural addictions are commonly associated with gambling, food, sexual intercourse, playing video games, exercise and shopping.

Gambling disorders

The gambling industry in Australia is associated with $23 billion dollars per annum in expenditure, and 41% of people seeking treatment for mental illness concurrently gamble (Victorian Responsible Gambling Foundation 2018). Gambling is associated with a range of mental health disorders including alcohol and other drug use, mood disorders, impulse control disorders and personality disorders (Victorian Responsible Gambling Foundation 2018). Two categories of gambling disorders exist: pathological gambling and problem gambling. 'Problem gambling' refers to lower, or intermediate, levels of gambling pathology that result in harm but do not necessarily meet criteria for a formal diagnosis of a gambling disorder (Chamberlain et al. 2017). 'Pathological gambling' refers to the more severe forms of gambling disorders where individuals experience of social, financial and occupational losses due to gambling (Grant et al. 2017).

Treatment for gambling disorders focuses primarily on psychological and psychosocial interventions. Similarly to substance use disorders, motivational interviewing, brief interventions and cognitive behaviour therapy (CBT) have been established as mainstay treatment options. Screening for gambling disorders can form the first step of a brief intervention (see Box 11.1).

There is now evidence to support using pharmacotherapy to treat pathological gambling. In particular, the opioid

Box 11.1 Problem Gambling Severity Index (PGSI)

The PGSI is the standardised measure of risk associated with problem gambling. The PGSI asks participants to self-assess gambling over the preceding 12 months.

SCORES

- Never = 0
- Rarely = 1
- Sometimes = 1
- Often = 2
- Always = 3

CATEGORIES

- Non-problem gambler (score: 0) – Non-problem gamblers gamble with no negative consequences.
- Low-risk gambler (score: 1–2) – Low-risk gamblers experience a low level of problems with few or no identified negative consequences (e.g. occasional spend over their limit or feel guilty for gambling).
- Moderate-risk gambler (score: 3–7) – Moderate-risk gamblers experience a moderate level of problems leading to some negative consequences (e.g. sometimes spending more than they can afford, lose track of time or feel guilty about their gambling).
- Problem gambler (score: 8 or above) – Problem gamblers gamble with negative consequences and a possible loss of control (e.g. often spending over their limit, gambling to win back money, feelings of stress associated with gambling).

It is important to note that these categories do not reflect a diagnosis, rather an identification of risk.

QUESTIONS

1. Have you bet more than you could really afford to lose?
   Never Sometimes Most of the time Always
2. Have you needed to gamble with larger amounts of money to get the same feeling of excitement?
   Never Sometimes Most of the time Always
3. Have you gone back on another day to try to win back the money you lost?
   Never Sometimes Most of the time Always
4. Have you borrowed money or sold anything to gamble?
   Never Sometimes Most of the time Always
5. Have you felt that you might have a problem with gambling?
   Never Sometimes Most of the time Always
6. Have people criticised your betting or told you that you had a gambling problem, whether or not you thought it was true?
   Never Sometimes Most of the time Always
7. Have you felt guilty about the way you gamble or what happens when you gamble?
   Never Sometimes Most of the time Always
8. Has gambling caused you any health problems, including stress or anxiety?
   Never Sometimes Most of the time Always
9. Has your gambling caused any financial problems for you or your household?
   Never Sometimes Most of the time Always

Source: Victorian Responsible Gambling Foundation 2018

antagonist naltrexone has been shown to improve psychosocial functioning and support abstinence from gambling when compared with placebo (Grant et al. 2014).

Prevalence

The difficulties associated with treating and managing co-occurring substance use and mental health disorders has been gaining prominence in drug and alcohol services, mental health services, gambling services and general health services over the past 30 years (Lai et al. 2015). There is strong evidence that substance use disorders occur more frequently among people with mental health disorders than among the general population (Lai et al. 2015). This has contributed to the high burden of disease for these co-occurring disorders worldwide (Lai et al. 2015).

There are causal relationships between alcohol consumption and more than 200 types of disease and injury. A significant proportion of the alcohol disease burden is due to road accidents, violence and suicides. In 2018, the harmful use of alcohol caused more than 5% of the total global burden of disease (approximately 3 million deaths) (WHO 2018b).

Alcohol consumption contributes to mortality early in life. Internationally, more than a quarter of all 15–19-year-olds are identified as being current drinkers (WHO 2018b). Women have been found to drink less often than men and, when they do drink, less quantities when compared with men (WHO 2018b).

Approximately 31 million people worldwide have a substance use disorder (United Nations Office on Drugs and Crime (UNODC) 2018a). In Australia, there has been a marked increase in the number of deaths associated with substance use, which peaked during 2016 at 1,808 deaths (UNODC 2018b). These drug-related deaths were primarily associated with prescription medications such as benzodiazepines and oxycodone, which is consistent with increasing concern internationally about the abuse of prescription drugs (UNODC 2018b).

AUSTRALIA

The use of alcohol, tobacco and other drugs continues to be a major cause of preventable disease in Australia (Australian Institute of Health and Welfare (AIHW) 2018a). The proportion of Australians drinking in excess across their lifetime has gradually declined since 2010 (AIHW 2017b). Nevertheless, most Australians aged over 14 years continue to consume alcohol, and alcohol remains the most commonly detected substance across all states and territories (AIHW 2017b).

Wastewater analysis in Australia provides estimates on drug use patterns by measuring concentrations of drug metabolites found in wastewater samples (AIHW 2018a). Alcohol and nicotine consistently remain the highest out of the substances tested for (AIHW 2018a). Despite this, the number of Australians who have never smoked tobacco in their lifetime is steadily increasing (AIHW 2018a).

The most commonly abused drug in Australia, after alcohol and tobacco, is cannabis (AIHW 2018b). However, the increased reporting of harm associated with methamphetamine use is concerning (AIHW 2018b). While the number of users of methamphetamine has actually decreased from 2.1% in 2013 to 1.4% in 2016, there has been a sharp increase in the number of deaths involving methamphetamine (AIHW 2017b). From 2013 to 2016 the percentage of methamphetamine users reporting mental health changes had also increased from 29% to 42% (AIHW 2017b). Amphetamine-based products are now reported to be less available with crystal methamphetamine ('ice') replacing powder (AIHW 2017b).

Similarly, the harms associated with using illicit opioids, primarily heroin, continue to increase. There has been a 25% increase in the number of hospitalisations associated with opioid poisoning from 2007–08 to 2017–18 (AIHW 2017b). The overall death rate attributable to heroin has increased gradually over the same period (AIHW 2017b).

Hospital emergency departments across the country continue to provide front-line treatment for a range of complications associated with substance use. Alcohol remains the drug of most significance in emergency departments and is associated with overdose, assaults, self-injury and vehicle accidents (Alfred 2015). Alcohol is also associated with the highest number of hospital admissions as a result of drug use. Due to the growing number of poly-drug users, in emergency departments it is imperative to consider the impact of multiple substance use, rather than focusing on one agent (e.g. crystal methamphetamine).

Finally, prescription drug use has steadily increased in Australia over the past decade. The rate of prescriptions being dispensed for pharmaceutical opioids has increased by 11% from 2012–13 to 2016–17 (AIHW 2017b). This data is consistent with international trends, which has highlighted the increase in the combination of prescription opioid and benzodiazepine use disorders (UNODC 2018b). This is of particular concern for nursing staff because many of these prescription drug use disorders begin within the hospital setting and as part of a therapeutic treatment regimen. In 2016, one in 20 Australians over the age of 14 years reported using prescription medication for non-medical purposes in the preceding 12 months (AIHW 2017b).

NEW ZEALAND

There has been an overall decline in alcohol drinking patterns across New Zealand; however, one in five adults still meet criteria for engaging in hazardous drinking (Ministry of Health 2018a). In 2015–16, 80% of adults reported drinking alcohol at least once in the previous year, with 31% indicating they had consumed alcohol at least twice in the previous week (Ministry of Health 2018).

Tobacco consumption has reduced significantly across New Zealand when compared with Australia. Nevertheless, despite the consistent decline in cigarette smoking, New

Zealand continues to struggle with an estimated 9% physical health loss directly attributable to tobacco use (Drug Foundation 2018).

Illicit substance use trends differ in New Zealand when compared with Australia. Cannabis is reported to be used by 15% of adult men and 8% of adult women (Ministry of Health 2015). Of those who regularly use cannabis, 42% report medicinal use (e.g. to treat pain), with older users (over 55 years) reporting higher rates of medicinal use (Ministry of Health 2015). Amphetamine use has not changed significantly over the past decade in New Zealand, remaining stable at around 1.1% of adults reporting use (Ministry of Health 2018a).

For a more detailed examination of multicultural differences between Australian and New Zealand populations, see Chapter 1.

Historical anecdote 11.1: Ancient remedies

Alcohol, cannabis and opium all have a long history of being prescribed for symptoms of mental ill health. Alcohol was a standard medical prescription up until the 1900s. In 1892 Dr Aldolphus Bridger (1852–1920) wrote: 'Depressed elderly should be given full bodied burgundy, high class claret, port, the better French, German and Italian wines ... A suitable form of alcohol will often do more to restore nervous health in old age than any medicine.'

Cannabis was regularly prescribed for patients who experienced depression or mania and widely marketed as a medication in England and Germany up until 1940. Opium, the milky juice of the unripe poppy, has been prescribed by physicians since the ancient Greeks. In the 1700 and 1800s private asylums that used opium to treat depression and anxiety became popular throughout Europe.

Read more about it: *Ishizuka H 2010 Carlyle's nervous dyspepsia: nervousness, indigestion and the experience of modernity in nineteenth-century Britain. In: Salisbury L, Shail A (Eds) Neurology and modernity: a cultural history of nervous systems, 1800–1950 (pp. 81–95). Palgrave Macmillan, London*

Substance use and misuse among specific populations

Indigenous Australians

Substance use and misuse among Indigenous Australians is a matter of the utmost concern. The health of Aboriginal and Torres Strait Islander people is improving in a number of areas; however, they continue to suffer from the results of colonisation causing significant health inequalities (AIHW 2015). Current data regarding alcohol and other drug use among Indigenous Australians is of poor quality and tends to be under-representative of the actual consumption rates (Brett et al. 2016).

Alcohol use is associated with significant social disruption, and approximately nine out of 10 Indigenous Australians who have had contact with the criminal justice system used alcohol that then contributed to their offence (AIHW 2017a; Brett et al. 2016). Across all indicators (rates of hospitalisation, mental health disorders, physical and social harms, and drug and alcohol use) Indigenous Australians are disproportionately affected.

The Goanna study was a large national survey of 2,877 Indigenous participants from across all states and territories of Australia and provides the most representative data regarding illicit substance use among Indigenous Australians (Bryant et al. 2016). Cannabis was found to be the most commonly used illicit substance, with around one in five reporting weekly or more frequent use (Bryant et al. 2016; Wand et al. 2016). The use of illicit substances other than cannabis was not common, with use being more prevalent in urban areas; this was attributed to increased ease of access (Bryant et al. 2016; Wand et al. 2016).

Indigenous Australians have less access to alcohol and other drug treatment programs. The gap in service availability is contributing to the ongoing harms experienced by Indigenous Australians (Brett et al. 2016).

An example of good outcomes in this area is the story of the Aboriginal women of Fitzroy Crossing. The group came together, with the support of many men, to ban full-strength takeaway alcohol in their community. A collaborative project about the achievements of their campaign brought together researchers, human rights advocates and the women themselves to produce a documentary and disseminate the findings (George Institute for Global Health 2015).

New Zealand Māori

The most recent data available on alcohol consumption and related harm among Māori show that Māori have similar rates of alcohol consumption as the total New Zealand population but that they have higher rates of hazardous drinking (this trend has remained consistent over the past 3 years) (Ministry of Health 2018b). This places them at high risk of short-term harm from alcohol use and contributes to statistics that demonstrate more alcohol-related harm occurring among Māori, particularly Māori women, than non-Māori (Ministry of Health 2018b).

Alcohol-related harm includes harm reported due to the alcohol use of others. Importantly, young people form a higher proportion of the Māori population than they do in the non-Māori population, and all data on substance use show increased prevalence of alcohol use among young people; this may contribute to the increased use and harm recorded in the Māori population (Ministry of Health 2018a).

A 2015 survey indicated that Māori men were 2.1 times more likely and Māori women were 2.3 times more likely to use cannabis compared with non-Māori (Ministry of Health 2015). Weekly cannabis use is higher in the most deprived areas of New Zealand (45%) compared with the least deprived areas (20%) (Ministry of Health 2015).

For a more detailed examination of Māori, Indigenous Australian and Torres Strait Islander mental health, see Chapter 1.

Pregnancy, lactation and parenting

The proportion of women consuming alcohol during pregnancy has been steadily declining since 2007 (AIHW 2017b). In 2016, the majority of women abstained from alcohol while they were pregnant (56%), and of those who continued to drink alcohol, 81% reported drinking monthly or less (AIHW 2017b). A much smaller proportion of women continued to use illicit substances after finding out that they were pregnant (1.8%) (AIHW 2017b).

There is a plethora of evidence demonstrating the link between heavy alcohol use in pregnancy and miscarriage, premature birth, stillbirth and the development of gestational hypertension (Cesconetto et al. 2016; Dumas et al. 2018; The Royal Women's Hospital 2018a). Alcohol passes rapidly through the placenta and into the baby's blood stream, which can lead to a deterioration, or malfunction, in the developing central nervous system (Cesconetto et al. 2016; The Royal Women's Hospital 2018a). At present there are no known safe levels of drinking during pregnancy and it is recommended that all women stop drinking before becoming pregnant (The Royal Women's Hospital 2018a).

Data collection regarding rates of alcohol use in the prenatal period is essential to identifying neonates at risk of developing fetal alcohol spectrum disorder (FASD) (Cesconetto et al. 2016). FASD is a chronic disorder that causes physical and/or neurodevelopment impairment as a result of fetal exposure to alcohol (NOFASD 2018). FASD is characterised by a range of neurodevelopmental problems, as well as facial and other physical abnormalities (although physical anomalies may not always be present; see Table 11.1 for diagnostic criteria and key features of a FASD assessment) (Bower & Elliot 2016).

Smoking during pregnancy has been identified as the single most common preventable risk factor for complications (AIHW 2018b). In 2016, one in 10 mothers smoked at some point during their pregnancy and those women were associated with fewer antenatal care visits than those who did not smoke (AIHW 2018b). Smoking tobacco during pregnancy is associated with a reduction in the supply of oxygen and blood to the developing baby (The Royal Women's Hospital 2018b). Nicotine causes an increase in heart rate in both the mother and fetus, which can contribute to the narrowing of blood vessels, thereby reducing the flow of blood through the umbilical cord (The Royal Women's Hospital 2018b). Smoking tobacco during pregnancy is associated with miscarriage, low birth weight and premature birth (The Royal Women's Hospital 2018b).

Although evidence is limited, universal screening for alcohol and other drug use in pregnancy (including tobacco) is recommended (Taplin et al. 2015; American College of Obstetricians and Gynaecologists 2017). This reduces targeted screening of groups that are marginalised, reduces stigma and reduces the under-identification of alcohol and other drug use in pregnancy. Pregnancy can be a very good time to address maternal alcohol and other drug use; however, any changes to substance use during pregnancy must be carefully considered due to the significant stress that a withdrawal syndrome can cause on the fetus.

Pharmacology of psychoactive drugs

Pharmacological aspects of addiction

When people take drugs, drink alcohol, eat, exercise, gamble or have sex, multiple neurotransmitters are released as part of the pleasure and reward feedback system in the brain. In particular, dopamine is released along the mesolimbic dopamine pathway in the ventral tegmental area (Berridge & Kringelbach 2015; Moore et al. 2014). The release of dopamine reinforces the behaviour by producing positive feelings and a sense of wellbeing. It is a central mechanism and communicates to the person that the activity is vital for survival and should be focused upon (Robertson et al. 2015). Importantly, it is the activation of the mesolimbic dopamine pathway by psychoactive substances and other behaviours not associated with the maintenance of life (e.g. gambling) that can lead to addiction. The repeated activation of this pathway contributes to the inability of people with substance use disorders and behavioural addictions to prioritise activities of daily living appropriately. Neurotransmission in the dependent person's brain is fundamentally different from that of the general population, creating a sense that their substance use, or other behaviour, is vital to their survival (Nutt et al. 2015).

This psychoactive effect includes changes in mood, arousal, perception, thinking and behaviour. Drugs may be produced in a laboratory (e.g. amphetamines, ecstasy) or extracted from plants (e.g. heroin, cocaine). They can be legal (e.g. alcohol) or illegal (e.g. cannabis). Utilising categories can greatly assist with identifying similar features of intoxication and withdrawal; for example,

TABLE 11.1 Fetal alcohol spectrum disorder

DIAGNOSTIC CRITERIA	DIAGNOSTIC CRITERIA	
	FASD WITH 3 SENTINEL FACIAL FEATURES	FASD WITH < 3 SENTINEL FACIAL FEATURES
• Prenatal alcohol exposure	Confirmed or unknown	Confirmed
Neurodevelopmental domains: • brain structure/neurology • motor skills • cognition • language • academic achievement • memory • attention • executive function including poor impulse control and hyperactivity • affect regulation • adaptive behaviour, social skills or social communication	Severe impairment in at least 3 neurodevelopmental domains	Severe impairment in at least 3 neurodevelopmental domains
Sentinel facial features: • short palpebral fissure • smooth philtrum • thin upper lip	Presence of 3 sentinel facial features	Presence of 0–2 sentinel facial features
Key features of FASD diagnostic assessment: • history: presenting concerns, obstetric, developmental, medical, mental health, behavioural, social • birth defects: dysmorphic facial features, other major and minor birth defects • adverse prenatal and postnatal exposures (including alcohol) • known medical conditions including genetic syndromes and other disorders • growth		
Adapted from FASD Hub 2016		

alcohol and benzodiazepines are both depressants so present very similarly during periods of acute intoxication. Some drugs have multiple actions and therefore can be placed in more than one category (Ries et al. 2014) (see Table 11.2 for the classification of substances based on their impact on the central nervous system). The common effect of all psychoactive drugs, at least in the early stages of use, is to produce euphoria and a change in mental state. Over time, many people describe little positive effect but rather a decrease in negative effect when they use, which is often associated with persistent use simply to mitigate against symptoms of withdrawal (Ries et al. 2014).

Novel psychoactive substances

The class of drugs known as 'novel psychoactive substances' (see Table 11.3) is structurally similar but not identical to psychoactive drugs that are currently available but illegal such as methamphetamines, cocaine, cannabis, ecstasy and depressants (Burns et al. 2014). Novel psychoactive substances may be known as 'legal highs', 'bath salts' or 'research chemicals' (UNODC 2019). These substances are constantly being developed and modified to stay ahead of legal restrictions. To avoid confusion, UNODC (2019) clearly defines these substances as: 'substances of abuse, either in a pure form or a preparation, that are not controlled by the 1961 Single Convention on Narcotic Drugs or the 1971 Convention on Psychotropic Substances, but which may post a public health threat'.

Determining the toxicity of this emerging class of drugs is challenging because it consists of many different substances that vary in their psychological and physiological effects and the drugs may be combined (Weaver et al. 2015).

Synthetic cannabinoids

Delta-9-tetrahydrocannabinol (THC) is the active component in natural cannabis and is a partial agonist of the CB1 and CB2 cannabinoid receptors (Akram et al. 2019). In contrast, synthetic cannabinoids tend to be full agonists at cannabinoid receptor sites that, as a result, causes them to be more potent than natural cannabis (Akram et al. 2019; Sud et al. 2018). This creates more intense symptoms during periods of intoxication and withdrawal, as well as placing users at higher risk of longer term psychological changes. Common street names for synthetic cannabinoids include 'Spice', 'K2', 'Kroc', 'Purple Haze' and 'Buddha' (Akram et al. 2019).

TABLE 11.2 Classification of substances

CATEGORY	DESCRIPTION	EXAMPLES
Depressants	Depressants are drugs that slow the activity of the brain and the central nervous system (it is important to note that this is not associated with mood). When used in small doses they can produce euphoria, relaxation or drowsiness. In larger doses they can produce a loss of consciousness similar to a deep sleep, impaired coordination, depression, coma and death by respiratory depression.	Alcohol (ethanol) Benzodiazepines (e.g. diazepam, alprazolam) Opioids (e.g. heroin, morphine, codeine) Barbiturates (e.g. phenobarbital) Volatile substances (e.g. solvents or petrol)
Stimulants	Stimulant drugs increase activity in the central nervous system and increase the body's level of arousal. Small doses increase awareness and concentration and decrease fatigue. Increasing amounts produce irritability, nervousness and insomnia. At high doses some people experience delusions and hallucinations. Toxic doses lead to convulsions and death via heart attack (myocardial infarction), stroke (cerebrovascular accident) or muscle meltdown (rhabdomyolysis) (Ries et al. 2014). Methamphetamine is broken down into three further categories: base, powder and crystal. Ecstasy previously contained only MDMA, however, is now being cut with a range of different adulterants, in particular, crystal methamphetamine.	Amphetamines (e.g. 'speed') Methamphetamine (e.g. crystal methamphetamine or 'ice') 3,4-methylenediozymethamphetamine Cocaine Nicotine Caffeine D-amphetamine (dexamphetamine) Methylphenidate (Ritalin)
Hallucinogens	Hallucinogens (also called 'psychedelics') share properties with depressants and stimulants. However, their specific function is to distort perception and consequently induce hallucinations (auditory, tactile and visual). In small doses, some hallucinogens reduce inhibitions and cause the user to become relaxed and feel more sociable. Some amphetamine derivatives such as MDMA (ecstasy) are chemically related to mescaline and have both stimulant and hallucinatory properties. These drugs may be placed in both categories for classification purposes.	Lysergic acid diethylamide (LSD) Psilocybin ('magic mushrooms') Mescaline (part of the Mexican cactus 'peyote') Datura ('angel's trumpet')
Other	Cannabis is often difficult to classify in pharmacological terms because it has a mixture of mood, cognitive, motor and perceptual effects and does not clearly belong with any one drug class (Kleinloog et al. 2014). Cannabis taken in low doses produces a mixture of stimulatory and depressant effects; at high doses the effects are mainly depressant. The effects of cannabis include euphoria, relaxation and a feeling of wellbeing, as well as perceptual distortions such as altered time sense. Memory, cognition and skilled task performance are impaired, although many users may feel confident and highly creative. Other physical effects include tachycardia, vasodilation and hypotension (Kleinloog et al. 2014; Martin-Santos et al. 2012). Cannabis stimulates the appetite and is also an antiemetic; people who have taken cannabis often experience 'the munchies', when they feel hungry and crave certain foods. As with all psychoactive drugs, the effects vary between people depending on the amount taken, the manner of administration, the frequency of use, concurrent use with other drugs, past exposure and the environment in which the drug is used (Kleinloog et al. 2014).	Cannabis Marijuana Hashish

TABLE 11.3 Novel psychoactive substances

DRUG	SIMILAR TO / EFFECTS	EXAMPLES
Aminoindanes	Similar to amphetamines and MDMA. Creates similar central nervous system activity as stimulants. Later versions of these drugs have been able to mimic empathogenic and entactogenic effects of drugs such MDMA.	'M-DAI Gold' (5,6-methylenedioxy-animoindane) 'Pink champagne' (2-aminoindane) Commonly found in powder form or crystals for ingestion.
Phencyclidine-type substances	Similar to central nervous system stimulants such as phencyclidine (PCP). Creates dissociative effects via modulation of NMDA receptors.	Limited information about PCP analogues; known as 'research chemicals'. Ketamine Ingestion is the most common route of administration for this class of substances. Ketamine is also intravenously and intramuscularly injected.
Phenethylamines	Includes amphetamines (methamphetamine/MDMA), amphetamine variations (2C series and D series drugs) and hallucinogen variations (stimulants with some hallucinogenic effects). These substances act as either central nervous system stimulants or as hallucinogens. This class includes synthetic analogues of mescaline (potent hallucinogens).	2C agents: 2C1, 2CB, 2CT, 2CE 'Europa', NBom, PMMA (para-Methoxy-N-methylamphetamine) '4-MMA' D Series: DOC, DOI Dihydrofuran substances: 'FLY', 'Dragonfly', 'Bromo-Dragonfly' Ingestion is the most common route of administration for this class of substances.
Piperazines	Similar effects to hallucinogens, with some stimulant activity. Termed 'failed pharmaceuticals' because some of the substances found in this class have been trialled as potential therapeutic agents.	BZP – trialled as an antidepressant, however, had similar properties to amphetamines. 'Pep pills'
Synthetic cannabinoids	Synthetic cannabinoids are added to plant material. Initially, these were synthetic analogues of delta-9-tetrahydroncannabinol; however, different groups of synthetic cannabinoids have since been developed with significant variance in chemical makeup.	'K2', 'Kroc', 'Black Mamba', 'Purple Haze', 'Spice', 'Genie' Smoking is the most common route of administration for this class of substances.
Synthetic cathinone	Chemically similar structure to amphetamine and methamphetamines. Cathinone is the principal agent in khat plant and is considered the basis on which many synthetic cathinones are developed.	Mephedrone, methadrone, methylone, meow, M-Cat, 'drone', 'bath salts', 'plant food' Ingestion is the most common route of administration for this class of substances.
Tryptamines	Primarily derivatives of hallucinogens such as psilocybin and DMT. These substances tend to mimic the effects of existing hallucinogens; however, they may also possess stimulant activity.	'Foxy-methoxy', 'alpha-o', '5-MEO' Ingestion is the most common route of administration for this class of substances.

Sources: *Musselman & Hampton 2014 and United Nations Office on Drugs and Crime 2019*

Synthetic cannabinoids are generally distributed as a green, leafy product that is sprayed with a chemical containing synthetic cannabinoids (Clancy et al. 2018). One of the major difficulties with the treatment and management of synthetic cannabinoids is that new variations are constantly being developed. Each chemical variation is associated with different risk factors and complications of use. Synthetic cannabinoid users present with a range of behavioural, affective and cognitive changes (Clancy et al. 2018). Acute effects may involve central nervous system depression presenting as lethargy and bradycardia (Sud et al. 2018). Synthetic cannabinoids have also been associated with an increased risk of seizures. Synthetic cannabinoids do not show up on conventional urine drug screens, so use has become more widespread among individuals in workplaces that require regular drug screening.

Contributing factors

The development of a substance use disorder is complex and multifaceted. Consideration must given to the interplay between the person's environment, social situation and genetic influences. Adolescents may turn to substance use in response to social isolation, peer pressure, poor academic achievement, family disruption, poor attachment or simple curiosity (Substance Abuse and Mental Health Services Administration (SAMSHA) 2017). This is further influenced by society and how various substances are portrayed in the media (e.g. the consequence-free use of drinking and smoking cigarettes in movies and television series) (SAMSHA 2017). Risk factors for developing a substance use disorder will vary significantly according to age, social/psychological development, ethnic/cultural background and environmental surroundings (SAMSHA 2017). SAMSHA (2017) advocates for a greater focus on protective factors against substance use (see Table 11.4).

During adolescence, the brain undergoes significant development; this increases a person's susceptibility to stress and high-risk behaviours. Direct causal mechanisms behind substance use are still relatively unknown; however, twin studies are starting to clearly demonstrate hereditary influences (Boisvert et al. 2019; Waaktaar et al. 2018).

Substance use disorders may also develop later in life in response to a range of stressors, although are often influenced by early life events. Alcohol use disorders are most common among this population and are frequently associated with retirement, age-related impairments that create difficulties with activities of daily living or the loss of a partner (Lehmann & Fingerhood 2018). Problems with prescription medication may also occur during adulthood and later life in the absence of earlier influencing factors. Chronic pain is more prevalent among older adults, and there is a tendency for adults to more easily access benzodiazepines in response to stressful life events (Lehmann & Fingerhood 2018).

The experience of a substance use disorder

The experience of a substance use disorder will vary significantly among individuals, and treatment approaches should be adjusted accordingly. No one treatment pathway will be the same, and nurses should adopt a flexible approach when working with someone with a substance use disorder. The concept of hope, and the idea that recovery is possible, is important. Health professionals can easily, and inadvertently, become frustrated at the rates of relapse associated with substance use disorders.

TABLE 11.4 Protective factors for adolescents

Individual factors	• Positive temperament • Social skills (e.g. problem solving, ability to stand up for beliefs and core values) • Positive social orientation (e.g. engaging in activities that contribute to healthy personal development, accepting rules and community values, identifying with school and choosing friends who don't use harmful substances) • Belief in one's ability to control what happens to adapt to change
Family factors	• Unity, warmth and attachment between parents and children • Parental supervision • Contact and communication between and among parents and children
Environmental factors	• Positive emotional support outside of the family such as friends, neighbours and elders • Supports and resources available to the family (e.g. crisis lines, programs for individuals with trauma experiences, stress management supports or family counselling) • Community and school norms, beliefs and standards regarding substance use • Access to education that focuses on commitment and achievement

Adapted from Substance Abuse and Mental Health Services Administration 2017

It is important to recognise these pre-existing judgements and work towards instilling hope and fostering self-efficacy because these can be powerful tools in working towards recovery (Glassman et al. 2013). See the following consumer stories for a range of client stories and experiences of substance use disorders.

CONSUMER'S STORY 11.1
Anonymous

Life for me has always been a huge struggle and I could never understand why. From a young age I stopped being able to process emotions like my friends and family could. I felt immense pain just being me. So, when drugs and alcohol came along at age 14, I thought I'd found my solution. But once I started, I couldn't stop, and my life got progressively worse and more unmanageable. After 8 years of a toxic spiral of feeling guilt, shame and remorse and then using again, I landed in a recovery rehab. It was my last option. Something had to change or I would eventually die.

I was introduced to community-based self-help groups. I was introduced to the solution. I now had a program to feel everything I had been so afraid to feel; and I didn't have to go through any of it alone. There was always a woman with more clean time who had been through what I had been through. I worked the recovery program and my self-esteem and self-worth started to grow. For the first time I started to create a relationship with myself by believing in a higher power. I am now nearly 9 months clean from all drugs and alcohol, and I've honestly never been happier.

CONSUMER'S STORY 11.2
Sari

I grew up in a small country town and was very much loved. I can only say that now looking back though, because at the time, despite presenting as a happy child who did well at school and sports, I often felt scared, sad, confused, unlovable and not good enough. My father had committed suicide when I was a baby, so I always felt different to everyone else. I do distinctly remember though, always hating drugs, wanting to do the right thing, and to be a good person. As a young adult I left the farm and became a nurse in the city, I loved my job, and helping others seemed to soothe that feeling of unworthiness.

In my early 20s I had a bad car accident and began to develop chronic pain. I was able to manage this mostly with over-the-counter pain relief; however, after my second child was born in my late 20s the pain became unbearable and my doctor put me onto a short course of oxycodone. Before I knew it this short course quickly became 3 years of hell. The first year I must admit was great. I could get everything done! I could function incredibly as a wife, mother, nurse, daughter, sister, friend, human being. I truly believed I had found the one thing that filled the vague hole in my chest. Unfortunately, after that first year things quickly went downhill. I was needing more and more to get me through, and I was withdrawing from life and everyone in it. All I wanted was to be alone with my drugs; I couldn't answer the phone, the door, or open my mail, and doctor shopping became a full-time job. I was consumed by my need for them and felt like I would die without them in my system. After only 3 short years my drug addiction had completely brought me to my knees, and I knew I could no longer live like this. I felt I was so broken that I had no choice but to finally ask for help and I began to pay attention to my faintly growing hope that there might possibly be a better way for me to live.

I went into rehab with the firm belief that this was just a physical condition that would resolve once I had detoxed and had a break, but I soon found out I was wrong. My addiction had changed me. The day I was to be discharged I was overwhelmed with absolute terror of – how on earth do I function without something in my system? It's hard to describe but it was like my skin had been ripped off and all my fears and secrets were there to be seen. I relapsed that very day on over-the-counter opiates just to quiet the intense anxiety I was feeling. I was back in that rehab within 2 weeks feeling even more ashamed, afraid and angry than ever before. I was truly broken now and willing to do anything at all to fix it. In the weeks prior, during my first stay in rehab, I'd been introduced to a 12-step fellowship and despite my medical background had become open to the idea that perhaps this wasn't just a physical problem but also a mental and spiritual illness. I knew that I felt deeply depressed, lost and hollow, but still with the slightest glimmer of hope that life could be better. I also came to understand that no one else could fix me and this was a journey that I could only take alone, with a full commitment to being open, honest and completely abstinent from all mood- and mind-altering drugs, including alcohol. This was a hard truth to accept – everyone else drinks! But I wasn't like everyone else anymore, I knew that my brain worked differently now, and I was highly susceptible to relapse.

I was incredibly lucky in the fact that the desire to use a drug left me very quickly, roughly within a week, but I did still have some residual physical withdrawal symptoms almost 3 months later. I should also add that I have never struggled with chronic pain since. I put this down to taking care of my physical health but also because I took the mental and spiritual aspect of the disease very seriously. I had never seen myself as someone who suffered from mental health issues before but since finding recovery it's something I must assess and monitor regularly. And despite my medical background I firmly believe that learning to care for my spiritual health is what saved my life. I no longer have that hole in my chest and on the most part feel content and happy within myself. If I hadn't been shown how to nurture all three aspects of my life then I wouldn't have a life worth living today, and if I neglect any one of them for too long then the other two will suffer soon after.

I'm certainly not proud of the places my addiction took me to, and having to swallow my pride, admit defeat and ask for help was possibly the hardest thing I've ever done. But I am forever grateful that I had faith in that little spark of hope and for the people who showed me that recovery was possible and forever within my grasp. I didn't choose to be an addict, but I do choose to recover and live my life to the best of my abilities. If there is one piece of advice I could ever give, it's that pride, fear and shame are powerful motivators to keep an addict sick in the cycle of misery. But willingness, honesty and hope are the keys to recovery and a new life. No one is ever completely hopeless or unworthy and recovery is possible for anyone.

CONSUMER'S STORY 11.3

Anonymous

I was trapped in the vicious cycle of addiction for 13 years. Being a young, carefree child was quickly ripped away and in crept relentless feelings of hopelessness and despair. Any hopes and dreams I had as a child seemed to have completely vanished from the horizon. I was resigned to the fact my life was effectively over; I really had thrown it all away and was destined to suffer a miserable existence. It was an incredibly painful and helpless place to be. From being in that place of utter despair, never would I have imagined it possible to be where I am today.

Today I am in recovery, 15 months clean and sober. I went to rehab for four and a half months and to supported accommodation from there. I was truly desperate to get clean and seek a better life for myself and my loved ones. Recovery is freedom like I never thought possible. Today I have a desire to live. I have hope, and I truly believe that if I remain clean and continue to say 'yes' to change I will have a future beyond my wildest dreams. Connection is the cornerstone of recovery and I would never have been able to do it without the help and love of others. Abstaining from drugs and alcohol was just the beginning; I had to change everything – my thinking, the way I dealt with my emotions and what I thought I already knew about life. I wouldn't have it any other way. I like the man I am becoming and I'm very proud. Recovery is a lifelong process and a work in progress. It must come first in my life, for all that I have depends on it. It has given me my life back and for that I'm eternally grateful.

Signs and symptoms

INTOXICATION

Acute intoxication on alcohol or other drugs can lead to an increased risk of aggression and disruptive behaviours. Intoxicated people can present in the clinical setting as frightened, disruptive and extremely upset at times. It is important to consider how we approach intoxicated clients to ensure the safety of the individual and those around them. Authoritarian approaches can provoke anger and aggression and should be avoided where possible.

When speaking with the client, ensure their name is used and speak in a slow, distinct speech with short, simple sentences. It is important to be genuine in your approach and to avoid using confusing or overly medical terminology. Maintain eye contact, without being intrusive, and do not attempt to engage in complex reasoning. (See Chapter 4 for useful skills in managing aggression and violence.)

It is important to consider the significant medical risks associated with acute intoxication on alcohol and other drugs (e.g. aspiration secondary to vomiting while acutely intoxicated on alcohol) (see Box 11.2 substance intoxication criteria). The presence of other organic contributing factors for an acute change in mental state should also be considered (e.g. the presence of an acute delirium). Airway management is the primary concern in those who are unconscious (see Box 11.3). Careful consideration must be given to using sedating medications (e.g. benzodiazepines) in those who are acutely intoxicated on central nervous system depressants due to the increased risk of respiratory depression.

WITHDRAWAL

The signs and symptoms of withdrawal will vary among the substance classes; however, in general they will present as the opposite of what occurs during the intoxicated state. For example, many heroin users experience chronic constipation, and one of the first signs of opioid withdrawal is diarrhoea. The dose and duration of drug use affects the withdrawal process in terms of symptoms experienced and the severity of the withdrawal syndrome (see Box 11.4

Box 11.2 Substance intoxication criteria

To constitute substance intoxication, the following four criteria must be met:

A – Recent ingestion of a substance

B – Clinically significant problematic behavioural and psychological changes (e.g. inappropriate sexual or aggressive behaviour, exaggerated changes in mood, or impaired judgement) that developed during or shortly after ingestion

C – One or more of the following signs or symptoms developing during or shortly after ingestion:
- slurred speech
- incoordination
- unsteady gait
- nystagmus
- impairment in attention or memory
- stupor or coma

D – The above signs or symptoms are not attributable to another medical condition and are not better explained by another mental disorder or intoxication from another substance.

Source: American Psychiatric Association 2013

Box 11.3 General principles of managing intoxication

- Maintenance of airway is a priority.
- Any patient presenting as confused, disoriented or drowsy should be treated as per head injury until proven otherwise.
- Intoxicated patients must be kept under observation until the level of intoxication diminishes.
- A thorough physical and mental status examination will assist with determining the level of intoxication.
- Patients who appear intoxicated may also be suffering from other concurrent conditions, so if the intoxication does not diminish with falling serum drug levels, the patient must be assessed for other possible causes of their condition.
- If an intoxicated person cannot walk, stand or get up from a chair they must be closely monitored.
- Intoxicated patients should be treated with respect. Speak slowly and simply. Treat them in a low-stimulus environment where possible and provide clear information to reduce the risk of further harm such as falls.
- Patients should be continually assessed for withdrawal. Alcohol withdrawal can occur before a zero-blood alcohol reading is noted.
- Multiple and concurrent substance use is becoming increasingly prevalent. It is important to consider the effect of multiple agents and subsequent interactions.
- Any patient presenting with seizures should be assessed for alcohol withdrawal, benzodiazepine withdrawal or stimulant intoxication, as well as other possible causes. The seizures must be treated according to policy and the patient observed for at least 4 hours after the seizure using the Glasgow Coma Scale score (see Table 11.12).

Adapted with permission from NSW Department of Health 2018.

Box 11.4 Diagnostic criteria for withdrawal

The essential feature of withdrawal is the development of a range of substance-specific behavioural, psychological and cognitive changes to the cessation, or acute reduction in, heavy and long-term substance use. Specifically, the following four criteria must be met:

A – Cessation of (or reduction) in use that has been heavy and prolonged
B – Two (or more) of the following, developing within several hours to a few days after the cessation (or reduction) of the substance:
- autonomic hyperactivity (e.g. sweating or racing heart; pulse greater than 100 bpm)
- insomnia (trouble sleeping)
- increased hand tremors
- nausea or vomiting
- psychomotor agitation
- anxiety
- seizures (usually generalised tonic–clonic type – rhythmic jerking movement, especially of the limbs)
- transient visual, tactile or auditory hallucinations or illusions

C – The signs or symptoms in criterion B cause clinically significant distress or impairment in social, occupational or other important areas of functioning
D – These symptoms are not attributable to another medical condition and are not better explained by another mental disorder including intoxication or withdrawal from another substance.

for diagnostic criteria for withdrawal) (see Table 11.5 for a summary of key features of withdrawal). Withdrawal can lead to significant and potentially life-threatening complications and, as such, requires close monitoring (Manning et al. 2018).

The treatment of withdrawal can occur in a range of different settings and is often driven by client preference. In Australia, there are three different environments in which withdrawal may occur – residential withdrawal units ('detox'), inpatient medical detoxification in a hospital or non-residential home-based withdrawal as an outpatient.

Alcohol withdrawal

The severity of an alcohol-related withdrawal syndrome is on a continuum from mild to severe (Manning et al. 2018). Withdrawal will begin anywhere from 6 to 24 hours after the person's last drink and will peak between 36 and 72 hours. Symptoms will generally resolve after 5–7 days (see Fig. 11.1). The presence of other medical conditions and multiple substance use disorders will vary the time course and severity of a withdrawal syndrome (Manning et al. 2018).

Assessment scales can assist with tracking the severity of a withdrawal syndrome and responses to treatment. Rating scales available include the Alcohol Withdrawal Scale (AWS) and the Clinical Institute Withdrawal Assessment for Alcohol (Revised) (CIWA-Ar). Caution must be exercised when using withdrawal scales because not all withdrawal syndromes will present in the same way and relying on completing a form does not replace the importance of observation and critical assessment of the client's symptoms (Bostwick & Lapid 2004).

Medically managing and treating an alcohol withdrawal syndrome generally involves using benzodiazepines (Manning et al. 2018). Diazepam is most commonly used benzodiazepine due to its long half-life, active metabolites and anticonvulsant properties (St Vincent's Hospital

TABLE 11.5 Key features of alcohol and other drug withdrawal syndromes

DRUG	ONSET	DURATION	CLINICAL FEATURES
Alcohol	Within 24 hours and up to 48 hours (depending on blood alcohol concentration (BAC), hours after last drink and level of neuroadaptation)	3–7 days (up to 14 in severe withdrawal)	Anxiety, agitation, sweating, tremors, nausea, vomiting, abdominal cramps, diarrhoea, craving, insomnia, elevated blood pressure, heart rate and temperature, headache, seizures, confusion, perceptual distortions, disorientation, hallucinations, seizures, delirium tremens, arrhythmias and Wernicke's encephalopathy
Nicotine	4–12 hours after last use	Peaks days 2–7 and continues in attenuated form for 2–4 weeks	Irritability, anger, anxiety, sadness, restlessness, sleep disturbance, increased hunger, sore throat, headache and difficulty concentrating
Cannabis	1–2 days after last use	Acute phase: 2–6 days, subsiding after 2–3 weeks May persist for some months	Anger, aggression, irritability, anxiety, nervousness, decreased appetite or weight loss, restlessness, sleep disturbances, chills, depressed mood, shakiness and sweating
Benzodiazepines	1–10 days (depending on half-life of drug) after last use	3–6 weeks (or longer depending on the half-life of the drug)	Anxiety, headache, insomnia, muscle aching twitching and cramping, nausea, vomiting, diarrhoea, perceptual changes, feelings of unreality, depersonalisation, seizures, agitation and confusion/psychosis
Opioids	Withdrawal from heroin and morphine can begin within 24 hours, while methadone and buprenorphine typically start later (days 3–5)	Heroin withdrawal typically peaks quickly (day 3), with more severe symptoms, subsiding fully within a week Methadone and buprenorphine withdrawal result in a more protracted withdrawal, with a less abrupt peak and longer duration of symptoms	Runny eyes and nose, sneezing and sweating, agitation, irritability, loss of appetite, craving, abdominal cramps, diarrhoea, anxiety, irritability, disturbed sleep, fatigue, joint and muscle aches, nausea/vomiting and moodiness
Stimulants	Crash phase: within hours of last use Withdrawal: 1–4 days after last use	2–4 days Acute phase: 7–10 days Subacute phase: a further 2–4 weeks	Cravings, dysphoria, anhedonia, increased appetite, fatigue, agitation, anxiety, increased sleep, vivid, unpleasant dreams and slowing of movement
Ketamine	Within 24 hours of last use	4–6 days	Cravings, decreased appetite or weight loss, fatigue, chills, sweating, restlessness, tremors, disturbed sleep, anxiety, depression and irregular or rapid heartbeat
GHB	Within 12 hours of last use	Up to 15 days	Confusion, agitation, anxiety, depression, paranoia, hallucinations, disturbed sleep, cramps, tremors, sweating and rapid heartbeat

Adapted from Manning et al. 2018

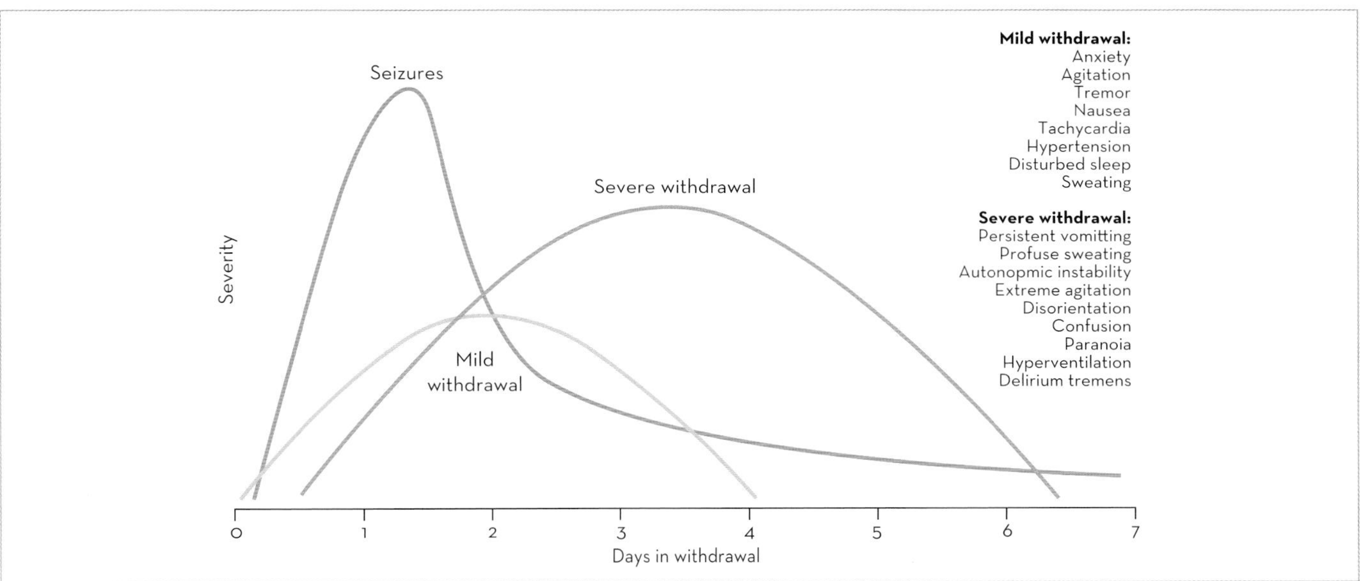

Figure 11.1
Alcohol withdrawal time course and symptoms
Adapted from NSW Department of Health 2008

Melbourne 2019). Shorter acting benzodiazepines such as oxazepam must be considered for those with compromised liver function or in the elderly (Manning et al. 2018) (see Table 11.6 for recommended medical and non-medical management options).

There are some factors that predict the likely severity of alcohol withdrawal syndrome. One is whether the client has a long history of regular heavy alcohol use – for example, drinking 4 L of wine every day for the past 20 years. Another is the use of other psychoactive drugs, particularly central nervous system depressants such as benzodiazepines. Further, if the person has a history of a complicated withdrawal syndrome – for example, delirium tremens or seizures – this places them at greater risk of withdrawal complications again in the future.

Benzodiazepine withdrawal

Benzodiazepine withdrawal will vary significantly depending on the duration of use and half-life of the benzodiazepine being used. Using short-acting benzodiazepines over an extended period can result in a complex withdrawal syndrome similar to that of alcohol, including similar risks of seizures and delirium (Manning et al. 2018). See Table 11.7 for a summary of expected withdrawal symptoms. Due to the variable nature of benzodiazepine withdrawal and potential complexities with concurrent other substance use, specialist consultation should be sought. Nurses should advocate for the continuation of regular benzodiazepines to avoid the onset of withdrawal until a planned taper can be developed in consultation with the client.

Opioid withdrawal

Opioid withdrawal varies significantly based on the substance being used, the route of administration, duration of use and the individual's general health (Manning et al. 2018). Longer acting opioid analgesics (e.g. methadone) are associated with a much slower onset of symptoms and an overall longer withdrawal syndrome when compared with short-acting opioids (e.g. heroin) (Manning et al. 2018). Specialist consultation should be sought for individuals with prescription opioid use disorders.

Withdrawal from heroin is not life threatening for those clients who have limited co-occurring disorders and who are provided with adequate hydration and electrolyte replacement (Manning et al. 2018). However, the risk of post-withdrawal relapse is very high in heroin users and withdrawal provides an opportunity to discuss opioid agonist treatment (e.g. methadone or buprenorphine). Heroin-related withdrawal will start 6–12 hours after the last use, peaks around 24–48 hours and subsides after 5–7 days (Manning et al. 2018). Withdrawal symptoms include runny eyes and nose, yawning, sweating, agitation, irritability, fevers, loss of appetite, muscle aches and joint pain, nausea/vomiting and cravings.

Encourage clients to consider opioid agonist treatment because this will rapidly diminish the symptoms of withdrawal and support longer term reductions in illegal or non-prescribed opioid use. Symptomatic treatment can be used but should be avoided where possible because multiple different agents are required to manage the withdrawal syndrome (e.g. metoclopramide for vomiting, loperamide

TABLE 11.6 Alcohol withdrawal treatment and management

Non-medical management	• Use an alcohol withdrawal scale (1–4-hourly reviews depending on the patient's needs and complexity). • Reduce external stimuli (e.g. visitors, light and noise from the television). • Use dim lighting at night-time to reduce the risk of misinterpreting the physical environment. • Provide regular reassurance and reorientation to the date, time and place. • Provide written orientation prompts (e.g. writing the current day and date on a board). • Provide ongoing explanations about symptoms and expected time course. • Consider risks (e.g. falls) when the patient is confused or delirious. • Provide regular observation given absconding risk (particularly if there is evidence of delirium).
Medication management	• Diazepam is the first-line treatment options for adults **without** concurrent severe liver dysfunction. • Shorter acting benzodiazepines such as oxazepam or lorazepam should be used in the elderly or those with severe liver dysfunction. • A maximum of 120 mg every 24 hours is generally sufficient to manage withdrawal. If doses exceed this, consult with specialist services. • Other underlying conditions should be considered when diazepam doses exceed 120 mg in 24 hours (e.g. delirium, hypoxia, Wernicke's encephalopathy, sepsis or paradoxical responses to medication). • Due to the long half-life and active metabolites of diazepam, prolonged dose tapering is not usually required (unless the patient is concurrently dependent on benzodiazepines). • Diazepam can generally be ceased within 72–96 hours. • Specialist services (e.g. addiction medicine) should be consulted when there is severe liver disease or other co-occurring substance use disorders. • People who are alcohol-dependent are likely to require higher than usual doses of diazepam to achieve clinically significant responses (e.g. 20 mg diazepam every 2–4 hours). • For excessive agitation, aggression or hallucinations, consider the use of low dose antipsychotics (e.g. olanzapine 2.5–5 mg 4/24 prn or haloperidol 1–2 mg PO/IMI 4/24).
Other medication	• Thiamine deficiency is a potentially serious complication of long-term, heavy alcohol use. • Thiamine should be administered parenterally for the first 3 days, 300 mg, three times per day. After 3 days the dose can be decreased to 100 mg, oral, daily. • High-dose thiamine is required (500 mg TDS), until resolution in symptoms, for those patients with a history of, or who are presenting with suspected, Wernicke's encephalopathy. • Thiamine 100–200 mg, twice per day, can be utilised when access intravenously is not possible. Clotting deficiencies must be excluded before beginning intramuscular thiamine. • Intravenous fluids if there is excessive sweating. • Electrolyte replacement (e.g. calcium, phosphate, magnesium and potassium). Consider the risk of a refeeding syndrome. • Hypomagnesaemia is common in those with alcohol use disorders. People with low magnesium appear to be at greater risk of a severe and complicated withdrawal syndrome. Thiamine absorption appears to be diminished in the presence of magnesium deficiency. • There is some evidence to support the use of beta-blockers to assist with reducing the severity of withdrawal symptoms. However, beta-blockers should be used with caution due to the suppression of symptoms that are monitored via alcohol withdrawal scales. • Current best practice does **not** support the use of alcohol in managing withdrawal for hospital inpatients.

Adapted from St Vincent's Hospital Melbourne 2019

for diarrhoea, hyoscine butylbromide for stomach and abdominal cramps, ibuprofen for muscle aches and pain, clonidine for excessive sweating, and benzodiazepines such as diazepam for anxiety and agitation) (Manning et al. 2018).

In contrast, a buprenorphine taper can be used and is the mainstay treatment for those not wanting to go onto opioid agonist treatment. Buprenorphine should not be administered for at least 12 hours after the last use of other shorter acting opioids due to the risk of precipitated withdrawal. Once withdrawal symptoms start to emerge a flexible approach should be adopted (see **Table 11.8** for an example dosing regimen). High doses of buprenorphine have not been found to more effectively manage symptoms of withdrawal and, as a result, clients generally do not require more than 6–8 mg per day (Manning et al. 2018).

Amphetamine withdrawal

Most people with amphetamine use disorders are able to undertake withdrawal in the community. The severity of the withdrawal syndrome is influenced by the amphetamine being used, the duration of use, the frequency of use, the method of administration and concurrent other substance use.

TABLE 11.7 Benzodiazepine withdrawal symptoms

STAGE OF WITHDRAWAL	PSYCHOLOGICAL SYMPTOMS	PHYSIOLOGICAL SYMPTOMS
Intoxication	Drowsiness, relaxation and sleepiness	Sedation and decreases in alertness and concentration
Acute withdrawal	Anxiety, panic attacks, depression, insomnia, poor memory/concentration, anger irritability and disordered perceptions	Agitation, tremor, headaches, weakness, dizziness, nausea, vomiting, diarrhoea, constipation, palpitations, fatigue and flu-like symptoms
Protracted withdrawal	Anxiety, depression, insomnia, irritability, muscle aches, restlessness, poor concentration and memory problems	Diarrhoea, constipation and bloating
Potential withdrawal complications	Transient hallucinations (visual, tactile, auditory), delirium and psychosis	Withdrawal seizures (1–2% of patients)

Source: Royal Australian College of General Practitioners 2015

TABLE 11.8 Buprenorphine dosing regimen

DAY	BUPRENORPHINE DOSE	RECOMMENDED TOTAL DAILY DOSE
Day 1	4 mg at onset of withdrawal 2–4 mg can be added at night as required	4 mg (max. 8 mg)
Day 2	4 mg in the morning 2–4 mg can be added at night as required	4 mg (max. 8 mg)
Day 3	4 mg in the morning 2 mg can be added at night as required	4 mg (max. 6 mg)
Day 4	2 mg in the morning 2 mg can be added at night as required	0 mg (max. 4 mg)
Day 5	2 mg as required	0 mg (max. 2 mg)

Source: Gowing et al. 2014

Amphetamine withdrawal generally starts 24 hours after the last use, will peak around 24–72 hours and slowly resolve over the following 7–10 days (Manning et al. 2018). Many amphetamine users experience protracted withdrawal symptoms such as poor sleep and mood instability, which can persist for up to 3 months after cessation. Amphetamine-related withdrawal can be broken into three distinct stages: the 'crash', acute withdrawal and protracted withdrawal. The crash phase is characterised by exhaustion, irritability, increased appetite, restlessness and anxiety. Acute withdrawal involves strong cravings, mood fluctuations, disturbed sleep, anhedonia, general aches and pains, headaches, muscle tension, poor concentration and disturbed thoughts, which may include paranoid ideations and hallucinations (Manning et al. 2018).

There are no standard guidelines for stimulant withdrawal and no clear replacement pharmacotherapies. The primary focus of treatment is on supportive management and symptom-triggered medication management. Benzodiazepines (e.g. diazepam) and antipsychotics (e.g. olanzapine) are often used to support acute withdrawal from amphetamines (Manning et al. 2018).

Historical anecdote 11.2: Cocaine and methamphetamine as medicine?

Cocaine has been used in South America since ancient times (processed from the leaves of the Erythroxylon cocoa plant). Sigmund Freud wrote about the mental health benefits of cocaine as an antidepressant, eventually developing an addiction to the drug. By the early 1900s it became hugely popular in America and was used as an active ingredient in many popular products including cocoa leaf cigarettes and the soft drink Coca-Cola. Methamphetamine was widely marketed by pharmaceutical companies as a powerful antidepressant. It was used by both the allied and German armies during World War II to improve soldiers' aggression and endurance. Adolph Hitler became addicted to methamphetamine and opium.

Read more about it: *Rasmussen N 2011 Medical science and the military: the Allies' use of amphetamine during World War II. Journal of Interdisciplinary History, 42(2): 205–33*

Cannabinoid withdrawal

Most clients withdrawing from cannabis do not require pharmacological treatment and can be managed at home. However, the severity of the withdrawal syndrome should be assessed carefully, with consideration of the individual's perception of how severe their withdrawal will be. Abrupt cessation of cannabis use after a period of regular, heavy use is associated with a clear withdrawal syndrome characterised by agitation, anxiety, irritability, flat mood, insomnia, vivid nightmares, poor appetite, tremors, sweating, fever and chills (Manning et al. 2018). Symptoms of withdrawal generally start 24 hours after the last use of cannabis, peak at 2–3 days and subside after 7 days (Manning et al. 2018).

Symptomatic treatment involves using long-acting benzodiazepines (e.g. diazepam), non-steroidal anti-inflammatories (e.g. paracetamol) and anti-emetics (e.g. metoclopramide) (Manning et al. 2018). Supportive therapies and relaxation techniques have been found to be very useful for some clients undergoing cannabinoid withdrawal.

Nicotine withdrawal

Nicotine withdrawal can impact on health care provision and should be carefully assessed. Using a rating scale such as the Fagerstrom nicotine dependence scale (see Table 11.9) can assist with treatment planning and the initiation of appropriate nicotine replacement therapy (NRT). Withdrawal will commence within 24 hours of a cessation, or reduction, in tobacco use. Symptoms include irritability, frustration, anxiety, poor concentration, restlessness, increase appetite, depressed mood, mood instability and insomnia (Manning et al. 2018). The mainstay treatment for nicotine withdrawal is NRT, for example, nicotine patches or lozenges (see Table 11.10). Many forms of NRT can be nurse initiated, however, this will vary depending on individual workplaces and settings.

TABLE 11.9 Fagerstrom test for nicotine dependence

QUESTION	ANSWER	SCORE
How soon after you wake up do you smoke your first cigarette?	Within 5 minutes	3
	6–30 minutes	2
	31–60 minutes	1
	After 60 minutes	0
Do you find it difficult to refrain from smoking in places where it is forbidden?	Yes	1
	No	0
Which cigarette would you hate to give up the most?	The first one in the morning	1
	All others	0
How many cigarettes per day you do you smoke?	10 or less	0
	11–20	1
	21–30	2
	31 or more	3
Do you smoke more frequently during the first hours after waking than during the rest of the day?	Yes	1
	No	0
Do you smoke if you are so ill that you are in bed most of the day?	Yes	1
	No	0
High dependence: 5 > Moderate dependence: 2–4 Low dependence: 1 Not dependent: 0		

Data from : Heatherton T, Kozlowski L, Frecker R, and Fagerström K. The Fagerström test for nicotine dependence: A revision of the Fagerström tolerance questionnaire. British Journal of Addiction, 1991; 86(9):1119–27

NURSE'S STORY 11.1

Maureen

The ultimate challenge and 'high' of working in drug and alcohol nursing is the experience of assisting a client and seeing them creating a happier life out of what is sometimes chaos. My part in providing the information and the skills that help that process of recovery gives me a sense of wellbeing and achievement about what I do.

I am only talking about small steps here. Every small step no matter how hesitant is cause for celebration and joy. You cannot do the client's work for them, but you can provide assistance to them on the journey they must make. That is where skill is needed. The skill is assessing where the client is on the motivational cycle and being able to provide assistance that helps them towards their recovery yet recognising that everyone has different recovery goals and that each person's needs are unique. So, the passion for me is in feeling that I am doing something to help people out of this mess. Even if it is only by offering my respect, recognition, skills and time.

The downside is that you cannot do it for them, and the struggle with addiction and dependence is a hard and lonely one. At those times when people give up on their goals, I remind myself that these problems were a long time developing and will be a long time in being resolved, and that a step back is just that, not the end of the game.

NURSE'S STORY 11.2

Inga

A question I get asked regularly, not only in the workplace but also at dinner parties, is: 'Why do you want to work with drug addicts?' To be honest I have never really been able to come up with a clear answer, but I will give it a go.

I have nursed in drug and alcohol for 15 years. I enjoy the job.

A skill learned early in my career was to engage clients honestly and openly with the expectation that this would be reciprocated. I find it a great privilege to be allowed into the complex layers of drug and alcohol dependency, allowing me the opportunity to offer solutions to health and social needs. There is great scope in working with clients holistically and not merely with their first presenting issue.

I have a very strong belief that as nurses we are not in a position to judge who is worthy of health care. Some of my colleagues treat drug-dependent clients with little respect and understanding. Part of my job is to challenge those beliefs, address fears, educate and assist clients in receiving non-discriminatory health care.

One rare gem that comes with drug and alcohol nursing is that of working with a team of people who know how to look after each other. Having a black sense of humour and being able to share a bottle of wine and many laughs keeps balance in your life and the ability to enjoy a fantastic career.

TABLE 11.10 Nicotine replacement therapy dosing guidelines

NRT PRODUCT	RECOMMENDED DOSE
Patch 24 hour: 21 mg, 14 mg, 7 mg 16 hour: 25 mg, 15 mg, 10 mg	Begin with full strength if smoking more than 10 cigarettes/day
Mouth spray 1 mg per spray	1–2 sprays every 30–60 mins, max 4 sprays/hour or 64 sprays per day
Lozenges 2 mg, 4 mg	2 mg and 4 mg: 9–15/day (4 mg if time to first cigarette < 30 mins)
Mini lozenges 1.5 mg, 4 mg	1.5 mg: 9–20/day 4 mg: 9–15/day (use 4 mg if time to first cigarette < 30 mins)
Gum 2 mg, 4 mg	2 mg: 8–20/day 4 mg 4–10/day (use 4 mg if time to first cigarette < 30 mins)
Inhalator 15 mg per cartridge	3–6 cartridges/day
NRT is contraindicated as a first-line treatment in those who have significant or active cardiovascular disease or sensitives to nicotine.	

Source: Mendelsohn et al. 2015

Physical health and substance use disorders

In Australia, the National Health and Medical Research Council (NHMRC) recommends an intake of no more than 20 g (two drinks) of alcohol on any day for men and women to reduce the lifetime risk of harm from alcohol-related disease or injury (NHMRC 2015). It also recommends that men and women should not drink more than four standard drinks on any occasion to reduce the risk of binge, or hazardous, drinking harm. The World Health Organization (2018b) estimates that alcohol use is associated with more than 200 different disease processes (see Table 11.11 for a summary of acute and chronic physical health consequences of substance use).

Assessment areas

Substance use disorders may occur in all settings of health care. Specific assessment tools and criteria are available to assist with obtaining accurate histories of substance use over time. It is important to carefully elicit alcohol and drug use to make a diagnosis so that an appropriate management strategy can be implemented. Many substance use problems are misdiagnosed or remain undetected, which can lead to significant negative outcomes.

Presentation and setting

The process of assessment depends on the nature of the presentation and the setting. Careful consideration for the environment must occur – this will assist with assessment processes and rapport development.

Substance use history

A client's substance use (prescribed and non-prescribed) must be measured to determine whether the level of use may cause harm or whether withdrawal is imminent. A recent substance use history will determine the type of substance used, the level of use, the frequency of use and whether a withdrawal state could occur, in order to ensure appropriate treatment planning occurs. This information is also important to identify triggers for initiating use,

TABLE 11.11 Physical health consequences of substance use

SUBSTANCE	ACUTE	CHRONIC
Alcohol	Dizziness Poor judgement Loss of coordination Memory loss Vomiting Headaches Accidental injury (e.g. road accidents, falls) Aggression/violence Alcohol poisoning/overdose (can lead to fatalities)	Decreased concentration Short-term and long-term memory impairments Increased risk of stroke Alcohol-related brain injury Alcohol-related dementia Alcohol-related psychosis Hypertension Tachycardia Cardiomyopathy Increased risk of acute myocardial infarction Liver cirrhosis Liver cancer Fatty liver Stomach ulcers Stomach and oesophageal cancer Oesophageal varices Gastro-oesophageal reflux disorder Gastritis Pancreatitis (acute and chronic) Reduction in testosterone, sperm counts and overall fertility in men Changes to menstruation in women Fetal alcohol spectrum disorder
Cannabis	Short-term effects are heavily influenced by the individual's prior experience and setting Short-term euphoria, poor concentration, psychomotor retardation, amotivation, anxiety Increased risk of car accidents Increased risk of relapse in psychotic illness Increased appetite, hyperemesis Reddening of eyes, decreased intraocular pressure Dry mouth	Impaired learning, impaired concentration, neurocognitive impairments, exacerbation of underlying psychosis, insomnia Poor appetite Cardiovascular disease Respiratory disease (associated with mechanism of administration)
Amphetamines	Pupil dilation, headache, bruxism Hyperventilation, dyspnoea, cough, chest pain, wheezing, exacerbation of asthma, pulmonary oedema Tachycardia, hypertension, palpitations, arrhythmia, acute myocardial infarction / cardiogenic shock Agitation, psychosis, tremor, hyperreflexia, muscle twitching, seizures, cerebral haemorrhage, cerebral oedema Nausea, vomiting, bowel infarction/perforation Diuresis, acute renal failure Mild fever, increased overall body temperature, malignant hyperthermia Increased sensory acuity, increased energy, increased motivation, increased concentration, decreased reaction time Increased risk of sexually transmitted infections (chem-sex) Amphetamine overdose Acute psychosis Rhabdomyolysis	Anxiety, confusion, insomnia, mood instability, aggression Chronic psychotic and mood disorders Impaired decision making, memory loss, poor concentration Weight loss, severe tooth decay, skin discolouration and sores Dilated cardiomyopathy Cardiovascular disease Chronic obstructive pulmonary disease and exacerbation of asthma (associated with mechanism of administration) Increased risk of blood-borne viruses (e.g. hepatitis C and HIV) in those who inject

TABLE 11.11 Physical health consequences of substance use—cont'd

SUBSTANCE	ACUTE	CHRONIC
Opioids	Euphoria, 'rush' Warm flushing, dry mouth, heaviness in extremities Nausea, vomiting, constipation Bradycardia, hypotension Opioid toxicity/overdose	Increased risk of mortality over time with doses exceeding 100 mg morphine equivalence Hypothalamic–pituitary–adrenal axis suppression Sleep apnoea Opioid induced hyperalgesia Constipation Immune suppression Prolongation of QT interval (particularly with long-term methadone treatment) Increased risk of blood borne viruses (e.g. hepatitis C and HIV) in those who inject
Hallucinogens	Tachycardia, hypertension Insomnia, tremor, poor coordination, psychomotor retardation Sparse or incoherent speech Respiratory depression Cardiac arrest Acute psychosis, anxiety, depression, violence, confusion, loss of control, lethargy, disorientation	Relatively unknown as there are very few long-term users of hallucinogens Anxiety, flashbacks and nightmares or 'bad trips'
Nicotine/ tobacco	Tachycardia Hypertension Dizziness Increased activity of the gastrointestinal tract Nausea Vomiting Reduction in appetite Alterations in taste Cough Asthma exacerbation Reduction in muscle tone Some relaxation effects	Stroke Cardiovascular disease Narrowing of blood vessels Persistent tachycardia Stroke Emboli Deep vein thrombosis Chronic obstructive pulmonary disease (emphysema and chronic bronchitis) Lung cancer Exacerbation of asthma Cancer (bladder, blood, cervix, colon and rectum, oesophagus, kidney and ureter, larynx, liver, oropharynx, pancreas, stomach, trachea and bronchus) Preterm delivery Stillbirth Low birth weight Sudden infant death syndrome Ectopic pregnancy Orofacial clefts in infants Miscarriage Reduction in male fertility Reduction in bone density Gum disease Increased risk of tooth loss Increased risk for cataracts Age-related macular degeneration Type 2 diabetes mellitus Rheumatoid arthritis Poor immune function

Sources: Cancer Council Victoria 2018, Centre for Disease Control and Prevention 2018, Government of South Australia 2019, Karila et al. 2014, Lawn et al. 2016, National Institute on Drug Abuse 2019, Substance Abuse and Mental Health Services Administration 2004, World Health Organisation 2018b

risk of relapse and to be able to implement an appropriate harm minimisation framework. A developmental and family history should be documented to identify the age at which the client first used a substance, how this use has developed over time, when the client thought the use became problematic, when there were periods of abstinence and when there were any changes to patterns of use (New South Wales Health 2013).

Taking a substance use history

When asking about substance use, approach the topic in an open way and speak of substance use as an accepted behaviour. Approach the assessment with a plan and consider the impact of any pre-existing judgements before entering the assessment. Ask questions about legal and more socially acceptable substances first (e.g. alcohol, tobacco and prescription medication) before asking about illicit drug use, which is often heavily stigmatised and stereotyped. This will be less confronting for the patient and help in developing rapport throughout the assessment.

In a substance use assessment, it is essential to cover the domains listed below. Individual health services may use standard substance use assessment forms that cover each of these elements. Systematic assessment of all patients should include a thorough examination of:

- indicators of risk (e.g. history of drink driving, loss of consciousness with multiple head strikes, overdose history)
- medical history (in particular, any history of medical problems associated with substance use such as pancreatitis secondary to chronic alcohol use, hepatitis C, HIV or infective endocarditis associated with injecting drug use)
- psychosocial issues (e.g. housing, social connections, domestic violence)
- physical signs and symptoms (e.g. ascites associated with alcohol use or extensive intravenous injection sites beyond the cubital fossa region)
- mental health status
- pathology results.

No single sign, symptom or pathology test is conclusive evidence of an alcohol or drug-related issue (New South Wales Health 2013).

Key elements of assessment

The following key elements should be clarified and explored as part of the assessment process:

- type of drug (if you are unfamiliar with the substance being used or the colloquial term being used, ask the patient to explain it further)
- types of beverage the client usually consumes (it is important with alcohol to distinguish what sort of alcohol is being consumed and what quantity it is being purchased such as drinking one 5 L cask of wine per day or a dozen 375 mL bottles of heavy beer).
- route of administration
- frequency of use
- dose (if you are unsure about the amount due to colloquial terms, ask the patient to explain the quantity they purchase their substance in and how long that lasts for, or ask them to explain their dosing system further)
- duration of use
- time and amount of the last dose (e.g. milligrams of methadone, grams of cannabis).

Note: It is important to ask the person if they are using more than one drug at a time and to record each substance separately. Poly-substance use can greatly increase the risk of complicated withdrawal and negative health consequences associated with use. It can be difficult for some people to discuss their substance use with someone they do not know; subsequently, developing rapport is a priority (see Box 11.5 for strategies to assist with the assessment process).

Observations

An assessment of a person's physical and mental state may reveal evidence of recent substance use such as the smell of alcohol or objective signs of withdrawal. A person who has misused substances for some time might have a decline in global functioning, which might be evidenced by a decline in health status and poor hygiene. An assessment should include the following:

- Assess their general appearance. Look for evidence of malnutrition (the person looking gaunt) and for signs of agitation, which might indicate stimulant use or withdrawal from a substance. People who regularly inject drugs will often wear long sleeves and long trousers, even in hot weather, in an attempt to cover up injection marks (see also Box 11.6).
- Look for signs of intoxication such as ataxia (lack of coordination of muscle movements), confused thinking, being argumentative or the smell of alcohol on the person's breath.
- Look for signs of withdrawal such as tremors and sweating, particularly of the hands and face. Consider objective signs of withdrawal rather than self-reported symptoms (e.g. bilateral tremor, diaphoresis and tachycardia versus the patient reporting that they feel sick).
- Look for stigmata such as abscesses at injection sites (see Box 11.6), inflammation of the nasal septum from snorting cocaine, bruising and scars unrelated to surgery, which might indicate accidents while under the influence of drugs and alcohol.
- Investigate pulse rate, blood pressure and evidence of head injury, which may indicate recent substance use (New South Wales Health 2013).

Box 11.5 Strategies to assist with obtaining an accurate substance use history

- Ensure the environment is as quiet and private as possible.
- If it is not possible to be completely private, speak quietly to encourage open discussion.
- When you are interviewing the client, note any inconsistencies in what you are being told.
- If the client becomes upset or distressed, leave the question and rephrase it later. Ensure the client is aware that they are driving the conversation and, if there are any topics they are not comfortable talking about, that these will not be discussed.
- A substance use history can also be elicited from the client's friends or family; however, this should be used with caution because may not always be an accurate reflection of current substance use patterns.
- How questions are posed is important. Clients may drink well in excess of recommended levels but not see their use as problematic. It is important to remain non-judgemental.
- Overestimate how much someone is using to encourage more accurate accounts of quantities. For example, ask: 'So, are you smoking around 25–30 cigarettes per day?' rather than asking the person to specify how much they are using on their own.
- Illegal substance use may elicit a range of emotions among healthcare providers. It is important to remember that substance use is a health issue, not a moral one. Although illicit substance use may be involved, the primary concern is the individual's health and not the legal aspects to their use.
- Phrase questions to evoke acceptance. For example, ask: 'What is your favourite drink?' or 'What do you like to drink?'.
- Phrase questions that assume the individual does drink or use substances. For example, 'So, how much cannabis would you smoke in a month?' or 'When was the last time you drank enough to be merry or even drunk?'.
- Use open-ended questions, summaries and validating statements to encourage discussion of topics: 'You were talking about how you used heroin in the past and have managed to stay clean for 2 years. That's brilliant. You must be proud of yourself for staying clean for so long. Talk me through what you did during that time.'

The Glasgow Coma Scale is a neurological scale that aims to give a reliable objective way of recording the conscious state of a person for initial as well as subsequent assessment and may be required for medical and trauma patients, particularly if they are intoxicated (see Table 11.12).

Box 11.6 Signs of intravenous drug use

- Puncture marks
- Cellulitis
- Phlebitis
- Skin abscesses
- Erosion or irritation around nostrils/septum
- Irritation around mouth or nose
- Tenderness or liver pain

Source: NSW Ministry of Health 2016

TABLE 11.12 Glasgow Coma Scale

Eye opening	Spontaneous	4
	To speech	3
	To pain	2
	None	1
Verbal response	Oriented	5
	Confused conversation	4
	Words (inappropriate)	3
	Sounds (incomprehensible)	2
	None	1
Best motor response	Obeys commands	6
	Localises pain	5
	Flexion withdrawal from pain	4
	Abnormal flexion to pain	3
	Extension to pain	2
	None	1
Total score	3/15–15/15	

Source: Rosenfeld 2012

Critical thinking challenge 11.1

1. When assessing a client for possible substance abuse, which of the following would alert the nurse to alcohol intoxication?
   A. pupillary constriction
   B. unsteady gait (ataxia)
   C. slurring of words
   D. a strong smell of alcohol on the person's breath
2. Which of the following would alert the nurse to possible opiate use?
   A. tremor and sweating
   B. wearing long sleeves and trousers on a very hot day
   C. inability to concentrate
   D. reddened eyes

Tests

MENTAL STATUS EXAMINATION

A mental status examination is essential (see Chapter 7), paying attention to:

- clouding of consciousness
- perceptual abnormalities, especially visual, auditory and tactile hallucinations (e.g. believing insects are crawling under the skin) – look for evidence of responding to perceptual disturbances (e.g. Do they look distracted? Are they picking at unseen stimulus? Are they muttering to themselves when no one is around?)
- thought abnormalities, especially paranoid ideation and changes to how the patient is expressing themselves (e.g. Are they making sense? Are they struggling to form their thoughts into a meaningful sentence?)
- suicidal ideation
- altered cognition.

LABORATORY TESTS

Laboratory tests may provide evidence of substance misuse. Physiological markers of consumption such as mean corpuscular volume and gamma glutamyl transferase are most widely used to verify a diagnosis of substance use; however, these should not be relied upon because progressed liver failure may significantly impact on enzyme production. Other reasons for alterations in these markers should always be considered. Consider blood alcohol levels and urine drug screens (with gas chromatography / mass spectrometry) for patients who are unable to provide a history.

Note: There is always a risk of false positives and false negatives with urine drug screening, so presumptive screening tests should always be interpreted with caution!

SCREENING TESTS

Screening tests may also be used and are not associated with urine drug screening. These instruments usually take the form of self-reported questionnaires and are used for diagnostic purposes. One of the most widely used screening instruments is the Alcohol Use Disorders Identification Test (AUDIT), which is designed to screen for a range of drinking problems, particularly harmful and hazardous use. It is especially suitable for primary healthcare settings and has reliability across cultural groups and a range of specific populations. The AUDIT is a self-report measure comprising 10 items, which are scored by totalling the items (see Box 11.7). The AUDIT is in the public domain and can be used without cost. There is an altered version of AUDIT called the Drug Use Disorders Identification Test (DUDIT), which is used to screen for a range of other substance use problems.

Another widely used screening tool is the ASSIST (Alcohol, Smoking and Substance Involvement Screening Test), a questionnaire developed by the World Health Organization. It screens for all levels of problem or risky substance use in adults (WHO 2015).

Interventions

Early and brief interventions

Studies have shown that early and brief interventions (talking to people at an early stage in their substance use) are an effective way to prevent later possible complications of substance use (Bien et al. 1993; Marsh et al. 2013; Moyer & Finney 2015; Vasilaki et al. 2006; Wild et al. 2007). Brief interventions for substance use involve sessions of 5–15 minutes and often include providing self-help materials such as pamphlets or substance use diaries. This may extend to a brief assessment and providing advice (in a one-off session), as well as assessing the client's readiness to change (motivational interview), harm reduction and follow-up.

The components of brief interventions include:

- assessment
- providing feedback to the client on risk or impairments due to drug use
- listening to the client's concerns and advising the client about the consequences of continued drug use
- defining treatment goals such as reducing or ceasing drug use
- discussing and implementing strategies for treatment (e.g. identifying triggers for drug use and strategies to overcome them and offering a follow-up session) (Marsh et al. 2013).

Brief interventions are recommended for clients experiencing relatively few problems related to their substance use and who have low levels of dependence. They are also recommended for clients with a dependence on nicotine, a low-to-moderate dependence on alcohol or a low-to-moderate dependence on cannabis. Brief interventions are not recommended for clients with severe dependence. If a brief intervention consists of only one session, it should include giving advice on how to reduce drug use or drinking to a safer level, providing harm-reduction information and discussing harm-reduction strategies (Bien et al. 1993; Marsh et al. 2013; Moyer & Finney 2015; Vasilaki et al. 2006; Wild et al. 2007).

Motivational interviewing

Motivational interviewing using the Transtheoretical Model of Change is an intervention developed by Prochaska, DiClemente and Miller to work with clients to assess and then enhance the motivation to change their level of substance use (Lundahl et al. 2013; Miller & Rollnick 2009; Prochaska & DiClemente 1984). Motivational interviewing is one of the most widely used interventions and has been adopted for a range of challenging behaviours beyond just substance use disorders. Nurse's story 11.3 provides a practical example of motivational interviewing in action

Box 11.7 Alcohol Use Disorders Identification Test (AUDIT) screening instrument

Please circle the answer that is correct for you.

1. How often do you have a drink containing alcohol?
   Never
   Monthly or less
   2–4 times a month
   2–3 times a week
   4 or more times a week
2. How many drinks containing alcohol do you have on a typical day when you are drinking?
   1 or 2
   3 or 4
   5 or 6
   7 to 9
   10 or more
3. How often do you have six or more drinks on one occasion?
   Never
   Less than monthly
   Monthly
   Weekly
   Daily or almost daily
4. How often have you found that you were not able to stop drinking once you had started?
   Never
   Less than monthly
   Monthly
   Weekly
   Daily or almost daily
5. How often during the last year have you failed to do what was normally expected of you because of drinking?
   Never
   Less than monthly
   Monthly
   Weekly
   Daily or almost daily
6. How often during the last year have you needed a first drink in the morning to get yourself going after a heavy drinking session?
   Never
   Less than monthly
   Monthly
   Weekly
   Daily or almost daily
7. How often during the last year have you had a feeling of guilt or remorse after drinking?
   Never
   Less than monthly
   Monthly
   Weekly
   Daily or almost daily
8. How often during the last year have you been unable to remember what happened the night before because you had been drinking?
   Never
   Less than monthly
   Monthly
   Weekly
   Daily or almost daily
9. Have you or someone else been injured as a result of your drinking?
   No
   Yes, but not in the last year
   Yes, during the last year
10. Has a relative or friend or a doctor or other health worker been concerned about your drinking or suggested you cut down?
    No
    Yes, but not in the last year
    Yes, during the last year

Source: World Health Organization 2001

(see Box 11.8 for more details about the stages of changes). Motivational interviewing also provides a framework for effectively interviewing clients abbreviated to 'OARS':

O – Open-ended questions
A – Affirmation. This involves acknowledging hard work and any difficulties the client may be having.
R – Reflective listening. Active listening is central to motivational interviewing and can demonstrate empathy, compassion and understanding.
S – Summary. Providing summary statements assists with demonstrating understanding and clarifying any areas of confusion. It will assist with ensuring that the client is aware that you are engaged and actively listening.

Cognitive behaviour therapy

CBT involves identifying self-destructive thoughts ('Everything has to be perfect', 'I always do the wrong thing') and replacing them with more realistic thoughts ('Not everything has to be perfect. Not always', 'I don't always do the wrong thing. Sometimes I do good things'). By replacing self-destructive thoughts with more realistic thoughts (cognitions), emotions and behaviour should change for the better as a result.

CBT may be effective for substance use and other co-occurring conditions including post-traumatic stress disorder and depression (McGovern et al. 2015; Riper et al. 2014). Motivational interviewing and CBT are important counselling approaches in the drug and alcohol field.

Detoxification

Detoxification is one of the first stages of treatment for people with substance use disorders. People enter into supervised treatment, either medical or non-medical, to

Box 11.8 The Transtheoretical Model of Change within motivational interviewing

PRE-CONTEMPLATION

The client has no intention of changing. They are in 'denial' about the need for change. The therapist works to increase the client's awareness of the problem while consistently remaining non-judgemental and respectful. The therapist provides information and consciousness raising at the same time. It is vitally important that the therapist does not disengage at this stage. The therapist needs to continue to try to connect with the client and raise awareness of the dangers of their alcohol and substance use even if the client does not initially show interest. Rapport is essential during this phase.

CONTEMPLATION

The client is aware of their problem but remains ambivalent about change. The therapist acknowledges the client's ambivalence while working to tip the decisional balance by weighing the pros and cons of change versus the risks and benefits of continuing substance use. Responsibility for change remains with the client.

PREPARATION

The client intends to change but might be confused about the best way to do so. The therapist inspires realistic hope, offers a menu of choices to help determine the best course of action and demystifies the change process. Both work to create a plan for change.

ACTION

Actual behaviour change commences. The client implements a collaborative, realistic plan. Both the therapist and the client monitor the client's progress, highlighting and valuing even small successes, and progressively problem solving.

MAINTENANCE

Behaviour change has been achieved and the client has developed a new lifestyle. The therapist and the client are vigilant to avoid relapse. They have realistic hopes and avoid exaggerated expectations.

Clients may slip back to a previous stage (e.g. from preparation to pre-contemplation) and work their way up again. This is an expected part of the process and relapses should be anticipated. The principle is to ascertain which stage of 'readiness to change' the client is at and then to provide information and support to move them on to the next stage. If the client understands what is occurring, they are more likely to change, and it is imperative that the therapist rolls with any resistance presented by the client along their pathway.

Source: Department of Health 2004

reduce the severity of the withdrawal syndrome and to manage any potential significant complications. It can take place in an inpatient unit or in the person's own home. The client may require medication, depending on the severity of the withdrawal and the client's wishes. Symptoms of withdrawal range in severity from mildly uncomfortable to life threatening; however, careful assessment and management can alleviate many of the symptoms. Nursing management of withdrawal focuses on five main areas:

- minimising progression to severe withdrawal
- decreasing risk of injury to self/others
- eliminating risk of dehydration, electrolyte and nutritional imbalance
- reducing risk of seizures
- identifying the presence of concurrent illness that masks/mimics withdrawal (New South Wales Health 2013).

Relapse prevention

There is a distinct difference between a lapse and a relapse. A lapse is a 'slip' in which the person uses a substance again, possibly a couple of times, then returns to their previous reduced level of use or abstinence. At this stage the person may decide to keep using or learn from their lapse and stop using. A relapse occurs when a person resumes substance use and is not able to maintain abstinence or their reduced level of use (Marsh et al. 2013). A lapse does not always result in a relapse, and clients should be encouraged to consider this during any relapse prevention work.

All clients should have a plan so that if they do lapse, they have support and strategies available to avoid the more dangerous relapse. A lapse should be viewed as a learning experience for both the client and the therapist. For example: What were the triggers that led to the lapse? How did the client manage to contain their substance use to a lapse and not relapse into old behaviours? Within a CBT or motivational interviewing framework the therapist explores the client's underlying thoughts and feelings that resulted in the lapse. The therapist's role is to assist the client to work through the thoughts that contributed to the lapse and replace them with less damaging thought processes for the future (Marsh et al. 2013).

Other healing approaches

It is always best to offer a wide spectrum of treatment approaches. Residential treatment services may be effective for some people. For others, pharmacotherapy such as acamprosate (Campral) and naltrexone decreases cravings to drink alcohol. For yet other clients, a 12-step program can be very effective; these are peer support programs such as Alcoholics Anonymous (AA) and Narcotics Anonymous (NA) (Alcoholics Anonymous 2001). These groups are based on an abstinence philosophy (Humphreys et al. 2014; Kelly et al. 2013).

Community drug and alcohol services provide a range of interventions including individual and group counselling, pharmacotherapies (e.g. methadone and buprenorphine maintenance for opiate-dependent clients), CBT and motivational interviewing.

Harm minimisation and harm reduction

Harm reduction is part of a three-pronged international approach to problematic substance use that allows agencies to provide an integrated and collaborative approach to care (National Drug Strategy 2015):

- supply-reduction strategies to disrupt the production and supply of illicit drugs and the control and regulation of licit substances
- demand-reduction strategies to prevent the uptake of harmful drug use, including abstinence-oriented strategies and treatments to reduce drug use
- harm-reduction strategies to reduce drug-related harm to individuals and communities. Harm-reduction strategies are those that reduce drug-related harm but do not necessarily address drug consumption.

Harm minimisation has been particularly successful in its contribution to containing the spread of HIV/AIDS (National Drug Strategy 2015) and encourages the acceptance that not all individuals are ready for abstinence. The successful use of harm minimisation strategies is one of the most powerful interventions for demonstrating acceptance and a non-judgemental approach. Ultimately, harm minimisation strategies aim to reduce the risk of medical and psychological problems associated with substance use for both the individual and the extended community. Harm minimisation strategies may include the following:

- needle and syringe programs. Primary needle and syringe programs extended beyond just providing sterile injecting equipment but also provide primary health care and a range of social support programs. Australia and New Zealand have well established needle and syringe programs, which has led to a significant reduction in spread of blood-borne viruses when compared with other Western countries.
- suggestions for alternative routes of drug administration, such as inhaling or oral use rather than intravenous use.
- alternative injecting sites – this is particularly useful for long-term injecting drug users who may have significantly damaged or impaired veins; it also assists users with understanding high-risk injecting high (e.g. the groin or neck) and how to avoid these areas
- take-home naloxone and associated training – naloxone is a rapid-acting opioid antagonist that has been used for a long time in emergency settings to reverse opioid overdoses (injecting drug users are now trained in administering naloxone, which can be lifesaving while awaiting emergency services)
- training in safe injecting practices such as using sterile equipment, filters, tourniquets and how to access emergency healthcare services
- medically supervised injecting facilities
- providing methadone and buprenorphine (opioid agonist treatment; see below)
- programs that inform alcohol drinkers of the dangers of driving while intoxicated, the advantages of having a designated driver and night-time transport schemes from hotels and nightclubs
- pill testing to assess purity of various illicit substances, particularly at festivals.

Another major harm-reduction strategy is opioid agonist treatment (previously known as opioid replacement therapy). The long-acting opioids methadone (24-hour dosing) and buprenorphine (24-, 48- or 72-hour dosing) are administered as substitution treatment for heroin or other opioid addiction and are considered 'essential medicines' for this purpose (WHO 2013). As substitution opioids have the potential to be diverted and intravenously injected, deterrent strategies have been introduced. Naloxone was added to buprenorphine, which created Suboxone (subutex + naloxone). Suboxone was marketed with the information that if the combination drug was injected, it would produce little euphoria but withdrawal symptoms in those already dependent, and this would deter diversion (Larance et al. 2014; Yokell et al. 2011). In 2011 in Australia, a sublingual film version of buprenorphine with naloxone was introduced to make dosing of buprenorphine easier to supervise and so reduce the risk of further diversion. It is important to note that despite these efforts, methadone, buprenorphine and suboxone are all able to be diverted. There are a range of non-for-profit harm-reduction organisations that can provide useful training and education for nursing staff – for example, Harm Reduction Victoria.

Co-occurring substance use disorders

Several terms are used to describe someone who has more than one disorder concurrently; mental health, alcohol and drug nurses tend to use the terms 'comorbid disorders', 'comorbidity', 'coexisting disorder' and 'dual diagnosis' interchangeably (Drake & Wallach 2000; Mills et al. 2008). However, more recently co-occurring substance use disorder has become the more accepted way of describing these presentations. Clients with a mental health problem are often drawn to alcohol and drugs with serious and sometimes fatal consequences (e.g. depression and alcohol, psychosis and methamphetamines, bipolar disorder and methamphetamines). There are many theories outlining this relationship, and no one model will definitively predict the relationship between mental health changes and substance use, but it can assist with treatment planning:

1. Direct causal relationship theory (one disorder produces the other disorder) – for example, a chronic crystal methamphetamine user might start to develop psychosis and the psychosis becomes the predominant problem. Alternatively, a mental illness may cause the drug use. Someone with depression may drink alcohol to relieve their symptoms of depression. The alcohol use then becomes the most debilitating problem.
2. Indirect causal relationship theory – for example, depression during childhood might lead to poor school results. This in turn might lead to a less satisfying career, frustration with one's life and subsequent drinking of alcohol to treat the depression. Depression causes the drinking but in an indirect way and as a result of multiple social influences.
3. Common causal factors – for example, traumatic experiences or a family history of mental illness and drug abuse produce both mental health and drug and alcohol problems, but one disorder does not directly initiate the other. Both disorders occur simultaneously as a result of the early trauma.

The client is one person, not two or more separate disorders. Nurses need to consider the impact of the substance use on each patient's overall treatment and as such be aware of treatment options. Unfortunately, there continues to be a 'silo' approach to treatment that can often create difficulties for people when attempting to access services (Allsop 2008; Baker & Vellman 2007).

Tobacco smoking is an important when considering co-occurring disorders. Features of schizophrenia include a lack of energy and a lack of interest in activities that would normally bring the individual pleasure (anhedonia). Sedation is also one of the side effects of antipsychotic medication used to treat psychosis. Stimulants provide energy (at least in the short term) and individuals with psychotic disorders may be drawn to the short-term energy enhancing effects of smoking.

Further, people with psychotic disorders have been found to have a greater number of nicotinic receptors with an increased affinity for nicotine. This has led to people with psychotic disorders smoking more heavily and over a longer period than the general population. The relationship between mental health changes and tobacco smoking needs to be considered carefully. Nicotine is well known to interact with and affect the metabolism of a range of medications, in particular neuroleptic medications such as clozapine, olanzapine and some benzodiazepines (Manning et al. 2018). Subsequently, serum levels of these medications can change with abrupt cessation of cigarette smoking.

Clinical significance of a co-occurring diagnosis

There is evidence to suggest that clients with co-occurring disorders have poorer outcomes than those with either a single mental health problem or a single substance use disorder. These patients can be more difficult to manage due to their complex health and social needs and have higher rates of non-adherence with treatment (Hughes et al. 2017; Wise et al. 2017). Clients with a comorbid diagnosis are more likely to have a chronic disability and consequently require more service utilisation (Hughes et al. 2017). These clients have fewer treatment options and increased risks of experiencing difficulties with relationships, poor employment prospects, social isolation, poor health and chronic financial difficulties (Roussy et al. 2017). These clients often have a number of surrounding issues that combine and add to the complexity of their treatment goals and outcomes – for example, children placed in care due to parental substance abuse, legal problems, housing difficulties and psychological problems (Marsh et al. 2013).

Managing clients with a co-occurring disorder

People with co-occurring substance use disorders and mental health changes can be difficult to treat. Nurses need to develop the ability to distinguish between a psychotic disorder that is part of a mental illness and one that is substance use related (see Box 11.9).

Patients with co-occurring disorders often evoke powerful and unpleasant feelings in health professionals that is commonly associated with the frequent attendances at hospital. There is often a lack of a clear pathway for clients attempting to access services. In addition, clients may feel stigmatised by a focus on abstinence within mental health settings that is in direct contrast to the harm-minimisation model supported by the drug and alcohol sector (Roussy et al. 2017).

The client group generally struggles to maintain simultaneous wellness with regard to both their mental health and substance use. Developing a collaborative therapeutic alliance is essential, and the nurse needs to adopt an empathetic and non-judgemental approach towards this patient population. Ideally, a client's mental state should be relatively stable before attempting detoxification or modifying use, although this is not always possible, and healthcare providers need to be flexible in their responses. Brief interventions can be used in both outpatient and inpatient settings. For management principles for clients with psychotic disorders and substance abuse, see Box 11.10.

As with all aspects of nursing care, safety is the main concern. If a client has been admitted to a mental health facility in a psychotic state it is essential that any acute risks are managed as a priority. If the client is at risk of withdrawal from one or more substances, withdrawal strategies as outlined earlier in this chapter need to be implemented immediately. Careful consideration should be taken regarding the expected severity of the withdrawal syndrome because it may not be appropriate for the

Box 11.9 Guidelines for differentiating between a primary psychotic disorder and a substance-induced disorder

- Substance-induced psychotic symptoms can result from intoxication, chronic use or withdrawal.
- Prolonged heavy use of psychostimulants (e.g. amphetamines) can produce a psychotic picture similar to schizophrenia.
- Hallucinogen-induced psychosis is usually transient but may persist if use is sustained.
- Heavy alcohol use has been associated with alcohol-related hallucinations.
- Psychotic symptoms can also occur during withdrawal (e.g. delirium tremens) and delirious states.
- A non-substance-induced psychotic disorder should be considered when:
  - psychosis preceded the onset of substance use
  - psychosis persists for longer than one month after acute withdrawal or severe intoxication
  - psychotic symptoms are not consistent with the substance used
  - there is a history of psychotic symptoms during periods of abstinence greater than one month
  - there is a personal or family history of a non-substance-induced psychotic disorder.

Source: Lubman & Sundram 2003 © Copyright The Medical Journal of Australia. *Reproduced with permission.*

Box 11.10 Management principles for clients with psychotic disorders and substance abuse

ASSESSMENT

- Screen clients with psychosis for substance misuse.
- Determine the severity of use and associated risk-taking behaviours (e.g. injecting practices, unsafe sex).
- Exclude organic illness or physical complications of substance misuse.
- Seek collateral history – family or close supports should be involved where possible.

TREATMENT

- First engage the client using a non-judgemental attitude.
- Educate the client.
- Give general advice about the harmful effects of substance misuse.
- Advise about safe and responsible levels of substance use.
- Support the individual to develop links between substance misuse and mental health changes (e.g. methamphetamine use and worsening paranoia).
- Educate the person about safer practices (e.g. safe sexual practices).
- Help the client to establish the advantages and disadvantages of current use and support consideration of change.
- With medical staff, evaluate the need for concurrent pharmacotherapy (e.g. methadone, acamprosate, nicotine replacement therapy).
- Refer the client to appropriate community services.
- Devise relapse-prevention strategies that address both psychosis and substance misuse.
- Identify triggers for relapse (e.g. meeting other drug users, family conflict) and explore alternative coping strategies.

Source: Lubman & Sundram 2003 © Copyright The Medical Journal of Australia. *Reproduced with permission.*

withdrawal process to occur within a mental health facility and the client may require more intensive support from medical teams. When the client is more settled, the nurse can begin to explore reasons for the client's substance use, including the relationship of the substance to the client's psychiatric symptoms, treatment for the client's mental illness and feelings of social isolation related to their negative symptoms.

The client's readiness to change for both their mental health and substance use disorder should be explored. If the client is not considering changing their substance use it is imperative that education is provided regarding harm minimisation strategies. Remember: clients may be at different stages of change regarding their problematic substance use and their mental illness, and interventions need to reflect this.

It is important to set small and achievable goals with this client population. Larger goals should be broken down into a series of steps that are manageable rather than focusing on larger and longer term goals (e.g. rather than obtaining employment focus on establishing a daily routine first). People frequently become isolated from family and friends during the course of their drug use. In feeling socially isolated they frequently become vulnerable to relapse if they lack the skills to form new and healthier friendship groups. The re-establishment of new social groups that are not associated with substance use is essential in relearning how to live without daily use.

NURSE'S STORY 11.3

Sue

I have found, from 25 years' experience working in a mental health unit, that almost every person admitted to a mental health unit has a co-occurring diagnosis or at least a problem with alcohol and/or drugs. My advice is: 'Don't be concerned – expect it as the norm.' Stop expecting to deal only with your 'bit' of the person. You need to be able to deal with the whole person. The mental health nurse has a responsibility to find out more about substance abuse, even if it is only how to recognise symptoms and how and when to refer to other services.

CASE STUDY 11.1

Helen

Helen has been a client of community health services for approximately 6 months receiving care for a leg ulcer, which is exacerbated by type 2 diabetes. She is 63 years old and lives by herself. Her husband died approximately 12 months ago. She has one married daughter and three grandchildren, who live overseas. On previous visits Helen was well groomed, her house was clean and she seemed pleased to see the community nurse, offering her cups of tea and cakes that she had cooked. Recently, though, Helen seemed to have lost interest in caring for herself. On the last visit she appeared unkempt; her clothes were wrinkled and had food stains on them. Her hygiene was poor, and the smell of urine and body odour was quite strong. The community nurse noticed two empty flagons of sherry on the table and a half-full sherry bottle. Helen was irritable and her words were slurred. She said that she felt lonely and bored without her daughter and husband, and that 'the sherry helps me to forget'. Helen denied any previous problems with alcohol or other substances, but she did say that sherry had helped her to cope with the death of her husband, and that the doctor had then given her some pills and gradually they had made her feel better. Helen thinks that she 'mostly remembers' to take her diabetes medication, but she does not know what all the fuss is about because there is 'nothing wrong' with her.

Critical thinking challenge 11.2

With reference to the case study about Helen (Case study 11.1), assume that you are working in a community mental health centre and have arranged to visit Helen. The community nurse has given you Helen's history in her referral letter.

1. How will you prioritise this situation?
2. What types of assessment will you initiate?
3. What questions might you ask?
4. Who will you discuss Helen's situation with?
5. What follow-up plan might you implement?

Chapter summary

Alcohol and other drug use is commonplace in Australia and New Zealand. Many people do not experience problems with their use, but some do and at harmful levels. People who have a co-occurring substance use disorders and mental health changes are at greatest risk. There is evidence that these people experience more social problems and have less positive treatment outcomes.

As a nurse it is important to assess every client for alcohol or other drug use and to offer timely and effective treatment. Careful assessment is the key to offering targeted treatment to those presenting with substance use disorders. It is imperative that appropriate withdrawal management is implemented early in a client's treatment program to reduce the risk of adverse events.

Treatment might take the form of brief interventions that can be offered in the alcohol and other drug or mental health setting. Alternatively, drug and alcohol and mental health services might need to find ways of working together to offer appropriate services to these clients.

Rates of tobacco use are high among clients with co-occurring disorders, and interventions should be made available to assist clients in reducing or ceasing their tobacco use as this can dramatically impact on treatment outcomes. Alcohol is still the most used substance and nurses need to undertake an accurate history and to follow area health service protocols to minimise the risk of withdrawal and associated complications.

Despite the high prevalence of co-occurring disorders, there is little evidence about the nature of best practice for this client group. However, early recommendations from the research literature suggest that a program that treats both disorders concurrently, with preference given to an integrated model of treatment, is most beneficial. Clients should be matched with treatments that work for them; there should be an emphasis on the relationship between the healthcare provider and the client. Clients are not separate diagnoses; they are a single person.

EXERCISES FOR CLASS ENGAGEMENT

1. Discuss the following questions with your group.
   A. What would you do if you were working on a ward or in a community setting where there were negative attitudes and feelings towards clients with alcohol and drug disorders? Would you challenge your colleagues or

refrain from commenting? What would you do if their attitudes impacted on client care? When would you challenge and what could you do?

B. How would you feel if you observed another nurse drinking vodka during a lunch break when you were both working together on a ward? What would you do?

C. The senior nurse on the ward invites you out for lunch at a nearby hotel. The senior has two strong alcoholic drinks in succession and the two of you return to the ward. You are due to be assessed by your senior later that week. Do you report your senior?

D. Are you aware of your own negative attitudes and feelings that might impede your interactions and therapeutic response to a client with a substance-related disorder? If you have such attitudes, how would you overcome them to establish a therapeutic relationship with the client?

E. What role does the Australian Health Professional Registration Authority (Ahpra) or the Nursing Council of New Zealand have in responding to a complaint about a nurse using substances when on duty?

2. A 36-year-old man is admitted with the following symptoms: T 38.1, P 106, R 28, BP 189/93, profuse perspiration and tremulousness. He appears highly agitated. A mental status examination reveals confusion, disorientation and visual and tactile hallucinations. His partner advises that he had been a heavy drinker, but he stopped 2 days ago. What substance-induced disorder is the client experiencing?
   A. substance-induced psychosis
   B. alcohol withdrawal syndrome
   C. delirium tremens
   D. substance-induced anxiety disorder
3. When the nurse does an initial admission interview on a client being admitted for detoxification, which of the following areas is it critical to assess?
   A. type(s) of drug used
   B. family history
   C. reason for admission
   D. physical history

Useful websites

Alcohol Advisory Council of New Zealand (AACNZ): http://www.alcohol.org.nz

AUDIT – the Alcohol Use Disorders Identification Test: http://www.who.int/substance_abuse/publications/alcohol/en

Australian alcohol guidelines: http://www.nhmrc.gov.au/health-topics/alcohol-guidelines

Australian Government National Drugs Campaign: http://www.drugs.health.gov.au

Cochrane Library, evidence-based healthcare decision making: http://www.cochranelibrary.com

Glasgow Structured Approach to Assessment of the Glasgow Coma Scale: http://www.glasgowcomascale.org

Harm Reduction Australia: http://www.harmreductionaustralia.org.au

Harm Reduction Victoria: http://www.hrvic.org.au

ICD-11: https://www.who.int/classifications/icd/en/

Matua Raki, National Addiction Workforce Development: http://www.matuaraki.org.nz

Mental Health Coordinating Council: http://www.mhcc.org.au

National Centre for Education and Training on Addictions: http://nceta.flinders.edu.au

National Drug and Alcohol Research Centre: https://ndarc.med.unsw.edu.au

National Drug Research Institute: http://ndri.curtin.edu.au

National Institute on Drug Abuse, the science of drug abuse and addiction: http://www.drugabuse.gov

New South Wales Health – Clinical guidelines for nursing and midwifery practice in NSW: https://www.health.nsw.gov.au/aod/professionals/Pages/clinical-guidelines-nursing-and-midwifery.aspx

Queensland Alcohol and Drug Research and Education Centre: https://public-health.uq.edu.au/queensland-alcohol-and-drug-research-and-education-centre

Substance Abuse and Mental Health Services Administration (SAMSHA): http://www.samhsa.gov

Te Pou o Te Whakaaro Nui, national centre of evidence-based workforce development for the mental health, addiction and disability sectors in New Zealand: http://www.tepou.co.nz

Thorne Harbour health: https://thorneharbour.org

Turning Point Alcohol and Drug Centre: http://www.turningpoint.org.au

United Nations Office on Drugs and Crime: http://www.unodc.org

Victorian Responsible Gambling Foundation: http://www.responsiblegambling.vic.gov.au

References

Akram, H., Mokrysz, C., Curran, H.V., 2019. What are the psychological effects of using synthetic cannabis? A systematic review. J. Psychopharmacol. 33 (3), 271–283.

Alcoholics Anonymous (AA) Australia, 2001. Alcoholics Anonymous world service. Available: www.alcoholicsanonymous.org.au/fact_me_membership.num.

Alfred, S., 2015. Methamphetamine management in the acute care setting. In: NCETA/SANDAS South Australian Methamphetamine Forum. Flinders University, Adelaide.

Allsop, S., 2008. Drug Use and Mental Health: Effective Responses to Co-Occurring Drug and Mental Health Problems. IP Publishing, Melbourne.

American College of Obstetricians and Gynaecologists (ACOG), 2017. Opioid use and opioid use disorder in pregnancy. ACOG 711, 1–14.

American Psychiatric Association, 2013. Diagnostic and Statistical Manual of Mental Disorders, fifth ed.

(DSM-5). American Psychiatric Association, Washington.

Australian Institute of Health and Welfare (AIHW), 2018a. Alcohol, tobacco & other drugs in Australia. Available: www.aihw.gov.au/reports/alcohol/alcohol-tobacco-other-drugs-australia/contents/.

Australian Institute of Health and Welfare (AIHW), 2018b. Australian mothers and babies 2016: in brief. Available: https://www.aihw.gov.au/reports/mothers-babies/australias-mothers-babies-2016-in-brief/contents/summary.

Australian Institute of Health and Welfare (AIHW), 2017a. Aboriginal and Torres Strait Islander health performance. Available: https://www.aihw.gov.au/reports/indigenous-health-welfare/health-performance-framework/contents/tier-2-determinants-of-health/2-16-risky-alcohol-consumption.

Australian Institute of Health and Welfare (AIHW), 2017b. National drug household survey 2016: detailed findings. Drug statistics series no. 31. Canberra, Australia.

Australian Institute of Health and Welfare (AIHW), 2015. The health and welfare of Australia's Aboriginal and Torres Strait Islander people. Available: https://www.aihw.gov.au/reports-data/health-welfare-overview/indigenous-health-welfare/overview.

Baker, A., Vellman, R., 2007. Clinical Handbook of Co-Existing Mental Health and Drug and Alcohol Problems. Routledge. Taylor & Francis, London.

Berridge, K.C., Kringelbach, M.L., 2015. Pleasure systems in the brain. Neuron 86 (3), 646–664.

Bien, T.H., Miller, W.R., Tonigan, J.S., 1993. Brief interventions for alcohol problems: a review. Addiction 88 (3), 315–335.

Boisvert, D.L., Connolly, E.J., Vaske, J.C., et al., 2019. Genetic and environmental overlap between substance use and delinquency in adolescence: an analysis by same-sex twins. Youth Violence Juv. Justice 17 (2), 154–173.

Bostwick, J., Lapid, M., 2004. False positives on the Clinical Institute Withdrawal Assessment for Alcohol-Revised: is this scale appropriate for use in the medically ill? Psychosomatics 45 (3), 256–261.

Bower, C., Elliot, E.J., 2016. Report to the Australian Government Department of Health: Australian guide to the diagnosis of fetal alcohol spectrum disorder (FASD). Available: https://www.fasdhub.org.au/siteassets/pdfs/australian-guide-to-diagnosis-of-fasd_all-appendices.pdf.

Brett, J., Lee, K., Gray, D., et al., 2016. Mind the gap: what is the difference between alcohol treatment need and access for Aboriginal and Torres Strait Islander Australians? Drug Alcohol Rev. 35, 456–460.

Bryant, J., Ward, J., Wand, H., et al., 2016. Illicit and injecting drug use among Indigenous young people in urban, regional and remote Australia. Drug Alcohol Rev. 35, 447–455.

Burns, L., Roxburgh, A., Matthews, A., et al., 2014. The rise of new psychoactive substance use in Australia. Drug Test. Anal. 6 (7–8), 846–849.

Cancer Council, 2018. Measures of tobacco dependence. Available: https://www.tobaccoinaustralia.org.au/chapter-6-addiction/6-12-measures-of-tobacco-dependence.

Cancer Council Victoria, 2018. Tobacco in Australia: Acute effects of nicotine on the body. Available: https://www.tobaccoinaustralia.org.au/chapter-6-addiction/6-10-acute-effects-of-nicotine-on-the-body.

Centre for Disease Control and Prevention, 2018. Health effects of cigarette smoking. Available: https://www.cdc.gov/tobacco/data_statistics/fact_sheets/health_effects/effects_cig_smoking/index.htm.

Cesconetto, P.A., Andrade, C.M., Cattani, D., et al., 2016. Maternal exposure to ethanol during pregnancy and lactation affects glutamatergic system and induces oxidative stress in offspring hippocampus. Alcohol. Clin. Exp. Res. 40 (1), 52–61.

Chamberlain, S.R., Stochl, J., Redden, S.A., et al., 2017. Latent class analysis of gambling sub-types and impulsive/compulsive associations: time to re-think diagnostic boundaries for gambling disorder? Addict. Behav. 72, 79–85.

Clancy, R.V., Hodgson, R.C., Kendurkar, A., et al., 2018. Synthetic cannabinoid use in an acute psychiatric inpatient unit. Int. J. Ment. Health Nurs. 27 (2), 600–607.

Department of Health, 2004. Working with young people on AOD issues: the stages of change model. Available: https://www.health.gov.au/internet/publications/publishing.nsf/Content/drugtreat-pubs-front9-wk-toc~drugtreat-pubs-front9-wk-secb~drugtreat-pubs-front9-wk-secb-3~drugtreat-pubs-front9-wk-secb-3-3.

Drake, R.E., Wallach, M.A., 2000. Dual diagnosis: 15 years of progress. Psychiatr. Serv. 51 (9), 1126–1129.

Drug Foundation, 2018. NZ Drug Foundation: Drug Index Tobacco. Available: https://www.drugfoundation.org.nz/info/drug-index/tobacco/.

Dumas, A., Toutain, S., Hill, C., et al., 2018. Warning about drinking during pregnancy: lessons from the French experience. Reprod. Health 15 (20), 1–9.

FASD Hub, 2016. FASD diagnosis: Australian guide to the diagnosis of FASD. Available: https://www.fasdhub.org.au/fasd-information/assessment-and-diagnosis/guide-to-diagnosis/.

George Institute for Global Health, 2015. Fighting for a future. The story of the women of Fitzroy Crossing. Available: www.georgeinstitute.org.au/projects/fighting-for-a-future-the-story-of-the-women-of-fitzroy-crossing. (Accessed 2 November 2015).

Glassman, S., Kottsieper, P., Zuckoff, A., et al., 2013. Motivational interviewing and recovery: experiences of hope, meaning and empowerment. Adv. Dual Diag. 6 (3), 106–120.

Government of South Australia, 2019. Adverse effects due to long-term opioids – medical staff information. Available: https://www.sahealth.sa.gov.au/wps/wcm/connect/f190e680499f905480cbde9b6ca12d15/Fact%2Bsheet.adverse%2Beffects%2Bdue%2Bto%2Blongterm%2Bopioids.medical.pdf?MOD=AJPERES&CACHE=NONE&CONTENTCACHE=NONE.

Gowing, L., Ali, R., Dunlop, A., et al., 2014. National guidelines for medication-assisted treatment of opioid dependence. Canberra: Department of Health. Available: http://www.nationaldrugstrategy.gov.au/internet/drugstrategy/Publishing.nsf/content/AD14DA97D8EE00E8CA257CD1001E0E5D/$File/National_Guidelines_2014.pdf.

Grant, J.E., Odlaug, B.L., Chamberlain, S.R., 2017. Gambling disorder, DSM-5 criteria and symptom severity. Compr. Psychiatry 75, 1–5.

Grant, J.E., Odlaug, B.L., Schreiber, L.R.N., 2014. Pharmacological treatment in pathological gambling. Br. J. Clin. Pharmacol. 77 (2), 375–381.

Hughes, J.A., Sheehan, M., Evans, J., 2017. Treatment and outcomes of patients presenting to an adult emergency department involuntarily with substance misuse. Int. J. Ment. Health Nurs. 27 (2), 593–599.

Humphreys, K., Blodgett, J.C., Wagner, T.H., 2014. Estimating the efficacy of Alcoholics Anonymous without self-selection bias: an instrumental variables re-analysis of randomized clinical trials. Alcohol. Clin. Exp. Res. 38 (11), 2688–2694.

Ishizuka, H., 2010. Carlyle's nervous dyspepsia: nervousness, indigestion and the experience of modernity in nineteenth-century Britain. In: Salisbury, L., Shail, A. (Eds.), Neurology and Modernity: A Cultural History of Nervous Systems, 1800–1950. Palgrave Macmillan, London, pp. 81–95.

Karila, L., Roux, P., Rolland, B., et al., 2014. Acute and long-term effects of cannabis us: a review. Curr. Pharm. Des. 20 (25), 4112–4118.

Kelly, J.F., Stout, R.L., Slaymaker, V., 2013. Emerging adults' treatment outcomes in relation to 12-step mutual-help attendance and active involvement. Drug Alcohol Depend. 129 (1–2), 151–157.

Kleinloog, D., Roozen, F., De Winter, W., et al., 2014. Profiling subjective effects of delta9-tetrahydrocannabinol using visual analogue scales. Int. J. Psychiatr. Res. 23 (2), 245–256.

Lai, H.M., Cleary, M., Sitharthan, T., et al., 2015. Prevalence of comorbid substance use, anxiety and mood disorders in epidemiological surveys, 1990–2014: a systematic review and meta-analysis. Drug Alcohol Depend. 154, 1–13.

Larance, B., Lintzeris, N., Ali, R., et al., 2014. The diversion and injection of a buprenorphine-naloxone soluble film formulation. Drug Alcohol Depend. 136, 21–27.

Lawn, W., Freeman, T.P., Pope, R.A., et al., 2016. Acute and chronic effects of cannabinoids on effort-related decision making and reward learning: an evaluation of cannabis amotivational hypotheses. Psychopharmacology (Berl) 233, 3537–3552.

Lehmann, S.W., Fingerhood, M., 2018. Substance-use disorders in later life. N. Engl. J. Med. 379 (24), 2351–2360.

Lubman, D., Sundram, S., 2003. Substance misuse in patients with schizophrenia: a primary care guide. Med. J. Aust. 178 (Suppl.May), 71–75.

Lundahl, B., Moleni, T., Burke, B.L., et al., 2013. Motivational interviewing in medical care settings: a systematic review and meta-analysis of randomized controlled trials. Patient Educ. Couns. 93 (2), 157–168.

Manning, V., Arunogiri, S., Frei, M., et al., 2018. Alcohol and Other Drug Withdrawal: Practice Guidelines, third ed. Turning Point, Richmond, Victoria.

Marsh, A., Dale, A., O'Toole, S., 2013. Addiction Counselling: Content and Process, second ed. IP Communications, Melbourne.

Martin-Santos, R., Crippa, J.A., Batalla, A., et al., 2012. Acute effects of a single, oral dose of delta9-tetrahydrocannabinol (THC) and cannabidiol (CBD) administration in healthy volunteers. Curr. Pharm. Des. 18 (2), 2966–4979.

McGovern, M.P., Lambert-Harris, C., Xie, H., et al., 2015. A randomized controlled trial of treatments for co-occurring substance use disorders and post-traumatic stress disorder. Addiction 110 (7), 1194–1204.

Mendelsohn, C.P., Kirby, D.P., Castle, D.J., 2015. Smoking and mental illness: an update for psychiatrists. Australas. Psychiatry 23 (1), 37–43.

Miller, W.R., Rollnick, S., 2009. Ten things that motivational interviewing is not. Behav. Cogn. Psychother. 37 (2), 129–140.

Mills, K., Deady, M., Proudfoot, H., et al., 2008. Guidelines on the Management of Co-Occurring Alcohol and Other Drug and Mental Health Conditions in Alcohol and Other Drug Treatment Settings. National Drug and Alcohol Research Centre, University of New South Wales, Sydney.

Ministry of Health, 2015. Cannabis Use 2012/13: New Zealand Health Survey. Ministry of Health, Wellington. Available: www.health.govt.nz/publication/cannabis-use-2012-13-new-zealand-health-survey.

Ministry of Health, 2018a. Alcohol Use in New Zealand: Key Results of the 2016/2017 New Zealand Alcohol and Drug Use Survey. Ministry of Health, Wellington.

Ministry of Health, 2018b. Alcohol and other drug use in New Zealand: key results 2017/2018. Available: https://minhealthnz.shinyapps.io/nz-health-survey-2017-18-annual-data-explorer/_w_0811ceee/_w_0eba45bd/#!/explore-topics.

Moore, T.J., Glenmullen, J., Mattison, D.R., 2014. Reports of pathological gambling, hypersexuality, and compulsive shopping associated with dopamine receptor agonist drugs. JAMA Intern. Med. 174 (12), 1930–1933.

Moyer, A., Finney, J.W., 2015. Brief interventions for alcohol misuse. CMAJ 187 (7), 502–506.

Musselman, M.E., Hampton, J.P., 2014. Not for human consumption: a review of emerging designer drugs. Pharmacotherapy 34 (7), 745–757.

National Drug Strategy, 2015. Intergovernmental committee on drugs: National Drug Strategy 2016–2025. Available: http://www.nationaldrugstrategy.gov.au/internet/drugstrategy/publishing.nsf/Content/draftnds.

National Health and Medical Research Council (NHMRC), 2015. Australian guidelines to reduce health risks from drinking alcohol. Commonwealth of Australia, Canberra. Available: www.nhmrc.gov.au/health-topics/alcohol-guidelines.

National Institute on Drug Abuse, 2019. Methamphetamine: What are the long-term effects of methamphetamine misuse? Available: https://www.drugabuse.gov/publications/methamphetamine/what-are-long-term-effects-methamphetamine-misuse.
New South Wales (NSW) Department of Health, 2008. NSW Drug and Alcohol Withdrawal Clinical Practice Guidelines. NSW Department of Health, Sydney.
New South Wales Health, 2013. Clinical guidelines for nursing and midwifery practice in NSW. In: Identifying and Responding to Drug and Alcohol Issues. NSW Health, Sydney. Available: https://www1.health.nsw.gov.au/pds/ActivePDSDocuments/GL2008_001.pdf.
NOFASD, 2018. FASD Definition. Available: https://www.nofasd.org.au/.
NSW Department of Health, 2018. Nursing & Midwifery Clinical Guidelines: identifying and responding to drug and alcohol issues. Available: https://www1.health.nsw.gov.au/pds/ActivePDSDocuments/GL2008_001.pdf.
Nutt, D.J., Lingford-Hughes, A., Erritzoe, D., et al., 2015. The dopamine theory of addiction: 40 years of highs and lows. Nat. Rev. Neurosci. 16 (5), 305–312.
Prochaska, J., DiClemente, C., 1984. The Transtheoretical Approach: Crossing Traditional Boundaries of Therapy. Dow/Jones Irwin, Homewood, Ill.
Rasmussen, N., 2011. Medical science and the military: the Allies' use of amphetamine during World War II. J. Interdiscip. Hist. 42 (2), 205–233.
Ries, R., Fiellin, D., Miller, S., et al., 2014. American Society of Addiction Medicine: Principles of Addiction Medicine. Wolters Kluwer, Philadelphia.
Riper, H., Andersson, G., Hunter, S.B., et al., 2014. Treatment of comorbid alcohol use disorders and depression with cognitive behavioural therapy and motivational interviewing: a meta-analysis. Addiction 109 (3), 394–406.
Robertson, C.L., Ishibashi, K., Mandelkern, M.A., et al., 2015. Striatal D1- and D2-type dopamine receptors are linked to motor response inhibition in human subjects. J. Neurosci. 35 (15), 5990–5997.
Rosenfeld, J.V., 2012. Practical Management of Head and Neck Injury. Churchill Livingstone, Sydney.
Roussy, V., Thomaco, N., Rudd, A., et al., 2017. Enhancing health-care workers' understanding and thinking about people living with co-occurring mental health and substance use issues through consumer-led training. Health Expect. 18 (5), 1567–1581.
Royal Australian College of General Practitioners (RACGP), 2015. Prescribing drugs of dependence in general practice, Part B: Benzodiazepines. Available: https://www.racgp.org.au/clinical-resources/clinical-guidelines/key-racgp-guidelines/view-all-racgp-guidelines/prescribing-drugs-of-dependence.
St Vincent's Hospital Melbourne, 2019. Alcohol Withdrawal Syndrome: Clinical Practice Guidelines. St Vincent's Hospital, Melbourne.
Substance Abuse and Mental Health Services Administration (SAMSHA), 2017. Focus on prevention: strategies and programs to prevent substance use. Available: https://store.samhsa.gov/system/files/sma10-4120.pdf.
Substance Abuse and Mental Health Services Administration (SAMSHA), 2004. Physical and psychological effects of substance use: Handout. Available: https://ncsacw.samhsa.gov/files/TrainingPackage/MOD2/PhysicalandPsychEffectsSubstanceUse.pdf.
Sud, P., Gordon, M., Tortora, L., et al., 2018. Retrospective chart review of synthetic cannabinoid intoxication with toxicologic analysis. West. J. Emerg. Med. 19 (3), 567–572.
Taplin, S., Richmond, G., McArthur, M., 2015. Identifying Alcohol and Other Use During Pregnancy. Outcomes for Women, Their Partners and Their Children. Institute of Child Protection Studies, Australian Catholic University, Canberra.
The Royal Women's Hospital, 2018a. Alcohol and pregnancy. Available: https://www.thewomens.org.au/health-professionals/maternity/womens-alcohol-and-drug-service.
The Royal Women's Hospital, 2018b. Cigarettes and tobacco. Available: https://thewomens.r.worldssl.net/images/uploads/fact-sheets/Cigarettes-and-tobacco-250818.pdf.
United Nations Office on Drugs and Crime (UNODC), 2018a. World Drug Report 2018: Executive summary – conclusions and policy implications. Available: www.unodc.org/wdr2018/en/exsum.html.
United Nations Office on Drugs and Crime (UNODC), 2018b. World Drug Report 2018: Global overview of drug demand and supply. Available: www.unodc.org/wdr2018/en/drug-demand-and-supply.html.
United Nations Office on Drugs and Crime (UNODC), 2019. UNODC Early warning advisory on new psychoactive substances. Available: https://www.unodc.org/LSS/Page/NPS.
Vasilaki, E.I., Hosier, S.G., Cox, W.M., 2006. The efficacy of motivational interviewing as a brief intervention for excessive drinking: a meta-analytic review. Alcohol 41 (3), 328–335.
Victorian Responsible Gambling Foundation, 2018. Problem gambling in people seeking treatment for mental illness. Available: www.responsiblegambling.vic.gov.au.
Waaktaar, T., Kan, K.J., Torgerson, S., 2018. The genetic and environmental architecture of substance use development from early adolescence into young adulthood: a longitudinal twin study of comorbidity of alcohol, tobacco and illicit drug use. Addiction 113 (4), 740–748.
Wand, H., Ward, J., Bryant, J., et al., 2016. Individual and population level impacts of illicit drug use, sexual risk behaviours on sexually transmitted infections among young Aboriginal and Torres Strait Islander people: results from the Goanna survey. BMC Public Health 16 (1), 1–9.
Weaver, M.F., Hopper, J.A., Gunderson, E.W., 2015. Designer drugs 2015: assessment and management. Addict. Sci. Clin. Pract. 10, 8.

Wild, T.C., Cunningham, J.A., Roberts, A.B., 2007. Controlled study of brief personalized assessment – feedback for drinkers interested in self-help. Addiction 102 (2), 241–250.

Wise, E.A., Streiner, D.L., Gallop, R.J., 2017. Predicting change in an integrated dual diagnosis substance abuse intensive outpatient program. Subst. Use Misuse 52 (7), 848–857.

World Health Organization (WHO), 2018a. International classification of diseases, 11th revision. Available: https://icd.who.int/en/.

World Health Organization (WHO), 2018b. Global status report on alcohol and health 2018. Available: www.who.int/substance_abuse/publications/global_alcohol_report/en.

World Health Organization (WHO), 2001. AUDIT: the Alcohol Use Disorders Identification Test. Guidelines for use in primary healthcare, 2nd edn. Available: http://whqlibdoc.who.int/hq/2001/who_msd_msb_01.6a.pdf.

World Health Organization (WHO), 2013. WHO model list of essential medicines. Available: http://apps.who.int/iris/bitstream/10665/93142/1/EML_18_eng.pdf.

World Health Organization (WHO), 2015. ASSIST (Alcohol Smoking and Substance Involvement Screening Test). Available: www.who.int/substance_abuse/activities/assist/en. (Accessed 1 June 2015).

Yokell, M.A., Zaller, N.D., Green, T.C., et al., 2011. Buprenorphine and buprenorphine/naloxone diversion, misuse, and illicit use: an international review. Curr. Drug Abuse Rev. 4 (1), 28–41.

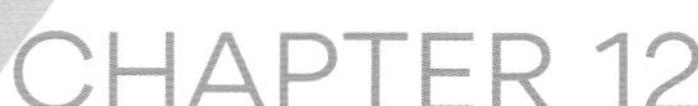

CHAPTER 12

Psychosis and schizophrenia

Toby Raeburn and Matthew Ball

KEY POINTS

- Most people diagnosed with psychotic disorders such as schizophrenia can recover if they are supported in ways they identify as most valuable.
- Mental health nurses who focus on working in partnership and compassionate, human-to-human relationships can be invaluable in supporting people labelled as psychotic.
- The etiology of schizophrenia is poorly understood. Despite this, theories are often promoted as explaining its origins.
- Trauma and social stressors can lead to experiences that result in a person being diagnosed with psychosis.
- Experiences of mental ill health that receive a diagnosis of a psychotic disorder such as schizophrenia can be understood by many people as meaningful responses to life experiences such as trauma and chronic misattunement to individual needs.

KEY TERMS

- Social determinants
- Language and labels
- Positive and negative symptoms
- Dominant models of understanding
- Alternative theories
- Psychotherapy and psychopharmacology
- Stigma and recovery

LEARNING OUTCOMES

The material in this chapter will assist you to:

- understand the prevalence and social determinants of people diagnosed with schizophrenia
- develop awareness of the influence of language, culture ideology and power embedded within current dominant approaches
- build familiarity with commonly used descriptions of signs and symptoms associated with psychosis and schizophrenia
- outline modern alternative approaches to working with psychosis including the Power Threat Meaning Framework, Open Dialogue and Intervoice: The International Hearing Voices Network
- describe five broad nursing interventions that may be useful for people experiencing psychosis or schizophrenia-related disorders.

Introduction

The human mind controls an amazing, relational and embodied process that regulates the flow of energy and information, processing millions of bits of information from myriad micro and macro experiences every day (Siegel 2009). Given its remarkable complexity, there should be little surprise that the mind is sensitive to anomalies. This chapter is concerned with how to provide nursing care to people whose minds experience distortions in perception, broadly referred to as psychosis and schizophrenia-related phenomena.

The word 'psychosis' stems from the ancient Greek term meaning 'illness of the mind', and records show that people have had such experiences ever since the beginning of recorded history (Porter 2002). In the modern era psychosis has become a term used to describe phenomena in which people experience a move away from regular perception into an inner world in which patterns of thinking, feeling and behaving become distorted. Many people experience psychosis as confusing, bizarre and frightening. For others, however, psychosis can actually be more bearable than their 'real world'.

Like other mental illnesses, experiences currently labelled as 'psychosis' and schizophrenia-type disorders do not have any laboratory tests or other diagnostic procedures that can either confirm or refute diagnoses. Often, psychosis is not only strange for the person who experiences it but also becomes confusing for people around them. Unfortunately, fear created by the confusion then leads people who receive diagnoses to be treated in discriminatory ways. Despite modern education campaigns, research reveals that people who have experienced psychosis feel the effects of stigma are as bad as or worse than the effects of the psychosis itself. People diagnosed with conditions such as schizophrenia are often considered unpredictable and dangerous. In fact, the reverse is true: people who experience psychosis have far higher chance of being victims of crime and violence (Khalifeh et al. 2015).

Many people fear that experiencing a psychotic episode means they will inevitably be burdened with a lifetime diagnosis of schizophrenia, but this is also not correct. Long-term studies have shown that more than 70% of people with a diagnosis of schizophrenia experience recovery (Torgalsbøen & Rund 2010; Zipursky & Agid 2015). Given such evidence, this chapter takes a recovery-oriented approach to understanding psychosis and schizophrenia-related phenomena. It is assumed that the focus of mental health nursing is working with the problems experienced by consumers whatever their diagnosis. The chapter addresses how people who receive a diagnosis such as 'psychosis' and 'schizophrenia' are understood and treated. Descriptions of common symptoms such as disorganisation, delusions and hallucinations are provided, along with alternative modern approaches to working with people who experience psychosis. This will familiarise nurses with signs of psychosis and enable them to consider a wide range of options in ways they endeavour to work with people who have experiences related to psychosis.

Prevalence and social determinants

Considerable variability in research design, geographic region, time of assessment, study setting, sample size and differing definitions of psychosis and schizophrenia-spectrum disorders across cultural groups make prevalence of psychosis hard to judge. Difficulties estimating prevalence were demonstrated in literature studied by Simeone et al. (2015), who noted that in Australia the *lifetime* prevalence of schizophrenia in 2010 was reported as being 0.75%, whereas the 12-month prevalence in New Zealand in 2008 was reported as being 0.1%. Chong et al. (2016) conducted a systematic review to discover the extent and economic burden of schizophrenia in the published literature of 24 countries and found that the prevalence of schizophrenia ranged from 0.26% to 0.67% of the population. Modern psychiatric literature such as the *Diagnostic and Statistical Manual for Mental Disorders*, 5th edition (DSM-5) (American Psychiatric Association (APA) 2013) estimates there is a lifetime prevalence of schizophrenia of approximately 0.3%–0.7%, and it rarely occurs before adolescence, with onset most common in the early to mid-20s. Unfortunately, due to stigma and historically poor care and approaches, people who experience psychosis and schizophrenia-type conditions are far more likely to experience disadvantage through poverty, incarceration and homelessness.

Burns et al. (2014) conducted a global systematic review of 26 countries and found there is a significant relationship between poverty and schizophrenia. A person is more likely to be diagnosed with schizophrenia, for example, if they grow up in an urban environment and belong to a lower socioeconomic group. Urbanisation presents a very clear and well-documented increased risk of developing schizophrenia. For example, China has recently undergone urbanisation at an unprecedented rate and scale, a process that was expected to increase the numbers of people with schizophrenia – and it did (Chan et al. 2015). As the cities doubled in size to house 600 million people, it was estimated that the numbers of people affected with schizophrenia rose from 3.09 million in 1990 to 7.16 million in 2010, a 132% increase, although the total population increased by only 18% (Chan et al. 2015).

Prison populations in Australia and New Zealand and similar populations overseas continue to have a disproportionately high number of people diagnosed with psychosis and schizophrenia-type conditions (Rautanen & Lauerma 2011). Studies of international prison populations indicate that 10–15% of offenders have a mental illness, and they are up to four times as likely to be experiencing psychotic illness than a person in the general community (Fazel & Seewald 2012). There could be mitigating circumstances; for example, a shoplifter might offend because of lapses of memory and concentration or because of confusion due to a psychotic episode, or comorbid drug or alcohol use. Nonetheless, the existence of an association between mental illness and crime contributes to the stigma that mentally ill people experience.

Cultural meaning and understanding are often overlooked when a person is labelled as being psychotic. This is despite the rich knowledge and understanding in many First Nations of the experiences we in the Western world call psychosis. The work of Taitimu et al. (2018) – *Ngā Whakāwhitinga (standing at the crossroads): How Māori understand what Western psychiatry calls 'schizophrenia'* is a fantastic example of how First Nation peoples understand the experience that modern approaches refer to as schizophrenia. Dr Lewis Mehl Madrona (2015) has also done work that provides rich understanding from Native American traditions in the United States and points to voices as a way of connecting to spirit in his integrative approach that embraces both traditional and Westernised knowledge. Although a comparative work on Aboriginal cultural and spiritual understandings of what we call schizophrenia has not yet been carried out in Australia, Aboriginal culture may hold deep ancient wisdom with potential to contribute to the wellbeing of both Aboriginal and non-Aboriginal wellbeing.

In OECD nations, psychotic disorders such as schizophrenia also tend to be more prevalent among the socially disadvantaged. The homeless population is one example where there are higher rates of the condition, and people of different cultural backgrounds, including Aboriginal and Torres Strait Islander people, have a higher prevalence (Grech & Raeburn 2019). The main societal costs related to psychosis are due to lost productivity caused by high unemployment and under-employment of people with mental illness, along with health service costs, which commonly include inpatient hospital, criminal justice system and community-based psychiatry costs (Kazdin & Blase 2011). For example, the annual costs for a person who experiences psychosis in Australia comprise $40,941 in lost productivity, $21,714 in health sector costs and $14,642 in other costs. Overall, this amounts to four times the cost in annual health expenditure for an average Australian adult (Neil et al. 2014). Understanding how nurses can assist people to overcome the challenges associated with psychosis is therefore an issue relevant not only to the wellbeing of individuals but to society as a whole.

The powerful role of language and labels

In many parts of society language is a tool that has been used to control, threaten and coerce people who experience mental ill health into line or to modify behaviours. Nurses need to be aware of the power of language, both verbal and non-verbal. At all times language needs to be respectful, honest and genuine in ways that enhance the process of growth. When considering modern terms used to describe signs and symptoms of phenomena commonly labelled as 'psychosis', mental health nurses need to keep in mind that, similar to other mental illnesses, no clear biological aetiology for psychosis or schizophrenia has ever been discovered.

History teaches that what is known in relation to mental health and illness is the result of society's ever-changing interpretation of the world around us. In the field of mental health very little purely rational, objective knowledge exists. An extreme example of this can be found in American history when, during the 1850s, diagnosistic label 'drapetomania' was developed by American doctor Samuel Cartwright to diagnose black slaves who tried to escape from their masters (Reich et al. 2008). In a publication entitled *Diseases and Peculiarities of the Negro Race*, Cartwright asserted that slaves should be submissive to their master and that if they weren't the slave should be treated as mentally ill. He asserted that drapetomania was a consequence of slave masters who were too kind to their slaves, and he suggested medical treatment. If slaves were identified as displaying symptoms of being dissatisfied without cause, he prescribed heavy whipping and making running a physical impossibility by removing both big toes. Dr Cartwright believed that if this medical advice was strictly followed, drapetomania could be completely eradicated. The diagnosis gained support from the Medical Association of Louisiana, and his publication was widely published.

The modern label 'schizophrenia' was coined in 1911 by Swiss psychiatrist Eugen Bleuler (1857–1939) as an amalgam of two Greek words: *schizo*, meaning 'split', and *phrenia*, meaning 'mind'. Bleuler intended the term to symbolise the schism between the external world of the individual and the internal conflict of the individual's mind (Stotz-Ingenlath 2000). His emphasis was on the lost connections between thoughts and those between thought, emotion and will. Despite this, a dominant societal myth that equates schizophrenia with a 'split personality' developed. This belief equated schizophrenia with a sort of 'Jekyll and Hyde' manifestation wherein an apparently 'normal' person may turn unpredictably into a person who is irrational and dangerous. Unfortunately, popular film and media characterisations of people who experience psychosis often fail to accurately depict the manifestations of the experience and more often than not perpetuate such common myths and stereotypes. Nurses need to keep in mind that labels such as drapetomania and schizophrenia are examples of how language has been used to construct psychological concepts that reflect attempts to understand human behaviour in the context of culture, ideology and power (Conrad & Barker 2010).

Descriptions of signs and symptoms of psychosis are therefore heavily reliant on cultural and linguistic terms. Such terms have been invented due to the neurotypical human desire to group experiences into clusters that appear to be similar. Despite the ever-changing language and lack of objectivity that surrounds how mental disorders such as psychosis are described it is nonetheless important for nurses to familiarise themselves with the current dominant ways of thinking and talking about mental ill health.

The signs and symptoms described in the section below are abridged descriptions from the 2013 DSM-5, which is the most used source for descriptors for symptoms of mental ill health in modern healthcare systems. These next two sections should be read with the concerns previously outlined regarding language, culture, ideology and power in mind.

Historical anecdote 12.1: Protest psychosis

An example of how labelling people with psychosis has been used to perpetuate power and ideology occurred in the 1960s in America when the second edition of the DSM was used to diagnose hundreds of African Americans with schizophrenia due to so-called symptoms that were called 'protest psychosis'. People who had been involved in protests campaigning for civil rights and an end to racism in America were diagnosed, admitted to hospital and treated for their 'condition' by nurses and doctors at Ionia State Hospital in Michigan. This was made possible by a change in wording in the DSM-II, which included 'hostility' and 'aggression' as signs of psychosis. This language enabled cultural difference and protest to be interpreted as a health problem.

Read more about it: *Metzl JM 2010 The protest psychosis: how schizophrenia became a black disease. Beacon Press, Boston*

Signs and symptoms

Psychotic disorders such as schizophrenia are currently understood as being characterised by one or more of the following five types of symptoms: delusions; hallucinations; disorganised thinking (speech); grossly disorganised or abnormal motor behaviour (including catatonia); or negative symptoms. Each of these states are outlined below.

Delusions are fixed beliefs that are not amenable to change in light of conflicting evidence. Their content may include a variety of themes (e.g. persecutory, referential, somatic, religious, grandiose). Examples include:

- paranoid delusions such as a belief that the person is being followed or monitored (e.g. 'My neighbour is plotting to kill me')
- grandiose delusions, where a person may believe they have special abilities or 'powers' (e.g. 'I can fly' or 'I'm on a mission from God')
- thought broadcasting, which is the belief that the person's thoughts are being broadcast to or heard by others.
- thought withdrawal, which is the belief that others are taking their thoughts
- thought insertion, which is the belief that thoughts are being placed in their mind against their will.

Hallucinations refer to distortions in perception. People with psychosis may experience hallucinations in any of the five senses, hearing, seeing, feeling, smelling or tasting sensations that do not appear to be real. Common hallucinations include:

- auditory hallucinations, which commonly include hearing voices talking to them or about them, or hearing music and other noises when there is no sound (e.g. hearing someone call their name when they are at home alone)
- visual hallucinations such as seeing things that are not there, or seeing things in a strange way (e.g. seeing unusual shapes, colours or lights, or seeing an image of someone standing before them)
- somatic hallucinations involving feeling something touch or something happening in their body when there is nothing there (e.g. feeling as though ants are crawling on their skin)
- olfactory hallucinations, which involve smelling things when there are no smells around (e.g. smelling rotting fish in the house, even though there are no fish there)
- gustatory hallucinations, which refer to tasting things in a strange way (e.g. tasting metal in their mouth).

Disorganised thinking is inferred from a person's speech. It is commonly characterised as including speech that switches rapidly from one topic to another; this may be described as 'derailment' or 'loose associations'. A person may reply to questions with answers that are tangential, which means they are oblique or unrelated. Sometimes speech may be incomprehensible, and it may be described as incoherent or 'word salad'. Nurses conducting a mental health assessment need to remember that mildly disorganised speech is common and non-specific, so symptoms must be severe enough to substantially impair effective communication. Severity of the impairment may be difficult to evaluate if the person making the diagnosis comes from a different linguistic background than that of the person being examined. Less severe disorganised thinking or speech may occur during the prodromal and residual periods of schizophrenia. Speech may include:

- 'neologisms', which involves using words that don't exist
- 'echolalia', which is repeating words/phrases used by other people in conversation
- 'perseveration', whereby the person uses excessive continuation/repetition of a single response or idea.

Disorganised behaviour may be exhibited in a variety of ways, ranging from childlike 'silliness' to unpredictable agitation. Problems may be noted in any form of goal-directed behaviour, leading to difficulties in performing activities of daily living. Catatonic behaviour is a marked decrease in reactivity to the environment. This can include:

- resistance to instructions (negativism)
- maintaining a rigid, inappropriate or bizarre posture
- a complete lack of verbal and motor responses (mutism and stupor)
- purposeless and excessive motor activity without obvious cause (catatonic excitement).

Other features include repeated stereotyped movements, staring, grimacing, mutism and the echoing of speech. Although catatonia has historically been associated with schizophrenia, catatonic symptoms are non-specific and may occur in other mental disorders (e.g. bipolar or depressive disorders with catatonia) and in medical conditions (catatonic disorder due to another medical condition).

Negative symptoms are absences or reductions of thought processes, emotions and behaviours that were present before the onset of the illness but have since diminished or are absent following the onset of the illness. These symptoms are substantial in schizophrenia but less common in other psychotic disorders.

Diminished emotional expression includes reductions in the expression of emotions in the face, eye contact, intonation of speech and movements of the hand, head and face that normally give an emotional emphasis to speech.

Avolition refers to a decrease in motivated self-initiated purposeful activities. The person may sit for long periods of time and show little interest in participating in work or social activities. Other negative symptoms include alogia, anhedonia and asociality:

- Alogia manifests in diminished speech output.
- Anhedonia is the decreased ability to experience pleasure from positive stimuli or a degradation in recalling pleasure previously experienced.
- Asociality refers to the apparent lack of interest in social interactions and may be associated with avolition, but it can also be a manifestation of limited opportunities for social interactions.

Symptoms of psychosis often contribute to deterioration in interpersonal relationships. Heightened levels of anxiety are experienced as the person identifies a perceived conflict between what is and what should be. Anger may occur when others appear to disregard what the person acknowledges as their reality and attempts are made to refocus and reorient. The person may feel their need for safety and security are threatened by their attempt to cope with an 'alien world.'

It is important to remember that the signs and symptoms described above are the opinion and view of the APA – the organisation that constructed the DSM-5. Such descriptions are therefore layered with cultural understandings from an American/Western point of view and, as previously stated, lack objective scientific evidence. When a person seeks to dispute the construct of schizophrenia, nurses can play a pivotal role in supporting and advocating for the legitimate views and experiences of the person in distress towards forming a collaborative understanding.

Types of psychosis and schizophrenia-related phenomena

As stated previously, experiences currently labelled as psychotic or schizophrenia-type disorders do not currently have any laboratory tests or other diagnostic procedures that can either confirm or refute a diagnosis. Making psychiatric diagnoses therefore relies heavily on detailed history taking, behavioural observation and opinion. Data gained from such processes are then measured against diagnostic criteria published by groups such as the APA (DSM-5) and the World Health Organization (the *International Classification of Diseases* 11th Revision, or 'ICD-11'). Groups such as these, in an attempt to increase effectiveness of assessment and treatment of mental ill health and allow clinicians to be consistent in language used to describe psychotic experiences, have grouped similar signs and symptoms into diagnostic categories. This is not an evidence-based approach but remains the dominant model. Common diagnostic terms currently used to describe psychotic disorders in modern health care include:

- substance-induced psychotic disorder
- brief intermittent psychosis
- delusional disorder
- schizophreniform disorder
- schizophrenia
- schizoaffective disorder.

Brief summaries below provide abridged versions of descriptions provided in *Schizophrenia Spectrum and Other Psychotic Disorders: DSM-5 Selections* (APA 2015).

Substance-induced psychotic disorder

To be diagnosed with substance-induced psychotic disorder a person needs to have experienced delusions or hallucinations and their health history, physical examination or laboratory findings need to indicate that psychosis developed during or soon after substance intoxication or withdrawal or after exposure to a medication capable of producing psychotic symptoms. The substance-induced psychosis needs to have caused substantial distress or impairment in social, occupational or other important areas of functioning. Other medical causes such as delirium need to be excluded, and it needs to be clear that the psychosis is not better explained by a pre-existing psychotic disorder that preceded the substance/medication use or that persists for a substantial period (at least a month) after the cessation of acute withdrawal or severe intoxication.

Brief intermittent psychosis

Brief intermittent psychosis is distinctive because it involves the sudden onset of psychosis and is strictly time-limited, lasting for more than a day but less than a month, with eventual full return to psychosocial functioning. To receive a diagnosis of brief intermittent psychosis a person needs to exhibit the presence of one (or more) of the following symptoms: delusions, hallucinations, disorganised speech (e.g. incoherence or frequent derailment), grossly disorganised behaviour or catatonic behaviour. Other experiences include mental disorders such as depression or bipolar disorder. The possibility that a person may be affected by drugs or other general medical conditions needs to be excluded. Specific description of a brief intermittent psychosis may also be added if it occurs in response to stressful events, during pregnancy or within 4 weeks' postpartum.

Delusional disorder

To be diagnosed with delusional disorder a person needs to have experienced the presence of one (or more) delusions for a month or longer. Second, on assessment it needs to be clarified that the person does not meet diagnostic criteria for schizophrenia, and if hallucinations are present, they must not be prominent or related to the delusional theme. Third, the person's behaviour needs to be interpreted as not being obviously odd or bizarre; social and occupational functioning needs not to have been markedly impaired. Fourth, if manic or major depressive episodes have occurred, these need to have been brief relative to the duration of the delusional periods. Fifth, other illnesses including mental disorders such as body dysmorphic disorder or obsessive-compulsive disorder or the possibility that the person may be affected by drugs or other general medical conditions needs to be excluded. On diagnosis the specific type of delusional psychosis should be described – for example, grandiose, jealous, persecutory, mixed or erotomanic.

Schizophreniform disorder

For a diagnosis of schizophreniform disorder, a person needs to have exhibited at least two of the following list of symptoms including at least one from a, b or c:

a. delusions
b. hallucinations
c. disorganised speech (e.g. frequent derailment or incoherence)
d. grossly disorganised behaviour
e. catatonic behaviour
f. negative symptoms (diminished emotional expression or avolition).

Symptoms must last for at least 1 month but less than 6 months. Other disorders such as schizoaffective disorder and depressive or bipolar disorder with psychotic features need to be excluded.

Schizophrenia

A diagnosis of schizophrenia requires a person to have experienced at least 6 months of a mixture of negative and positive symptoms. Negative symptoms are characterised by a marked disturbance level of functioning in one or more major areas such as work, interpersonal relations or self-care and is markedly below the level achieved before the onset (or when the onset is in childhood or adolescence, there is failure to achieve the expected level of interpersonal, academic or occupational functioning). Within the 6-month period the person also needs to have experienced at least 1 month of positive symptoms for a substantial period, with at least one of a, b or c being present.

a. delusions
b. hallucinations
c. disorganised speech (e.g. frequent derailment or incoherence)
d. grossly disorganised or catatonic behaviour
e. negative symptoms (i.e. diminished emotional expression or avolition).

Other conditions such as schizoaffective disorder and depressive or bipolar disorder need to be excluded and the symptoms must not be attributable to any other physiological cause or substance use.

Schizoaffective disorder

Schizoaffective disorder describes a long-term condition in which a person experiences a mood episode (major depression or mania) along with symptoms fulfilling the primary criteria for schizophrenia. Diagnoses must exclude the effects of a substance (a drug of abuse, a medication) and other medical conditions as causative. If a manic episode is part of the presentation the schizoaffective disorder may be specified as 'bipolar type'. If major depressive episodes occur, it may be classified as 'depressive type'.

Alternative approaches to psychosis and schizophrenia-related phenomena

While the definitions listed above tend to be the dominant descriptions used in modern health services, it is important for nurses to know that there is a growing disquiet regarding the lack of effectiveness, overly biomedical and concrete nature of such diagnostic terms. Frustration with systems such as the DSM-5 has led people working with allied health professionals and people with lived experience of mental ill health to develop a range of emerging, alternative approaches to understanding experiences currently labelled as psychosis and schizophrenia. Brief summaries of four promising modern alternative approaches are outlined as follows.

The Power Threat Meaning Framework

Published by the British Psychological Society, the PTM framework provides a conceptual and intellectual alternative to diagnostic and medicalised thinking and practice in the treatment of mental ill health. PTM seeks to provide an entirely new approach to assessment and diagnosis that considers aspects of human experience such as the operation of power, the links between threats and fear responses, and the autonomy of people within personal, social, economic and material environments. PTM highlights that personal stories and meaning-making offer rich and meaningful alternatives to psychiatric diagnosis.

Considering the highly debatable nature of psychosis and schizophrenia-related phenomena, the PTM framework provides a more pragmatic way to develop a collaborative formulation of people's experiences, empowering individuals to formulate their own meaning and sense of whether they have a disorder or not. Language associated with schizophrenia diagnosis has become something of a chimera of the psychiatric paradigm, heavily embedded in the power imbalance of psychiatric relationships. Nurses may therefore find the PTM framework useful to understand the negative experience of power in a people's lives and the potential for the positive use of power when a person is supported to find meaning in the context of threat.

Dissociachotic theory

Developed by mental health nurse practitioner (co-author of this chapter) Matthew Ball, dissociachotic theory provides an alternative way of understanding experiences traditionally referred to as psychosis. Dissociachotic theory contends that experiences currently mistakenly labelled as psychotic disorders are in fact meaningful forms of dissociation that serve to create experiential separation from perceived threats. Building on the seminal work of Corstens et al. (2008) on working with voices and the polyvagal theory developed by Porges (2011), dissociachotic theory contends that extraordinary experiential realities are often mislabelled as abhorrent symptoms like hallucinations and delusions. The theory suggests such phenomena should be viewed as meaningful human coping strategies, designed to satisfy the innate human need for social, emotional and physical safety.

Traditionally psychological theories have suggested that threat responses generally emerge from one of three instinctual coping strategies known as fight, flight or freeze responses. Dissociachotic theory proposes that as the human brain has evolved and the prefrontal cortex has become increasingly linked to executive function, a fourth instinctual threat response known as 'dissociachotic phenomena' has developed. The theory contends that experiences currently labelled as psychotic symptoms are in fact dissociachotic phenomena, which provide animated meaningful responses to threatening experiences.

Early work indicates that when dissociachotic theory is put into practice the role of nurses and other supporters becomes focused on uncovering the meaning that dissociachotic phenomena holds for people and using therapeutic communication to explore and remedy the sense of threat and need for safety experienced by the individual concerned. As a reduction in sense of threat and increase in safety is achieved, the theory suggests that dissociachotic phenomena subside, thereby explaining the episodic nature of such phenomena. Dissociachotic theory is consistent with nursing approaches that emphasise the importance of interpersonal relationships and is supported by social constructionist philosophy that legitimises the differences in reality experienced by every individual.

Open dialogue

Open dialogue therapy (ODT) is a promising new therapeutic technique developed in Scandinavia for treating psychosis. The primary goal of ODT is increased engagement of a person's social network/family in therapy, with a view to creating a more open dialogue about experiences related to psychosis in the home environment.

Seven core principles are embedded in ODT. The first is a requirement for providing immediate help, meaning that access to health services must occur within 24 hours of the first contact between the health team and the patient, family or referral service and thereafter the person must receive immediate support from health professionals during any crisis.

The second principle involves the ongoing inclusion of a social network within the therapeutic sessions. This social network is selected by the client and may consist of relatives, friends, neighbours, employers, co-workers or other care agencies and, as such, is fundamental to the therapy sessions through sharing stories of the patient. As well as listening to one another, the patient and the health team providing treatment, this social network also provides support to the patient.

The third principle of ODT is flexibility and mobility, which refers to the need for services to be flexible and thus adapt to the changing requirements of the patient and the support network. In practice this allows a range of psychotherapeutic approaches to be adapted to the needs of the client such as psychodynamic theory, systemic family therapy and dialogical theory, as well as pharmacological and social constructionism. Meetings are preferably conducted within the patient's home with the consent of the client and their family.

The fourth and fifth principles of ODT are responsibility and psychological continuity. These refer to the importance of the initial team that assesses the client coordinating treatment throughout the entire process so that psychological continuity of therapy is maintained.

The final two principles of ODT are tolerance of uncertainty and dialogism (Seikkula et al 2001). Tolerance of uncertainty refers to the fact that the recovery journey is full of ups and downs and that all involved need to be willing to accept risks that are included in recovery. Dialogism refers to the openness that is needed between the client, their social network and clinicians as they move along their recovery journey. Family connectedness is improved as they discuss the client's 'difficulties and problems'. Rather than a formal interview approach, the team adapts to the language and way of speaking the family is used to (Hetherington 2015).

Intervoice: The International Hearing Voices Network

Developments in understanding the impact of trauma on the brain has led to the creation of the International Hearing Voices Network (www.intervoiceonline.org). Founded by Professor Marius Romme and a group of people with lived experience, Intervoice reasons that psychotic experiences such as voices (also known as auditory hallucinations) need to be understood from the perspective of their meaning for the person who experiences them. The network also supports theories that traumatic experiences can often be the origin of voice hearing rather than interpreting voices as being an aberrant symptom of schizophrenia (Longden 2013). In Consumer's story 12.1, Matthew talks about how he found validation for his experiences in the 'hearing voices' movement, which is an example of the emerging influence of consumer-led understandings and involvement. International Hearing Voices Network groups operate at a wide variety of locations in Australia, New Zealand and overseas. Relevant weblinks can be found in the 'Useful websites' list at the end of this chapter.

CONSUMER'S STORY 12.1
Matthew Ball

I had used illicit drugs since my early teens. I had lived overseas and experienced homelessness, and I could see little future in my life when at the age of 21 I went with my mother to see a GP. The GP was concerned about my focus on suicide, sense of hopelessness and reported drug use, so following liaison with the mental health team, he arranged for a direct admission to a psychiatric hospital. Although I had many friends growing up, I had few functional relationships in my life at this time and my family was very concerned about my wellbeing. They had little knowledge about mental health problems at this stage.

Although I was assessed by a consultant psychiatrist and a nurse, I felt that the nurse heard me most clearly and appeared to be less concerned by my diagnosis and more concerned with who I might be and the experiences that might have contributed to my condition. I was started on antipsychotic and antidepressant medication and discharged 6 weeks later to my mother's home, with planned GP follow-up. One of the friends I made in hospital killed himself shortly after I left hospital, and not long after this I made an attempt on my own life. I told people I was hearing voices saying that I was worthless and should kill myself. I also heard the voice of a man saying that he was watching me through video cameras at all times, and I became very frightened. I did not try to end my life because the voices were telling me to. I was suicidal in the context of despair and homelessness that was exacerbated by the system's responses.

Several admissions followed during which I had stopped using illicit drugs, yet I still heard derogatory voices and felt a sense that the world and myself were being controlled by an external 'force'. I was suicidal and I tried to kill myself, following through on a plan I had made. Other frightening psychotic experiences included seeing a cat who I believed attempted to kill me, which led to my imprisoning myself for 3 days until I knew that the cat had gone. I experienced a sense of being an incompetent human being and searched for potential explanations for my experiences, exploring my sexuality and seeking religious justifications. I was admitted to hospital five times, but I felt that the nursing and medical teams never discovered what caused my experiences of psychosis. My unusual realities were considered part of a biomedically informed rationale for a psychotic disorder, and the possibility of my suffering from schizophrenia was not excluded. Nurses spent a lot of time with me in the unit, but they were task-oriented. I believe that they could have used basic mental health nursing skills, such as building a therapeutic relationship, to develop a more meaningful understanding of the events that contributed to my experiencing psychosis. Treatment focused on medications and electroconvulsive therapy. I was prescribed a concoction of antipsychotic, antidepressant and mood-stabilising medications. I feel now that, as my primary healthcare workers, nurses could have been more assertive in identifying for me the side effects of my medication and their negative impact. A proactive approach on their part might have prevented or addressed a number of the difficulties and problems that arose. I gained 50 kg in 18 months, probably due to medication, a poor diet and reduced exercise, and I became increasingly socially isolated: all of which were perceived by nursing staff as the usual negative symptoms of a psychotic illness. No-one talked about recovery, and the concept of a positive personal and clinical journey was not easy to imagine.

During my fifth admission I commenced 2 years of psychotherapy because medication and hospitalisation had not led to an improvement in my symptoms. I went to live in a nurse-led housing community of eight residents with mental health problems, where the person-centred emphasis was less on diagnosis and disease and more on the acceptance of my own experiences and reality, and support for my journey towards my future. I made a number of friends in the mental health system, and that mutual acceptance between peers proved to be a significant factor in making sense of the whole experience, and finally, in accepting myself.

Over time the voices and other psychotic phenomena impacted my life less, and I worked with a psychiatrist to reduce, then stop, all medications. I worked as a volunteer then found paid employment before moving into my own accommodation. Since the 4-year period when I was 'treated' by the mental health system for a psychotic disorder I have spent 15 years following my life journey, being part of a beautiful family as a husband and a father to three children, and developing a successful career in mental health nursing and therapy. Especially valuable in helping me to interpret the cause of the voices that I experienced has been the 'hearing voices' approach towards making sense of and understanding psychosis.

Theories of causation/aetiology

To date, research has failed to demonstrate the aetiology/cause of psychotic disorders. Despite this, many theories have attempted to explain them. Three commonly posited biological theories are brain anatomy, genetics and brain biochemistry. It would be erroneous to consider these three factors as mutually exclusive, and it may be more likely that there is a relationship between the three. Schizophrenia has often been referred to as a 'neuropsychological disorder', which implies that the origins of the psychological disturbance lie in the neurological structure and function of the brain. Modern imaging techniques have been used to suggest lower brain tissue volume and higher cerebrospinal volumes in people with schizophrenia, but these findings are not conclusive, and these factors are now being demonstrated as being a side effect of antipsychotic medication. A great deal more research exploring weather there are links between brain anatomy and schizophrenia is required and the cause–effect relationship remains inconclusive (Boos et al. 2011). Despite more than 50 years of seeking understanding of the biogenetic model of schizophrenia no conclusive evidence has been shown to support biological aetiological theories.

There is, however, a growing body of modern evidence related to the influence of traumatic life experiences in developing psychotic disorders. Recognising the dose response between adverse childhood experiences and reduced health and social outcomes is important (Brown et al. 2009). Research examining adverse childhood experiences data covers many mental health, physical health and social domains and has revealed a dose response between the number of childhood traumas and the likelihood of being labelled as psychotic, with more traumatic experiences in childhood increasing the risk of being labelled as psychotic. The work of Read et al. (2014) proposes that psychosis should be understood as a response to adversity. They refer to the 'trauma-genic neurodevelopmental model of psychosis' that demonstrates, through functional magnetic resonance imaging, five primary changes in brain chemistry and structure that are used to justify similar states to schizophrenia are also found in people who have experienced cumulative childhood trauma (Read et al. 2014).

The stress-vulnerability-protective factors model (Weisman 2005) is a framework that attempts to integrate environmental, biological and traumagenic theories, suggesting that people are exposed to stressful events in the course of their lives and that these events may precipitate symptoms in some people who have a biological predisposition to mental ill health (Jones & Fernyhough 2007). Essential to this theory is the notion that some people are more vulnerable to mental ill health than others. In the case of psychosis and schizophrenia the theory suggests that vulnerability may be related to a combination of environmental and biological factors (Van Heeringen et al. 2000). Weisman (2005) explored of the role of family as part of a person's environment and culture, finding that a person's family and home environment have the potential to affect the course of psychosis. More specifically, people with lived experience of psychosis from families that showed high levels of expressed emotion typified by excessive criticism, hostility or emotional over-involvement, appeared to struggle more than people with lived experience who were from families with patterns of relating that were not high in expressed emotion (Kopelowicz et al. 2003).

Nursing interventions

Any mental health nursing intervention should focus on the holistic understanding of the person seeking support. This is often overlooked, and disorder-specific approaches are then developed. As outlined previously, using psychiatric approaches to psychosis and schizophrenia-related phenomena are generally thought to share the common characteristics of severe disturbances in perception, cognition and thinking. While the term 'psychosis' is most strongly associated with schizophrenia, it may also be a feature of other disorders such as bipolar disorder, depression, dementia and delirium. When conducting health assessments nurses need to be aware the current approaches that seek to assess mental disorders such as psychosis and schizophrenia are highly questionable and contentious. Seven common interventions nurses deliver in the process of caring for people who experience psychosis and schizophrenia-related phenomena include assessment, therapeutic communication, psychopharmacology, physical health promotion, social advocacy, relapse prevention and recovery-oriented care planning. Each of these interventions are briefly discussed as follows.

Assessment

Because mental health has no objective scientific instruments or tests to rely upon (such as a blood tests or x-rays), the assessment process is heavily influenced by the knowledge and understanding of the person conducting the assessment. Any assessor's knowledge is limited, meaning that the safest way to conduct mental health assessment is to collaborate with the person being assessed in an attempt to identify strengths and challenges and to assist them and the people they live with towards a more satisfying life. Nurses need to be as interested in people's abilities and activities as they are in indicators that suggest mental ill health. It is crucial for nurses to remember that:

- a mental health assessment should never be a mental illness assessment
- assessment can be helpful or unhelpful
- assessment is a process not a single event
- assessment can be an intervention in itself
- misinformation can misinform future actions
- incomplete or ill-informed assessment may be considered worse than no assessment.

Fusar-Poli et al. (2020) indicates the presence of low-grade (subthreshold) psychotic symptoms, poor functioning, depression and disorganisation as predictors of an overt psychotic episode. In addition, comorbid features such as substance abuse and depression should not be overlooked. Because the onset of schizophrenia may occur during adolescence or in early adulthood, this constellation of negative symptoms tends to interfere with education, employment and the development of meaningful connections with others in a social setting. Negative symptoms may sometimes cause conversations to be limited and responses to be short, often monosyllabic. Symptoms such as alogia and avolition (described previously) leave the person feeling numb and unable to respond to the demands of daily living. There is often a significant loss of drive and the person has difficulty initiating and completing activities. Both the illness and the treatment can introduce impairments such as difficulty learning new concepts and disturbances in attention, which further impact on treatment and rehabilitation efforts since they undermine the acquisition of new skills. It is important to remember that assessment focuses on the hypothesis distilled into the DSM-5 symptomology and is not a scientific approach.

The early phase of a psychotic disorder may sometimes be confused by parents as a 'normal' one because parents are aware that adolescent children are known to need increased privacy and to seek separation from parental surveillance. Limited social engagement means the person finds it difficult to develop and sustain stimulating and rewarding social relationships and partnerships at a time when most people are socialising, seeking life partners and training for their future careers. Instead of beginning to earn an income and seek personal independence, a person who is developing schizophrenia might find themselves hospitalised or dependent on their parents for help with personal hygiene, nutrition and motivation to undertake physical activity.

Course and outcome cannot be reliably predicted for every person, but a variable course with sometimes lengthy periods of remission and intermittent relapses is common, although the illness can become chronic in a proportion of people. Early onset is associated with poorer outcomes and later onset results in better outcomes; for most people, negative symptoms predominate later in the course of the illness (APA 2013). Factors associated with a better prognosis include:

- a good level of premorbid adjustment
- sudden and later onset
- self-awareness and resilience
- having identifiable triggers for episodes
- concurrent mood disturbance
- short periods of acute illness
- higher levels of functioning between episodes
- fewer residual symptoms
- good neurological function.

With reference to schizophrenia, the DSM-5 (APA 2013) no longer specifically refers to a 'chronic phase', instead specifying whether the symptoms are 'continuous' or in 'full' or 'partial' remission. Continuous symptoms 'fulfil the diagnostic symptom criteria of the disorder for the majority of the illness course' (APA 2013, p. 100). A long-term course appears to be favourable in about 20% of people with schizophrenia, and a small number of these recover completely. Of the other 80%, most will need help with daily living; many remain chronically ill, with exacerbations and remissions of active symptoms; and others experience a course of progressive deterioration. Psychotic symptoms usually diminish over time, but negative symptoms and cognitive deficits, which are closely related to prognosis, tend to persist (APA 2013, p. 102). It is important to note that there is a bias in the DSM-5 to support its own argument, with most commentators or professional associations recognising that the recovery rate is significantly higher.

Although nurses are taught to use the mental state examination, this is especially problematic in the context of psychotic disorders. The key aspects of assessing 'insight' and 'judgement' of an individuals delegitimise the experience of the person, dismissing the possibility they may experience alternative realities. Such an approach rarely facilitates meaningful outcomes. Instead, nursing assessment should focus on principles of mutual leaning and sharing the experience of being human as described by mental health nursing theorists Joyce Travelbee (1971) and Gertude Schwing (1954). Schwing skilfully demonstrated the value of human connection and creating an environment that the person could be in human relationship, supporting the view of Blueler that 'the only treatment of schizophrenia that is to be taken seriously is the psychological one' (Schwing 1954, p. 34).

Historical anecdote 12.2: Pseudo-patients

Lack of objectivity in diagnoses related to psychosis was exposed by an experiment conducted by a group of psychologists in 1968. Led by University of Stanford psychology professor David Rosenhan and published by the journal *Science* in 1973, the experiment involved three women and five men (including Rosenhan himself) who briefly acted as pseudo-patients feigning auditory hallucinations in an attempt to gain admission to psychiatric hospitals in five different states in North America. Despite none of them really being ill, all of the pseudo-patients were admitted and diagnosed with psychiatric disorders. After admission each pseudo-patient began to act normally and informed staff that they felt fine and were no longer experiencing any further psychosis. Despite this, to be released all pseudo-patients were forced to agree they had a mental illness and to take antipsychotic drugs as a condition of discharge. The average time that the pseudo-patients were kept in hospital for treatment was 19 days. Following the experiment one of the hospitals involved challenged Rosenhan to send pseudo-patients to its facility, whom it guaranteed its staff would then detect. Rosenhan agreed and, in the following weeks, out of 193 new patients, hospital staff identified 41 people as pseudo-patients, with 19 of them receiving suspicion from at least one psychiatrist and one other staff member. In fact, Rosenhan had sent no further pseudo-patients to the hospital.

Read more about it: *Rosenhan DL 1973 On being sane in insane places. Science 179(4070): 250–8*

Therapeutic communication

Overcoming mental ill health can be intense. Like a rollercoaster ride, movement towards recovery can bring with it lots of highs and lows. As part of this process nurses may adopt a range of modes of communication in the process of delivering individual assistance including approaches such as counselling, giving feedback and teaching new thinking and coping skills. How nurses communicate with people who experience psychosis and schizophrenia-type conditions plays a vitally important role in their recovery. People with positive relationships with their nurses and other carers are more likely to experience recovery outcome (Cleary et al. 2012).

There are a number of nursing behaviours that might assist in building a therapeutic alliance such as listening empathically, validating the client's experience and engaging in a collaborative approach with the person in need of care. Working together as a team and using statements like 'we' and 'us' will help inspire collaboration. A formal or 'stiff' approach has been shown to be negatively related to effectiveness (Mårtensson et al. 2014).

Nurses have the most frequent and regular contact with people who experience psychosis and schizophrenia, their family and other support people, so nurses are in the best position to assist them with stressors, provide education and establish a therapeutic relationship. Nurses can learn effective communication strategies that will enable them better to 'be with' the person with schizophrenia or psychotic disorders. For example, the advice offered by the New Zealand Early Intervention in Psychosis Society (www.earlypsychosis.org.nz/index.php/about-psychosis/support-from-family-friends) could be useful if the person is distracted by their symptoms, experiencing difficulties with attention and concentration and/or distressed and isolated. This advice includes:

- Respect the person's privacy and autonomy.
- Keep communication and choices clear.
- Check that the person and nurse have a shared understanding about what has been said.
- Do not dismiss them, even if what they are saying sounds unusual or doesn't make sense to you.
- Recognise what the person says seems very real to them.
- Listen respectfully to what they are saying.
- Avoid arguing or getting into a debate unless safety is an issue.

At times, much of nurse's use of therapeutic communication may need to focus on the so-called negative symptoms (lack of motivation, blunted emotions, loss of drive, social withdrawal and inattention) that are major determinants of social disability. A person having experiences described as 'psychotic' usually struggles to function at a level that they might previously have achieved. Early manifestations might include poor or deteriorating school performance, poor social relations, decreased self-care and a failure to achieve expected developmental milestones. In addition to the decline in social and occupational performance common to the prodromal phase of the illness, the person may present with all or some of the symptoms listed in Table 12.1.

Cognitive behavioural interventions may be suited to some people in later stages of recovery or as maintenance when they are well. The underlying assumption behind cognitive behaviour therapy (CBT) is that people can positively influence their symptoms by changing their thinking and behaviour. Moreover, the symptoms currently experienced are the result of habits in thinking and behaviour learned in the past and have a detrimental effect in the present. The approach to therapy is therefore to unlearn the destructive ways of the past and to replace them with more constructive approaches for the future. Unlike antipsychotic medication, CBT has no adverse effects and has the potential to improve a person's quality of life long after treatment ceases.

For example, a person who hears frightening hallucinations while travelling on public transport may

TABLE 12.1 Adverse effects of antipsychotic medications and nursing interventions

ADVERSE EFFECT	NURSING INTERVENTION
Weight gain, especially with clozapine, olanzapine and chlorpromazine	Stress the importance of activity and exercise and accompany the person, if possible, to overcome lethargy. Assess current dietary intake and suggest modifications if required. Be aware not to blame the person for the challenges in managing the effects of medication.
Parkinsonian effects: blank, mask-like expression, drooling, tremor, muscle rigidity, stiffness and shuffling gait	Reassure the person that these adverse reactions subside with time. Monitor for parkinsonian effects and administer anticholinergics as prescribed and prn. Be open with the person about the limited value of additional medication in managing some side effects.
Akathisia, which may disturb both sleep and rest with the incessant urge to move the limb and to change position	Report this to the medicine prescriber, who might need to review the antipsychotic if adverse reactions cannot be tolerated. Anticholinergics might ameliorate adverse reactions.
Neuroleptic malignant syndrome, which is serious and life-threatening; usually develops quickly but could occur any time the person is taking a higher potency typical antipsychotic (e.g. haloperidol)	This is a medical emergency that literature suggests has a mortality rate between 3% and 27%, with a lowering trend since the advent of atypical antipsychotic medications (Modi et al. 2016). Symptoms are hyperthermia, severe motor rigidity, disturbances in levels of consciousness, cardiovascular functioning, blood pressure, sweating, pyrexia, hypotension, tachycardia, stupor and muscular rigidity. Cease antipsychotic immediately and refer to a medical practitioner. Nursing care consists of vigilance for the syndrome in those who are taking high-potency drugs such as haloperidol; hydration; monitoring; and reduction of body temperature.
Tardive dyskinesia (TD; 'late-occurring movement disorder'), a devastating, irreversible adverse reaction to long-term conventional antipsychotic medication (e.g. haloperidol) but less frequently atypical antipsychotics	Effects range in severity from mild to incapacitating and include: uncontrollable coarse tremor; spasm-like movements of the body, arms and legs; rolling of the tongue; and smacking of the lips. TD continues after cessation of antipsychotics and is often made worse by administering antiparkinsonian drugs such as benztropine. Refer involuntary movements to the medical practitioner to cease, lower or taper off the dose and assess.
Acute dystonic reaction (spasm) – muscle spasms in the trunk and neck (opisthotonos and torticollis); eyes can roll up uncontrollably (oculogyric crisis); life-threatening when muscles of the larynx spasm and occlude the airway	This is a medical emergency demanding swift nursing intervention. Acute dystonic reactions respond swiftly to intravenous, intramuscular or oral (route depends on the level of acuity) administration of antiparkinsonian drugs such as benztropine, followed by careful observation. In the case of laryngeal spasm, the person may require airway support and oxygen therapy until it resolves.

discover that listening to music through headphones and a portable device can drown out the voices, and no one can detect that they are talking to 'voices' if they speak into a mobile phone. In addition, the person can be encouraged to view the hallucinations as part of an illness that can be managed and that these voices are harmless. People experiencing delusional thinking can be encouraged to explore the content of these delusions.

So-labelled 'delusional' thinking may involve the belief that the neighbours are spying on them, so the person might be encouraged to modify their thinking so they view their neighbours' actions as being motivated by concern rather than malice. Getting to know and trust the neighbours could be a solution. It must be acknowledged that, because of the nature of delusional thinking, this approach may or may not be successful and, in all likelihood, success might take significant time to achieve (see Table 12.2). It should also be noted that so-labelled delusions often have an origin in real events and the risks of attempting to correct 'faulty thinking' is that we may well be denying the truth of a person and could engage the negation reflex. This is whereby a person will try to

TABLE 12.2 Nursing approaches to psychotic disorders

ISSUE	NURSING RESPONSE
Delusional thinking	• Attempt to understand the content of the delusional thinking. Delusional ideas can often provide a clue to themes occurring in the person's thinking. Consider alternative language (preferably adopting the language of the person) and acknowledge that you believe the delusions are real to the person concerned. This conveys a concerned understanding and helps develop trust. • Be authentic in acknowledging that you and the person may have different experiences and views of a situation or reality – this is not collusion but a demonstration that you accept the person's experience of reality. • Collaborate with the person to identify different aspects of the environment that may be valuable to adjust to create a safer experience for the individual.
Auditory hallucinations	• Engage with the person to understand their realities. • If the voices are suggesting certain actions, explore the resources the person has to make choices over their own actions. Voices may suggest a person takes actions that impact on personal safety – work with the person to understand that the voices may have important metaphorical meaning related to past distress and that they are distinct from the individual in terms of choice in acting on the voices. • Discuss and explore the potential value of increased support from the nurse, a peer worker or other person to manage any distress being caused by the voices. • Work with the person to identify activities that appear to stimulate hallucinations and devise ways of coping with such situations. • In partnership with the person, identify actions that reduce the impact of hallucinations such as listening to music through headphones, rituals, play or creativity. • When in acute distress, a person may value prn medication; this should be considered in collaboration with the individual.
Fear/anxiety/paranoia	• Reflect on any fear, anxiety or paranoia the person may be experiencing. • Discuss fears and experiences and consider any supports that might be of value. • Be aware of your own behaviour and how it could be misinterpreted. Ensure your approach is quietly confident and mindful of the person's need for generous personal space. • Physical contact should always be by consent and should only be considered as an approach to reassurance and support in collaboration with the person. Considering the likely presentation as a stress/trauma response will support such consideration. • Always seek to work in partnership with the person as a mutual human being.
Disordered thinking	• Spend time exploring experiences with the person. • Reflect on the impact of disordered thinking in the person's life. • In collaboration with the person, consider if medication may be useful, but be mindful not to suppress the individual's personal expression. • Consider physical activity as a mechanism for assisting the person to regain a sense of ownership over their body and personal sense of safety. • Working with the person reflect on any factors that may be increasing the feelings of unsafety.
Stress/trauma response	• Consider a stress/trauma-related response as a common reason for a person being in distress experiencing a 'psychotic' state. • Understanding what has happened, not what is wrong, is vital in collaborating on the most supportive approach from a nurse. • Consider the impact of distress of any psychotic experiences, especially on daily living and broader acute and chronic wellbeing.

convince the professional of the validity of their 'delusion' and in doing so be labelled as having increased 'delusions' (Arnold & Vakhrusheva 2016).

Sometimes family members have mixed feelings about their relative's mental disorder or, conversely, the person may have suffered abuse from a family member and would not wish that person to be involved with their treatment. Relatives and the person with schizophrenia or a psychotic illness might all have to deal with conflicting emotions, but O'Brien and Cole (2004) found that generally relatives find exclusion to be a source of stress and they would rather be included in the person's care than not. Kennedy et al. (2009) concluded that more education should be offered to carers, relatives and guardians in the early stages of psychotic disorders because the consumer might be too acutely unwell to offer meaningful feedback, and psychotic disorders are stressful for both the consumer and their support systems. Make an effort in every case to find out the help that relatives and carers want from the treating team, as well as the level of contribution they are prepared to commit, since their knowledge and resources are vital to care planning if their cooperation and involvement can be secured. Families and caregivers might benefit from education about coping strategies that work, problem solving, communication skills and the impact of medication (Andrews et al. 2014). Family psycho-education programs are both highly effective and very much underutilised (Lamberti 2001).

Psychopharmacology

Antipsychotics first began to be used during the 1950s. Depending on strength and dose they have a strong tranquilising effect, producing sedation. They are said to reduce psychotic symptoms such as hallucinations and delusions, although this is not true for many individuals. Every medication can have advantages and disadvantages. Some work faster than others; some remain in the bloodstream longer. Nurses need to make sure they understand the positives and negatives of common psychotropics and maintain open communication with consumers and prescribing clinicians regarding any concerns about medication.

In most cases it is best to adopt a 'Stay low and go slow' approach with psychotropic medication. 'Staying low' means using medication only after other approaches such as psychotherapy and social advocacy have been tried and a need for medication becomes absolutely clear. 'Go slow' refers to taking a cautious gradual approach to increasing the dose of medication as needed. When it comes time to stop medication, it is also important to withdraw from use slowly. Ideally, changes in medication dosage should be done in close consultation with a person's prescribing clinician. This should be their decision, however, because staying on psychotropic medication generally detrimentally affects a person's physical health in the long term.

The evidence to support the mechanism of action of antipsychotics and their outcomes is limited and, through a personal recovery lens, the notion of treating experiences as symptoms may well miss the hopes, meaning and dreams of the person concerned, who may prefer to live with phenomena referred to as psychosis. Additionally, any choice of medication should be made in meaningful collaboration with each individual. This has been skilfully described by psychiatrist Joanna Moncrieff (2013), who refers to a drug-based, not diagnosis-based approach that invites the person to describe the way they would like to feel if they were to take medication and avoid suggesting that the medication specifically targets 'disease', explaining that this idea cannot be objectively proven. Such an approach reflects interpersonal and ethical nursing values.

SIDE EFFECTS

People experience a wide range of negative side effects caused by antipsychotics. It is common for these medications to have peripheral nervous system side effects such as dry mouth, headaches, constipation, urinary hesitancy, photophobia, decreased lacrimation (tear production) and sexual dysfunction. Central nervous system side effects may include sedation, parkinsonian effects, akathisia and lowered seizure threshold. Other unwanted side effects include photosensitivity, retinal deterioration and hormonal interference. The most commonly experienced symptoms in schizophrenia are negative symptoms. Unfortunately, antipsychotic medications are largely ineffective against negative symptoms and can actually make them worse, giving rise to the so-called neuroleptic-induced deficit syndrome, which includes apathy, lack of initiative, indifference, blunted affect and reduced insight into their experiences (Ueda et al. 2016).

Other severe adverse reactions are acute dystonic reaction, agranulocytosis, neuroleptic malignancy syndrome and tardive dyskinesia. Acute dystonic reactions are painful muscle spasms in the face, neck, trunk, pelvis or extremities that may last for either short or long periods. Although treatable with anticholinergics and rarely life-threatening, the spasms cause substantial distress. Agranulocytosis is a potentially fatal blood disorder with prodromal signs similar to those observed in influenza. Symptoms include sudden fever, chills, sore throat, muscle weakness and sore mouth. Early recognition is essential and is facilitated through monitoring of laboratory findings. Stopping antipsychotic medication immediately is mandatory if agranulocytosis develops. Common symptoms of neuroleptic malignancy syndrome include high body temperature (fever), excessive sweating and mouth saliva, muscle stiffness, altered mental status and big swings in blood pressure. Early recognition is essential, and stopping antipsychotic medication immediately is mandatory if neuroleptic malignancy syndrome is identified. Tardive dyskinesia is a syndrome involving gross motor movements of the entire muscular system. Characteristically, the client displays hyperkinetic activity of the mouth, such as sucking/smacking of the lips and protrusion of the tongue, along with side-to-side movements of the chin. Facial grimaces, tics and spastic distortions are also evidenced. This condition usually appears in patients after long-term therapy and is irreversible.

Anticholinergic medications (also known as antiparkinsonian agents) are a group of drugs that have been found helpful to counteract the negative side effects of antipsychotics. As outlined above these can include muscle rigidity, akinesia, tremor, akathisia and a range of others. Anticholinergics work by blocking acetylcholine in neural synapses. Three common anticholinergic agents are benztropine mesylate, trihexyphenidyl and biperiden. The objective of treatment is to provide maximum relief of uncomfortable symptoms and to promote normal physical function. Unfortunately, when anticholinergics are started, many people experience dry mouth dizziness, blurred vision, nausea and increased nervousness. Other problems can include constipation, tachycardia, urinary hesitancy or retention, drowsiness, weakness, vomiting and headache. In addition, these medications can increase central nervous system stimulation, which is usually manifested by increased restlessness and agitation, disorientation, memory loss, confusion, delirium or visual hallucinations.

IATROGENESIS

The term 'iatrogenesis' refers to harm or unintended adverse outcome caused by a healthcare intervention that is not normally considered part of the natural course of the illness being treated. Modern-day health services tend to maintain biomedical approaches to mental health treatment that emphasise the use of long-term antipsychotic medication, which places nurses in a challenging position regarding administration of antipsychotic drugs. Research shows that people with lived experience of schizophrenia experience very poor physical health and have a life expectancy that is significantly shorter, living 15 years shorter than the general population (van Os & Kapur 2009). Reasons include weight gain, diabetes, metabolic syndrome and cardiovascular and pulmonary disease, which are known to be caused by long-term administration of medications administered to 'treat' schizophrenia and psychosis. With the extraordinary rates of polypharmacy and high doses in Australia and other Western nations, the risks increase. Given the substantial physical health side effects of modern psychopharmacology, avoiding antipsychotic medication may be a rational and skilful decision and one that nurses should consider before seeking to necessarily convince a person to take medication that may not have any positive effects, and may well have many negative impacts on a person's life including, for many, early death.

Table 12.1 lists what the nurse can do to help a person who is experiencing some of the more common side effects caused by antipsychotics. Chapter 19 includes a comprehensive section on antipsychotic or neuroleptic drugs, which is an excellent guide for students seeking more information. A further useful resource is, 'A critical literature review of the direct, adverse effects of neuroleptics' (Dorozenko & Martin 2017). The report provides both a literature review in academic format and guide for individuals and supporters who are prescribed antipsychotic medication.

Physical health promotion

An Australia-wide study by Morgan et al. (2014) collected data nationally from 1,642 participants with psychotic disorders to present estimates of 'treated prevalence and lifetime morbid risk of psychosis, and to describe the cognitive, physical health and substance use profiles of participants' (p. 2,163). The results were alarming, and the study concluded that people with psychotic illness needed a comprehensive, integrative recovery model to improve their health and quality of life. The investigators found that 60.8% of the participants had metabolic syndrome, 65.9% were smokers, 47.4% were obese, 32.4% were sedentary, 49.8% had a lifetime history of alcohol abuse and/or dependence and 50.8% had lifetime cannabis abuse/dependence (Morgan et al. 2014). 'People with psychosis continue to experience poor physical health, even though many of their risk factors are modifiable and despite public health campaigns aimed at these very risk factors (Morgan et al. 2014, p. 2,171).

Very similar results were found by Mitchell et al. (2013) when they conducted a meta-analysis of publications examining medical comorbidity and cardiovascular risk factors in people diagnosed with schizophrenia. The highest rates of metabolic syndrome were found in those prescribed olanzapine (Mitchell et al. 2013, p. 306). Obesity is known to be compounded by drugs such as clozapine, which can be responsible for significant weight gain (van Os & Kapur 2009). Laugharne et al. (2016) surveyed Australian psychiatrists to find out what they did to discover and treat metabolic syndrome in their patients who were prescribed antipsychotic drugs. Fewer than one-third responded; of these, 55% had no established routine to screen for metabolic syndrome and 13% said they did not know how to detect it. Fewer than 50% checked patients' weight, fasting glucose or lipids, and basic monitoring equipment was absent in 50% of cases. Nonetheless, 83% of respondents admitted a medicolegal responsibility to monitor for the condition (Laugharne et al. 2016). Other related issues are the patient's responsibility and include poor engagement in health maintenance behaviours (e.g. cancer screening and exercise), cigarette smoking and poor diet (APA 2013, p. 105).

For many people who have experienced a harsh outcome to their battle with experiences labelled as schizophrenia or psychotic illness, especially the homeless and the destitute, access to much-needed health care remains a major issue. Of those who can access mental health services, many experience difficulties arising from the often serious and debilitating adverse effects of medications required to manage their illness. Adherence with treatment is often problematic, and many choose to cease taking medication, which often results in a return to clinician perceptions of mental illness and repeated admissions. This tragic pattern is often referred to in mental health contexts as the 'revolving-door syndrome'. It is important to be aware of the contexts of revolving-door syndrome, which can include nurses (in collaboration with psychiatrists) limiting the potential for alternatives to medication and hospital. It is also important to understand nonadherence as a legitimate right of any person to the opinion of a prescriber. In people who experience psychosis, this legitimate right is often overlooked and limited by professionals who take a single-minded risk-focused perspective that has limited evidence.

Social advocacy

People who have experiences labelled as psychosis or schizophrenia often confront social challenges. These impact on issues of everyday life, which the unaffected person seems to carry out with relative ease. Impacts may include misinterpreting one's external social environment accurately, resulting in feelings of threat or peril, social isolation, poor self-esteem and challenges with expressing emotions and understanding how others accept these expressions. The role of social advocacy in supporting a person to manage impacts arising from their experience is just as important as treating symptoms and is central to any treatment. A nurse's ability to provide useful social advocacy relies on establishing a therapeutic relationship that addresses individual needs.

Work, education and socioeconomic status are key aspects of most people's lives, and those who have experiences with psychosis and or schizophrenia often suffer significant disruption and disadvantage. Lack of employment opportunities represents a form of social exclusion facing those experiencing the effects of schizophrenia. Unemployment rates are very high in people who experience psychoses, and of those who are engaged in employment, a significantly large period of time is lost to sick leave. There is a great need for research into the area of the beneficial effects of work on those who experience schizophrenia, as well as the factors that either facilitate or inhibit finding work or returning to work. Often the transition back into work is easier if voluntary work is undertaken initially. Each Australian state has disability discrimination legislation that may have a bearing on the type of assistance the workplace is required to undertake. In most cases the employer is responsible for providing a workplace that is both safe and free from adverse responses from the employer and other employees. This is often difficult given the societal stigma that a disorder such as schizophrenia carries.

Having a safe home that is conducive to a sense of security and wellbeing is an essential human need, yet this need goes unmet for a great number of people who are diagnosed with schizophrenia, a common mental illness among people who are homeless. Studies have shown that psychosis and homelessness are interrelated in several ways and intersected with trauma and adversity, gender, race and other social determinants (Grech & Raeburn 2019). Unusual realities can result in the disruption of home life and the destruction of relationships. So-called positive symptoms may affect the relationship between a person with schizophrenia who is a tenant and the owner of a property, in some cases resulting in eviction of the individual with the disorder. This is of course a form of discrimination and perpetuates stigma and lack of knowledge and awareness by the public. Negative symptoms often affect the person's ability to form and maintain attachments with others. Coupled with negative symptoms are the everyday challenges of work, which may result in failure to meet commitments associated with tenancy and housing repayments.

However, this is not the only way in which mental illness and homelessness are related. For some, mental illness develops after the person becomes homeless and is probably associated with the immense stress associated with the conditions of homelessness: frequent assaults, rapes, robberies, malnourishment, lack of support and lack of access to health services. Clearly, suffering from schizophrenia and being homeless is destructive. According to the literature, the death rate for those who find themselves in both situations is four times that of the general population and twice that of those experiencing schizophrenia but who have a home (Ayano et al. 2019). The great challenge for mental health policymakers and clinicians is to provide comprehensive health care to the homeless mentally ill and to promote access to housing and health agencies for people who are diagnosed with schizophrenia.

Relapse prevention

Longer lasting forms of psychotic disorders such as schizophrenia are usually episodic, relapsing and remitting, with periods of acute psychosis alternating with periods of relative stability. Up to 40% of all people experience a relapse of acute episode within a year of being hospitalised, so it is essential to be able to detect the early signs and triggers of a potential relapse and to support a person to finding meaningful ways to support themselves in different environments and relationships to reduce the likely re-experiencing of threat and distress. Lamberti (2001) was an early pioneer in the field of relapse prevention in schizophrenia and his work is seminal. Lamberti found that the key to relapse prevention was working closely with families and other supporters, who are often more likely than consumers to detect the onset of relapse. This approach of course needs to be collaboratively agreed with the individual.

Relapse prevention involves several steps: establishing a therapeutic relationship and ongoing education; identifying the early signs of relapse; monitoring for signs of relapse; and intervening early when or if these signs are observed. It is important to engage the person, their family and their supports in the process and to have a positive relationship to ensure accuracy and honesty (Andrews et al. 2014). Unfortunately, family and carers are often overlooked as allies in patient care. O'Brien and Cole (2004) studied an acute mental healthcare facility in Australia and found that relatives and carers expected to be included in care planning as a good source of information about the consumer but instead felt they were 'actively distanced', resented by nurses and made to feel irrelevant.

Recovery-oriented care planning

Recovery-oriented care planning is a means of avoiding, or at least reducing, coercive interventions by recording consumers' care preferences. It may take the form of an advance directive, which documents the consumer's wishes in the event of a mental health emergency (Weller 2010). Acute increased distress might require nurses to respond to crises including suicidality, severe neglect, cognitive disorganisation and other risks. Once a mental health crisis has developed, options for negotiated care become more challenging to the professional, with a greater likelihood that people will be hospitalised and treated under mental health legislation. Advance care plans are negotiated with consumers when their distress has reduced and they are able to communicate their care preferences more intentionally and skilfully.

A recovery plan might specify medication the consumer does or does not wish to receive, who should be contacted for support and what strategies have been found helpful in past crises. Consumers need to be supported in developing their recovery care plan, usually by a friend or family member. They may also wish to involve a lawyer. The plan should be discussed with the consumer's treatment team and a copy kept in the consumer's file. Nurses can assist consumers to initiate advance care plans and can advocate for advance care plans to be incorporated into the consumer's treatment plan. Nurses also need to be aware of the content of recovery care plans and of their ethical responsibility to respect the choices recorded (Coffey et al. 2017). Recovery care plans are not binding on clinicians, but every attempt should be made to provide care that is in keeping with the consumer's expressed wishes. It should also be made clear to a person developing an advance care plan that mental health legislation will be used over a care plan should a clinician make that decision, and the person does not have a legal right to refuse that decision.

NURSE'S STORY 12.1

Kay

I was 18 in the 1970s when I started psychiatric nursing at a clinic in Sydney. A friend had started her training there and she said that her job was simply to talk to people all the time; it sounded wonderful after being in an office where we weren't allowed to talk at all! The clinic was an unusually progressive place with no locked wards, and nurses were expected not to spend time in the office unless they were writing reports at the end of the day, but to be relating to the patients all throughout the day. It sounded simple: we played cards, chess, basketball or tennis, walked and went to the movies with the patients. We dispensed medications, talked, listened and built relationships. I was not an extrovert, but I had to overcome that and approach people who were alone or agitated or angry or burrowed under the bedclothes, and sometimes bluntly rejecting contact.

The most confronting patients were those who were actively psychotic because they were different from anyone I had ever encountered before. Psychotic patients were also acutely attuned to feelings, so any fearfulness or avoidance on my part would be quickly detected, and rejection, sometimes abuse, would ensue. Experienced nurses said it was not the symptoms but the underlying feelings that I needed to respond to; after all, if the person thought that they were being spied on, their thoughts were being interfered with by others, or the voices in their head were saying abusive things about them, they would probably feel vulnerable, fearful and defensive. Instead of reasoning or arguments, what they needed was humanity and consideration, and to be helped to feel more safe and secure. We call it 'reflection' and 'empathy' nowadays, and it always worked.

In our second year I was assigned my own group of patients in the day hospital. I learned to conduct large and small therapy groups, to play basketball with my group and to dispense their medications. I learned to do relaxation therapy and report my progress to expert supervisors and to learn supervision in turn. In my third year I staffed the clinic's drop-in psychiatric help centre in the local shopping centre, placed there so people who were out shopping, such as young mothers with babies, could drop in and talk about problems. I also performed crisis assessment and follow-up visits to discharged patients in the community, with the domiciliary team.

Professional relationships among the staff from the psychiatrists to the students were the most democratic and mutually helpful that I have ever known, and that equality was reflected in our relationships with the patients. Students were continuously and ungrudgingly mentored by registered nurses who taught us everything they knew: medications and how to check for compliance and side effects; how to run a group so people felt safe and supported; how to interpret devastating personal attacks as symptoms of the patient's distress; how to encourage a person to talk or just 'be with' them silently if they didn't want to interact; and how to work on different levels simultaneously and turn a card game into a comfortable, inclusive therapy session.

I believe that the most revelatory skill I learned was how to suppress the expectation that a 'conversation' should be two-way – to be receptive to confidences without being judgemental and without letting myself, my feelings, my beliefs and my needs intrude. I often reflect upon the hands-on education I received and contrast it with what we teach and students learn nowadays in universities, and some aspects of the change continue to disturb me. Nurses develop a better academic understanding but receive a narrower and shallower mental health skills base in the 'comprehensive' undergraduate education system. We delivered more holistic care, and we were more competent in the past before occupational therapists, social workers and psychologists took over many of the roles once performed by mental health nurses. Yet the consumer today is represented by recovery and consumer empowerment movements, so they at least are often better served despite a national health service that seems to accept lowered standards of care for people in the interests of economy.

Final word regarding stigma

Many people who receive a diagnosis of schizophrenia labour under the stigma associated with the illness and as a result have poor self-esteem. While medical and nursing organisations and governments attempt to demystify the illness, various media portrayals often use the term 'schizophrenic' to describe difficult and socially inappropriate behaviours that happen in the community. The term is used by the layperson as a way of conceptualising aberrant behaviour that they may not fully understand. This is a means of explaining behaviours that they find difficult or impossible to understand by any other means.

When a person is experiencing psychotic behaviour (e.g. hallucinations and delusions) in a way that affects others in the community (by being intrusive or aggressive), the media tends to sensationalise such events to titillate the public. Furthermore, Nairn (2005) analysed mass media in a study and found that few ever reported the views of those with mental illness. According to Nairn, consumers' views are seldom heard. Lee (2002) noted that even if psychiatric stigma is concealed, it remains a constant source of psychic pain to people diagnosed with schizophrenia. In the depths of their illness the person can rarely concentrate on societal norms such as appropriate dress, social etiquette and personal hygiene because of the intensity of their symptoms. In addition, some of the medications used to treat schizophrenia have unsightly adverse effects, which serve to further identify and alienate the person experiencing the illness.

The news media have an enormous influence on the way people view mental illness, and even when no harm is intended, the words 'schizophrenic', 'crazy' or 'insane' are inappropriately used as terms of description. SANE Australia maintains the Stigma Watch website (www.sane.org/services/stigmawatch), which highlights instances of mockery or vilification such as occasions on which people who have committed violent or horrible crimes are stated by news media to have a mental illness before any diagnosis has been made. SANE Australia believes that these repetitive references add to the general public's confusion and lack of clarity about mental illness.

Other social media environments seek to provide alternative understandings to reduce stigma and increase public knowledge of the disorder. 'Mad in America' (www.madinamerica.com) is an example of social media that hosts people with lived experience and clinical professionals to publish ideas and concepts and commentate on latest research and ideas. One example is an article about ISPS Australia's response to Schizophrenia Awareness Week titled 'Drop the label' (Ball 2018). ISPS Australia is the Australian chapter of ISPS International that campaigns for psychological and social approaches to schizophrenia.

Chapter summary

Psychosis and schizophrenia-related phenomena refer to experiences that are often debilitating and affect around 1% of the population. These experiences often occur early in a person's adult life and can affect perception, behaviour, mood, thinking ability and social and occupational functioning. Despite their prevalence and impact, psychosis and schizophrenia-related phenomena have yet to be fully understood. They continue to be erroneously associated with 'split personality' or 'multiple personality', and people who are diagnosed with schizophrenia or psychotic disorders are often mistrusted, feared and discriminated against. Aetiology is probably due to a melange of causes including social, environmental, psychological and biological factors; all are current focuses of research and theory development. The consumer movement has greatly influenced the ways in which the aetiology, terminology, prognosis and recovery from schizophrenia and psychotic disorders are viewed. Strong advocacy of capable consumers is necessary when the stigma of violence and dangerousness is overemphasised by a great many in society, compounding the difficulties faced by people experiencing the clinical manifestations of these illnesses.

Nurses play an important role in assisting people who experience psychosis and schizophrenia-related phenomena to recover from illness, maintain their health and achieve their optimal level of wellness. Nurses use the information gained from mental health assessment, including both subjective and objective data, to plan and implement care designed to assist people to predict and prevent relapse and to take responsibility for their own style of recovery. The great challenge to improve the lives of those who experience these illnesses is far from over. Understanding schizophrenia and psychotic disorders, the symptoms and some ways in which the people who experience such conditions can be assisted, enables the nurse to contribute to meeting this challenge.

Useful websites

Australian Government Department of Health: https://www1.health.gov.au/internet/publications/publishing.nsf/Content/mental-pubs-f-plan09-toc - mental -pubs-f-plan09-ap1.

International Hearing Voices Network:.

- http://hvna.net.au.
- http://hearingvoiceswa.org.au.
- http://voicesnsw.com.au.
- https://hearingvoicesnetworkanz.wordpress.com.
- https://hearingvoicesnetworkanz.wordpress.com/support-groups.
- www.intervoiceonline.org.

New Zealand Early Intervention in Psychosis Society: www.earlypsychosis.org.nz/index.php.

NSW Schizophrenia Fellowship: www.sfnsw.org.au.

SANE Australia: www.sane.org/mental-health-and-illness/facts-and-guides.

- StigmaWatch: www.sane.org/mental-health-and-illness/facts-and-guides/reducing-stigma.
- Discussion regarding schizophrenia: www.sane.org/mental-health-and-illness/facts-and-guides/schizophrenia.

Second Life virtual world was utilised in a study by Australian Professor Peter Yellowlees designed as an educational tool to simulate the frightening experiences of hallucinations associated with mental illness in order to develop greater understanding among non-sufferers: www.youtube.com/watch?v=P4-PUF3ScLo.

Surviving Schizophrenia is a video in which Elyn Saks, Debra Lampshire and Paris Williams, all world experts on mental health, use their personal experiences and work in their respective fields to debunk the myths and stigma surrounding schizophrenia: http://attitudelive.com/documentary/surviving-schizophrenia.

Voice hearer and psychologist Eleanor Longden talks about her journey back to mental health and makes the case that it was through learning to listen to her voices that she was able to survive: www.ted.com/talks/eleanor_longden_the_voices_in_my_head.

References

American Psychiatric Association (APA), 2015. Schizophrenia Spectrum and Other Psychotic Disorders: DSM-5 Selections. American Psychiatric Publishing, Washington DC.

American Psychiatric Association (APA), 2013. Diagnostic and Statistical Manual of Mental Disorders, fifth ed. APA, Washington DC.

Andrews, G., Dean, K., Genderson, M., et al., 2014. Management of Mental Disorders, fifth ed. Clinical Research Unit for Anxiety and Depression, University of New South Wales School of Psychiatry, Darlinghurst.

Arnold, K., Vakhrusheva, J., 2016. Resist the negation reflex: minimizing reactance in psychotherapy of delusions. Psychosis 8 (2), 166–175.

Ayano, G., Tesfaw, G., Shumet, S., 2019. The prevalence of schizophrenia and other psychotic disorders among homeless people: a systematic review and meta-analysis. BMC Psychiatry 19 (1), 370.

Ball, M., 2018. ISPS Australia's Response to Schizophrenia Awareness Week: Drop the Label! https://www.madinamerica.com/2018/05/isps-australias-response-to-schizophrenia-awareness-week-drop-the-label/. (Accessed 22 April 2019).

Boos, H., Cahn, W., van Haren, N., et al., 2011. Focal and global brain measurements in siblings of patients with schizophrenia. Schizophr. Bull. 17, 1–12.

Brown, D.W., Anda, R.F., Tiemeier, H., et al., 2009. Adverse childhood experiences and the risk of premature mortality. Am. J. Prev. Med. 37 (5), 389–396.

Burns, J.K., Tomita, A., Kapadia, A.S., 2014. Income inequality and schizophrenia: increased schizophrenia incidence in countries with high levels of income inequality. Int. J. Soc. Psychiatry 60 (2), 185–196.

Chan, K.Y., Zhao, F., Meng, S., et al., 2015. Urbanization and the prevalence of schizophrenia in China between 1990 and 2010. World Psychiatry 14 (2), 251–252.

Chong, H.Y., Teoh, S.L., Bin-Chia Wu, D., et al., 2016. Global economic burden of schizophrenia: a systematic review. Neuropsychiatr. Dis. Treat. 12, 357–373.

Cleary, M., Hunt, G.E., Horsfall, J., et al., 2012. Nurse-patient interaction in acute adult inpatient mental health units: a review and synthesis of qualitative studies. Issues Ment. Health Nurs. 33 (2), 66–79.

Coffey, M., Hannigan, B., Simpson, A. 2017. Care planning and co-ordination: imperfect solutions in a complex world. J. Psychiatr. Ment. Health Nurs. 24 (6), 333–334.

Conrad, P., Barker, K.K., 2010. The social construction of illness: key insights and policy implications. J. Health Soc. Behav. 51 (Suppl. 1), S67–S79.

Corstens, D., Escher, S., Romme, M., 2008. Accepting and working with voices: the Maastricht approach. In: Moskowitz, A., Schäfer, I., Dorahy, M.J. (Eds.), Psychosis, Trauma and Dissociation: Emerging Perspectives on Severe Psychopathology. Wiley-Blackwell, Chichester, West Sussex, pp. 319–332.

Dorozenko, K., Martin, R., 2017. A critical literature review of the direct, adverse effects of neuroleptics. In: Curtin University. Report prepared for the National Mental Health Consumer & Carer Forum. Available from: https://nmhccf.org. au/sites/default/files/docs/nmhccf_-_clr_-_web_accessible_version_-_final_-_august_2017_0.pdf. (Accessed 2 December 2017).

Fazel, S., Seewald, K., 2012. Severe mental illness in 33,588 prisoners worldwide: systematic review and meta-regression analysis. Br. J. Psychiatry 200, 364–373.

Fusar-Poli, P., de Pablo, G.S., Correll, C.U., et al., 2020. Prevention of psychosis: advances in detection, prognosis, and intervention. JAMA Psychiatry. doi: 10.1001/jamapsychiatry.2019.4779. Online ahead of print.

Grech, E., Raeburn, T., 2019. Experiences of hospitalised homeless adults and their health care providers in OECD nations: a literature review. Collegian 26, 204–211.

Hetherington, J., 2015. Peer-supported open dialogue. Ther. Today 26 (10), 26–29.

Jones, S.R., Fernyhough, C., 2007. A new look at the neural diathesis–stress model of schizophrenia: the primacy of social-evaluative and uncontrollable situations. Schizophr. Bull. 33 (5), 1171–1177.

Kazdin, A.E., Blase, S.L., 2011. Rebooting psychotherapy research and practice to reduce the burden of mental illness. Perspect. Psychol. Sci. 6 (1), 21–37.

Kennedy, M., Dornan, J., Rutledge, E., et al., 2009. Extra information about treatment is too much for the patient with psychosis. Int. J. Law Psychiatry 32, 369–376.

Khalifeh, H., Johnson, S., Howard, L., et al., 2015. Violent and non-violent crime against adults with severe mental illness. Br. J. Psychiatry 206 (4), 275–282.

Kopelowicz, A., Liberman, R.P., Wallace, C.J., 2003. Psychiatric rehabilitation for schizophrenia. Int. J. Psychol. Psychol. Ther. 3 (2), 283–298.

Lamberti, J.S., 2001. Seven keys to relapse prevention in schizophrenia. J. Psychiatr. Pract. 7 (4), 253–259.

Laugharne, J., Waterreus, A.J., Castle, D.J., et al., 2016. Screening for the metabolic syndrome in Australia: a national survey of psychiatrists' attitudes and reported practice in patients prescribed antipsychotic drugs. Australas. Psychiatry 24 (1), 62–66.

Lee, S., 2002. The stigma of schizophrenia: a transcultural problem. Curr. Opin. Psychiatry 15 (1), 37–41.

Longden, E., 2013. The voices in my head. Available: www.ted.com/talks/eleanor_longden_the_voices_in_my_head/transcript?language=en.

Mårtensson, G., Jacobsson, J.W., Engström, M., 2014. Mental health nursing staff's attitudes towards mental illness: an analysis of related factors. J. Psychiatr. Ment. Health Nurs. 21 (9), 782–788.

Mehl Madrona, L., 2015. Remapping Your Mind: The Neuroscience of Self-Transformation Through Story. Bear & Company, Rochester.

Metzl, J.M., 2010. The Protest Psychosis: How Schizophrenia Became a Black Disease. Beacon Press, Boston.

Mitchell, A.J., Vancampfort, D., Sweers, K., et al., 2013. Prevalence of metabolic syndrome and metabolic abnormalities in schizophrenia and related disorders – a systematic review and meta-analysis. Schizophr. Bull. 39 (2), 306–318.

Modi, S., Dharaiya, D., Schultz, L., et al., 2016. Neuroleptic malignant syndrome: complications, outcomes, and mortality. Neurocrit. Care 24 (1), 97–103.

Moncrieff, J., Cohen, D., Porter, S., 2013. The psychoactive effects of psychiatric medication: the elephant in the room. J. Psychoactive Drugs 45 (5), 409–415.

Morgan, V.A., McGrath, J.J., Jablensky, A., et al., 2014. Psychosis prevalence and physical, metabolic and cognitive co-morbidity: data from the second Australian national survey of psychosis. Psychol. Med. 44 (10), 2163–2176.

Nairn, R.G., Coverdale, J.H., 2005. People never see us living well: an appraisal of the personal stories about mental illness in a prospective print media sample. Aust. N. Z. J. Psychiatry 39 (4), 281–287.

Neil, A.L., Carr, V.J., Mihalopoulos, C., et al., 2014. Costs of psychosis in 2010: findings from the second Australian national survey of psychosis. Aust. N. Z. J. Psychiatry 48 (2), 169–182.

O'Brien, L., Cole, R., 2004. Mental health nursing practice in acute psychiatric close-observation areas. Int. J. Ment. Health Nurs. 13 (2), 89–99.

Porges, S., 2011. The Polyvagal Theory: Neurophysiological Foundations of Emotions, Attachment, Communication, and Self-Regulation. W. W. Norton & Company, New York.

Porter, R., 2002. Madness: A Brief History. Oxford University Press, London.

Rautanen, M., Lauerma, H., 2011. Imprisonment and diagnostic delay among male offenders with schizophrenia. Crim. Behav. Ment. Health 21 (4), 259–264.

Read, J., Fosse, R., Moskowitz, A., et al., 2014. The traumagenic neurodevelopmental model of psychosis revisited. Neuropsychiatry 4 (1), 65–79.

Reich, S.M., Pinkard, T., Davidson, H., 2008. Including history in the study of psychological and political power. J. Community Psychol. 36 (2), 173–186.

Rosenhan, D.L., 1973. On being sane in insane places. Science 179 (4070), 250–258.

Schwing, G., 1954. A Way to the Soul of the Mentally Ill. International Universities Press, New York.

Seikkula, J., Alakare, B., Aaltonen, J., 2001. Open dialogue in psychosis I: an introduction and case illustration. J. Constr. Psychol. 14 (4), 247–265.

Siegel, D., 2009. Mindsight. Scribe, Sydney.

Simeone, J.C., Ward, A.J., Rotella, P., et al., 2015. An evaluation of variation in published estimates of schizophrenia prevalence from 1990–2013: a systematic literature review. BMC Psychiatry 15, 193–207.

Stotz-Ingenlath, G., 2000. Epistemological aspects of Eugen Bleuler's conception of schizophrenia in 1911. Med. Health Care Philos. 3 (2), 153–159.

Taitimu, M., Read, J., McIntosh, T., 2018. Ngā Whakāwhitinga (standing at the crossroads): how Māori understand what Western psychiatry calls 'schizophrenia'. Transcult. Psychiatry 55 (2), 153–177.

Torgalsbøen, A., Rund, B., 2010. Maintenance of recovery from schizophrenia at 20-year follow-up: what happened? Psychiatry 73 (1), 70–83.

Travelbee, J., 1971. Interpersonal Aspects of Nursing. FA Davis. Co., Philadelphia.

Ueda, S., Sakayori, T., Omori, A., et al., 2016. Neuroleptic-induced deficit syndrome in bipolar disorder with psychosis. Neuropsychiatr. Dis. Treat. 12, 265–268.

Van Heeringen, C., Hawton, K., Williams, J.M.G., 2000. Pathways to suicide: an integrative approach. In: Hawton, K., Van Heeringen, C. (Eds.), The International Handbook on Suicide and Attempted Suicide. John Wiley & Sons, Hoboken, NJ, pp. 223–234.

van Os, J., Kapur, S., 2009. Schizophrenia. Lancet 374 (9690), 635–645.

Weisman, A., Rosales, G., Kymalainen, J., et al., 2005. Ethnicity, family cohesion, religiosity and general emotional distress in patients with schizophrenia and their relatives. J. Nerv. Ment. Dis. 193 (6), 359–368.

Weller, P., 2010. Psychiatric advance directives and human rights. Psychiatry Psych. Law 17 (2), 218–229.

Zipursky, R.B., Agid, O., 2015. Recovery, not progressive deterioration, should be the expectation in schizophrenia. World Psychiatry 14 (1), 94.

CHAPTER 13

Eating disorders

Peta Marks and Bridget Mulvey

KEY POINTS

- Eating disorders are mental illnesses associated with significant morbidity and mortality; anorexia nervosa has the highest mortality rate of any mental illness.
- Recovery is always possible, and outcomes improve with early identification, intervention and appropriate treatment.
- Many myths and stereotypes are associated with eating disorders. Nurses need to be aware of their own values, attitudes and biases that may impact on their capacity to work effectively with the person.
- Psychological distress associated with eating disorders is high; ambivalence and resistance to treatment are part of the illness and are to be expected.
- Nurses working across all clinical settings need an understanding of eating disorders because patients will present to varied clinical settings (primary care and inpatient or outpatient mental health services) with complex medical and psychiatric complications.

KEY TERMS

- Anorexia nervosa
- Binge eating disorder
- Body image disturbance
- Bulimia nervosa
- Cognitive behaviour therapy
- Family-based therapy
- Motivational interventions
- Nutritional rehabilitation
- Other specified feeding or eating disorder (OSFED)
- Psychoeducation
- Refeeding syndrome
- Specialist supportive clinical management
- Therapeutic meal support

LEARNING OUTCOMES

The material in this chapter will assist you to:

- develop an understanding of eating disorders and disordered eating behaviours, within individual, family and social contexts
- identify areas of health and wellbeing – including physical health, mental health, nutritional status, social and behavioural patterns – affected by eating disorders, and to understand the genuine struggle with ambivalence to treatment typically experienced by a person with an eating disorder
- understand the importance of a collaborative and compassionate nursing approach to positive clinical outcomes across all treatment settings and describe important aspects of nursing care for hospitalised patients with anorexia nervosa
- identify various approaches to treatment including specialist supportive clinical management, cognitive behaviour therapy, interpersonal therapy, motivational interventions, family-based therapy, psychoeducation and pharmacotherapy.

Introduction

This chapter discusses the eating disorders including anorexia nervosa, bulimia nervosa, binge eating disorder and other specified feeding or eating disorder (OSFED). Eating disorder symptoms are known to exist on a continuum from risk-taking behaviours such as disordered eating and dietary restriction, to moderately serious, higher prevalence illnesses (e.g. bulimia nervosa and binge eating disorder) to very serious relatively low prevalence disorders (e.g. anorexia nervosa).

While a person cannot be simultaneously diagnosed with anorexia nervosa, bulimia nervosa and OSFED, disordered eating behaviours can fluctuate between these illnesses over time. OSFED is a more recently defined category of eating disorder (American Psychiatric Association 2013) and, as such, has not been well described in the research literature. However, OSFED's predecessor, 'eating disorder not otherwise specified', which differed from OSFED in that it included binge eating disorder (which has now been categorised separately), was well researched, demonstrating that subclinical disorders can also have a significant impact on health, wellbeing, quality of life, morbidity and mortality (Mitchison et al. 2017).

Eating disorders are characterised by one or more seriously disturbed eating behaviours, such as food restriction or recurrent episodes of uncontrolled eating, and weight-control behaviours including self-induced vomiting, excessive exercising or the misuse of laxatives or diuretics. A person with an eating disorder is preoccupied with their weight, and their self-worth is dependent largely, or even exclusively, on their shape and weight and their ability to control them. Because of stigma and because eating disorders are often hidden, many people in the community who experience them do not seek treatment. As such, there is substantial unmet need regarding awareness and identification, diagnosis and treatment (Kornstein 2017).

Nurses across all clinical settings need to develop an evidence-based understanding of the development and maintenance of eating disorders, identifying those at risk and gaining the skills required to intervene early and to work with people towards their recovery. Educating the community, providing effective person-centred treatment and supporting better outcomes for people and their families are the focus. As with all other physical and mental health disorders, 'early recognition and timely intervention based on a developmentally appropriate, evidence-based, multidisciplinary team approach (medical, psychological & nutritional) is the ideal standard of care' (Academy for Eating Disorders 2016).

Eating disorders are among the most serious and misunderstood of all mental illnesses, with myths and stereotypes impacting significantly on those who experience them (Bannatyne & Abel 2015). Eating disorders are not lifestyle choices driven by vanity or a desire for attention. They are complex and potentially lethal illnesses that generally require long-term treatment. People with eating disorders do not bring the illness on themselves and cannot simply choose to stop dieting or change the negative self-destructive behaviours that form part of the illness. As well as having significant negative health effects, eating disorders are associated with significant quality of life impairment and impact on a person's personal, work/education and social/emotional life.

Types of eating disorders

Anorexia nervosa

Anorexia nervosa is a complex and serious mental illness that has impairment outcomes comparable to people with schizophrenia and high rates of psychiatric comorbidity, medical morbidity and mortality. Low body weight or low body mass index (BMI) is the central feature and it is characterised by intense fear (and avoidance of) weight gain or of being 'fat', which motivates persistent and severe dietary restriction and other weight loss behaviours. Anorexia nervosa usually starts in early to middle adolescence (but it can emerge at any age) and begins with dieting or restricting food that is perceived to be fattening or 'unhealthy' (e.g. 'clean eating'). This dietary restriction becomes more rigid and extreme as the illness progresses and is generally accompanied by worsening depressed mood, cognitive impairment, increasing anxiety and obsessive-compulsive features.

Common weight-loss behaviours include excluding entire food groups (e.g. carbs), excessive exercise, self-induced vomiting or purging and, less commonly, using appetite suppressants or diuretics. Young people who develop anorexia nervosa may fail to make expected weight gains or maintain normal developmental trajectories (as opposed to losing weight). If the onset of anorexia nervosa is pre-pubertal, the sequence of pubertal events will be delayed or even arrested (e.g. in girls the breasts do not develop and there is primary amenorrhoea, and in boys the genitals remain juvenile) and menstruation in women may or may not occur. In the *Diagnostic and Statistical Manual of Mental Disorders*, 5th Edition (DSM-5), BMI is used to stage severity of illness – that is, BMI < 15 kg/m^2 = extreme; BMI 15–15.99 kg/m^2 = severe; BMI 16–16.99 kg/m^2 = moderate; and BMI > 17 kg/m^2 = mild (Zipfel et al. 2015).

Consumer's story 13.1 describes the early development of an eating disorder.

People experiencing anorexia nervosa often feel that their identity becomes synonymous with the eating disorder and through the disorder they experience a sense of control over their environment or satisfaction at achieving weight-loss goals. This is despite the significant nutritional compromise and life-threatening medical complications the person experiences as a result of weight loss and malnutrition, and the often-debilitating psychological distress that accompanies the illness (Mehler & Brown

2015). There are real feelings of body weight and shape distortion, where the person feels globally overweight or focuses on particular body parts (particularly, buttocks, thighs or abdomen) as being 'too fat'. The idea of weight gain is seen as an unacceptable failure of self-control, so regardless of how underweight a person with anorexia nervosa may become (or how unwell they may be feeling), there remains an overwhelming fear of becoming fat, a desire to lose more weight and an increasing preoccupation with strategising for continued weight loss.

CONSUMER'S STORY 13.1

Rebecca

Rebecca is a 16-year-old in Year 11, living with her parents and older sister, and doing her Higher School Certificate. Rebecca has lost a significant amount of weight over the past few months by engaging in very restrictive eating and excessive exercise behaviours, but she remains at the lower healthy weight range. She was previously sporty, sociable and a high academic achiever but this year has struggled with changes to her peer group at school, as well as bullying by exclusion and having shame-inducing comments posted to her Facebook page, which has caused her to feel anxious, embarrassed, sad and very distressed at times. Her mother, a dietician, has tried to help Rebecca to eat healthily, but this has been ineffective, and she is worried her daughter has an eating disorder. When Rebecca fainted at school, her mum took her to a GP. The GP found that Rebecca had lost 8–10 kg over the preceding 2 months and was medically unstable (low body temperature, low pulse, blood pressure changes on standing and an irregular ECG) and referred her immediately to the local hospital emergency department for further assessment.

At the hospital, the triage nurse was overheard telling the doctor: *I've got a 16-year-old in bed 5 who is medically unstable for you to see. She doesn't look skinny, but apparently the GP and mother are worried she's got an eating disorder. I really don't get people who starve themselves to be beauty queens.*

LEARNING POINT

Stereotyping, stigma and discrimination can affect a practitioner's attitude and approach, which in turn impacts on a consumer's help-seeking behaviour and potentially their health outcome. It is important to share your knowledge with other health practitioners, in an effort to dispel some of the myths and stereotypes that surround eating disorders.

Bulimia nervosa

Bulimia nervosa is characterised by regular, overwhelming urges to overeat large amounts of food (binge), followed by undertaking compensatory behaviours to avoid weight gain such as self-induced vomiting, excessive exercise, food avoidance or laxative misuse. Like people with anorexia nervosa, people with bulimia nervosa overvalue their weight and shape and fear weight gain. They often experience symptoms of anxiety and depression. The word 'binge' is often used inaccurately – a 'binge' is defined as eating an excessive amount of food that is definitely larger than most individuals would eat, over a similar period of time, under similar circumstances. There is always a sense of lack of control associated with binge eating (Levinson et al. 2017).

One of the main triggers for binge eating is hunger; a cycle is often established where food is restricted during the day and binge eating behaviour occurs in the afternoon/evening. Other triggers can be interpersonal stressors, intense emotions, boredom or negative feelings related to self-worth, body weight and shape. Binge eating continues until the person is uncomfortably or painfully full and leads to feelings of guilt, self-recrimination and self-disgust. Fear of weight gain triggers vomiting or other compensatory behaviours, further reinforcing the person's poor sense of self-worth and, as they resolve to do better with 'dieting' the next day, helps maintain the bulimic cycle.

The key feature distinguishing bulimia nervosa from anorexia nervosa is weight: people with bulimia nervosa are likely to have normal or near-normal body weight. People with bulimia nervosa are less likely to require refeeding in inpatient hospitalisation; however, that is not to say that bulimia nervosa is a harmless illness. In fact, the fluid and electrolyte disturbances created by purging can create serious and potentially fatal medical problems (e.g. cardiac arrhythmias, oesophageal tears, gastric rupture) that may require treatment in hospital.

Consumer's story 13.2 describes a consumer presenting to her GP with a request for laxatives, but where the issue is disordered eating and elimination patterns.

CONSUMER'S STORY 13.2

Mandy

Mandy is a 25-year-old who presented to a new GP for a laxative prescription because her usual doctor was unavailable. She was booked in to see the nurse first because it had been some time since she'd visited a doctor. Mandy reported that she had been having problems with abdominal pain, said she was constipated and wanted to see the doctor for a stronger laxative. She had tried most over-the-counter laxatives, but they were not effective. Mandy admitted she had problems with stress, controlling her weight and managing her diet. She thought she had been suffering from food allergies – probably lactose and gluten intolerance (she avoided both in her diet). She had just started a new job, was not eating regularly and was skipping meals. She also experienced tiredness, moodiness and erratic menstrual periods. She was thin and pale but was not clinically constipated on examination.

The primary care nurse said: *Mandy, I don't see any clinical signs of constipation when I feel your tummy, so let's have a think about what else might be going on. Some people who worry about constipation say they have difficulties with their eating. Would you say that this is an issue for you?*

LEARNING POINT

Asking about disordered eating behaviours in a matter-of-fact, non-judgemental way is important for early identification and intervention. The SCOFF is a simple evidence-based screening tool that can be used in any clinical setting. It involves five simple questions:

S Do you make yourself **S**ick because you feel uncomfortably full?
C Do you worry you have lost **C**ontrol over how much you eat?
O Have you recently lost **O**ver 6 kg in a 3-month period?
F Do you believe yourself to be **F**at when others say you are too thin?
F Would you say **F**ood dominates your life?

An answer of 'yes' to two or more of these questions indicates the need for a more comprehensive assessment around eating and dieting practices. In addition, asking the two questions below has been shown to indicate a high sensitivity and specificity for bulimia nervosa (which is more common in older adolescents and young adults):

1. Are you satisfied with your eating patterns?
2. Do you ever eat in secret?

Source: Hill et al. 2010

Binge eating disorder

Binge eating disorder is the most common eating disorder and has demonstrated impacts on a person's health and quality of life. Someone with binge eating disorder experiences recurrent episodes of binge eating but without the use of compensatory behaviours. Similar to people with other eating disorders, binge eating is accompanied by a sense of lack of self-control while eating and, after a binge, marked distress (guilt, disgust) and feelings of anxiety and depression. Binge eating disorder can occur in people who are normal weight, overweight or obese. Not all people who are obese engage in binge eating, but those who do experience greater functional impairment, poorer quality of life, greater subjective distress and psychiatric comorbidity than those who do not. Nearly three-quarters of people who experience binge eating disorder have a co-occurring mental disorder – this significant psychiatric comorbidity is comparable with anorexia and bulimia nervosa (Erskine & Whiteford 2018).

Other specified feeding or eating disorder

At times, people experience eating disorders that cause clinically significant distress or impairment in important areas of functioning (e.g. social, occupational) but that do not meet the full criteria for diagnosis as an eating disorder. Examples include a person who meets all of the criteria for anorexia nervosa but whose weight is within or above the normal range, or someone who meets all the criteria for bulimia nervosa or binge eating disorder, except the criteria around frequency of binge eating or other compensatory behaviours. OSFED also includes purging disorder, where a person purges without binge eating, and night eating syndrome. The UK's National Institute for Health and Care Excellence published a guideline recommending treatment should be the same as the eating disorder the person is most closely experiencing (Riesco et al. 2018).

In addition, there are a number of eating or feeding disorders that are identified but will not be discussed in this chapter because they are not focused on body weight and shape concerns: avoidant/restrictive food intake disorder (ARFID), whereby the person restricts their eating due to a lack of interest in food, textural issues or as a response to a previously upsetting food-related experience; PICA, where the person craves and eats non-food substances such as dirt; and Rumination disorder, where the person regurgitates, re-chews and swallows food.

Incidence and prevalence

Incidence and prevalence rates for eating disorders are difficult to determine and are not known in many parts of the world (Hoek 2016). Lack of insight, denial, shame, secrecy and stigma about the disorders may contribute to this lack of data around epidemiology (Mitchison & Mond 2015) but also reflects a lack of investment in epidemiological eating disorder research.

The Australian InsideOut Institute for Eating Disorders (www.insideout.org.au) states that approximately 5% of Australians are affected by eating disorders over their lifetime – that equates to 83,500 Australians currently living with anorexia nervosa, 120,000 Australians currently living with bulimia nervosa and around 1 million Australians currently living with binge eating disorder. A large 2015 Australian population-based study found that one in six people (16.3%) had a clinical eating disorder – with atypical types more common – and adolescent cohort studies in the Australian community indicate point prevalence of all DSM-5 eating disorders may be as high as 15% in females and 3% in males (Hay et al. 2015). We also know that eating disorder behaviours such as binge eating and very restrictive eating have increased four- to fivefold over the past 20 years and in even greater rates in people who are overweight (Da Luz et al. 2017). Australia's Child and Adolescent Survey of Mental Health and Wellbeing (2012–2013) estimated 2.4% of 11–17-year-olds experience problem eating behaviours (3.5% females and 1.4% males) (Lawrence et al. 2015). While the peak age of onset of eating disorders usually occurs between 13 and 18 years, early onset prepubertal eating disorders (i.e. middle childhood) do occur (Zerwas et al. 2015). Bulimia nervosa and binge eating disorder are more likely to first occur in later adolescence or early adulthood, although people with these disorders may not present for treatment until much later in life.

Worryingly, recent Australian research found that only 13% of males and 20% of females with eating disorders (both adolescents and adults) were engaged in treatment (Thapliyal et al. 2017), which means that most people who experience an eating disorder are not diagnosed and do not receive treatment.

Eating disorders and gender

Most people who experience eating disorders are female; however, eating disorders also occur in boys and men. Eating disorders occur in pregnant women, in older adults, in lesbians, gay men and transgender and non-conforming adults, in people across all age and cultural groups and across the socioeconomic spectrum, in people with other mental health problems, in people with other physical health problems and in people who are over their most healthy weight or living in a larger body.

Eating disorders and disordered eating behaviours are increasingly occurring in males, who are underdiagnosed and under-represented in eating disorder research and clinical practice (Mitchison & Mond 2015; Zayas et al. 2018) (see Consumer's story 13.3). Some researchers state that eating disorders tend to be diagnosed earlier for males than females (Zerwas et al. 2015); however, there is population-based data showing no sex differences in age of onset (including for those under 14 years). Other research has found onset of eating disorders is later for males (Mitchison & Mond 2015). A recent review found that binge eating disorder is the most common eating disorder experienced in adult males (at almost equal prevalence as females), followed by bulimia nervosa and anorexia nervosa.

CONSUMER'S STORY 13.3

Vahid

Vahid grew up in a bigger body and always felt self-conscious and ashamed because he was fat. Teased at school, he turned to food as a coping mechanism, for comfort. By the time he was 25, he decided that he would diet and exercise, losing a significant amount of weight through extreme dietary restriction and trying to bulk up his muscles at the gym. Despite having what his friends thought of as an 'ideal' body, 28-year-old Vahid was miserable. The rigid dieting became too much and Vahid began to binge eat, in secret, especially if he'd had a few drinks at a party and his guard was down. He felt so guilty and distressed about what he'd eaten that he would sometimes vomit and sometimes just double down at the gym and not eat for a few days at a time, to avoid putting on weight. Although he thought that he probably needed help to stop the binge-purge-starve cycle that he found himself in, Vahid also felt ashamed that he had a 'girl's' problem and feared that nobody would believe him.

Significant differences may exist between males and females in terms of predisposing, precipitating and perpetuating factors for an eating disorder. For example, males who have an eating disorder are more likely to have been premorbidly mild to moderate obesity, whereas women tend to have a normal weight history but *feel* fat before losing weight; males with bulimia nervosa, binge eating or binge eating disorder are less likely to engage in vomiting or laxative abuse and more likely to use excessive exercise as a compensatory behaviour than women. Men report that anger can trigger a binge, whereas suppressing anger is a more likely trigger for women (Strother et al. 2012). Internalisation of the thin ideal, weight-based self-worth, food restriction and body dissatisfaction have been reported in lesbian women, gay men, transgender and non-conforming adults (Bell et al. 2018; Cervantes-Luna et al. 2019). And transgender youth are reported to experience increased internalisation, body surveillance, disordered eating and body shame (Wong & Lawrence 2015).

Body dysmorphic disorder (listed within the 'Obsessive compulsive and related disorders' section of DSM-5 rather than in the 'Eating disorders' section) and anorexia nervosa share a number of significant overlaps – 'sociodemographic characteristics, severity of body image concerns, level of body dissatisfaction and preoccupation, degree of perfectionism, altered experience of emotion, degree of obsessive-compulsive disorder comorbidity and deficits in body size estimation' (Phillipou et al. 2019, p. 136). And muscle dysmorphia, a subtype of body dysmorphic disorder, is widely thought to be more prevalent in males than females. It is characterised by a preoccupation with muscularity and achieving a low degree of body fat and is associated with eating disorder symptoms (like body checking, body avoidance), as well as greater psychopathology, psychosocial impairment and suicide risk than other body dysmorphic disorders.

The clinical features of eating disorders specific to males, and associated with malnutrition, include a decrease in spontaneous early morning erections and nocturnal emissions, lower testosterone levels and higher rates of alcohol dependence. However, impairment in quality of life, lost productivity and psychological distress related to eating disorders do not significantly differ between males and females (Mitchison & Mond 2015).

Historical anecdote 13.1: Eating disorders effect all genders

Descriptions of disordered eating practices can be found in ancient religious texts. Puritanical Christian groups in the 1600s promoted fasting methods for spiritual enlightenment, suggesting starvation could be used to assert control over bodily desires for purification and a more spiritual life. Interestingly, early descriptions of eating disorders rarely viewed them as conditions experienced by males. Dr William Gull, who coined the term 'anorexia nervosa' as early as 1873, described it as a condition in 'females between the ages of fifteen and twenty-three characterised by extreme emaciation'. Early treatment approaches focused on separating women who experienced anorexia nervosa from their family because they were viewed as 'thin-blooded and emotional', causing distress within the family unit. It wasn't until the aftermath of the First World War and the increasing emergence of several war-related mental health conditions such as 'shell-shock' (post-traumatic stress disorder) that mental health clinicians began to accept that 'male anorexia' was also a condition that needed attention.

Read more about it: *Zhang C 2014 What can we learn from the history of male anorexia nervosa? Journal of Eating Disorders, 2(1): 138.*

Eating disorders in children and adolescents

Children with eating disorders can get sicker more quickly than adults. Emaciation and medical complications can occur more rapidly because young people have lower energy stores and dehydrate sooner. As a result, rapid weight loss in children is more likely to result in life-threatening complications (DerMarderosian et al. 2018; Royal College of Psychiatrists 2012).

Children under 12 years of age who present with an eating disorder may present with similar psychological symptoms as adolescents and adults. However, they are less likely to report fear of fatness or weight gain, less likely to appreciate just how severe the illness is, more likely to present with non-specific symptoms, more likely to be boys and more likely to have lost weight rapidly (Hay et al. 2014). They are also less likely to vomit or abuse laxatives and more likely to be diagnosed with an unspecified feeding or eating disorder (Hay et al. 2014).

Early and more aggressive nutritional rehabilitation is needed for children and adolescents with eating disorders to prevent potentially irreversible complications affecting development, such as growth retardation, delayed pubertal maturation and irreversible and long-term effects on bone development, as well as structural and morphological changes in different organ systems (including the brain), pubertal delay/arrest and chronicity of illness (Campbell & Peebles 2014; DerMarderosian et al. 2018).

Critical thinking challenge 1

1. How would you describe a 'normal' interest in body image, eating and dieting versus an 'obsessive' interest?
2. Is your answer different for males and females?
3. Does age affect what you consider to be 'normal'?
4. Severe dieting is the single biggest risk factor for the onset of an eating disorder. There is also a focus on preventing obesity and a high incidence of dieting behaviour in the community. How might it be possible to balance these messages of risk and prevention?

Contributing factors

There are several factors that increase a person's vulnerability to developing an eating disorder. Some of these are modifiable risk factors, others are not. For example, being female, 10–25 years old and living in an industrialised society are the top three unmodifiable risk factors; genetic predisposition, a perfectionistic temperament and a history of traumatic life experiences are also unmodifiable.

Dieting, disordered eating behaviours and excessive exercise, as well as body dissatisfaction, are modifiable risk factors – variables that are potentially a focus for targeted prevention activities (McLean & Paxton 2019). In terms of risk, high-frequency (or severe) dieting is the strongest predictor for developing any eating disorder (Hilbert et al. 2014), and early onset of dieting is associated with poorer physical and mental health, more disordered eating, extreme body dissatisfaction and more frequent general health problems such as reduced bone mineral density, as well as family conflict and depressed mood in adolescents (Chung et al. 2017; Hinchcliff et al. 2016; Hohman et al. 2018).

A number of risk factors are described below. Remember, though, that most people are exposed to many of these factors and do not develop an eating disorder, so it is likely that an intricate interplay exists between the risk and protective factors, and that for each individual, the illness develops in a unique way.

Biological and genetic factors

Anorexia nervosa, bulimia nervosa and binge eating disorder are all heritable conditions influenced by genetic and environmental factors (Hoek 2016; Yilmaz et al. 2015). Recent research has identified that anorexia nervosa is a complex heritable phenotype (i.e. it has characteristics that result from interaction of genes with environment) that has significant genetic correlations with other psychiatric disorders (e.g. obsessive-compulsive disorder), with educational attainment and with multiple metabolic traits (Duncan et al. 2017; Thornton et al. 2018; Zipfel et al. 2015). First-degree relatives of people who have had anorexia nervosa are up to 11 times more likely to develop the disorder than someone from the general population and are significantly more likely to develop an eating disorder in general. Maternal eating disorders have also been linked with negative pregnancy effects (e.g. diabetes, pre-eclampsia and gestational hypertension), complications during delivery (e.g. prolonged labour, induced delivery), impacts on prenatal and neonatal growth (Watson et al. 2018) and poor respiratory outcomes (Popovic et al. 2018).

Biological sequalae that occur as a result of dietary restriction and disordered eating, or of excessive exercise, as well as weight loss associated with physical illness or the presence of an illness such as diabetes mellitus (which requires dietary restriction), also increase the risk of developing an eating disorder.

Individual psychological factors

Impaired interpersonal functioning and negative affect have been noted as risk factors for all people with eating disorders. People with anorexia nervosa commonly present with personality traits including low self-esteem, perfectionism, obsessionality, alexithymia and intimacy concerns, along with a sense of not feeling in control of their life. A range of emotion regulation difficulties are also common, including feelings of guilt, disgust and shame, avoidance and negative problem solving, comparing themselves with others and submissive behaviours, worry and rumination, and using emotional suppression to avoid conflict (Oldershaw et al. 2015).

Personality traits more common to people with bulimia nervosa include impulsivity, mood lability and self-criticism (Merlotti et al. 2013). People with bulimia nervosa or binge eating disorder may be impulsive, experience difficulty with emotional regulation and at times experience dissociation as a self-harming behaviour or even as an addictive behaviour (Haynos et al. 2017; Lavender et al. 2015). Bulimia nervosa and binge eating disorder have been associated with physical, sexual and emotional abuse, while neglect and other traumatic experiences (e.g. criticism, teasing, bullying around weight and shape, loss and grief) in childhood have all been associated with eating disorders (Caslini et al. 2016; Guillaume et al. 2017).

Social theories about eating disorders are explored in Box 13.1.

Box 13.1 Social theories about eating disorders

Cognitive behaviour theory suggests the restriction of food and other characteristic behaviours are related to the person's beliefs about weight and eating and that these beliefs reinforce the overvaluation of restrained eating, as well as the underlying body shape and weight concerns. *Sociocultural theories* of eating disorders relate to the environmental factors that impact on how people view themselves and comparisons with others, and how prevailing social norms (e.g. the thin ideal) are internalised. *Feminist theories* see eating disorders in relation to the messages women receive from society about their bodies and the relationship with success, admiration and control – and that the thin ideal is society's attempt to fight against increasing independence and power of women. From a *psychodynamic theoretical perspective*, issues of separation and autonomy, involving enmeshed relationships, as well as difficulties with the expression of anger and psychosexual development, are described (Smolak & Levine 2015).

Sociocultural and environmental influences

Sociocultural influences include unrealistically thin media (and social media) images, the stigmatisation of people who are overweight – stereotyping them as lazy and unintelligent – as well as the increasing use of cosmetic surgery by people seeking a 'perfect' body and the cultural acceptance of thinness as being more highly valued than almost any other strength or quality. Low self-esteem and concerns about appearance and body image are exacerbated for many people by this social and cultural pressure to conform to a particular 'thin' ideal of beauty. Comparing one's body with others (e.g. peers, family, famous people or Instagram 'influencers') and appearance-related bullying/teasing and 'fat shaming' are recognised as factors contributing to body dissatisfaction, dieting and symptoms of disordered eating. There is a strong and consistent association between the use of social media and body image and eating concerns in adolescents and young women, with the use of social networking sites that utilise photo-posting and 'liking' activities:

- contributing to body comparison and dissatisfaction
- driving a desire for thinness, dietary restraint and disordered eating
- reinforcing the internalisation of thinness ideals (de Vries et al. 2016; Hummel & Smith 2015; McLean et al. 2015; Sidani et al. 2016; Tiggemann & Slater 2016).

For middle-aged women, menopausal status and anxiety around ageing are also associated with body image dissatisfaction and for developing or exacerbating eating disorder symptoms (Thompson & Bardone-Cone 2019).

In recent years, pressure has been applied to the fashion, media, marketing and advertising industries to encourage the employment of models with a greater diversity of more realistic weight and body shapes. As a result, several 'real body' campaigns have been launched and promoted. The French government joined Israel, Spain and Italy in legislating against excessively underweight models working in the fashion industry. Whether these changes will impact in any way on lowering future incidence and prevalence rates of eating disorders is unknown. Given the rise and impact of social media, where unhealthy images (including those that are pro-anorexia (pro-Ana) or 'thinspiration/thinspo' and 'fitspo') and nutritional advice can be promulgated by anyone (including people who promote 'clean eating'), it would seem more likely that targeted social media literacy would make a greater impact (McLean et al. 2017).

Sports, hobbies or careers where body weight, shape and appearance are emphasised (e.g. modelling, gymnastics, body building and ballet dancing) are high-risk activities, particularly for those in the at-risk population (Treasure et al. 2010).

Interpersonal relationships

FAMILY RELATIONSHIPS

Some family factors can play a role in the genesis or maintenance of eating disorders; however, this does not mean that families are to blame for the eating disorder – there is no research that proves a causative link between family functioning and the onset of eating disorders (Schaumberg et al. 2017). Some of the family issues that will be explored in treatment may include any significant changes in parental structure, parenting and communication styles, conflict around mealtimes, modelling eating-disordered behaviours (e.g. dieting, compulsive exercise) and eating disorder attitudes (e.g. body dissatisfaction). Any issues identified during assessment or treatment will be addressed as part of treatment. Eating disorders place incredible stress on families – including impacting on their health. Families need reassurance and assistance to develop the knowledge and skills they will need to support their loved one to recover. In most instances, the person's family are the primary resource – the support and understanding they can provide are very often vital to the recovery process. Evidence shows that family involvement is useful in reducing psychological and medical morbidity, especially for children and younger adolescents but also with older adolescents and emerging adults – particularly those with a short duration of illness (less than 3 years) (Brown et al. 2016).

Historical anecdote 13.2: Jane Fonda

French doctor Pierre Janet first described people exhibiting bulimic behaviours in 1903, but it was not until 1979 that Gerald Russell published the first formal paper on bulimia nervosa. He described it as a distinct variant of anorexia. In 1987, the DSM-III-R listed bulimia as a separate disorder for the first time. Jane Fonda, a pioneer of the women's fitness and fashion industry, struggled with body image and bulimia from her early teenage years in the 1960s. Although she grew up in a physically safe home, Fonda has described emotional pressure from her father and the society she grew up in to 'look perfect'. Such pressure had a major impact on her self-concept. She battled low self-esteem and poor self-image during adolescence and her struggles soon morphed into bulimia, which she failed to finally overcome until middle age.

Read more about it: *Bosworth P 2011 Jane Fonda: the private life of a public woman. Houghton Mifflin Harcourt, Boston*

PEER AND OTHER IMPORTANT RELATIONSHIPS

Adolescence is a time when the relationships that develop within peer groups begin to overshadow the importance of family for many young people. It is important to consider the impact of all peers, including friends and connections that young people have in their online community – the increasing use of social media by young people means they are particularly vulnerable to online disinhibition (e.g. saying and doing things in an online space that they wouldn't do in person and may later regret); research has shown that overuse can have negative effects on wellbeing and mental health (Oberst et al. 2016). Access to and the impact of relationships developed in the context of the 'pro-Ana' movement, which exist across all social media platforms, are also particularly influential and potentially dangerous, where 'thinspiration tips and tricks' of weight loss are shared and the 'community' support each other to maintain focus and motivation on extreme thinness – claiming anorexia nervosa as a lifestyle choice, not an illness (Bert et al. 2016).

Peer groups that have a high level of body-related competitiveness, or where there is pressure to diet or to be thin, people of influence (e.g. a weight-focused coach or personal trainer) can reinforce the overvaluation of appearance that some young people experience and are vulnerable to. Bullying or teasing around appearance is related to shame and body dissatisfaction – this can be online or in person. Peer groups that diet together and compare body weight and shape (whether overtly or covertly) are extremely influential for young people. Body comparison is a common behaviour among young people and in social media, but it contributes to peer competition and comparison and is associated with negative outcomes (Ferguson et al. 2014). For example, we know that posting selfies, particularly where there is significant investment in taking and editing the selfie, is associated with body dissatisfaction, overvaluation of shape and weight (the internalisation of the thin ideal) and dietary restraint

(Lonergan et al. 2019; McLean et al. 2015). In the more recent 'fitspiration' and 'clean eating' movement on Instagram and other social media platforms, images of a thin, muscular body ideal are promoted, often including inspirational quotes (of which 11.3% are dysfunctional) (Tiggemann & Zaccardo 2018). Research has demonstrated that fitspo inspires people to improve fitness and eat more healthily but is also associated with significant increases in body dissatisfaction (Tiggemann & Zaccardo 2015). Almost a fifth (17.5%) of women who post on fitspiration are thought to be at risk for a clinical eating disorder (Holland & Tiggemann 2017).

Prevention and protective factors

Given the significant life impact, illness severity and treatment complexity of eating disorders, prevention is an important public health goal. Individual protective factors include good social and emotional skill development (emotional wellbeing), assertiveness, being self-directed and having a positive coping style – developing resilience. Media literacy and the ability to critically process media images are also important. Protective family factors may include family connectedness, being part of a family where the emphasis is on recognising strengths and skills unrelated to weight and appearance (rather than being weight and physical appearance focused), and a harmonious, consistent, parenting approach. One of the simplest and best protective behaviours for families, across eating disorders and a range of other mental health concerns, is to have shared family meals (Utter et al. 2017). From an environmental and sociocultural perspective, a climate where a range of body shapes and sizes are accepted, where performance is valued over physical attractiveness and where relationships (e.g. peers, teachers, community members) are supportive and caring, rather than competitive and critical, may be protective (Breithaupt et al. 2017).

Critical thinking challenge 2

1. Think about your personal body image, weight and shape perception. What do you notice about these aspects of how you view yourself?
2. What do you believe have been the major influencers on your own body image, or weight and shape perception?
3. To what extent have images in the media, including social media, affected your body image?
4. How might your own body image, weight and shape beliefs impact on how you provide nursing care and a therapeutic relationship with a person who has an eating disorder?

Signs and symptoms

Physical health

Measures of weight or BMI are not necessarily good indicators of the degree of potential medical compromise. People who lose weight rapidly can become medically compromised at higher weights than those who lose weight slowly over time, even if they are still at high BMIs. It is important to note that many potentially life-threatening medical sequelae are difficult to detect or are nondetectable with medical testing, and patients who die from medical complications of their illness often have normal laboratory test values (DerMarderosian et al. 2018).

Malnutrition affects every organ in the body, and the related medical complications can be life-threatening. Acute complications of anorexia nervosa include bradycardia and cardiac compromise, hypotension, hypothermia, electrolyte disturbance (generally associated with purging, dehydration, starvation), gastrointestinal motility disturbances, renal problems, infertility and perinatal complications. Most of the medical complications of anorexia nervosa (except osteoporosis and necrotic bowel) can be reversed with nutritional rehabilitation and maintenance of a healthy weight range. However, the long-term effect of malnutrition on cognition and brain structure and functioning requires further research (Zipfel et al. 2015).

The abnormalities seen in a person with bulimia nervosa, particularly electrolyte disturbances, are usually related to frequent vomiting or laxative and diuretic misuse. Binge eating disorder carries similar medical risks and long-term consequences to those seen in obesity, such as hypertension, high blood cholesterol, heart disease and increased risk of diabetes and stroke (Table 13.1).

Mental health

The psychological and emotional aspects of eating disorders are significant and can be devastating for the person and their family.

The underlying psychological and emotional issues that are related to the onset and maintenance of the eating disorder will be the issues that will need to be addressed over longer term treatment. Most people with eating disorders experience comorbid mental health issues; lifetime comorbidity is high, particularly with major depressive disorder, anxiety disorder, obsessive-compulsive disorder, substance abuse/dependence, post-traumatic stress disorder and personality disorder. Anxiety disorders frequently predate the onset of an eating disorder and anxiety may also develop or worsen as treatment progresses and weight is restored. It is important to remember that the cognitive and psychological effects of starvation and the symptoms of the illnesses themselves can complicate the mental health picture. For example, symptoms of depression such as low mood, irritability and social withdrawal are common in very underweight people and are the result of malnutrition. These symptoms

TABLE 13.1 Effects of malnutrition

BODY SYSTEM/ORGAN	EFFECTS
Cardiovascular effects	• Bradycardia, hypotension and cardiac arrhythmias • ECG abnormalities – prolonged QTc interval and non-specific ST segment depression or T wave changes – are associated with electrolyte disturbances and malnutrition • Cardiac arrest can result from arrhythmias • **Hospitalisation and cardiac monitoring are recommended for people presenting with bradycardia or a prolonged QTc interval on ECG (see** Fig. 13.1**)**
Electrolyte abnormalities	• Electrolyte abnormalities – including low potassium, chloride and sodium levels – in bulimia nervosa and people with anorexia nervosa who purge • Frequent vomiting can result in metabolic alkalosis and hypokalaemia, whereas laxative misuse can lead to metabolic acidosis, hyponatraemia and hypokalaemia • **Refeeding syndrome can be fatal**
Renal dysfunction	• Reduced glomerular filtration rate, elevated serum urea nitrogen and hypovolaemia can occur in both anorexia and bulimia nervosa • Reduced urine production can indicate severe dehydration or progressive renal insufficiency • Associated renal failure is sometimes seen in adult patients, especially in those whose illness has become chronic
Gastrointestinal effects	• Feeling bloated or full even after eating small amounts of food can indicate shrinking of the stomach or delayed gastric emptying • Binge eating can lead to gastric dilation and, in rare cases, stomach rupture or death • Diarrhoea can be a sign of laxative abuse; constipation can result from inadequate food (and fibre) intake, dehydration or decrease in gastric motility • Common household food supplies such as artificial sweeteners, chewing gum and diet drinks can have laxative effects • Recurrent vomiting can lead to enlarged parotid and salivary glands, oesophagitis or oesophageal or gastric tears • Abdominal pain or involuntary regurgitation of food can be associated with both the trauma and the frequency of vomiting
Endocrine effects	• Irregular menstrual periods or amenorrhoea due to chaotic eating and/or the effect of malnutrition on central regulatory structures such as the pituitary gland and the hypothalamus, in combination with decreased secretion of leptin, a hormone secreted by fat cells • Decreased serum testosterone levels and accompanying loss of libido are commonly found in underweight males • Thyroid function (in particular, T_3 levels) may be depressed in people with anorexia nervosa and is consistent with clinical findings such as dry skin and brittle hair, fatigue and cold intolerance
Musculoskeletal effects	• Osteopenia, osteoporosis and associated risk of fractures are common in long-term/severe anorexia nervosa • Irreversibly decreased bone mineral density is associated with prolonged malnutrition, low oestrogen levels and amenorrhoea for longer than 6 months, and decreased muscle mass • A dual-energy x-ray absorptiometry (DEXA) scan is generally ordered to assess bone mineral density when a woman with an eating disorder has experienced amenorrhoea for longer than 6 consecutive months • Linear growth retardation can occur in children when the onset of an eating disorder occurs before closure of the epiphyses
Dental and oral effects	• Dental erosion and subsequent cavities can occur with recurrent self-induced vomiting • Riboflavin deficiency may cause fissures of the lips, especially in the corners of the mouth, and iron and zinc deficiencies cause glossitis and loss of taste sensation
Skin/integumentary effects	• Malnutrition leads to loss of subcutaneous fat • Lanugo – a fine, downy hair that grows on the face and body – is often seen and is believed to be an adaptation to loss of body fat and it functions to help preserve body temperature • Cool hands and feet with bluish discolouration (peripheral cyanosis), calluses on the dorsum of the dominant hand due to repeated self-induced vomiting, brittle nails and dry skin are commonly seen

TABLE 13.1 Effects of malnutrition—cont'd

BODY SYSTEM/ORGAN	EFFECTS
Neurological effects	• Structural and functional changes have been reported in anorexia nervosa; some reverse with refeeding and maintenance of normal weight, while others persist beyond recovery • Structural changes in the brain including loss of brain volume, cerebral atrophy and ventricular dilation have been reported in anorexia nervosa • Reduced total white matter volume and global grey matter volume are consistently reported; grey matter volume atrophy has been reported in a range of areas of the brain including the frontal lobe (responsible for executive functions) and temporal lobe (involved in memory, language, emotion and integration of sensory information), which are both critical for flexible eating, reward and motivation
Cognitive effects	• Impaired concentration and memory • Cognitive inflexibility, characterised by perseverative, rigid, circular and inflexible thinking with significant deficits in the ability to use 'bigger picture thinking' or holistic thinking strategies • A pervasive preoccupation with food, body shape and weight-related issues, one of the core diagnostic criterion of anorexia nervosa • In children and adolescents, poor concentration can lead to difficulties keeping up with schoolwork, and special consideration should be requested from education departments for exams and assessments and amounts of classroom time may need to be tailored to the individual's stage of recovery • The profound effects on cognitive function, and in particular executive functioning, impair the person's ability to engage in psychological interventions; this impairment underscores the need for nutritional rehabilitation beyond a minimum healthy weight such that the person is able to engage in, and make effective use of, psychological interventions and, ultimately, reach physical, emotional and psychological recovery

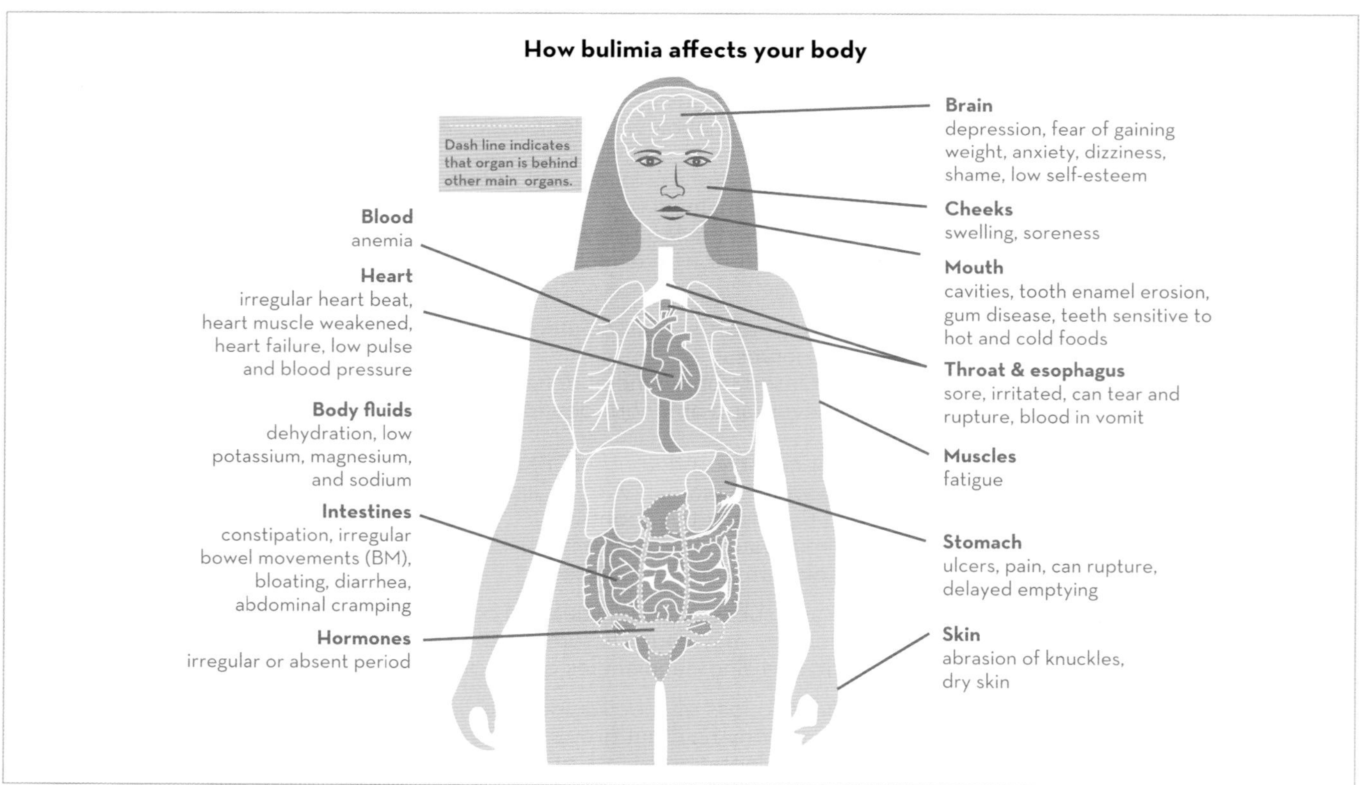

Figure 13.1
Medical complications of anorexia nervosa
Courtesy Of National Women's Health Information Center

do not necessarily warrant a separate diagnosis of major depression because they often reverse with nutritional rehabilitation.

The increased anxiety and emotional distress that accompanies treatment (requiring weight gain, normalising eating and addressing underlying psychological issues) can be harrowing for the person and their family. Supportive nursing interventions including validation, empathy, externalising the illness and working collaboratively with the person and their family are therefore very important.

Assessment

A comprehensive multidisciplinary assessment will determine whether the criteria for diagnosis of a specific eating disorder are met and identifies symptoms and behaviours that require intervention in the person's treatment program. This is also the opportunity for clinicians to establish rapport with the person and to get to know them as an individual. A collaborative approach to assessment and treatment planning is an important part of engaging the person with recovery.

Physical assessment

The physical assessment, including blood chemistry, urinalysis and ECG, helps detect any significant medical complications. It is also important to exclude other causes of weight loss. A medical examination includes weight and height measures, vital signs, cardiovascular and peripheral vascular function, metabolic status, dermatological manifestations and evidence of self-harm.

Medical complications develop at higher weights in those who lose weight rapidly and recording the history of highest and lowest weights helps assess the rapidity and course of weight loss and estimate healthy weight range for an individual. It is also useful to note any significant relationships between life events and weight loss because this gives insight into potential contributing factors that can be addressed in treatment. In adults, height and weight are used to calculate BMI (see Box 13.2), which helps determine the degree of starvation. Children and adolescents younger than 16 years of age are assessed on percentage of ideal body weight or gender-specific standardised growth charts.

Mental health assessment

A mental health assessment will confirm the specific diagnosis, identify comorbid mental illness and exclude possible differential diagnoses such as major depression, which can present as loss of appetite and weight loss, without the body image disturbance and fear of weight gain seen in eating disorders. Other aspects of the person's mental health status that influence the clinical course and outcome will be assessed, including mood and anxiety, substance use, motivation to engage with treatment, personality traits and family support (Hay et al. 2014).

Box 13.2 Calculation of body mass index

To calculate BMI, divide the person's weight (in kilograms) by their height (in metres squared). For example, an adult who is 163 cm (1.63 m) tall and weighs 55 kg would have a body mass index of 20.70, which is within the normal range. To calculate:

$$1.63 \times 1.63 = 2.656$$

$$55 \div 2.656 = \text{a BMI of } 20.70$$

An online calculator can be accessed at: www.heartfoundation.org.au/healthy-eating/Pages/bmi-calculator.aspx

BMI percentile (rather than just BMI) is used to determine expected height, weight and growth trajectories in children and teenagers (see https://www.cdc.gov/healthyweight/bmi/resultgraph.html).

A mental state assessment should be conducted and cognitive changes that may have occurred due to starvation should be identified – in particular, slowed thought processes, short-term memory impairments, changes in cognitive flexibility, difficulty with attention and poor concentration. Psychosocial factors that should be reviewed in the mental health assessment include the person's family history (including eating disorders and other mental illness in family members), attachment and developmental issues, any interpersonal problems or relationship issues that are particularly impacting on the person, as well as trauma or significant life events (Hay et al. 2014).

Denial of illness and minimisation of symptoms are common in people with anorexia nervosa and can complicate the assessment process. Parents or carers of children and adolescents are generally interviewed as part of the assessment to help validate findings and provide a family history that is helpful in identifying risk and protective factors.

Body image assessment

It is useful to understand the person's perception of their weight and to identify any significant events that might have triggered negative responses to body image, such as teasing, bullying or criticism about weight or body shape. Assessing the degree and nature of body image disturbance and fear of weight gain assists in diagnosis, in understanding the severity of the disorder and in guiding treatment. Assessment of body image has several components:

1. **Body image distortion:** a multidimensional phenomenon consisting of perceptual disturbance, cognitive-affective and behavioural components in which people describe their body or parts of it as large or fat despite concrete evidence to the contrary (Smolak & Levine 2015).

2. **Body image dissatisfaction:** a disturbance of cognition and affect that leads to a negative evaluation of physical appearance. Body image dissatisfaction may be considered 'normative' because it is highly prevalent in the general community, not just in people with eating disorders. However, this is not to say that it is harmless. Even in women without eating disorders, body image dissatisfaction is associated with significant quality of life impairment and impacts on mental health, psychosocial functioning and physical health (Mond et al. 2013).
3. **Body-related avoidance:** avoidance behaviours can be personal or situational. Avoiding confrontation with one's own body (e.g. by not looking in mirrors or avoiding taking baths where the body is clearly visible) is thought to be related to body image distortion (Vossbeck-Elsebusch et al. 2014). Body-related avoidance behaviour significantly contributes to body size overestimation. Situational avoidance involves avoiding environments or social situations that provoke anxiety about the body, like going to the beach.
4. **Body checking behaviours** such as feeling bones, weighing oneself many times a day, checking the body's silhouette in the mirror, or only looking at one part of the body, may also be assessed.

Simple questions that can provide insight into the person's body image include:

- 'When I look at you, I can see that you are very thin. How do you see yourself?'
- 'People often *feel* fat, even when they are not. How do you feel about your body?'
- 'Some people weigh themselves many times a day. Do you do this?'
- 'When you look in the mirror, do you focus on one particular part of your body or look at your body as a whole?'
- 'What weight do you think is the right weight for you? What weight would you like to be?'

Suicide assessment

People with eating disorders are at risk of suicide and self-harm, with some disorders conferring more risk than others. In particular, anorexia nervosa is associated with high rates of death by suicide (Bodell et al. 2019), and about 20% of people with anorexia nervosa engage in non-suicidal self-injury (Bodell et al. 2019; Davico et al. 2019). Self-injurious behaviours are also common in people with other eating disorders: they are more frequent in adolescents, those with comorbid mental health problems and those whose eating disorder includes binge and purge symptoms (Kostro et al. 2014). Asking the person about suicidal ideation and active self-harm is important. Questions like, 'Have things been so bad with the eating that you have wanted to harm yourself in any way?' will not trigger the person towards suicidal or self-harm behaviours. More likely, the person will be relieved to know that someone understands how severe the disorder has become and how bad they are feeling. Nurses need to respond to all expressions of suicidality in this very high-risk group. See Chapter 7 for further information on suicide assessment.

Nutritional and exercise assessment

A dietary history is used to identify specific deficiencies and should include information about the person's nutritional (food and fluid) intake, as well as any behaviours designed to reduce or control appetite (e.g. caffeine, smoking), alcohol use, use of supplements (e.g. vitamins, herbal preparations) and frequency of self-measurement of weight. Energy input and output are assessed, including the amount and types of food eaten and avoided, and the degree of any compensatory behaviours including over-exercising, bingeing and purging used to control weight gain. Many people with eating disorders avoid whole food groups (typically meat protein, dairy products and/or carbohydrates). Because of the person's beliefs about uncontrollable weight gain, some foods can be considered 'fear foods'.

Excessive exercise is estimated to occur in 30–80% of people with eating disorders (Renz et al. 2017), more commonly in those with anorexia than bulimia nervosa (Dittmer et al. 2018). It can be used as a compensatory behaviour to avoid weight gain, or as a weight loss mechanism. Excessive exercise can be identified where a person experiences negative emotionality (e.g. intense guilt) when exercise is missed or postponed, or where hard exercise is focused primarily on influencing weight or shape (instead of on enjoyment). Asking people what the goal of their exercise is will help determine if it is excessive and associated with the eating disorder and help develop a graded approach to return to exercise during nutritional and psychological recovery (Dobinson et al. 2019).

Assessing disordered eating behaviours and rituals

Disordered eating behaviours are driven by fear of weight gain. In inpatient settings, nurses can assess the extent of the person's struggle with food when observing mealtime behaviours. Box 13.3 provides examples of some frequently observed eating disorder behaviours.

People with eating disorders sometimes utilise excessive amounts of some condiments or foods that they perceive may be of benefit in terms of weight loss. Large quantities of fluid can help suppress hunger, and it is not unusual for a person with an eating disorder to drink copious amounts of fluid if they perceive this as helpful in avoiding weight gain. Drinking just prior to being weighed (water loading) may occur in an attempt to give the impression of weight gain.

Box 13.3 Examples of eating disorder behaviours

- Refusing to eat
- Cutting out particular foods (e.g. cake, cheese, chocolate) or whole food groups (e.g. carbohydrates, fats, proteins)
- Cutting up food into tiny pieces and then eating the pieces individually, or by colour, or in groups of numbers (e.g. two peas followed by two pieces of carrot)
- Attempting to remove any oil and fats from food (e.g. pressing food into absorbent serviettes and scraping butter from sandwiches)
- Restricting foods so as to eat the same thing every day
- Fear of touching food or having different food groups touch on the plate
- Eating painfully slowly and without enjoyment
- Constantly fidgeting at the table – this could be related to anxiety or to the physical hyperactivity that can be activated by starvation
- Obsessive kilojoule counting and/or measuring of all food quantities
- Leaving the table during or immediately after the meal to purge or throw away food hidden during the meal
- Excessive use of diet foods or diet products
- Excessive preoccupation with the preparation and serving of food to others, but not eating it
- Avoiding eating with others in a social context
- Binge eating (eating more than someone else would eating within a specific period of time)
- Using compensatory behaviours such as vomiting, laxatives or excessive exercise to 'earn' food

People with bulimia nervosa commonly skip breakfast and lunch and then binge eat at night in response to the body's hunger signals. Bingeing can be spontaneous or planned, and it can occur in a ritualistic manner; for example, the binge may occur at the same time and place every day, or it may only happen on certain nights of the week when there is no one else around, or the binge may progress with foods in a particular order. It can cause great anxiety to a person if their planned binge episode is prevented or interrupted, or events outside their control impact on them carrying out the ritual. Some people with bulimia will, over time, choose food that is easily regurgitated or food that is economical if they cannot finance their binges (which can be very expensive). A binge episode is usually terminated in response to abdominal fullness, distension and pain, running out of food and/or social interruptions.

Self-induced vomiting usually follows a binge episode, and techniques used to induce vomiting include putting the fingers or another implement like a toothbrush down the throat, or regurgitation after eating may be spontaneous. Signs that vomiting may be occurring in people with anorexia nervosa include weight loss or no weight gain despite apparent adherence to a prescribed nutritional program, leaving the dining table immediately after a meal to go to the shower or toilet, or the smell or presence of vomit in the toilet, sink or shower. Low potassium or raised amylase can indicate purging.

Diuretics cause fluid loss and laxatives work on the large bowel – after most of the nutrients from food have already been absorbed in the small intestine (Kiela et al. 2016).

It is important for nurses to approach discussing disordered eating behaviours and rituals sensitively and in a curious and non-judgemental way. The person may be deeply embarrassed by some of their behaviours, which they may perceive as disgusting; they may also be protective of the behaviours as part of the disorder or worried that they will be forced to change what they are doing immediately, causing massive weight gain. Asking questions about disordered eating behaviours can be made less threatening by using statements that indicate that other people also experience similar issues; for example, 'Many people who experience an eating disorder do things that they feel help them to control their eating or weight, like vomiting or using other ways of getting rid of food. Has this ever been something that you have tried?'

Family assessment

When undertaking a family assessment, it is important to assess the quality of family relationships, the level of support available within the family, the way family members communicate with each other, family attitudes towards eating and appearance, and the effect the eating disorder has on family and social relationships. A family history of eating disorder, mental illness or substance use may have implications for treatment. During the assessment, be mindful that many families and carers are emotionally exhausted by their own struggle to help their family member to manage the eating disorder, and that feelings of guilt, failure, anger, blame and fear are common. Feeling blamed is harmful and could impair the desire, willingness and capacity to participate actively and constructively in the process of treatment and recovery, so it is important to convey a warm, encouraging, non-judgemental and collaborative approach.

While family involvement is strongly encouraged, confidentiality issues must be considered for both adolescents and adults, and these should be clearly discussed during the assessment period. The decision to involve families, spouses and/or partners of adult patients should be made in consultation with the patient.

The importance of the nurse's role in supporting families through the treatment process cannot be overstated. At the family assessment stage, providing information around the eating disorder and helping family members to understand the challenges and opportunities that are associated with the disorder can be useful.

Interventions

Recovery from an eating disorder is always possible and should be the goal. The illness duration can range from less than a year in children and adolescents who are identified and treated early, to a long-term illness, with remission and relapse of symptoms occurring.

Treating people with eating disorders occurs in primary care, outpatient and day patient programs and inpatient care in medical, paediatric or mental health settings. Determining the most appropriate treatment service will depend on the person's age and their physical and mental health, as well as the availability of expert local healthcare providers. A multidisciplinary team approach is needed as medical and nursing care, nutritional rehabilitation, psychological therapy and, particularly in children and adolescents, family-based therapy are all integral parts of treatment. The priorities for treating someone with an eating disorder, regardless of the practice setting, includes:

- engaging with the person using a non-judgemental, inclusive, empathic and curious approach
- engaging with the person's family and enlisting their support in appealing to the 'healthy' part of their loved one
- conducting a thorough assessment as outlined above
- providing information about normal eating (including healthy nutrition and eating patterns) and supporting the person to establish regular eating, which reverses the cognitive effects of starvation
- monitoring medical stability and responding to medical complications
- providing structured psychological treatment, including support and psychoeducation, building the therapeutic relationship in the first instance, and later, when the person is sufficiently stabilised from a medical/nutritional/cognitive perspective in terms of the effects of starvation, individualised therapy (Hay et al. 2014).

People with binge eating disorder are generally treated in a community setting through primary care. The aims of treatment include normalising eating patterns, reducing or eliminating binge episodes, stabilising weight within a healthy weight range, effectively treating any underlying psychopathology and preventing relapse.

Hospitalisation

People with an eating disorder are generally admitted to hospital when they require nursing care. They may be at imminent risk of serious medical sequelae or complications of the illness, they may be experiencing significant mental health symptoms associated with the illness, or outpatient treatment may not be working (Hay et al. 2014).

People with anorexia nervosa or OSFED are more likely to become medically compromised and require hospitalisation than those with bulimia nervosa. Indicators for admission include medical instability, significant risk of self-harm or suicide, psychiatric symptoms (severe low mood, suicidality, psychosis) and severe family dysfunction or abusive relationships. Compulsory treatment may be used where necessary. All nurses should be aware of the local policies related to admission for people with eating disorders.

Treating someone in a hospital setting includes:

- safely refeeding the person – avoiding refeeding syndrome (see later in the chapter) and underfeeding
- reducing and eliminating (where possible) binge eating and purging behaviours
- medical stabilisation and treating physical complications
- supporting and enhancing the person's ability to restore healthy eating patterns and engage fully with treatment
- helping the person to assess and address the psychological aspects of the illness (including their thoughts, feelings, attitudes, beliefs, motives, conflicts)
- treating a co-occurring mental health issue, including anxiety or mood disorder, and addressing issues such as impulse control, emotion regulation and other self-esteem and behavioural issues that contribute to maintaining the illness
- discharge treatment planning that involves psychological therapy, regular monitoring by a GP and dietetic support
- engaging with the person's family or significant others to enlist their support
- providing psychoeducation, family therapy or individual counselling where possible and appropriate.

In public hospitals in Australia and New Zealand, inpatient admission generally consists of either a short-term admission for medical stabilisation or a longer admission for weight restoration and normalisation of eating. Restoration of weight to a minimum healthy BMI is recommended because this facilitates the person's ability to cognitively engage in ongoing outpatient psychotherapy. A brief admission for 24–48 hours for medical stabilisation only is not conducive to recovery and may be likely to result in rapid readmission with the person in a worse physical or psychological condition. A longer admission to a medical or paediatric unit in a general hospital for medical stabilisation and initiation of nutritional rehabilitation does occur, both in Australia and New Zealand. Ideally, this should include meal support and psychological support from consultation-liaison mental health nurses as well as dietetic and psychiatric support.

Specialist inpatient programs aim to provide a structured yet nurturing environment that includes behavioural modification strategies targeted towards weight gain and challenging and addressing abnormal eating behaviours. Behavioural programs are usually based on an activity 'level system', through which the patient progresses as they are nutritionally rehabilitated. These programs usually incorporate strict bed rest while the person is physically compromised, ambulation on then off the ward and then increasing the time out of hospital to practise normal eating behaviours in the home and community environment. When the person is medically stable, increasing levels of supervised activity/physiotherapy, including stretching and strengthening exercises, help the person to regain muscle and bone health. For children and adolescents, ongoing school education during hospitalisation is incorporated into the inpatient program whenever possible.

It is essential to have realistic expectations and clear goals for the admission. It is important for everyone to understand that hospitalisation is just one part of the recovery process: no one leaves hospital 'cured' from an eating disorder – recovery can be a long process involving ongoing weight restoration, normalisation of eating patterns and talking therapy. Ideally, when someone leaves hospital, they will be medically stable, on the way towards weight restoration and, as a result, have a greater cognitive capacity to engage effectively with a psychotherapeutic intervention, be that individual or family-based (or both).

Like any mental illness, recovery from an eating disorder is a challenging personal journey that takes time and courage. It requires self-knowledge, self-compassion and the support of friends, family and health professionals. Return of symptoms and multiple admissions to hospital are not uncommon (see Consumer's story 13.4). To avoid the person feeling defeated and like a failure, or becoming helpless and institutionalised after several admissions, it is particularly important that every hospitalisation involves collaboratively developing a plan for the admission that includes clearly defined goals. Nurses also need to be mindful of their approach and how important this is to how a person feels about the admission and what they can achieve. Nurses need to be aware of any attitudes, beliefs or values that they hold that may impact on (or impair) their clinical efficacy.

CONSUMER'S STORY 13.4
Lizzie

Lizzie is a 24-year-old woman who has been admitted to the acute mental health unit for the third time in 18 months. She has a 10-year history of anorexia nervosa and, although she has spent most of the last 10 years out of hospital and has completed her university studies, she has not been able to achieve a healthy weight since she was first diagnosed. Lizzie has been having individual psychotherapy on and off for the past 5 years and is estranged from her family. Two years ago Lizzie was sexually assaulted one night on the way home from the library. She has been extremely unwell since that time.

Lizzie is admitted, having lost all the weight she put on at the last hospital admission. She is very medically compromised, tearful, defeated and psychologically unwell, requiring one-to-one nursing care. She struggles desperately with the eating disorder and, by her own admission, hides food, tampers with the nasogastric tube (even though she has agreed to have it inserted) and exercises in secret when she gets an opportunity. Lizzie says that she wants to recover and feels like nobody can help her.

NURSING RESPONSE OPTION 1

The staff roll their eyes when they hear that Lizzie is back. 'What a surprise ... She's never going to get better. I don't know why we bother! I don't know why she bothers! She's such a difficult patient. What a waste of a bed. Don't give her to me – I just don't get it'.

NURSING RESPONSE OPTION 2

The nursing staff in the handover empathise with Lizzie's struggle. They know how difficult Lizzie is finding recovery; they are cognisant of the trauma she has experienced and the toll the illness is taking on her physical and mental health. They understand that recovery from anorexia nervosa can be a long-term process. They are keen to know why the discharge plan didn't adequately support Lizzie to maintain her weight after discharge. They are determined to support Lizzie to pick up the pieces and they hold hope for her recovery. 'Lizzie must be feeling so defeated being back here so soon. I wonder what happened when she left here last time?'

REFLECTION

1. What do you envisage might be the impact on Lizzie of the two different nursing responses outlined above?
2. How would you respond to staff who were expressing the type of response seen in option 2?

Nursing care of people who are medically unstable

Nurses working with people who have severe and complex eating disorders and who are medically unstable require both medical and mental health knowledge and skills. Medical resuscitation and stabilisation of any medical instability always take priority if the patient has been admitted to hospital with life-threatening complications. If the patient is bradycardic on admission, continuous cardiac monitoring and daily 12-lead ECGs are recommended. Four-hourly vital sign measures including heart rate, temperature and blood pressure are recorded until normal readings are sustained for at least a minimum of 72 hours. Overnight vital sign measurements and blood sugar levels, taken when the body is most at rest, provide invaluable insight into the body's ability to maintain homeostasis. Nasogastric feeds administered either continuously or overnight are vital in reversing medical instability when patients are unable to consume enough kilojoules orally.

Examples of nursing responsibilities in this situation include:

- monitoring the patient's physical safety
- documenting vital signs and acting as per local protocols when vital signs indicate medical instability – every service treating people with eating disorders needs to have clear guidelines for managing medical instability
- empathising with any distress the person expresses and validating their experience

- initiating and encouraging the prescribed refeeding process
- inserting and ensuring the patency of any nasogastric tubes and acting to prevent the patient from tampering with feeds
- documenting nutritional intake
- monitoring for clinical signs of refeeding syndrome
- observing for and managing challenging behaviours such as covert exercise, weight manipulation, vomiting, hiding food in an empathic and supportive way
- talking with the person about their emotional response to admission and providing therapeutic support and psychoeducation to help contain the anxiety and distress of both the patient and their family
- administering prescribed medication.

Psychological and emotional care of the person requires that nurses:

- understand that eating disorder behaviours are driven by fear of weight gain and overwhelming anxiety
- work with the person and their family to develop skills to contain anxiety and distress
- facilitate and encourage motivation to change, rather than imposing or enforcing behavioural change – getting to know the person, their plans for the future, hopes, dreams and desires will help them (and you) to see the bigger picture
- provide supportive meal supervision designed to achieve nutritional rehabilitation, normalised eating behaviours and reduction in compensatory behaviours
- consistently adhere to the plan of care
- ensuring all limits set have a clear and transparent purpose and are discussed with the person at the outset
- attend multidisciplinary case reviews to contribute to treatment planning.

REFEEDING SYNDROME

Refeeding syndrome is a rare but potentially fatal complication that can occur in the first 1–2 weeks of commencing refeeding for people who are severely malnourished. It is important for nurses in all clinical settings to be vigilant for the signs and symptoms of refeeding syndrome, which is a medical emergency that can be variable, unpredictable and may occur without warning.

Refeeding syndrome involves disturbances in insulin and serum electrolytes, specifically changes in phosphate, potassium and magnesium, vitamin deficiencies and sodium and fluid retention. If serum phosphate levels drop significantly, especially during the first week of refeeding, this can cause cardiac, neurological and haematological complications and sudden death. Electrolyte abnormalities should be monitored daily until they have stabilised within normal ranges.

People with eating disorders who are particularly at risk of refeeding syndrome include those who have:

- severe malnutrition, particularly where it has been prolonged
- rapid weight loss greater than 1 kg per week over several weeks
- a very low BMI (less than 14, although the syndrome has been reported in patients with a normal BMI)
- abnormal electrolytes prior to refeeding
- a history of severe dietary restraint or not eating for a week or more
- vomiting, laxative misuse or bingeing
- concurrent medical conditions such as diabetes, infection or major organ failure (Royal College of Psychiatrists 2012).

During the first 1–2 weeks of refeeding, nurses monitor for clinical signs of refeeding syndrome (confusion, delirium or other mental status changes, seizures, cardiac arrhythmias, fluid retention and oedema) and ensure prophylactic phosphate and vitamin and mineral supplements are administered. If signs of refeeding syndrome become evident, urgent medical consultation should be sought to normalise electrolyte levels and prevent cardiovascular and other organ system failure and death. Prophylactic phosphate supplements, carefully prescribed rates of refeeding and daily monitoring of electrolyte levels during the first 1–2 weeks of starting refeeding minimise the risk of a patient developing refeeding syndrome. Ideally, the patient will ultimately obtain all their vitamin and mineral requirements through food, but initially vitamin and mineral supplements are routinely prescribed.

Therapeutic relationships

Effective nursing management requires developing a therapeutic alliance *with* the person and *against* the eating disorder. Without this, it is likely that the person will see the eating disorder as their ally or their only friend and feel that their parents, friends and health practitioners are all against them. The therapeutic alliance is enhanced by validating the person's experience ('recovery is really hard'), empathetic discussion, consistent positive regard, reassurance, motivational enhancement and supporting the person to develop new insights and accept change. Nurse's story 13.1 describes the experience of providing nursing care for adolescents with anorexia nervosa.

Positive regard for the person can be displayed by 'externalising' the eating-disordered thoughts and behaviours as separate from the person; for example, 'Is *the anorexia* making it really difficult for you to eat today?', 'I know it's hard for you to eat when *the anorexia* is telling you not to. How can I best help you to fight *those eating disorder* thoughts'? Putting this distance between the illness and the person is a very important first step towards helping the person see that the things they value (e.g. health, friendships, doing well at school, having a great career) are incompatible with the long-term maintenance of an eating disorder. It is also very useful for families to learn to identify and externalise the person's disordered eating thoughts and behaviours as part of their illness rather than as wilful behaviour on the part of their child or family member.

Unless a particular situation is life-threatening, confrontation and invasion of privacy (e.g. observing a patient in the bathroom) are generally unnecessary and are destructive for both developing therapeutic relationships and for promoting the person's self-responsibility and motivation for change. Even if these behaviours are necessary, it is possible to address them in a collaborative (rather than demoralising) way and to provide choice wherever possible. For example, 'Lucy, I know that you find it difficult to resist the eating disorder when it demands you exercise in the shower. I'd like to help you regain control of that. Let's look at the options ...'

Food avoidance and the use of compensatory behaviours will be reflected to a great extent in the person's pattern of weight gain (and in their blood and urine test results). Generally, if they fail to gain the expected amount of weight each week in hospital, they have either restricted their oral intake or participated in compensatory behaviours. Invading privacy or engaging in confrontation will result in an angry eating-disordered response rather than encouraging positive growth and motivation for change. The following statement is an example of a comment that would lead to an angry eating disordered response: 'Lucy, it's pretty clear by your weight loss that you've been cheating on the program. You're never going to get out of here if that's your approach.' Taking control of eating and ceasing compensatory behaviours are ultimately the responsibility of the patient. The goal for nurses is therefore not to enforce change but to gradually encourage the person's motivation to change by exploring and challenging their individual perspective on, and experience of, their disordered eating behaviours. For example: 'Lucy, your weight has gone down today and I'm wondering if we can talk about that? Usually, weight loss is either from not eating enough, or from exercising or vomiting. I'm wondering if you have felt so bad in the last few days, or so pushed around by the eating disorder, that you've been doing any of those things?'

Younger children, however, may need a more directive approach than adolescents and adults, especially when they have not yet developed abstract thought processes. For example: 'Jenny, your weight has gone down and we need to sort that out ... because to get better, you need to get back into a healthy weight range. I've noticed you haven't been finishing all your meals. You need to do that to get better. How can we help you to make sure that you finish all your meals?'

NURSE'S STORY 13.1

Gail

When I first started working with adolescents who have anorexia nervosa, I was scared that I would say or do the wrong thing. As a paediatric nurse, I didn't understand the complexity of the illness or why it was so difficult for them to eat normally and maintain a healthy weight.

Previously, I had always tried to meet my patients' needs and advocate for them, but I could see that if I supported the disordered eating behaviours, I would collude with the illness and the person would only lose more weight. When I first tried to talk to them about the behaviours, they would lie to me or get angry, and I initially found this hard to understand and quite frustrating.

Luckily, I work with a great team and was able to learn 'on the job'. My senior nursing colleagues spent a lot of time teaching me about the illness and about how the behaviours I was seeing were not directed at me personally, but rather reflected the strength of the anorexic thoughts and the person's overwhelming fear of change.

I realised that I wasn't responsible for making the person gain weight. Rather, I tried to understand what it was like for them to experience the illness, work collaboratively with them to see the illness for what it is, and help them to increase their motivation and capacity to recover. I soon found that by taking a different approach, I could encourage patients to better manage their fears and start taking responsibility for making small but positive changes in their behaviours.

Now that I understand just how difficult it is for people who experience eating disorders to change, I am better able to support them in managing their anxiety, I am better at working collaboratively and I am able to gain the person's trust so they communicate honestly with me.

Along with a greater understanding of people who experience eating disorders came a sense of confidence in my role as a nurse and a feeling of satisfaction with my job, rather than frustration. I enjoy my work with these young people now and feel that I am making a positive difference in their lives.

Nutritional rehabilitation, normalising eating patterns and meal support

The cornerstones of nutritional treatment are education, meal planning, establishing regular eating patterns and discouraging dieting. Everyone with an eating disorder will be fearful of weight gain, particularly in the early stages of treatment, where regular eating is initiated, and often there is heightened distress as a person approaches weight milestones. Psychoeducation about the effects of extreme dietary restriction/starvation, bingeing, purging, disordered eating and the need to reverse these is important.

Depending on the treatment setting and the type of eating disorder, a meal plan designed to achieve a prescribed weekly weight gain or to normalise eating behaviours should be developed. The meal plan will be individualised and takes into consideration the person's tastes, their cultural background, their physical needs and their clinical picture. It will also identify portion sizes and gradually introduce foods that have been avoided. The aim is that the diet will include all the food groups and that fear foods have been habituated, with nursing staff providing reassurance and encouragement and validating how difficult the recovery process can feel.

For those who are struggling with their intake, nutritional supplementation may be required. These are given either as a drink or via a nasogastric tube, which is usually considered when the person is medically compromised and is not able to eat enough food to reverse the medical complications and achieve adequate nutritional rehabilitation. When initiated, nasogastric feeds should initially be given slowly enough so as not to cause refeeding syndrome, but not so slowly as to underfeed the person. Continuous feeding over a 24-hour period helps to avoid low blood sugar levels from the effects of delayed insulin phase and metabolic changes and the supplemental feed should restrict the percentage of daily energy provided by carbohydrate to help mitigate against the risk of refeeding syndrome (Madden et al. 2015).

People's reactions to nasogastric feeds are varied. Some express relief that they do not have to eat what they perceive to be enormous amounts of food required for weight gain and view positively the fact that the initial responsibility for weight gain has been taken away from them. Others struggle with the invasive nature of the tube and the lack of control they feel they have over their nutritional intake. 'Nasogastric feeding is less likely to be perceived negatively if the procedure has been fully explained, demystified and medicalised' (Robinson & Nicholls 2015, p. 22). Regardless of how they are delivered, nutritional supplements are given for the shortest possible time – ultimately, the person needs to relearn how to eat food normally – and so the goal is always transition to an oral meal plan as soon as possible. Transition to a full oral diet including three meals and three snacks needs to occur before discharge.

Supporting the person to cope with the distressing thoughts that accompany nutritional rehabilitation is an important role for nurses. This will include helping the person to develop a range of strategies that help – for example, distraction, cognitive challenging and mindfulness. In inpatient settings, nurses can help by providing therapeutic meal support, having clear boundaries around expected mealtime behaviours and acting as a role model for healthy eating behaviour. The goals of meal support are to help the person to normalise their eating behaviours, begin the process of weight gain or at least ensure weight maintenance, reintroduce the concept of eating as a pleasant social experience, assist the person to address and decrease food rituals, and increase their ability and confidence in making healthy food choices and eating a 'normal' amount.

THE 3-HOUR RULE

People who have eating disorders need to understand that if they undereat or restrict their food intake, have lost an understanding of hunger and satiety, or engage in non-hungry eating, then working to establish a regular eating pattern and introducing the 3-hour rule will be important. The 3-hour rule simply means eating something every 3 hours and eliminating dieting. Since hunger is the primary trigger for binge eating, maintaining consistent intake is the first step in ceasing binge/purge behaviours. Establishing a pattern of eating something every 3 hours often creates anxiety and fear of rapid, uncontrolled weight gain in many patients. Nurses need to reassure the person that research and clinical experience demonstrate that this does not occur, and that in fact, the body's metabolism increases with regular eating.

MONITORING INTAKE AND WEIGHT GAIN

Monitoring dietary intake is an important tool that helps identify food/eating patterns and gives the person and the team an overview of what and how much the person is really eating. In hospital, monitoring will generally be done by the nursing staff, but the person may also do this themselves, provided the record is accurate.

Monitoring the person's thoughts and feelings in response to their dietary intake can also be a helpful tool for nurses and other health professionals to review with them. These forms (or online tools) ask the person to identify their thoughts and feelings in association with their eating or restricting behaviours, exposing how the person responds to emotions like guilt, anger and sadness through their intake, and identifying how the eating disorder bullies them into behaving in a certain way. The Recovery Record App also enables the primary therapist to prescribe evidence-based strategies to help the person manage these responses, and to observe intake in real time.

As weight restoration (or partial weight restoration) is the primary goal of treatment for someone who has anorexia nervosa or who is underweight, and demonstrating that regular eating does not necessarily lead to weight gain as a person with bulimia nervosa or binge eating disorder may fear, weight needs to be regularly and accurately monitored. Patients are often highly anxious about being weighed and so weighing should be done in a sensitive and straightforward manner. Describing a person's weight as 'the number on the scale' rather than 'your weight' is a cognitive behaviour therapy (CBT) technique designed to help the person separate that number from how they feel about themselves – particularly because every scale is different and certain behaviours, such as drinking water, can change the number within a matter of minutes. Because symptoms of starvation include perseveration and rigid thinking, it is not helpful to have an emphasis on a 'goal weight' that a patient will likely become fixated on. Instead, advise that reviewing medical parameters such as improved cardiovascular status and blood results and ultimately the return of ovulation and a normal menstrual cycle, as well as psychological recovery in terms of the person's mood and thinking, will inform ongoing nutritional rehabilitation.

Most treatment facilities aim for an average weekly weight gain of 1–2 kg in inpatient settings and 0.5 kg in outpatient settings. The frequency of weighing, or monitoring of expected weight gain, varies between treatment settings, but twice a week is enough to monitor and reward progress. In an outpatient setting any team member can undertake monitoring of weight gain, but in the hospital environment it is generally a nurse's responsibility. Patients are usually weighed early in the morning wearing only a hospital gown and before consuming any food or drink. At times, patients who are struggling use techniques to falsely increase their weight, including drinking large amounts of water just prior to weighing and hiding weights on their body. Therefore, patients are usually asked to empty their bladder just before weighing and urinalysis will identify if water loading (if the specific gravity is low (< 1.010)) or purging (if a high pH (8–9) is recorded) has occurred. A sudden increase in weight, or an increase that is inconsistent with the observed eating behaviour, will alert you that weight manipulation may be occurring, and discussion should ensue about possible behaviours that may account for this. A random (unexpected/spot) weight measurement can be undertaken outside the normal weighing time if there is concern that the person is manipulating their real weight.

It is important to remember that if someone is attempting to manipulate their weight, they are doing so out of fear and distress and because they are really struggling with the ambivalence that the eating disorder generates. They will probably be feeling very anxious that their behaviours will be detected but at the same time will be relieved when the secret is out. Nurses need to respond in a sensitive, respectful and empathic way when discussing these issues with the person, to avoid them feeling humiliated, judged and hopeless. For example: 'I can see by this spot weigh that your weight is actually quite a lot lower than what it was yesterday. I'm guessing that you have felt really worried about weigh days because you've been struggling so much with the eating ... is that right? Can you tell me what you've been doing to keep your weight measurements going up?'

Psychotherapeutic techniques and treatments

General principles of treatment for people with eating disorders, regardless of the type include (Hay et al. 2014):

- person-centred informed decision making
- involving a person's family and significant others
- recovery-oriented practice
- least restrictive treatment context
- multidisciplinary approach
- stepped and seamless care
- a dimensional and culturally informed approach to diagnosis and treatment.

Examples of some of the psychotherapeutic techniques and treatments currently used in managing people with an eating disorder are discussed below. In clinical practice, a combination of these therapies, or other psychotherapies not described below (e.g. psychodynamic psychotherapy, dialectical behaviour therapy and narrative therapy), may be used. When considering therapy for an eating disorder, the person's medical status, age, family supports, cognitive capacity, duration of illness and the accessibility of services are all considered. Nurses story 13.2 describes the role of a primary care mental health nurse.

NURSE'S STORY 13.2

Peta

I am a credentialled mental health nurse and family therapist who specialises in working with people who have eating disorders – mostly anorexia nervosa but also those with OSFED or people with severe bulimia nervosa complicated by another physical or mental health condition. I have undertaken relevant postgraduate training in family therapy and have done a lot of professional development (cognitive behaviour for eating disorders, acceptance and commitment therapy, dialectical behaviour therapy, family-based therapy for eating disorders) and studied some manualised eating disorder treatments – there is always more to learn. This is definitely an area of practice that really challenges the mental health nurse to use the breadth of mental health nursing knowledge and skills. Our background in biological science means we also have the knowledge and skills to assess and respond to a person's physical health status and monitor the impact of medications.

COGNITIVE BEHAVIOUR THERAPY

Enhanced CBT for eating disorders (CBT-E) is structured to focus on the processes associated with maintenance of the eating disorder. CBT-E uses a variety of cognitive and behavioural interventions but uses strategic behaviour change to modify thinking, rather than the direct cognitive restructuring usual in other forms of CBT. CBT-E is delivered in three stages, typically over 40 sessions. The first stage involves engaging the person in treatment and change, jointly creating the formulation, establishing self-monitoring practices, weekly weighing, establishing regular patterns of eating and providing education to the person and significant others. Stage 2 is brief and incorporates a review of stage 1 and planning for stage 3. The final stage is the main body of treatment, where the over-evaluation of shape and weight, dieting rules, interpersonal problems, perfectionism and self-esteem issues are addressed. The focus here is on eliminating dieting, problem solving and modifying thoughts that link body and weight with self-esteem, as well as relapse prevention and developing skills to manage stressors. CBT-E is an effective treatment for many outpatients with eating disorder (Fairburn et al. 2015).

There is only tentative evidence that usual CBT is effective for relapse reduction after weight restoration in anorexia nervosa, and it is not an appropriate treatment for those with anorexia nervosa who are not weight restored. However, evidence for using CBT with people who have bulimia nervosa is strong (when used to address the cycle of dieting, binge eating and purging or other extreme weight-control behaviours). CBT has also been developmentally adapted for adolescents with binge eating disorder and bulimia nervosa.

FAMILY-BASED TREATMENT

There is moderate research to support family therapy as an effective treatment for younger children and adolescents who live with their families and whose have experienced anorexia nervosa for less than 3 years (Hay et al. 2014). The focus of family therapy approaches varies, but the general theme is that the family are involved in treatment and support weight restoration and recovery. Models of family intervention have been developed for adults and couples, but these have not been evaluated. Family therapy is the treatment of choice for most children and adolescents with anorexia nervosa but is not demonstrably effective for those over 18 years of age (Hay et al. 2014).

Families play an important role in the assessment and treatment of young people with eating disorders. Unless contraindicated, families are best placed to support their loved one to manage the burden of the illness. Families need to understand the illness and be involved and engaged as an important resource by the treating team. To facilitate change, families need to develop effective coping strategies for managing the behaviours that support and maintain the illness and adopt interactional patterns that accommodate the young person's normal growth and development.

Sometimes families can inadvertently reinforce the eating disorder (particularly when the person's distress around eating is so intense) by giving into, accommodating or colluding with the eating disordered behaviours (e.g. making family meals consisting only of 'safe' foods). If families of children and adolescents are not engaged with, and committed to, the treatment program, or are unable to work together to provide clear, firm boundaries regarding food and disordered eating behaviours, relapse is more likely.

One particular model of family therapy designed for children and adolescents with anorexia nervosa, Maudsley family-based therapy, has proven to be effective for some families. This therapy is delivered in three phrases. The first phase involves the parents taking control of their child's eating until 90% of ideal body weight is achieved; the second phase involves the family gradually giving control over eating back to the young person while continuing to supervise them until they reach their healthy weight range; and the final phase involves supporting the young person to address any unresolved individual concerns, as well as assisting the family to return to the normal family life cycle by addressing any unresolved family or marital interactional problems.

Family-based therapy has also been adapted for use with families who have a young person with bulimia nervosa, prodromal presentations of anorexia nervosa, paediatric obesity and ARFID. The emphasis shifts from weight restoration to normalisation of eating, eating new/fear foods, regular family meals and supporting parents to model healthy eating (Rienecke 2017).

MANTRA (MAUDSLEY MODEL OF ANOREXIA NERVOSA TREATMENT FOR ADULTS)

MANTRA is a cognitive-interpersonal manual-based outpatient treatment for adults with anorexia nervosa developed by the Maudsley Hospital team in London designed to address the underlying worries the person experiences, including interpersonal difficulties, fear of rejection, negative perception of self and the experience of negative emotions (Schmidt et al. 2014). It uses a motivational interviewing approach that is highly strategic in looking out for and creating 'teachable moments' that will support the person to shift the balance towards change and recovery.

INTERPERSONAL THERAPY

Interpersonal therapy for people with eating disorders is based on the premise that interpersonal difficulties result in the development of disturbances in self-esteem and mood, which then give rise to eating disorder symptoms. Interpersonal therapy is a structured, time-limited psychotherapy that focuses on resolving interpersonal difficulties and encouraging the development of affirming relationships, thereby providing a viable alternative to the eating disorder in attaining positive self-esteem, affect and problem-solving skills. The symptoms of the eating disorder are not themselves the focus of therapy. Interpersonal therapy appears to have long-term efficacy for those with bulimia nervosa and people with binge eating disorder (Reas & Grilo 2014).

MOTIVATIONAL INTERVENTIONS

Motivation is a key issue for people with eating disorders. In particular, a person's motivation to change at the outset of treatment is thought to be helpful in predicting outcome (Clausen & Jones 2014). Motivational interventions typically target denial, ambivalence and resistance to change. They are commonly used with people who have eating disorders – either before they participate in other psychological interventions or as a key element of other therapies such as MANTRA. Understanding motivation and where a person is at in terms of their motivation is important because delivering interventions or elements of treatment that are targeted towards a person in the action stage are likely to be ineffective if the person is pre-contemplative and denying that there is a problem. This can create difficulties where action is required to ensure a person's medical safety, but the person does not believe there is a problem. For this reason, collaboration with the person and targeting issues that they see as important is essential, as is taking a respectful approach. Acknowledge that changing, when you're not that convinced there is a problem, is very challenging, and support the person using motivational interviewing techniques to begin to develop an understanding of the impact of the illness.

PSYCHOEDUCATION

Psychoeducation involves providing information about the eating disorder to enable the person with an eating disorder (and their families/carers) to better understand the illness and its effects and to develop more effective coping strategies to overcome difficulties they are experiencing. Psychoeducation is an essential part of treatment for all types of eating disorder. It is much easier for people with eating disorders to change the eating disorder behaviours when they understand the interplay between the behaviours and the illness and their dual role in keeping them trapped.

Some examples of psychoeducation topics are:

- the short- and long-term medical and psychological effects of starvation
- the biological factors that regulate weight – this includes discussion of how dieting largely works against the body's weight regulators, causing stress to both physical and psychological functioning
- the physical side effects of vomiting and laxative and diuretic abuse
- the binge–purge cycle and how it affects self-esteem – nurses can help the person to identify and manage cues for bingeing and purging behaviours, learn distraction or relaxation techniques to decrease the urge to vomit immediately after meals and understand the benefits of eating regularly throughout the day, thereby reducing the physical and psychological drive to binge in the evenings
- the importance of establishing a healthy pattern of exercise based on enjoyment and focusing on muscle strengthening and bone health, rather than focusing on burning up kilojoules for weight control or controlling body shape
- the effects of anxiety on the body and techniques for coping (e.g. mindfulness practices, cognitive challenging).

The Western Australian Centre for Clinical Interventions (www.cci.health.wa.gov.au) provides a range of psycho-education materials specific to eating disorders for use in clinical practice.

Psychoeducation on an individual or a group basis can also be extremely useful for engaging parents and family members in the treatment program, increasing their understanding of the complexity of the illness, developing realistic expectations and facilitating useful strategies to better manage the person's disordered eating behaviours. The more informed families are, the less anxious or blaming they become and the more open they will be to making positive changes that can support and improve the person's health outcome.

There are many web-based resources available for families, as well as state-based eating disorders associations, that provide parent and carer support programs throughout Australia and New Zealand. See the list of useful websites at the end of this chapter.

SPECIALIST SUPPORTIVE CLINICAL MANAGEMENT

Specialist supportive clinical management combines features of supportive psychotherapy and clinical management to establish a 'supportive therapeutic context'. The person is encouraged to explore issues that impact on and promote change and they are encouraged to actively make changes to core symptoms by increasing their weight, eating less restrictively and decreasing the use of inappropriate compensatory behaviours. The process focuses on facilitating normal eating, weight restoration and psychoeducation about anorexia nervosa as well as addressing other life issues that may be identified by the person as relevant to the eating disorder. Supportive psychotherapy is a generalised therapy that has been used in to treat people with eating disorders and can be implemented in primary care and general mental health settings. Techniques like active listening, verbal and non-verbal attending, using open-ended questioning, encouraging reflection, providing reassurance and praise are key. Advice giving and therapist self-disclosure are also used. Specific components of supportive therapy include reassurance, explanation, guidance, suggestion, encouragement and permission for catharsis or sharing of pent-up feelings such as fear, grief, sorrow, concern and frustration.

SELF-HELP PROGRAMS

Evidence-based self-help programs are now recommended as a possible first-stage intervention for bulimia nervosa and binge eating disorder in people aged 18 years or older (National Institute for Health and Care Excellence 2017). Self-help programs that include direct support from health professionals are termed 'guided' or 'supported' self-help. They have been found to have better adherence and treatment outcomes than 'pure' self-help (Beinther et al. 2014). There is less evidence available on the effectiveness of self-help and supported self-help for underweight people with anorexia nervosa and with adolescents and younger people.

PHARMACOTHERAPY

Pharmacotherapy is not used as a first-line treatment for people with anorexia nervosa. Evidence for pharmacological treatment is weak, but low-dose antipsychotics (e.g. olanzapine) may be helpful for some people to reduce anxiety, rumination and obsessive thinking (Hay et al. 2014) and have shown promise in diminishing thought intrusions and distorted body image. Selective serotonin reuptake inhibitors are not indicated in the acute or maintenance stages of anorexia nervosa for young people (Hay et al. 2014). The potential role of anxiolytics and antidepressants is best assessed after nutritional rehabilitation in low-weight patients with anorexia nervosa, as food and nutritional rehabilitation can be the best 'medicine' for improving mood.

Pharmacotherapy has been shown to be a helpful adjunctive treatment (along with CBT-E) for people with bulimia nervosa and binge eating disorder (Hay et al. 2014). If psychological therapy is not readily available, pharmacological treatment for people with bulimia/binge eating disorder is supported by evidence. However, the first-line treatment for both disorders is therapist-led CBT or CBT-E (Hay et al. 2014).

A final word on the nurse's role

Nurses in all clinical settings are ideally placed to make a significant impact on the health and mental health of the many Australian children, young people, women and men who experience eating disorders. Nurses have the skills required to work holistically and collaboratively, to empathise, to validate and to support people with eating disorders through this complex and challenging life experience. Recovery is always possible, at any stage of the illness. What is required is that, as nurses, we are kind and hold hope for the person when they are not able to hold hope for themselves; we understand the difficulties the person is experiencing in their struggle to recover, we support families who are frightened and bewildered and questioning themselves, and we critically reflect on our own practice to ensure we are offering high-quality evidence-informed practice that supports the person's recovery and optimises their outcome.

Working with people who have eating disorders is a rewarding professional experience – these are complex illnesses that stretch our knowledge and skills and require us to reflect on the impact of our values and attitudes on our nursing practice. Nurses who choose to specialise in working with people who have eating disorders undertake additional training and professional development and engage in regular clinical supervision (e.g. credentialled mental health nurses, mental health nurse practitioners working in primary care or private practice may provide psychological therapy, family-based therapy, CBT-E or other specialised treatment).

The following is an extract from a letter written by a recovering young adult:

> It's now been six years since I was first diagnosed with anorexia nervosa. I know I still have many years ahead to learn about life and to learn from my mistakes and experiences, but this recovery process has taught me so much about confronting myself, challenging myself and training my mind to think positively and it does work. Thank you for firmly confronting my disorder when I couldn't and for hanging in with me, keeping me alive and supporting me long enough for me to finally get to the point where I feel strong enough as a person to not need or want this illness any more.
>
> Source: Private communication with paediatric nurse Gail Anderson

Professional aspects of working with a person who has an eating disorder in an inpatient setting include:

- maintaining clear professional boundaries, which includes not being over-involved, or dismissive and under-involved
- developing and regularly reviewing an evidence-based local behavioural program for patients that is achievable for nurses within their specific work environment
- having realistic expectations regarding what can be achieved during a hospital admission given the complexity and chronicity of the illness; this includes the awareness that relapse and readmission are common and are not a sign of failure but an opportunity to review the relapse plan
- being aware of one's own personal emotional wellbeing and participating in adequate clinical supervision and support
- enjoying the challenge of caring for individuals with an eating disorder and assisting them to understand and care for themselves in more healthy ways
- validating the person's experience and maintaining positive regard for the person in the face of their ambivalence and resistance to treatment.

Chapter summary

This chapter has provided an introduction to the eating disorders encountered in nursing practice and has included a focus on psychological factors, medical complications, assessment and treatment. Eating disorders are complex, multidimensional illnesses that encompass a range of psychological and physical health issues. Although there is a relatively low but increasing incidence of eating disorders, the severity of impact of these disorders in terms of quality of life, morbidity and mortality is high. Many sufferers encounter difficulties in accessing appropriate services and this difficulty, coupled with the shame, denial and ambivalence to treatment commonly associated with these disorders, can result in delayed treatment. This is of particular concern because of the known effectiveness of early treatment in preventing or reducing progression to severe and chronic illness.

So, what of the future? In modern Western societies there seems to be an ever-increasing concern with body image, weight, shape and appearance for both women and men. For some this leads to severe distress, disruption and diagnosis with one of a growing list of disorders including the eating disorders. A greater emphasis on primary prevention strategies, particularly targeting the self-esteem, body image and resilience of the very young, both males and females, is needed.

A multidisciplinary approach to treatment of eating disorders is crucial and nurses committed to caring for people with an eating disorder have much to contribute in inpatient, outpatient, community and primary care treatment settings. Patients are admitted to hospital when they require 24-hour nursing care – this might be in mental health, paediatric, cardiac care, emergency department or general medical settings. In order that optimal care is provided, it is essential that all nurses understand and develop skills to manage the biopsychosocial complexity of these very challenging illnesses, relative to their scope of practice and clinical setting.

More research is needed to better understand the relative importance of biological and psychosocial risk and protective factors, and to continue developing more effective treatments. One needs only to look at the outcome data to see that new therapeutic treatments need to be developed to enhance outcomes and decrease the high levels of associated morbidity and mortality. Furthermore, more emphasis needs to be placed on early and more aggressive nutritional rehabilitation to enable those with an eating disorder to cognitively engage in therapeutic psychological interventions. Nurses are in a key position to undertake research designed to better understand eating disorders and promote evidence-based effective nursing strategies that will enhance care and outcomes for people experiencing an eating disorder.

EXERCISES FOR CLASS ENGAGEMENT

1. In a group, discuss the influence of the media, marketing, the advertising industry and popular role models on the development of eating disorders among young women and men.
2. Discuss the reasons why body image dissatisfaction tends to increase during adolescence.
3. Do a search on the internet for Ancel Keys' 1950s Starvation Study. Identify the physical, psychological, social and emotional aspects that relate to starvation, which people with eating disorders commonly experience. Some people think that eating disorders are self-inflicted and purposeful, or that they are a type of personality disorder. Having reviewed this study, what aspects of it challenge these kinds of assumptions?
4. Working with the person to find their strengths is an important part of recovery from an eating disorder. Make a table with two columns. In one column, list the self-defeating thoughts that a person with an eating disorder may experience. In the other column, suggest alternatives that are self-supporting behaviours and thoughts.
5. 'Fat talk' has been said to be a common motif of female culture, particularly with young women in developed countries. Girls and women are encouraged to aspire to the thin 'ideal' body type and often say self-disparaging things or communicate with others around this theme. Consider the following commonly heard statement: 'I feel so fat today'. This expression is made more commonly by young women than men and is repeated over and over. But, in fact, the person is actually feeling another emotion, such as worry, guilt, anger or frustration. The expression of emotion is covered up by referring instead to an outward physical presence (being fat). So 'fat talk' is actually a metaphor for a feeling. When this notion is identified as a metaphor, it is possible for it to be challenged and replaced. What are some more productive metaphors or statements that you could suggest young women could make to help them to express their emotions more accurately?
6. Some health practitioners say that people with eating disorders engage in manipulative and 'splitting' behaviours. We know that 'splitting' is actually a process whereby a team of practitioners fails to be consistent or to work collaboratively towards shared goals. We also know that words like 'manipulative' can be very damaging and labelling. How will you protect yourself against taking up judgemental and non-therapeutic language and ideas when you are working as a clinical nurse?

Useful websites

Australian and New Zealand Academy for Eating Disorders: http://www.anzaed.org.au/

Bridges Eating Disorder Association of WA: http://www.bridges.net.au/

Butterfly Foundation for Eating Disorders: https://www.thebutterflyfoundation.org.au/

Eating Disorders Association of New Zealand: https://www.ed.org.nz/

Eating Disorders Queensland: https://eatingdisordersqueensland.org.au/

Eating Disorders Victoria: https://www.eatingdisorders.org.au/
InsideOut Institute for Eating Disorder Research: https://insideoutinstitute.org.au/
Journal of Eating Disorders – peer-reviewed journal publishing leading research in the science and practice of eating disorders: https://jeatdisord.biomedcentral.com/
National Eating Disorders Collaboration (NEDC): http://nedc.com.au/
South Australia Statewide Eating Disorder Service (SEDS): https://www.sahealth.sa.gov.au/
The Victorian Centre for Excellence in Eating Disorders (CEED): http://ceed.org.au

Other resources

National ED Helpline: 1800 ED HOPE/1800 33 4673
Email: support@thebutterflyfoundation.org.au or phone the helpline to speak to a counsellor 8 am to midnight 7 days a week.

References

Academy for Eating Disorders, 2016. Eating disorders: a guide to medical care. Critical points for early recognition and medical risk. Available at: www.aed.org. (Viewed 12 December 2019).
American Psychiatric Association, 2013. Diagnostic and Statistical Manual of Mental Disorders, fifth ed. APA, Washington, DC.
Bannatyne, A.J., Abel, L.M., 2015. Can we fight stigma with science? The effect of aetiological framing on attitudes towards anorexia nervosa and the impact on volitional stigma. Aust. J. Psychol. 67, 38–46.
Bell, K., Rieger, E., Hirsch, J.K., 2018. Eating disorder symptoms and proneness in gay men, lesbian women and transgender and non-conforming adults: comparative levels and a proposed mediational model. Front. Psychol. 9, 2692.
Beinther, I., Jacobi, C., Schidt, U.H., 2014. Participation and outcome in manualized self-help for bulimia nervosa and binge eating disorder – a systematic review and metaregression analysis. Clin. Psychol. Rev. 34 (2), 158–176.
Bert, F., Gualano, M.R., Camussi, E., et al., 2016. Risks and threats of social media websites: twitter and the Proana movement. Cyberpsychol. Behav. Soc. Netw. 19, 4. https://doi.org/10.1089/cyber.2015.0553. [published online].
Bodell, L.P., Cheng, Y., Wildes, J.E., 2019. Psychological impairment as a predictor of suicide ideation in individuals with anorexia nervosa. Suicide Life Threat. Behav. 49 (2), 520–528.
Bosworth, P., 2011. Jane Fonda: The Private Life of a Public Woman. Houghton Mifflin Harcourt, Boston.
Breithaupt, L., Eickman, L., Byrne, C.E., et al., 2017. Enhancing empowerment in eating disorder prevention: another examination of the REbeL peer education model. Eat. Behav. 25, 38–41.
Brown, A., McClelland, J., Boysen, E., et al., 2016. The FREED Project (first episode and rapid early intervention in eating disorders): service model, feasibility and acceptability. Early Interv. Psychiatry 12, 250–257.
Campbell, K., Peebles, R., 2014. Eating disorders in children and adolescents: state of the art review. Pediatrics 134 (3), 582–593.
Caslini, M., Bartoli, F., Crocamo, C., et al., 2016. Disentangling the associations between child abuse and eating disorders: a systematic review and meta-analysis. Psychosom. Med. 78 (1), 79–90.
Cervantes-Luna, B.S., Ponce de Leon, C.S., Ruiz, E.J.C., et al., 2019. Aesthetic ideals, body image, eating attitudes and behaviors in men with different sexual orientation. Rev. Mex. Trastor. Aliment. (Mex. J. Eat. Disord.) 10 (1), 66–74.
Chung, Y.I., Kim, J.K., Lee, J.H., et al., 2017. Onset of dieting in childhood and adolescence: implications for personality, psychopathology, eating attitudes and behaviours of women with eating disorder. Eat. Weight Disord. Stud. Anorexia Bulimia Obes. 22 (3), 491–497.
Clausen, L., Jones, A., 2014. A systematic review of the frequency, duration, type and effect of involuntary treatment for people with anorexia nervosa, and an analysis of patient characteristics. J. Eat. Disord. 2, 29.
Da Luz, F.Q., Sainsbury, A., Mannan, H., et al., 2017. Prevalence of obesity and comorbid eating disorder behaviors in South Australia from 1995 to 2015. Int. J. Obes. 41 (7), 1148–1153.
Davico, C., Amianto, F., Gaiotti, F., et al., 2019. Clinical and personality characteristics of adolescents with anorexia nervosa with or without non-suicidal self-injurious behavior. Compr. Psychiatry 94, https://doi.org/10.1016/j.comppsych.2019.152115. 152115.
DerMarderosian, D., Chapman, H.A., Tortolani, C., et al., 2018. Medical considerations in children and adolescents with eating disorders. Child Adolesc. Psychiatr. Clin. N. Am. 27, 1–14.
de Vries, D.A., Peter, J., de Graaf, H., et al., 2016. Adolescents' social network site use, peer appearance-related feedback, and body dissatisfaction: testing a mediation model. J. Youth Adolesc. 45, 211–224.
Dittmer, N., Jacobi, C., Voderholzer, U., 2018. Compulsive exercise in eating disorders: proposal for a definition and clinical assessment. J. Eat. Disord. 6 (42), https://doi.org/10.1186/s40337-018-0219-x.
Dobinson, A., Cooper, M., Quesnel, D., 2019. The Safe Exercise at Every Stage (SEES) guideline: a clinical tool for treating and managing dysfunctional exercise in eating disorders. Available: www.safeexerciseateverystage.com.
Duncan, L., Yilmaz, Y., Bulik, C., 2017. Genome-wide association study reveals first locus for anorexia nervosa and metabolic correlations. Am. J. Psychiatry 174 (9), 850–858.
Erskine, H.E., Whiteford, H.A., 2018. Epidemiology of binge eating disorder. Curr. Opin. Psychiatry 31 (6), 462–470.

Fairburn, C.G., Bailey-Straebler, S., Basden, S., et al., 2015. A transdiagnostic comparison of enhanced cognitive behaviour therapy (CBT-E) and interpersonal therapy in the treatment of eating disorders. Behav. Res. Ther. 70, 64–71.
Ferguson, C.J., Munoz, M.E., Garza, A., et al., 2014. Concurrent and prospective analyses of peer, television and social media influences on body dissatisfaction, eating disorder symptoms and life satisfaction in adolescent girls. J. Youth Adolesc. 43, 1–14.
Guillaume, S., Jaussent, I., Maimoun, L., et al., 2017. Associations between adverse childhood experiences and clinical characteristics of eating disorders. Nature. Sci. Rep. 6, 35761.
Hay, P., Girosi, F., Mond, J., 2015. Prevalence and sociodemographic correlates of DSM-5 eating disorders in the Australian population. J. Eat. Disord. 3 (19), 1–7.
Hay, P., Chinn, D., Forbes, D., et al., 2014. Royal Australian and New Zealand College of Psychiatrists clinical practice guidelines for the treatment of eating disorders. Aust. N. Z. J. Psychiatry 48 (11), 977–1008.
Haynos, A.F., Pearson, C.M., Utzinger, L.M., et al., 2017. Empirically derived personality subtyping for predicting clinical symptoms and treatment response in bulimia nervosa. Int. J. Eat. Disord. 50, 506–514.
Hilbert, A., Pike, K., Goldschmidt, A., et al., 2014. Risk factors across the eating disorders. Psychiatry Res. 220 (1–2), 500–506.
Hill, L.S., Reid, F., Morgan, J.F., et al., 2010. SCOFF, the development of an eating disorder screening questionnaire. Int. J. Eat. Disord. 43 (4), 344–351.
Hinchcliff, G.L.M., Kelly, A.B., Chan, G.C.K., et al., 2016. Risky dieting amongst adolescent girls: associations with family relationship problems and depressed mood. Eat. Behav. 22, 222–224.
Hoek, H.W., 2016. Review of the worldwide epidemiology of eating disorders. Curr. Opin. Psychiatry 29 (6), 336–339.
Hohman, E.E., Balantekin, K.N., Birch, L.L., et al., 2018. Dieting is associated with reduced bone mineral accrual in a longitudinal cohort of girls. BMC Public Health 18, 1285.
Holland, G., Tiggemann, M., 2017. 'Strong beats skinny every time': disordered eating and compulsive exercise in women who post fispiration on Instagram. Int. J. Eat. Disord. 50 (1), 76–79.
Hummel, A.C., Smith, A.R., 2015. Ask and you shall receive: desire and receipt of feedback via Facebook predicts disordered eating concerns. Int. J. Eat. Disord. 48, 436–442.
Kiela, P.R., Gishan, F.K., 2016. Physiology of intestinal absorption and secretion. Best Pract. Res. Clin. Gastroentorol. 30 (2), 145–159.
Kornstein, S.G., 2017. Epidemiology and recognition of binge-eating disorder in psychiatry and primary care. J. Clin. Psychiatry 78 (Suppl. 1), 3–8.
Kostro, K., Lerman, J.B., Attia, E., 2014. The current status of suicide and self-injury in eating disorders: a narrative review. J. Eat. Disord. 2, 19.
Lawrence, D., Johnson, S., Hafekost, J., et al., 2015. The mental health of children and adolescents. Report on the second Australian Child and Adolescent Survey of Mental Health and Wellbeing. Canberra: Department of Health.
Lavender, J.M., Wonderlich, S.A., Engel, S.G., et al., 2015. Dimensions of emotion dysregulation in anorexia nervosa and bulimia nervosa: a conceptual review of the empirical literature. Clin. Psychol. Rev. 40, 111–122.
Levinson, C.A., Zerwas, S., Calebs, B., et al., 2017. The core symptoms of bulimia nervosa, anxiety, and depression: a network analysis. J. Abnorm. Psychol. 126 (3), 340–354.
Lonergan, A.R., Bussey, K., Mond, M., et al., 2019. Me, my selfie, and I: the relationship between editing and posting selfies and body dissatisfaction in men and women. Body Image 28, 39–43.
Madden, S., Miskovic-Wheatley, J., Clarke, S., et al., 2015. Outcomes of a rapid refeeding protocol in adolescent anorexia nervosa. J. Eat. Disord. 3, 8.
Mehler, P.S., Brown, C., 2015. Anorexia nervosa: medical complications. J. Eat. Disord. 3, 11.
McLean, S.A., Paxton, S.J., 2019. Body image in the context of eating disorders. Psychiatr. Clin. North Am. 42, 145–156.
McLean, S.A., Wertheim, E.H., Masters, J., et al., 2017. A pilot evaluation of a social media literacy intervention to reduce risk factors for eating disorders. Int. J. Eat. Disord. 50 (7), 847–851.
McLean, S.A., Paxton, S.J., Wertheim, E.H., et al., 2015. Photoshopping the selfie: self photo editing and photo investment are associated with body dissatisfaction in adolescent girls. Int. J. Eat. Disord. 48, 1132–1140.
Merlotti, E., Mucci, A., Volpe, U., et al., 2013. Impulsiveness in patients with bulimia nervosa: electrophysiological evidence of reduced inhibitory control. Neuropsychobiology 68, 116–123.
Mitchison, D., Hay, P., Griffiths, S., et al., 2017. Disentangling body image: the relative associations of overvaluation, dissatisfaction, and preoccupation with psychological distress and eating disorder behaviors in male and female adolescents. Int. J. Eat. Disord. 50 (2), 118–126.
Mitchison, D., Mond, J., 2015. Epidemiology of eating disorders, eating disordered behaviour, and body image disturbance in males: a narrative review. J. Eat. Disord. 3, 20.
National Institute for Health and Care Excellence, 2017. Eating disorders: recognition and treatment. In: NICE Guideline NG69. NICE, London.
Mond, J.M., Mitchison, D., Latner, J., et al., 2013. Quality of life impairment associated with body dissatisfaction in a general population sample of women. BMC Public Health 3 (13), 920.
Oberst, U., Wegmann, E., Stodt, B., et al., 2016. Negative consequences from heavy social networking in adolescents: the mediating role of fear of missing out. J. Adolesc. 55, 51–60.
Oldershaw, A., Lavender, T., Sallis, H., et al., 2015. Emotion generation and regulation in anorexia nervosa: a

systematic review and meta-analysis of self-report data. Clin. Psychol. Rev. 39, 83–95.

Popovic, M., Pizzi, C., Rusconi, F., et al., 2018. The role of maternal anorexia nervosa and bulimia nervosa before and during pregnancy in early childhood wheezing: findings from the NINEFA birth cohort study. Int. J. Eat. Disord. 51 (8), 842–851.

Phillipou, A., Castle, D.J., Rossell, S.L., 2019. Direct comparisons of anorexia nervosa and body dysmorphic disorder: a systematic review. Psychiatry Res. 274, 129–137.

Reas, D.L., Grilo, C.M., 2014. Current and emerging drug treatments for binge eating disorder. Expert Opin. Emerg. Drugs 19 (1), 99142.

Renz, J.A., Fisher, M., Vidair, H.B., et al., 2017. Excessive exercise among adolescents with eating disorders: examination of psychological and demographic variables. Int. J. Adolesc. Med. Health 31 (4), https://doi.org/10.1515/ijamh-2017-0032.

Rienecke, R., 2017. Family-based treatment of eating disorders in adolescents: current insights. Adolesc. Health Med. Ther. 8, 69–79.

Riesco, N., Aguera, Z., Granero, R., et al., 2018. Other specified feeding or eating disorders (OSFED): clinical heterogeneity and cognitive-behavioural therapy outcome. Eur. Psychiatry 54, 109–116.

Robinson, P.H., Nicholls, D., 2015. Critical Care for Anorexia Nervosa: The MARSIPAN Guidelines in Practice. Springer., London.

Royal College of Psychiatrists, 2012. Junior MARSIPAN: Management of Really Sick Patients under 18 with Anorexia Nervosa. Council Report CR168. Royal College of Psychiatrists, London.

Schaumberg, K., Welch, E., Breithaupt, L., et al., 2017. The science behind the Academy for Eating Disorders' nine truths about eating disorders. Eur. Eat. Disord. Rev. 25 (6), 432–450.

Schmidt, U., Wade, T.D., Treasure, J., 2014. The Maudsley model of anorexia Nervosa treatment for adults (MANTRA): development, key features, and preliminary evidence. J. Cogn. Psychother. 28 (1), 48–71.

Sidani, J.E., Shensa, A., Hoffman, B., et al., 2016. The association between social media use and eating concerns among US young adults. J. Acad. Nutr. Diet. 116 (9), 1465–1472.

Smolak, L., Levine, M.P., 2015. The Wiley Handbook of Eating Disorders, Assessment, Prevention, Treatment, Policy, and Future Directions. John Wiley & Sons, Chichester.

Strother, E., Lemberg, R., Stanford, S.C., et al., 2012. Eating disorders in men: underdiagnosed, undertreated and misunderstood. Eat. Disord. 20 (5), 346–355.

Thapliyal, P., Mitchison, D., Miller, C., et al., 2017. Comparison of mental health treatment status and use of antidepressants in men and women with eating disorders. Eat. Disord. 26, 248–262.

Thompson, K.A., Bardone-Cone, A.M., 2019. Disordered eating behaviours and attitudes and their correlates among a community sample of older women. Eat. Behav. 34, 101301.

Thornton, L.M., Munn-Chernoff, M.A., Baker, J.H., et al., 2018. The Anorexia Nervosa genetics initiative (ANGI): overview and methods. Contemp. Clin. Trials 74, 61–69.

Tiggemann, M., Slater, A., 2016. Facebook and body image concern in adolescent girls: a prospective study. Int. J. Eat. Disord. 50 (1), 80–83.

Tiggemann, M., Zaccardo, M., 2018. 'Strong is the new skinny': a content analysis of #fitspiration images on Instagram. J. Health Psychol. 23 (8), 1003–1011.

Tiggemann, M., Zaccardo, M., 2015. 'Exercise to be fit, not skinny': the effect of fitspiration imagery on women's body image. Body Image 15, 61–67.

Treasure, J., Claudino, A.M., Zucker, N., 2010. Eating disorders. Lancet 375, 583–593.

Utter, J., Denny, S., Peiris-John, R., et al., 2017. Family meals and adolescent emotional well-being: findings from a national study. J. Nutr. Edu. Behav. 49 (1), 67–72.

Vossbeck-Elsebusch, A.N., Waldorf, M., Legenbauer, T., et al., 2014. Overestimation of body size in eating disorders and its association to body-related avoidance behaviour. Eat. Weight Disord. 20 (2), 173–178.

Watson, H.J., Zerwas, S., Torgersen, L., et al., 2018. Maternal eating disorders and perinatal outcomes: a three-generational study in the Norwegian mother and child cohort study. J. Abnorm. Psychol. 126 (5), 552–564.

Wong, W., Lawrence, F.N., 2015. Am I man/woman enough: using trans-youth 'self-portrait drawing' to analyse their body image. In: Fisher, R., Howard, L., Monteith, K. (Eds.), The Gender & Sexuality Hub. Online: http://www.inter-disciplinary.net/critical-issues. (Accessed 4 December 2019). Gender & love: A Critical Issues research and publications project.

Yilmaz, Z., Hardaway, J.A., Bulik, C.M., 2015. Genetics and epigenetics of eating disorders. Adv. Genomics Genet. 5, 131–150.

Zayas, L.V., Wang, S.B., Coniglio, K., et al., 2018. Gender differences in eating disorder psychopathology across DSM-5 severity categories of anorexia nervosa and bulimia nervosa. Int. J. Eat. Disord. 51 (9), 1098–1102.

Zerwas, S., Larsen, J.T., Petersen, L., et al., 2015. The incidence of eating disorders in a Danish nationwide register study: associations with suicide risk and mortality. J. Psychiatr. Res. 65, 16–22.

Zhang, C., 2014. What can we learn from the history of male anorexia nervosa? J. Eat. Disord. 2 (1), 138.

Zipfel, S., Giel, K.E., Bulik, C.M., et al., 2015. Anorexia nervosa: aetiology, assessment and treatment. Lancet Psychiatry 2 (12), 1099–1111.

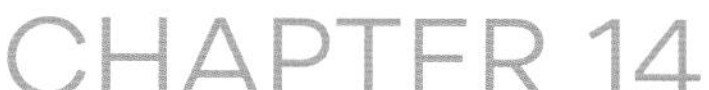

CHAPTER 14

Personality disorders

Toby Raeburn and Marika Van Ooyen

KEY POINTS

- Personality disorders are common conditions, with borderline personality disorder being the most likely of these disorders that nurses will encounter in their practice.
- A wide range of terms are used to describe personality disorders. Section 2 of the *Diagnostic and Statistical Manual of Mental Disorders*, 5th edition (DSM-5) groups personality disorders into three broad clusters: (A) odd or eccentric; (B) dramatic, emotional or erratic; and (C) anxious or fearful. In acknowledgement of the diagnostic complexity of personality disorders, section 3 of DSM-5 presents a refined group of seven disorders designed to guide future research and improve the acceptance of personality disorders as a homogenous group.
- Effective nursing care of people with a personality disorder involves developing a therapeutic relationship and setting clear boundaries.
- Staff education and clinical supervision helps nurses to reflect on their practice and to gain insight and understanding into the person's behaviour.

KEY TERMS

- Behaviour
- Borderline
- Diagnosis
- Dialectical
- Disorder
- Family
- Hospital
- Mood
- Personality
- Recovery
- Trauma

LEARNING OUTCOMES

The material in this chapter will assist you to:

- discuss personality
- identify the main characteristics of each of the three clusters of personality disorders
- develop an understanding of responses that nurses and other health professionals may experience when working with people who have a personality disorder
- identify effective nursing approaches to work with people who have a personality disorder.

Introduction

People with a personality disorder exhibit behaviours, thoughts and feelings that interfere with their ability to experience satisfying relationships with others and to achieve success at work and socially. They are unlikely to seek treatment to change their personality, although they frequently present for help with depression, anxiety and substance abuse. Nurses caring for people with a personality disorder need appropriate education and training to be able to engage therapeutically.

Research suggests that many people diagnosed with a personality disorder have experienced childhood physical or sexual abuse (Commons Treloar 2009; Leichsenring et al. 2011; National Health and Medical Research Council (NHMRC) 2012). Rates are difficult to pin down, but high numbers of people with a diagnosis of borderline personality disorder (BPD) have a history of repeated emotional, sexual or physical trauma and/or emotional neglect in their childhood. According to Leichsenring et al. (2011) approximately 39% of people with BPD have a comorbid diagnosis of post-traumatic stress disorder. Experiencing childhood sexual assault and beatings, witnessing violence against their mother, suffering torture, teenage rape, relentless ridicule and living with addicted parents whose interests and focus are frequently elsewhere are all examples of a recipe for indelible trauma. These ongoing abuses can result in boundary confusion, fear, impulsivity, shame, self-hatred, powerlessness, guilt, an incoherent sense of self, emotional chaos and other out-of-control feelings (Koekkoek et al. 2010; Vermetten & Spiegel 2014). Acknowledging and empathising with the effect that trauma may have had in the lives of people with personality disorders is therefore essential. There are national practice recommendations for providing trauma-informed care for mental health services and these principles include: promoting safety; role-modelling interpersonal relationships that heal; understanding culture; advocating for person control, choice and autonomy; understanding trauma and its impact; sharing power; inspiring hope and supporting recovery; integrating care; and sharing power and governance (see Bateman et al. 2013; Cleary & Hungerford 2015). For clinicians working with people with personality disorder these principles can be embedded in everyday practice by remembering the key concepts of safety, trustworthiness, choice, collaboration and empowerment (Kezelman & Stavropoulos 2012).

This chapter describes how personality disorders are currently categorised and identifies the defining characteristics of different types of personality disorder according to the *Diagnostic and Statistical Manual of Mental Disorders*, 5th edition (DSM-5) (American Psychiatric Association 2013). Some of the challenges in making a diagnosis of personality disorder are also discussed. The chapter focuses on assessing and intervening in BPD, a cluster B disorder, because it is the disorder nurses are most likely to encounter in practice. For people using psychiatric services, the prevalence of BPD is greater than 20% in community patient populations and around 40% for inpatient populations (NHMRC 2012).

What is personality?

Each of us has a personality and a commonsense understanding of what that means. We may describe others as 'outgoing', 'assertive', 'withdrawn' or 'shy', for example. Sometimes the terms we use to describe ourselves are not the ones that would be chosen by those who know us. Some individuals have personalities that seem to draw people to them – they may be described as charismatic, outgoing, friendly, good team players, helpful or kind. Others seem to have difficulty attracting others or maintaining relationships – they appear to be unreceptive, cold, aloof, isolative, eccentric or perhaps moody, aggressive or reckless. Our personality may be thought of as the expression of our feelings, thoughts and patterns of behaviour that evolve over time. Genetics, family, life events, culture and the society we live in all contribute to shaping our personality. Personality manifests via our general disposition, behavioural patterns and approach to the world and is especially evident during interactions with others.

It is our range of enduring and recognisable personality characteristics that makes us unique and enables us to respond to the experiences that life presents us with. Features that distinguish one person's personality from another's may be apparent in one's outlook on life, the way we respond and adapt to challenges and how circumstances are interpreted (Kern et al. 2014). Different historical periods, societies and cultures describe personalities differently and encourage or discourage certain personality types. For example, people raised in regimes such as the former East Germany, where the secret police network was widespread and intruded into families, would be more likely to be secretive, suspicious of others and unforthcoming. Similarly, contemporary indigenous cultures that are group-oriented may endorse mutual friendliness, sharing and fitting in at the expense of competitiveness and individualism.

Types of personality disorder

Enduring aspects or features of our personality are referred to as 'personality traits' and these traits are what differentiate us from one other. Social mores provide unwritten boundaries for what constitutes a 'normal' personality trait. For example, if a student expresses concern at having to present their work to the class because they are shy and public speaking makes them nervous, most people would understand their difficulties. With perseverance and support, most students will incrementally gain confidence and participate in tutorials regardless of some level of continuing discomfort. However, some people are so averse to public speaking that they will eventually avoid social situations where this might be required of them, to the extent of dropping out of an interesting course or a good job or from contact with friendship groups. Such extreme behaviour is beyond what is socially regarded as shyness. The personality trait has moved beyond normal boundaries to a point where it may be understood in terms of psychopathology. Some people display personality traits that seem to be beyond the scope of what is considered reasonable as observed by their behaviour and attitudes to others, and this creates practical and social problems for them and others in activities of daily living.

When these personality manifestations interfere significantly with a person's life or the lives of those close to them, the person may be diagnosed with a personality disorder. As with personality types, traits associated with personality disorders are often apparent in childhood and persist through adolescence to adulthood. The difference is largely of degree: the characteristics associated with a personality disorder are more inflexible and are underpinned by low self-esteem. The person's responses to stressors are maladaptive and include self-centredness and lack of empathy for others. The characteristics of people with a personality disorder involve extreme and persistent problems across emotional, interpersonal, behavioural and cognitive domains, as well as difficulties with sense of self (Bateman 2012; Feigenbaum 2010).

The questions for anyone involved with a person displaying extreme, persistent behaviours that ultimately work against their own interests relate to determining what behaviours are problematic for the person and others, and what can be done. The challenge for nurses, and indeed for anyone involved with such a person, lies in determining appropriate behaviour, given that norms relating to behaviour are socially and culturally constructed. When is the expression of someone's personality to be considered disordered?

Personality disorders can be recognised as enduring patterns of behaviour that are often damaging to the individual and others and are nearly always characterised by maladaptive and inflexible ways of coping with stress. People with a personality disorder often have an intense impact on those around them. Section 2 of the DSM-5 groups personality disorders into three clusters: A, B and C. Cluster A is composed of the disorders of an odd or eccentric nature; cluster B includes dramatic, erratic and emotional disorders; and cluster C comprises the anxious and fearful group (American Psychiatric Association 2013). Table 14.1 summarises the disorders covered by each cluster along with the diagnostic criteria used in clinical settings. However, it can be challenging to assess and diagnose personality disorders because a person who exhibits symptoms of one type of personality disorder invariably also exhibits symptoms of other disorders. In an effort to address the difficulty of categorically defining people's problems as one personality disorder or another, the DSM-5 has introduced new information contained in section 3 that seeks to guide research that may improve the clarity and evidence base for personality disorders. The simplified suggested classifications reduce the number of personality disorder types to seven (see Table 14.2).

Some of the criteria in Tables 14.1 and 14.2 overlap, and there are many people who could be diagnosed with more than one personality disorder. In the past, the most common clinically documented personality disorder diagnosis was that of the residual category, 'Not otherwise specified', which means that the clinician cannot decide between two or more possibilities (Horn et al. 2014). This may not reflect a limitation in the clinician's diagnostic ability but rather a realistic acknowledgement that the styles of interaction with someone with a personality disorder can change noticeably under different circumstances.

Prevalence

Personality disorders are reasonably common. Huang et al. (2009) investigated the prevalence of DSM-IV personality disorder clusters in 13 countries (n = 21,162) using the International Personality Disorder Examination. They estimated the prevalence to be 6.1% for any personality disorder and 3.6%, 1.5% and 2.7% for clusters A, B and C respectively. They found rates of personality disorders were higher among males (cluster C), people who were separated or divorced (cluster C), the unemployed (cluster C), the young (clusters A and B) and the poorly educated (clusters A, B and C) (Huang et al. 2009).

It has been estimated that more than half of people with a history of attempted suicide and half of all psychiatric outpatients have a personality disorder (Ansell et al. 2015; Soloff & Chiappetta 2012). Kim and Tyrer (2010) report that 40% or more of community mental health clients have a coexisting personality disorder, while in tertiary psychiatric services and prisons prevalence rates are between 70% and 90%. Many people who require long-term, assertive treatment have a personality disorder alongside a substance abuse, anxiety, mood or psychotic disorder (Newton-Howes et al. 2010). When people experience psychosis and a personality disorder, the latter might not be diagnosed, which may explain some of the engagement and treatment difficulties that contribute to poor outcomes (Newton-Howes et al. 2010).

In both men and women, the prevalence of personality disorders appears to decrease with age (Cooper et al. 2014; Debast et al. 2014). As currently classified, evidence shows that personality disorder affects around 6% of the world's population, with no consistent variation or differences between countries (Tyrer et al. 2010). Other reviews of epidemiological studies in different populations achieved consistent estimates of personality disorders: the median prevalence rate for 'any personality disorder' was 10.65% and the mean rate was 11.39%, indicating that one in 10 people have a diagnosable personality disorder (Samuels et al. 2002; Torgersen et al. 2001; Tyrer et al. 2015). Lamont and Brunero (2009) reviewed studies of prevalence rates of personality disorder and found they ranged from 5%

TABLE 14.1 Criteria for classifying personality disorders

CLUSTER A (ODD OR ECCENTRIC)	CRITERIA
Paranoid personality disorder	The person: • has expectations of being harmed or exploited without sufficient reason • is preoccupied with unjustified doubts • is unwilling to confide in others • perceives hidden, demeaning or threatening messages in innocent remarks or comments by others • tends to bear grudges • perceives attacks upon their character or reputation that are not apparent to others • suspects their spouse or partner of infidelity.
Schizoid personality disorder	The person: • neither enjoys nor desires close relationships • prefers solitary activities • has little interest in sexual activity • is indifferent to either praise or criticism • shows emotional frigidity.
Schizotypal personality disorder	The person: • exhibits evidence that they are experiencing ideas of reference • expresses odd beliefs and thinking in their speech and is odd in their appearance • shows evidence of some paranoid ideation • has social anxiety • lacks a social network/friends.
CLUSTER B (DRAMATIC, ERRATIC AND EMOTIONAL)	CRITERIA
Antisocial personality disorder	The person: • is at least 18 years old • may have expressed a conduct disorder before age 15 years • exhibits a disregard for the law • exhibits reckless, aggressive, deceitful and impulsive behaviour • does not show remorse • is unable to sustain employment/study.
Borderline personality disorder	The person: • is terrified of abandonment and actively attempts to avoid it • experiences intense and unstable moods • forms intense and unstable relationships • experiences disturbances of identity • engages in impulsive self-destructive behaviours • exhibits recurrent suicidal behaviour • experiences chronic feelings of emptiness and transient paranoia.
Histrionic personality disorder	The person: • craves being the centre of attention and engages in self-dramatisation and/or uses physical appearance to attain this • displays inappropriately sexually seductive behaviour • uses speech to impress others but is lacking in depth • is prone to exaggeration and dramatic expression of emotion • tends to exaggerate the degree of intimacy they share with others • tends to be easily led by others.
Narcissistic personality disorder	The person: • brims with self-importance and grandiosity • is preoccupied with fantasies of success, power, genius or beauty • has a profound belief that they are special and therefore exude a sense of entitlement (i.e. are deserving of special treatment and favours) • displays arrogance • needs to be admired • lacks empathy • tends to exploit others for their own benefit.

TABLE 14.1 Criteria for classifying personality disorders—cont'd

CLUSTER C (ANXIOUS AND FEARFUL)	CRITERIA
Avoidant personality disorder	The person: • fears disapproval, rejection and ridicule and so avoids occupations and social situations where this may occur • avoids intimate relationships due to the same fears • is preoccupied with the fear of shame, rejection and ridicule • is embarrassed or anxious in social situations • feels inferior • is very reluctant to take risks.
Dependent personality disorder	The person: • is unable to make decisions or initiate projects without considerable advice, reassurance and direction • has difficulty with expressing disapproval • experiences discomfort when alone and fears isolation • lacks confidence and will go to extraordinary lengths to obtain support from others • has an urgent need to establish a new relationship for support and care when an existing relationship ends.
Obsessive-compulsive personality disorder	The person: • is preoccupied with details, rules, schedules and organisation; perfectionism interferes with the completion of tasks • is overly conscientiousness, inflexible, rigid and stubborn • tends to hoard possessions and is reluctant to spend • tends to prefer to work rather than socialise.
PERSONALITY DISORDER NOT OTHERWISE SPECIFIED	CRITERIA
	• The person displays features of more than one disorder, without meeting the full criteria in one or more areas of functioning.

Adapted from American Psychiatric Association 2013

TABLE 14.2 Classification suggestions for future research into personality disorders

CLASSIFICATION	CRITERIA
Schizotypal personality disorder	People who exhibit eccentric behaviour, distort communication with others and are uncomfortable in close relationships may exhibit chronic mistrust and negative interpretations of others' actions.
Antisocial personality disorder	People who disregard and persistently violate the rights of others.
Borderline personality disorder	People who struggle with emotional regulation and impulsiveness.
Narcissistic personality disorder	People who chronically overestimate their own importance and lack empathy towards others.
Avoidant personality disorder	People who struggle socially due to persistent feelings of inadequacy and are hypersensitive to the views of others.
Obsessive-compulsive personality disorder	People preoccupied with order and control.
Personality disorder trait specified (PD-TS)	For when a personality disorder is considered present, but the criteria for a specific personality disorder are not fully met.

Adapted from American Psychiatric Association 2013

to 10% (one in 10 in the United States, one in 15 in Australia and one in 20 in the United Kingdom).

The most common and most complex personality disorder encountered in the clinical setting is BPD. The prevalence of BPD in other countries among the general population is estimated at approximately 1–4%, and prevalence rates of BPD among people who use psychiatric services is estimated at up to 23% for outpatients and up to 43% for inpatient populations (NHMRC 2012). Among adolescents, BPD rates have been estimated at 1–14% (NHMRC 2012). Australian estimates suggest that the prevalence of BPD among Australians aged 24–25 years is approximately 3.5%, noting that no prevalence data exist for Australian adolescents (NHMRC 2012).

Contributing factors

The causes of personality disorder are not known, but there are a range of theories. Research consistently reveals that people who have experienced childhood physical, emotional or sexual abuse or emotional neglect, as well as those raised in families characterised by withdrawal or violence, are much more likely to display behaviours consistent with a personality disorder diagnosis than those who have not been abused or neglected (NHMRC 2012). Contemporary aetiological explanations are predicated on a combination of biological, psychological and social risk factors, including heredity, life experiences and environmental factors that determine whether personality traits become rigid and show potential to undermine the self. Cloninger and Svrakic suggest it is reasonable to assume that the 'temperament and character components of PD are all moderately heritable' (Cloninger & Svrakic 2008, p. 471), and there is also support for the view that it results from a combination of adverse biological and environmental events/factors (NHMRC 2012). Research suggests that about half of the symptoms of BPD (the most frequently studied personality disorder) are long term and characterological in nature, and the other half are acute and usually respond well to treatment (Crawford et al. 2011; Zanarini 2009).

Historical anecdote 14.1: Different does not equal disordered

Georgina Weldon was a British professional singer who, in the early 1870s, lived in Tavistock House where she ran an orphanage using music lessons to rehabilitate street children. Georgina was a spiritualist who believed the soul of her dead mother lived in the body of her pet rabbit. By 1875 her husband Harry Weldon had grown tired of his wife's orphanage and enlisted the help of two doctors to use her spiritual beliefs to suggest she was insane and have her locked in a lunatic asylum. When staff from the asylum arrived to take her away by force, Georgina escaped and evaded capture. She went to Bow Street Magistrates Court to press charges for assault, which was unusual in the Victorian era. Having been proven sane in a court of law, Mrs Weldon went on to successfully sue her husband for his mistreatment.

Read more about it: *Wise S 2013 Inconvenient people: lunacy, liberty, and the mad-doctors in England. Counterpoint Press, Berkeley*

The experience of personality disorders

People are rarely admitted to inpatient mental health settings simply because of their personality disorder. Rather, they are admitted because of conditions coexisting with their disorder, such as anxiety, depression or substance misuse, or for assessment due to extreme behaviours, including self-harming or suicidal intent. Impulsive behaviours, self-harming and abuse of drugs and alcohol tend to bring people with personality disorders into contact with healthcare services. Very often their admissions are accompanied by a sense of drama/crisis, broken relationships and the consequences of struggling to cope with the stresses of life.

Research reveals that large numbers of people in general psychiatric samples have a coexisting personality disorder (see Friborg et al. 2013; 2014). People with a diagnosis from cluster A, odd and eccentric personality disorders, are the least likely to seek treatment. Those with cluster C, anxious and fearful disorders, more frequently require treatment. It is those with cluster B, dramatic and emotional personality disorders, who most frequently find themselves the recipients of care from mental health clinicians. When one reviews the characteristics of people who have these disorders, it is easy to appreciate why this may be so. Reckless behaviour, impulsivity, sexual risk-taking and self-harming and self-mutilating behaviour tend to bring them into contact with legal and/or healthcare services. Other behaviours that may draw attention include shoplifting and abuse of drugs and alcohol.

Signs and symptoms

Since people with personality disorders demonstrate repetitive patterns of behaviour stemming from their personality, the individual experiences problems in living, rather than specific symptoms as with other psychiatric disorders. The type of maladjusted behaviour evidenced indicates that the observable pathology is outwardly directed towards and against others. Common signs of personality disorder include but are not limited to one or more of the following:

- unsatisfying, dysfunctional interpersonal relationships
- difficulty regulating emotions
- difficulty experiencing empathy
- easily distractible
- low levels of self-motivation
- marked lack of persistence except in areas of self-gratification
- limited ability to tolerate stress
- impulsivity
- regular episodes of verbally or physically explosive behaviour, especially when feeling challenged
- lacking in ability to reflect linked to ongoing difficulty in learning from experience
- lacking foresight
- difficulty maintaining any moral code or value system
- behaviour is often self-protective, self-defeating or destructive and can appear deceptive.

Personality disorders include myriad conditions covering a wide array of personality, character and behavioural maladjustments in living. For more information on the specific conditions please see refer back to Table 14.1. Skodol et al. (2011) note that although symptoms vary in severity, people with personality disorder commonly present as being devoid of concern for others and as extremely egocentric; they will also lie to either explain or excuse their own behaviour or to gain sympathy. Given that these people characteristically have no or little insight into their problems, they have a pronounced tendency to blame others for problems of their own making, which further impairs their already strained relationships with others. Since they also tend not to learn from their mistakes in their relationships and in other aspects of life, they often repeat these errors over and over. So, for example, people with BPD fear being abandoned, yet they continue to behave in ways that tend to drive others away. This, coupled with the fact that their tolerance for emotional pain is low, inevitably leads many to experience low self-esteem, which they may deal with by self-medicating with alcohol or other drugs or engaging in self-harming behaviour such as cutting, or they may develop eating disorders or be sexually promiscuous.

Such maladaptive behaviours are examples of ways in which these people may deal with the feelings they experience. Signs and symptoms that also need to be considered include harmful drug and alcohol use, self-harm or mutilation, suicidal ideation and/or attempts, instances of aggression or violence, unexplained visible injuries to the body, risky sexual activity and problems with family and workplace relationships. An established pattern in one or more of the high-risk behaviours, such as illicit drug abuse or violence, may indicate that the person has come to the attention of the police. Outstanding fines or impending legal proceedings further complicate the lives of people with a personality disorder.

Self-harm and personality disorders

One range of behaviours that is especially difficult for nurses to countenance and work with in people who enact these behaviours is self-harm. People with various personality disorders may exhibit these behaviours, but one of the main reasons that BPD has become a negative and stigmatising label is that self-harm is more prevalent among people with this diagnosis. Self-harming behaviours include, but are not limited to, cutting the skin of the wrist, head banging, deep scratching with or without an implement and self-burning with cigarettes. These self-harming behaviours are also a significant risk factor for suicide (Crawford et al. 2009).

Self-harming behaviours are confronting and distressing and undoubtedly contribute to negative attitudes towards people with BPD and feed into stigmatisation (Commons Treloar 2009; Fanaian et al. 2013; Koekkoek et al. 2010; Purves & Sands 2009). Understanding the reasons for self-harm may help nurses and other mental health clinicians to face their own human reactions of disbelief, horror, fear, shock or disgust and to interact with people in more humane, professional and therapeutic ways. In other words, increased understanding of both the person and the self are required to work effectively with this group of people.

Reasons for self-harming include:

- regaining some self-control
- providing emotional relief
- relieving tension build-up
- alleviating feelings of emptiness
- escaping flashbacks and returning to reality
- expressing forbidden anger against self or others
- releasing self-hatred arising from experiencing violence
- decreasing alienation from others (Booth et al. 2014; Turner et al. 2012).

Research shows that self-harm is a strategy used by some people to attempt to deal with overwhelming emotional distress and pain (Feigenbaum 2010; Holm et al. 2009; Holm & Severinsson 2011). As Feigenbaum (2010, p. 115) succinctly states, from a person's perspective self-harm is 'the solution not the problem'. Needless to say, many clinicians continue to see self-harm as the problem, not a part of the solution, and with good treatment, a temporary or interim solution. The reality is that expecting people to simply give up self-harming actions can precipitate intense panic and anxiety because they are effectively being asked to give up a tried and true way of managing rage, shame and alienation from self and others that works for them.

Historical anecdote 14.2: On the 'border'

Use of the term 'borderline' to describe people's mental state began in the early 20th century. Professor Carl Pelman (1838–1916) at Bonn University in Germany wrote a paper using the term 'borderline' to describe a range of mental health problems that did not fit a description of 'psychosis', which was the dominant diagnostic category back then. By 1938 the term 'borderline' had begun to be associated with personality when psychoanalysts began describing people who failed to fit into either the psychotic or psychoneurotic groups, which were the two main diagnostic categories of the time. The phrase 'borderline' was therefore used to describe dominant symptoms such as narcissism and insecurity. The diagnostic term we associate with borderline personality disorder today has changed and modernised in various editions of the DSM.

Read more about it: *Howell E 2018 From hysteria to chronic relational trauma disorder: the history of borderline personality disorder and its connection to trauma, dissociation, and psychosis. In: Moskowitz A, Dorahy MJ, Schäfer I (eds) Psychosis, trauma and dissociation: evolving perspectives on severe psychopathology. John Wiley & Sons, Hoboken, pp. 83–95*

Assessment areas

One of the greatest difficulties for people with a personality disorder is attachment – satisfying emotional involvement with others – to people in general and health professionals in particular (Koekkoek et al. 2010). Hence, the central challenges for clinicians are engagement and building rapport (Crawford et al. 2009), which depend on establishing a therapeutic relationship with the person by being open-minded, self-aware, patient and persevering. This means that engagement, the therapeutic relationship and assessment are ongoing.

Initial assessment should exclude conditions such as hyperthyroidism, Cushing's syndrome, mood/anxiety disorder, post-traumatic stress disorder, substance abuse or an organic disorder that may explain some symptoms. If an organic cause is suspected, further investigations may be ordered and, in some cases, testing of blood alcohol levels and a drug screen may be indicated. Indeed, substance or alcohol abuse often coexists with personality disorders and with BPD in particular (Di Pierro et al. 2014; Whitbeck et al. 2015). Taking a drug (legal or illegal, prescribed or over the counter) or withdrawing from one is likely to change the person's mental status and behaviours. Aggression, agitation or changing mood states (lability) due to withdrawal may be misinterpreted as signs of personality disorder; side effects of steroid abuse may manifest similarly. The single most significant criterion for differentiating between medical conditions, substance abuse and side effects of prescription medication is a comparison of the person's presenting behaviour with their usual ongoing behaviour. Personality disorders are characterised by pervasive long-term patterns of behaviour, whereas other conditions usually involve abrupt inconsistent behavioural changes.

Nurses need to be aware of all these potentialities when assessing and caring for people with a personality disorder. Assessment is a continuous process that often requires lengthy interviews drawing on high-level communication and listening skills, and keen observation. It needs to be holistic, taking into account the person's present relationships as well as childhood experiences and traumatic events. Even then, the findings may be considered provisional, at least until further corroborating material is gathered. An empathetic approach during assessment is required in order to build a therapeutic relationship with people who have personality disorders and often have difficulty establishing and maintaining both professional and personal relationships. With the growing implementation of trauma-informed care as a guiding principle for delivering mental health care there is a focus on framing assessments and ongoing treatment from the enquiring premise 'What happened to you?' rather than the more blaming, problem-focused question 'What's wrong with you?' (Kezelman & Stavropoulos 2012). (See Chapter 7 for more about assessment.)

Furthermore, given the multicultural nature of contemporary society, it is very important for nurses to be sensitive to cultural differences. A behaviour that seems incongruent to a nurse of Anglo-Celtic origin may in fact be the norm for the cultural background of the person. For example, in some cultures, interactions between women and men, the young and the elderly are governed by certain conventions that serve to maintain respect and mirror the power differentials in relationships. Their behaviours, such as eye contact, physical proximity and turn-taking during interactions, may be different from what you are accustomed to, and your behaviours may seem odd to them.

While the layperson might be excused for believing that diagnoses are clear-cut, nurses need to be aware that all psychiatric diagnoses lack clarity in some situations and overlap at times. This means that debates about whether a given person has a specified disorder are often legitimate. Psychiatry is an inexact science, and even when a definitive personality disorder diagnosis can be made, the optimal approach to treatment is not always clear (Tyrer et al. 2015). As in previous editions, the DSM-5 (American Psychiatric Association 2013) issues a cautionary statement to clinicians about interpreting its diagnostic categories; indeed, they are advised that specific diagnostic criteria serve only to inform professional judgement, not to override it. This is especially the case in personality disorder, where the diagnosis is often debated.

Historically, psychiatric diagnoses have often become pejorative labels, where those bearing the descriptors have been prejudged and stereotyped, especially by health professionals (Flaskerud 2012; Tyrer et al. 2015). At different times, hysteria and BPD have been used to negatively evaluate people. As a result, people have felt that they were treated negatively because of their diagnosis (Horsfall et al. 2010). The current diagnosis of BPD is tantamount to negative labelling because it is often experienced as unhelpful and stigmatising. Nursing staff often develop negative feelings and perceptions about this person group (Westwood & Baker 2010). It is therefore important that nurses work in partnership with people in a person-centred, recovery-oriented way to avoid actively or passively assisting the person to internalise stigma (Horsfall et al. 2010).

The current taxonomy of personality disorders, alongside the use of checklists and abstract diagnostic criteria, is generally considered inadequate because it leads to narrow, subjective assessments that ignore life events, the person's history and their social circumstances (Kim & Tyrer 2010; Tyrer et al. 2015). A series of articles published in *The Lancet* in 2015 relate to personality disorder, including classification and assessment – see www.thelancet.com/series/personality-disorder.

Interventions

Service providers report that people with BPD are moderately to very difficult to work with effectively (Westwood & Baker 2010), but increasing evidence is emerging for the effectiveness of a range of treatment modalities that will make it easier to work with people who experience personality disorders (NHMRC 2012; Stoffers et al. 2012). Change is likely to be slow and piecemeal, and nurses need personal resilience and staying power, as well as highly developed interpersonal communication skills, to work productively with people with a personality disorder. Developing a therapeutic relationship underpins all the treatment approaches. Trust is fundamental – conveying hope and optimism and being respectful during all interactions. To develop an optimistic and trusting relationship it is important to work with people in 'an open, engaging and non-judgmental manner, and [to] be consistent and reliable' (National Collaborating Centre for Mental Health (NCCMH) 2009, p. 99). The needs and preferences of the person should also be considered so that people with a personality disorder can make choices about their care and treatment in an informed way (NCCMH 2009).

Research by McGrath and Dowling (2012) on psychiatric nurses' responses to people with a diagnosis of BPD revealed the following four themes:

- challenging and difficult
- deceptive, destructive and threatening behaviour
- preying on the vulnerable, resulting in splitting staff and other service users
- boundaries and structure.

The theme of 'challenging and difficult' related to the symptoms that people with BPD display, along with the perception that they seldom take responsibility for their behaviours. Staff were often pessimistic about peoples' prognosis and therefore felt helpless and hopeless. The theme of 'manipulative, destructive and threatening behaviour' referred to the perception that people with BPD often have hidden motivations and commonly use violent or self-harming behaviour to elicit responses from others, including nurses. 'Preying on the vulnerable resulting in splitting staff and other service users' referred to people with BPD who were perceived to have manipulated relationships between staff or other consumers. The final theme of 'boundaries and structure' described nurses' need for strong boundaries when working with people with BPD. Overall, it was common for nurses to struggle with feelings of anger, frustration and fear while delivering care to people with BPD (McGrath & Dowling 2012).

Thus, there is a need for clearer principles to guide practice as well as further training and education (e.g. motivational techniques, trauma, supervision) to improve the skills of professionals (Fanaian et al. 2013; McGrath & Dowling 2012). To work effectively with people with a personality disorder, clinicians need to consider the following 'preventable errors', which they can potentially change in themselves:

- loss of professional objectivity and perspective, often characterised by strong emotions (positive or negative) termed countertransference
- perpetuating the myth that a person with a personality disorder cannot recover, which is stigmatising and can create a self-fulfilling prophecy
- giving direct advice on personal and social problems, which can create dependence, noncompliance or resentment (Lawn & McMahon 2015).

Crisis intervention

Crisis intervention and stabilisation are the first priorities in responding to acute distress in people with BPD (NHMRC 2012). Dealing with the presenting problem that has precipitated the admission or emergency home visit (if possible) is a good beginning, as this may fix something practical or calm the person sufficiently to be able to engage adequately with them. Nurses need to actively involve the person with a personality disorder in all decision making so decisions are based on an explicit, joint understanding and the person is encouraged to consider the various treatment options and negative outcomes associated with poor choices made in response to distress (NCCMH 2009). Goal setting and problem solving should start as soon as the person is able to communicate and negotiate collaboratively.

Limit setting

Because people with personality disorders have underdeveloped self-control in a range of social, emotional and behavioural domains, clear limit setting is also among the first priorities – to clearly communicate what behaviours are acceptable in the therapeutic relationship and what are not. Limit setting provides a degree of externally reinforced control over the behaviours people have difficulty controlling. There must be consensus among team members about how behaviours are to be managed. Clear and frequent communication among team members will assist this. Firm, fair and consistent limit setting enacted with a non-judgemental attitude should be continually strived for.

Limit setting aims to offer people with personality disorders a degree of control over their behaviour. Whenever limit setting is employed, the person should know in advance the behaviours expected, as well as the consequences for breaches. As far as is practicable, the person should be involved in setting these limits and determining the consequences. When limit setting is carried out consistently by a team that communicates well, behaviours of seduction, dependency, rejection, agenda setting, collusion and staff splitting may be avoided (Fanaian et al. 2013). In a hospital setting, using 'time-outs' (where the person is offered monitored time in a quiet, private, low-stimulus environment until the urge to self-harm passes) has been found to be a useful tool in practice because it encourages the person to attempt to deal with maladaptive behaviours in a more positive and acceptable way. Sensory interventions are often used in inpatient settings as a way of adapting healthier coping strategies that help to regulate distress and intense emotions. Sensory approaches aim to stimulate the senses as a method of self-soothing; strategies include using weighted blankets, massage chairs, calming lights and pictures, kinetic sand and fidget toys, and aromatherapy (Scanlan & Novak 2015). Many inpatient mental health settings have sensory/'comfort' rooms or sensory kits for patients to access during times of distress (Novak et al. 2012).

Self-management

It is clear from this discussion that nurses and other members of the healthcare team face a range of personal, interpersonal and professional challenges that are not easy to address constructively. Some of the personal–professional tensions to be acknowledged, reflected upon and managed carefully are:

- flexibility and adaptability to individual needs regarding control and safety
- emotional connection vis-a-vis functional professional objectivity
- calmness in the face of anxiety-creating behaviours
- believing people's stories versus disbelief that such things can happen
- developing trust in a situation of fear.

A trusting and optimistic relationship is the cornerstone for working effectively with people with a personality disorder. This is why education and clinical supervision are essential (Lawn & McMahon 2015; NCCMH 2009). Interestingly, Zanarini (2009) says that any interactive treatment modality can be effective, provided it is done by a reasonable person with a thoughtful, insightful and caring approach – meaning that learning a specific technique is not the key, but understanding the person and ourselves is.

Interactive therapies

Given that many people with a personality disorder are prone to treatment non-adherence (for a range of reasons), the challenges for both the person and clinician are obvious. In a systematic review of 25 studies of treatment for people with a personality disorder, the non-completion rate was 37%, and a range of person and environment factors were associated with this (McMurran et al. 2010). Thus, active engagement is crucial. Crawford et al. (2009) studied engagement and retention in 10 specialist services for people with a personality disorder (1,186 referrals) and found that although most people engaged, men and younger people were less likely to complete the package of care.

Cognitive behaviour therapy (CBT) uses aspects of both cognitive therapy (which targets unhelpful beliefs) and behavioural therapy (which aims to change non-constructive or damaging behaviours). CBT aims to help people to develop more effective coping mechanisms by equipping them with strategies that promote realistic ways of thinking about and responding to everyday situations (Matusiewicz et al. 2010). Research generally supports the conclusion that CBT is an effective treatment modality for people with a range of personality disorders (Matusiewicz et al. 2010).

Dialectical behaviour therapy (DBT) is based on CBT, and research shows it is useful for people with BPD (Koekkoek et al. 2010). DBT actively incorporates social skills training. The focus of this therapy is: (1) the attenuation of parasuicidal and life-threatening behaviours; (2) the attenuation of behaviours that hinder therapy; and (3) the attenuation of behaviours that frustrate the person's ability to improve their quality of life. Essentially, this therapy, developed by Marsha Linehan (1998; 2000), conceptualises people with personality disorders as having significant problems regulating their emotions and behaving in accordance with social norms, often as a result of unsupportive, socially chaotic or traumatic life histories (Harned et al. 2012). DBT involves an intensive, highly structured approach to treatment including both individual and group sessions that focus on identifying strengths and overcoming negative coping habits. Therapy teaches new skills and facilitates practice of replacement behaviours in a range of social contexts. Common components of a DBT program include:

- individual therapy – focused on strengths identification, reflecting on recent challenges and using the therapist–person relationship as a template for practising new coping skills
- group therapy and teaching sessions – focused on four core themes of interpersonal effectiveness, distress tolerance, emotion regulation and mindfulness
- role-playing – behaviour rehearsals practised in either individual or group therapy sessions

- homework – often involving practising social skills in real-life contexts
- telephone therapy – unlike many other approaches, telephone contact between therapist and person is encouraged in between individual sessions (Booth et al. 2014; O'Connell & Dowling 2014).

DBT has a growing body of evidence, including randomised controlled trials and systematic literature reviews, that suggest it can be useful for a range of personality disorders (McMain et al. 2014; O'Connell & Dowling 2014; Pasieczny & Connor 2011).

CONSUMER'S STORY 14.1

Mark

Mark is a 19-year-old who was admitted to a public hospital after having severely beaten both of his parents while under the influence of alcohol. His parents reported that 'he was always a problem' and was continuously in and out of trouble at school. At the age of 14, Mark was with his friend in a stolen car when they were stopped by the police who, according to Mark, later 'beat them' and brought them to a juvenile detention home. Subsequently, Mark was placed on probation for 2 and a half years.

Mark developed an animosity towards the police and believes the police are 'doing wrong and not doing justice to the people'. He has had several confrontations with police, but he refused to elaborate on the specific incidents. However, in talking with nurses on the ward, he did relate portions of some of these experiences. He admits to having robbed the homes of some elderly people. He stated that in his conscience he does not feel that there is anything wrong with this. 'After all,' he said, 'I didn't steal from our neighbours'. He further commented, 'This is a dog-eat-dog world. I was brought up on the streets'. He admitted that he started to drink at the age of 16. Since that time he has had many episodes of excessive drinking and, when he came home, he was, according to his parents, violent, hostile and unmanageable. One year ago, he related that he struck his father for the first time and later he also struck his mother. His mother said she is 'scared of him'. A few months ago, Mark left his parents' home and went to live in an apartment with a friend. He worked sporadically at various odd jobs but never for very long. Mark describes himself as 'a good worker, who deserves more than what I get paid' and 'a good friend with people I get along with'.

His parents voiced concern about their son's behaviour, stating that they had tried different ways to reach him in an effort to prevent his drinking habit but were not successful. They thought they had the solution when he came home on the day of the attack, drunk and threatening. They called the police. But by the time the police arrived, Mark had severely beaten both his parents. He was taken to the city jail and later transferred to hospital. His parents were treated at a nearby emergency department and released. They have hopes that perhaps this hospitalisation will help him find a morally and socially acceptable way of life. In the hospital, Mark made new friends and became more interested in politics. He made several statements about the conditions in the United States, and his room is full of political literature, most of it leftist, for example, *Quotations from Chairman Mao Zedong* and *Mass Line*, a newspaper of the American Communist Workers Movement. He says that he is trying to find a life on his own, that he is not yet a Communist but is learning and trying to understand what is going on. He wrote a letter to his parents in which he tried to convince them of his new political views and tried to explain what these things mean to him. He wrote:

> The nation is run by the government and the government is run by the rich. All of the masses of the working people are the backbone of the country. In a matter of years, not many, there will be a revolution and there will be a great change in government and all Fascist courts, police, judges and other unrealistic forces trained in using the great masses of the people then will no longer be.

In the same letter, he described some of his experiences at the hospital:

> When I enquired about the purpose of the pills which they had given to me, they would say they were 'to keep me calm and from being nervous and upset'. Since then, they have asked, 'Don't you sleep much better since you have taken the pills in the daytime?', although I have taken none all of this time, but two.

During various therapy sessions Mark's mood changed from time to time. Sometimes he was very cooperative and friendly, talking freely, logically and coherently about his personal problems and his personal life history. When his drinking habits were discussed, he repeatedly stated he felt he was old enough and adult enough to take the responsibility of this and said he was able to stop himself from becoming drunk, but he also said he gets pleasure from being drunk and wants to do it again. He describes himself as 'a lumpen proletarian who belongs to the proletariat but prefers an easy way of life if possible with luxury, pleasure, et cetera'. He says he 'likes to have everything the best'. If he has to choose, he wants to have 'the best car, the best home, the best suit, the best shoes and everything the best. I want to enjoy a family and have at least one boy and a daughter, but no more than four children'. He says that he does not like a normal way of education and does not like to work in a factory – he prefers to be 'the man who delivers and carries things on the truck'. He further characterises himself as having 'a hot temper and one who acts easily and quickly'. He demonstrated this aspect of his personality in several of the sessions by jumping up, waving his arms and talking in a loud voice when the topics focused on issues or subjects he disliked.

He enjoys going to occupational and recreational therapy and spends much of his time talking politics with other patients, especially those younger than him. Periodically, he insists that he has to be released as soon as possible. He is becoming slightly more critical of his drinking habits and says he is sorry for hitting his parents. He believes he is ready to go home, return to his family and to try to start a new life.

EXERCISE FOR CLASS ENGAGEMENT

After reading Mark's story, discuss the following questions with your group:

1. Based on the information provided, what diagnoses would you consider for Mark?
2. What extra information would be needed to make a diagnosis?
3. What potential problems might a person like Mark present for nursing staff in terms of treatment?

NURSE'S STORY 14.1

Vanessa

Vanessa, the credentialled mental health nurse leading the DBT program at a community health centre, felt an immediate empathy for Mark because he reminded her of her brother Steven. Vanessa engaged Mark in regular one-to-one therapy and psychotherapy using a DBT approach and provided oversight for group sessions run by a psychologist at the centre. Vanessa also monitored Mark's continuation on the antidepressant medication prescribed by the referring psychiatrist.

Early in therapy Vanessa encouraged Mark to make a commitment to avoid further visits to his parents' home to facilitate his grieving and to allow adaptation to his recovery journey. Mark agreed and immediately warmed to Vanessa's empathetic approach, telling her that she was, 'The best counsellor I've ever met ... way better than the psychiatrist who is only interested in what pills I am taking'. While Vanessa appreciated Mark's enthusiasm, she was aware of the way that people with personality disorders can exhibit dependent traits and so made a mental note to reflect on and discuss Mark's case during her monthly clinical supervision session.

Despite Mark's enthusiasm and assurances, within a couple of months he began returning to his parents' home, abusing them in moments of stress. This led to further police involvement and culminated in a court order. Vanessa found the weeks when Mark behaved in this way extremely difficult because she couldn't stop thinking about the relationship problems she had experienced with her brother Steven. Vanessa often found herself drinking extra wine and struggling to sleep following workdays that involved such sessions with Mark.

Overall therapy proved to be such slow progress that Vanessa often felt as if they were taking a step back for every two steps forward. However, after two years of support Mark slowly developed more mature and adaptive emotional regulatory skills. He slowly became more aware of his tendency to idealise others and his fears of rejection. He continued to battle with urges to act impulsively when he became angry but got involved in a gym that appeared to be providing a healthier outlet for his feelings. As she observed incremental improvements in Mark, Vanessa also found reflecting on Mark's case self-enlightening as she continued to learn more about her psychotherapeutic capacity through clinical supervision.

Nursing approaches

Nursing people who have a personality disorder or other illnesses should be integrated and wherever possible the same nurse and treatment team should provide ongoing care for both the personality disorder and the co-occurring mental illness (NHMRC 2012). If this is not possible, the nurse or service providing treatment for the co-occurring condition should collaborate with the clinician who is responsible for managing the person's care (NHMRC 2012). Team-based approaches need to be supported by high-quality training and education that supports staff development in areas such as engagement skills, communication skills and the ability to use reflection so that all team members are able to operationalise a similar understanding and skill set and provide therapeutic care (Bowen & Mason 2012). On initial encounter, people with personality disorders often give the impression of being intelligent, charming, pleasant, friendly and functional people. However, closer scrutiny of the behaviour and verbal comments such as those made by Mark in the consumer's/nurse's story indicate that the facade is often misleading. In planning therapy for patients with personality disorders nurses will find the some of the principles in Box 14.1 useful.

Nurses should keep in mind that people with personality disorders seldom see themselves as needing help. They view themselves as being in step and consider the rest of the world in contention with them. They tend to be consummate actors attempting to fool others and, in the process, end up fooling themselves instead. They play at life and living, many times never fully realising what it is that they are missing. They commonly miss one of life's most unique experiences – loving and being loved.

Pharmacological interventions

Reviewers of treatments conclude that there is limited evidence to justify using medication in people with a personality disorder (NHMRC 2012). However, doctors do use some psychotropic medications to ameliorate symptoms and enable people to undertake the therapies in this chapter. Particular symptoms targeted include mood dysregulation

Box 14.1 Principles of working with people with a personality disorder

- Explore treatment options with a hopeful, optimistic recovery orientation.
- Bear in mind that many will have experienced abuse, rejection and/or stigma.
- Ensure the person is actively involved in problem solving and choices.
- Involve the person in setting limits and determining consequences.
- Remember that life involves constant risk and clinicians need to avoid 'assuming' all responsibility for risk.
- Stressful life situations tend to increase aberrant behaviour.
- Symptoms are often used to mask feelings of inadequacy, worthlessness and fear.
- Impulsive acting-out often emerges in response to frustration.
- Deceptive and aggressive behaviour are used by people with a personality disorder to avoid meaningful relationships.
- Limit setting and consistent structuring of the environment enhance opportunities to learn socially acceptable responses.
- Limits should be set according to the person's ability to accept responsibility for themselves.
- A direct, honest approach reinforces positive behaviour.
- Consistency in staff responses promotes realistic self-awareness.
- Entrapment can occur when unrealistic goals are set and promises are made that cannot be kept.
- Compliance with the therapeutic regimen is achieved through collaboration and sharing with the person.
- The nurse–patient relationship should incorporate learning experiences directed towards self-regulation.
- Use rational authority that permits freedom and experimentation within clear limits.
- Provide opportunities for experimentation along with assistance towards realistic self-evaluation by the person.
- Recognise that people with personality disorders will frequently attempt to place responsibility for the satisfaction of their needs on other people.
- Inability to recognise or control personal feelings towards the patient will impede a nurse's therapeutic relationship.

Adapted from National Collaborating Centre for Mental Health 2009

(selective serotonin reuptake inhibitors), impulsivity (mood stabilisers, anticonvulsants, carbamazepine), limited sociability (atypical neuroleptics) and cognitive distortions (atypical neuroleptics) (NHMRC 2012). Chapter 19 provides more information about these medications.

Chapter summary

People diagnosed with a personality disorder present major challenges for mental health service providers. Nurses and others need training, education and staff support to deal with the challenges posed by this patient group. Some of the new treatments emerging show evidence of efficacy, and in the not-too-distant future it is reasonable to hope that personality disorder will be better defined, identified and appropriately managed without stigma (Kim & Tyrer 2010). There is also a need to develop best practice programs that can be integrated into clinical practice by non-specialised health professionals (Koekkoek et al. 2010). In fact, Gunderson (2009) advocates for developing centres of excellence for personality disorders to support new generations of clinicians and researchers, as has been previously developed for treating people with other mental disorders. Studies need to be developed around structured and systematic strategies to provide empirical evidence upon which to base practice. The principles of trauma-informed care – safety, trustworthiness, choice, collaboration and empowerment – assist nurses and others to work in collaboration with this group of people (Kezelman & Stavropoulos 2012). Consistency, self-awareness and reflection, and a focus on hope, can make working with this cohort an extremely rewarding experience.

Useful websites

National Health and Medical Research Council: www.nhmrc.gov.au/guidelines-publications/mh25.

National Institute for Health and Care Excellence – borderline personality disorder treatment and management: www.nice.org.uk/guidance/cg78.

National Institute for Health and Care Excellence – personality disorders overview: http://pathways.nice.org.uk/pathways/personality-disorders.

National Institute of Mental Health: www.nimh.nih.gov/health/publications/borderline-personality-disorder/index.shtml.

Project Air: https://www.projectairstrategy.org/index.html.

Royal College of Psychiatrists: www.rcpsych.ac.uk/healthadvice/problemsdisorders/personalitydisorder.aspx.

References

American Psychiatric Association, 2013. Diagnostic and Statistical Manual of Mental Disorders, fifth ed. APA, Washington DC.

Ansell, E.B., Wright, A.G., Markowitz, J.C., et al., 2015. Personality disorder risk factors for suicide attempts over 10 years of follow-up. Personal. Disord. 6 (2), 161.

Bateman, A.W., 2012. Treating borderline personality disorder in clinical practice. Am. J. Psychiatry 169 (6), 560–563.

Bateman, J., Henderson, C., Kezelman, C., 2013. Trauma-informed care and practice: towards a cultural shift in policy reform across mental health and human services in Australia. A National Strategic Direction,

Position Paper and Recommendations of the National Trauma-Informed Care and Practice Advisory Working Group. Mental Health Coordinating Council, Sydney.

Booth, R., Keogh, K., Doyle, J., et al., 2014. Living through distress: a skills training group for reducing deliberate self-harm. Behav. Cogn. Psychother. 42 (2), 156–165.

Bowen, M., Mason, T., 2012. Forensic and non-forensic psychiatric nursing skills and competencies for psychopathic and personality disordered patients. J. Clin. Nurs. 21 (23–24), 3556–3564.

Cleary, M., Hungerford, C., 2015. Trauma-informed care and the research literature: how can mental health nurses take the lead to support women who have survived sexual assault? Issues Ment. Health Nurs. 36, 370–378.

Cloninger, R., Svrakic, D., 2008. Personality disorders. In: Fatemi, S., Clayton, P. (Eds.), The Medical Basis of Psychiatry. Humana Press, Totowa, NJ, pp. 471–483.

Commons Treloar, A.J., 2009. Effectiveness of education programs in changing clinicians' attitudes toward treating borderline personality disorder. Psychiatr. Serv. 60 (8), 1128–1131.

Cooper, L.D., Balsis, S., Oltmanns, T.F., 2014. Aging: empirical contribution. A longitudinal analysis of personality disorder dimensions and personality traits in a community sample of older adults: perspectives from selves and informants. J. Personal. Disord. 28 (1), 151.

Crawford, M., Price, K., Gordon, F., et al., 2009. Engagement and retention in specialist services for people with personality disorder. Acta Psychiatr. Scand. 119 (4), 304–311.

Crawford, M.J., Koldobsky, N., Mulder, R., et al., 2011. Classifying personality disorder according to severity. J. Personal. Disord. 25 (3), 321–330.

Debast, I., van Alphen, S.P., Rossi, G., et al., 2014. Personality traits and personality disorders in late middle and old age: do they remain stable? A literature review. Clin. Gerontol. 37 (3), 253–271.

Di Pierro, R., Preti, E., Vurro, N., et al., 2014. Dimensions of personality structure among patients with substance use disorders and co-occurring personality disorders: a comparison with psychiatric outpatients and healthy controls. Compr. Psychiatry 55 (6), 1398–1404.

Fanaian, M., Lewis, K.L., Grenyer, B.F., 2013. Improving services for people with personality disorders: views of experienced clinicians. Int. J. Ment. Health Nurs. 22 (5), 465–471.

Feigenbaum, J., 2010. Self-harm – the solution not the problem: the dialectical behaviour therapy model. Psychoanal. Psychother. 24 (2), 115–134.

Flaskerud, J.H., 2012. DSM-5: implications for mental health nursing education. Issues Ment. Health Nurs. 33 (9), 568–576.

Friborg, O., Martinsen, E.W., Martinussen, M., et al., 2014. Comorbidity of personality disorders in mood disorders: a meta-analytic review of 122 studies from 1988 to 2010. J. Affect. Disord. 152, 1–11.

Friborg, O., Martinussen, M., Kaiser, S., et al., 2013. Comorbidity of personality disorders in anxiety disorders: a meta-analysis of 30 years of research. J. Affect. Disord. 145 (2), 143–155.

Gunderson, J.G., 2009. Borderline personality disorder: ontogeny of a diagnosis. Am. J. Psychiatry 166 (5), 530–539.

Harned, M.S., Korslund, K.E., Foa, E.B., et al., 2012. Treating PTSD in suicidal and self-injuring women with borderline personality disorder: development and preliminary evaluation of a dialectical behavior therapy prolonged exposure protocol. Behav. Res. Ther. 50 (6), 381–386.

Holm, A.L., Berg, A., Severinsson, E., 2009. Longing for reconciliation: a challenge for women with borderline personality disorder. Issues Ment. Health Nurs. 30 (9), 560–568.

Holm, A.L., Severinsson, E., 2011. Struggling to recover by changing suicidal behaviour: narratives from women with borderline personality disorder. Int. J. Ment. Health Nurs. 20 (3), 165–173.

Horn, E.K., Bartak, A., Meerman, A.M., et al., 2014. Effectiveness of psychotherapy in personality disorders not otherwise specified: a comparison of different treatment modalities. Clin. Psychol. Psychother. 22, 426–442.

Horsfall, J., Cleary, M., Hunt, G.E., 2010. Stigma in mental health: persons and professionals. Issues Ment. Health Nurs. 31 (7), 450–455.

Howell, E., 2018. From hysteria to chronic relational trauma disorder: the history of borderline personality disorder and its connection to trauma, dissociation, and psychosis. In: Moskowitz, A., Dorahy, M.J., Schäfer, I. (Eds.), Psychosis, Trauma and Dissociation: Evolving Perspectives on Severe Psychopathology. John Wiley & Sons, Hoboken, pp. 83–95.

Huang, Y., Kotov, R., De Girolamo, G., et al., 2009. DSM-IV personality disorders in the WHO world mental health surveys. Br. J. Psychiatry 195 (1), 46–53.

Kern, M.L., Della Porta, S.S., Friedman, H.S., 2014. Lifelong pathways to longevity: personality, relationships, flourishing, and health. J. Pers. 82 (6), 72–84.

Kezelman, C., Stavropoulos, P., 2012. Practice Guidelines for Treatment of Complex Trauma and Trauma Informed Care and Service Delivery. Adults Surviving Child Abuse, Kirribilli.

Kim, Y.R., Tyrer, P., 2010. Controversies surrounding classification of personality disorder. Psychiatry Investig. 7 (1), 1–8.

Koekkoek, B., Van Der Snoek, R., Oosterwijk, K., et al., 2010. Preventive psychiatric admission for patients with borderline personality disorder: a pilot study. Perspect. Psychiatr. Care 46 (2), 127–134.

Lamont, S., Brunero, S., 2009. Personality disorder prevalence and treatment outcomes: a literature review. Issues Ment. Health Nurs. 30 (10), 631–637.

Lawn, S., McMahon, J., 2015. Experiences of care by Australians with a diagnosis of borderline personality disorder. J. Psychiatr. Ment. Health Nurs. 22 (7), 510–521.

Leichsenring, F., Leibing, E., Kruse, J., et al., 2011. Borderline personality disorder. Lancet 377 (9759), 74–84.

Linehan, M.M., 1998. An illustration of dialectical behavior therapy. In Session. Psychother. Pract. 4 (2), 21–44.
Linehan, M.M., 2000. Commentary on innovations in dialectical behavior therapy. Cogn. Behav. Pract. 7 (4), 478–481.
Matusiewicz, A.K., Hopwood, C.J., Banducci, A.N., et al., 2010. The effectiveness of cognitive behavioral therapy for personality disorders. Psychiatr. Clin. North Am. 33 (3), 657–685.
McGrath, B., Dowling, M., 2012. Exploring registered psychiatric nurses' responses towards service users with a diagnosis of borderline personality disorder. Nurs. Res. Pract. doi:10.1155/2012/601918.
McMain, S.F., Guimond, T., Streiner, D.L., et al., 2014. Dialectical behavior therapy compared with general psychiatric management for borderline personality disorder: clinical outcomes and functioning over a 2-year follow-up. Am. J. Psychiatry 169 (6), 650–661.
McMurran, M., Huband, N., Overton, E., 2010. Non-completion of personality disorder treatments: a systematic review of correlates, consequences, and interventions. Clin. Psychol. Rev. 30 (3), 277–287.
National Collaborating Centre for Mental Health (NCCMH), 2009. Borderline personality disorder: treatment and management. National Clinical Practice Guideline Number 78. The British Psychological Society and The Royal College of Psychiatrists, Leicester.
National Health and Medical Research Council (NHMRC), 2012. Clinical Practice Guideline for the Management of Borderline Personality Disorder. National Health and Medical Research Council, Melbourne.
Newton-Howes, G., Tyrer, P., Anagnostakis, K., et al., 2010. The prevalence of personality disorder, its comorbidity with mental state disorders, and its clinical significance in community mental health teams. Soc. Psychiatry Psychiatr. Epidemiol. 45 (4), 453–460.
Novak, T., Scanlan, J., McCaul, D., et al., 2012. Pilot study of a sensory room in an acute inpatient psychiatric unit. Australas. Psychiatry 20 (5), 401–406.
O'Connell, B., Dowling, M., 2014. Dialectical behaviour therapy (DBT) in the treatment of borderline personality disorder. J. Psychiatr. Ment. Health Nurs. 21 (6), 518–525.
Pasieczny, N., Connor, J., 2011. The effectiveness of dialectical behaviour therapy in routine public mental health settings: an Australian controlled trial. Behav. Res. Ther. 49 (1), 4–10.
Purves, D., Sands, N., 2009. Crisis and triage clinicians' attitudes toward working with people with personality disorder. Perspect. Psychiatr. Care 45 (3), 208–215.
Samuels, J., Eaton, W.W., Bienvenu, O.J., et al., 2002. Prevalence and correlates of personality disorders in a community sample. Br. J. Psychiatry 180 (6), 536–542.
Scanlan, J.N., Novak, T., 2015. Sensory approaches in mental health: a scoping review. Aust. Occup. Ther. J. 62 (5), 277–285.
Skodol, A.E., Bender, D.S., Oldham, J.M., et al., 2011. Proposed changes in personality and personality disorder assessment and diagnosis for DSM-5 part II: clinical application. Personal. Disord. 2 (1), 23–40.
Soloff, P.H., Chiappetta, L., 2012. Subtyping borderline personality disorder by suicidal behavior. J. Personal. Disord. 26 (3), 468.
Stoffers, J.M., Völlm, B.A., Rücker, G., et al., 2012. Psychological therapies for people with borderline personality disorder. Cochrane Database Syst. Rev. (2), CD005652.
Torgersen, S., Kringlen, E., Cramer, V., 2001. The prevalence of personality disorders in a community sample. Arch. Gen. Psychiatry 58 (6), 590–596.
Turner, B.J., Chapman, A.L., Layden, B.K., 2012. Intrapersonal and interpersonal functions of non-suicidal self-injury: associations with emotional and social functioning. Suicide Life Threat. Behav. 42 (1), 36–55.
Tyrer, P., Mulder, R., Crawford, M., et al., 2010. Personality disorder: a new global perspective. World Psychiatry 9 (1), 56–60.
Tyrer, P., Reed, G.M., Crawford, M.J., 2015. Classification, assessment, prevalence, and effect of personality disorder. Lancet 385 (9969), 717–726.
Vermetten, E., Spiegel, D., 2014. Trauma and dissociation: implications for borderline personality disorder. Curr. Psychiatry Rep. 16 (2), 1–10.
Westwood, L., Baker, J., 2010. Attitudes and perceptions of mental health nurses towards borderline personality disorder persons in acute mental health settings: a review of the literature. J. Psychiatr. Ment. Health Nurs. 17 (7), 657–662.
Whitbeck, L.B., Armenta, B.E., Welch-Lazoritz, M.L., 2015. Borderline personality disorder and axis I psychiatric and substance use disorders among women experiencing homelessness in three US cities. Soc. Psychiatry Psychiatr. Epidemiol. 50 (8), 1285–1291.
Wise, S., 2013. Inconvenient People: Lunacy, Liberty, and the Mad-Doctors in England. Counterpoint Press, Berkeley.
Zanarini, M.C., 2009. Psychotherapy of borderline personality disorder. Acta Psychiatr. Scand. 120 (5), 373–377.

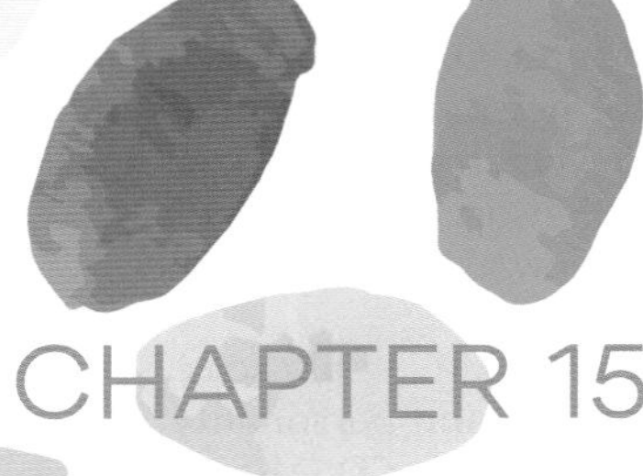

CHAPTER 15

Mental disorders of childhood and adolescence

Lucie Ramjan and Greg Clark

KEY POINTS

- The term 'childhood' spans the period from birth to adolescence. According to the World Health Organization, adolescents are aged 10–19 years. Some health services cater to young people up to the age of 25 years, as such within this chapter the combined group aged 0–25 years will at times be referred to collectively as 'children and young people'.
- The prevalence of mental health conditions in the early years of life can range from 10% to 20% internationally, including in Australia and New Zealand.
- In adolescence, anxiety and depression are among the most common mental health problems.
- Half of all mental disorders arise before the age of 14 but often go undetected. Although the highest prevalence of mental health problems occurs in the 18–24 age group, precursors to serious mental illness that are identified and managed during childhood and adolescence can serve to reduce this statistic.
- Mental health problems do not occur in isolation from other aspects of young people's lives.
- Evidence of a child or an adolescent experiencing behavioural or emotional problems may be indicative of difficulties with family, peers or school.
- It is essential to clarify the individual's perception of the problem they are experiencing and their goals for 'treatment', as well as their parents' perceptions and desired outcomes while working safely to protect the young person's right to confidentiality.
- 'Engagement' is the establishment of a therapeutic alliance, or rapport, in collaboration with the young person and their family to achieve desired outcomes and goals. This occurs from the initial interview. Understanding young people's language and their style of communicating is integral to effectively engaging with them.
- Nurses involved in the care of children and adolescents may have to deal with legal issues relating to duty of care, child protection and mental health legislation.

KEY TERMS

- Assessment
- Depression
- Engagement
- Gillick competence
- Internalising and externalising problems
- Psychoeducation
- Psychosis
- Resocialisation
- Suicide

LEARNING OUTCOMES

The material in this chapter will assist you to:

- develop an introductory understanding of childhood and adolescent mental health problems and disorders
- gain awareness of the extent of childhood and adolescent mental health problems in Australia and New Zealand and internationally
- appreciate the range of mental health services available to children and adolescents
- explore the role of nurses working with children and adolescents with mental health needs and supporting their families.

Introduction

Children and adolescents cannot simply be considered as 'little adults'. Within the field of mental health there are distinct differences between early life and adulthood. In recognition of the specific needs of children and young people, youth services (including mental health services) often extend their age range to include young adults up to 25 years of age.

This chapter introduces the field of child and adolescent mental health nursing. It explores the role of nurses and, using case studies from clinical practice, provides examples of disorders experienced by children and adolescents. Furthermore, it describes interventions that nurses can implement to assist young people and their families.

Although some disorders are intergenerational, they may differ in their form of presentation during different developmental stages. For example, children with depression may present as agitated or with a variety of somatic symptoms, whereas adolescents with depression might appear antisocial, aggressive or withdrawn or become involved in substance use (Rey et al. 2015). Some problems that are common to adults may start in childhood or be influenced by events that occurred early in life. Some problems may resolve with neurological development, emotional maturity or a stable, supportive environment. Likewise, with effective intervention and treatment there will be problems from which the young person can achieve a complete recovery.

Anxiety, depression and self-harm are among the most common mental health problems experienced during adolescence (World Health Organization 2019). More than 75% of people with serious mental illness such as schizophrenia or bipolar disorder have their first episode before the age of 25 (Layard & Hagell 2015) and at least half of all mental health problems emerge by the age of 14 (World Health Organization 2019). The highest prevalence of all mental health problems, including substance disorders, occurs in the 16–24 age group, with suicide being the third highest cause of death worldwide (Gore et al. 2011; Naghavi 2019). In Australia, 12.7% of people aged 16–24 are reported to have a substance use disorder, with rates higher in young men (Australian Institute of Health and Welfare 2011). With statistics such as these, it is crucial that the mental health of children and young people be a priority for society as a whole.

An important factor in considering the effect of any kind of illness on young people is the disruption it may bring to their development and education. In adulthood our lives can be dramatically impacted through illness, yet we have usually completed the basic developmental tasks of life and have finished the foundations of education. For a child or adolescent, however, various problems may develop simply due to the interruption caused by illness. Similarly, a child's experiences during early development and onwards can influence subsequent developmental progress, mental health and wellbeing, giving rise to problems in adolescence and later life.

Despite the prevalence of child and adolescent mental health disorders, mental health issues continue to go unrecognised and untreated in children and young people, leading to poorer outcomes in areas such as health, education and occupation. This can result in a vast economic cost to society. Specialised child and adolescent mental health services are frequently unavailable in more remote areas of Australasia, many young people are therefore unable to access appropriate early recognition and support (Morris et al. 2011). It is with this in mind that health service policy, planning and models of care for children and young people should be targeted at strategies such as health promotion, prevention and early intervention to support tomorrow's adults and reduce the associated financial burden (Erskine et al. 2015; World Health Organization 2014; 2019).

Diagnosis in child and adolescent mental healthcare

Unlike previous editions of the American Psychiatric Association's *Diagnostic and Statistical Manual of Mental Disorders*, the fifth edition (2013) places greater emphasis on a developmental and lifespan perspective, accepting that a significant proportion of mental health problems begin in childhood and adolescence. Symptoms exhibited by young people may be transient, dynamic and changing over time and may not always fall easily into a diagnostic category. While acknowledging that these problems are not limited to a specific age group, there is a higher frequency of occurrence during periods such as early childhood, middle childhood and adolescence. Table 15.1 provides an overview of mental health issues typically experienced in childhood and adolescence.

The child behaviour checklist (see Box 15.1) places stronger emphasis on behaviour and problems rather than categories. Viewing problems within such a framework helps us understand young people as having issues related to predominant personality traits, developmental factors or incidents and influences within their family and wider social environment. By contrast, static diagnostic systems can mask the fluid, changing and reorganising nature of young people's experience as they progress towards adulthood, and may also run the risk of encouraging a focus on one 'problem' in isolation, rather than exploring a child's functioning in different settings and from different sources of information (Achenbach & Ndetei 2015; Thompson et al. 2012). For this reason, this chapter describes mental health problems in the context in which symptoms are observed, rather than in relation to categorical diagnostic criteria.

Incidence

Writers in various Western countries have often expressed concern about the prevalence of emotional problems in

TABLE 15.1 Overview of mental health issues in children and young people

NEURODEVELOPMENTAL DISORDERS	ELIMINATION DISORDERS	DEPRESSIVE AND BIPOLAR DISORDERS	ANXIETY DISORDERS
Attention deficit hyperactivity disorder Autism spectrum disorder Communication disorders Specific learning disorder Tic disorder	Encopresis Enuresis	Bipolar disorder Disruptive mood dysregulation disorder Major depressive disorder Persistent depressive disorder	Agoraphobia Generalised anxiety disorder Panic disorder Selective mutism Separation anxiety Social anxiety Specific phobia
DISRUPTIVE, IMPULSE CONTROL AND CONDUCT DISORDERS	**TRAUMA AND STRESSOR-RELATED DISORDERS**	**SCHIZOPHRENIA SPECTRUM AND OTHER PSYCHOTIC DISORDERS**	**FEEDING AND EATING DISORDERS**
Conduct disorder Intermittent explosive disorder Oppositional defiant disorder	Acute stress disorder Adjustment disorder Disinhibited social engagement disorder Post-traumatic stress disorder Reactive attachment disorder	Brief psychotic disorder Delusional disorder Schizoaffective disorder Schizophrenia	Anorexia nervosa Avoidant/restrictive food intake disorder Binge-eating disorder Bulimia nervosa Other specified feeding or eating disorder Pica

Adapted from American Psychiatric Association 2013

Box 15.1 Child behaviour checklist

GENERAL AREAS

- **Internalising problems:** inhibited or over-controlled behaviours such as anxiety or depression
- **Externalising problems:** antisocial or under-controlled behaviours such as delinquency or aggression

SPECIFIC AREAS

- **Somatic complaints:** recurring physical problems that have no known cause or cannot be medically verified; these may include headaches or a tendency to develop signs and symptoms of a medical disorder
- **Delinquent behaviour:** behaviour where rules set by parents or communities are broken, such as property damage, theft of cars and other items
- **Attention problems:** concentration difficulties and an inability to sit still, including school performance problems
- **Aggressive behaviour:** bullying, teasing, fighting and temper tantrums
- **Social problems:** where individuals have impairment of their relationships with peers
- **Withdrawal:** where the individual is specifically inhibited by shyness and being socially isolated
- **Anxious/depressed behaviour:** a range of feelings of loneliness, sadness, feeling unloved, a sense of worthlessness, anxiety and generalised fears
- **Thought disorders:** what might be seen as bizarre behaviour or thinking

Adapted from Sawyer et al. 2007

the earlier years of life. Within countries surveyed, the incidence ranges from 10% to 20% (World Health Organization 2018). This pattern is already reflected in Australasia, with the Second Australian Child and Adolescent Survey of Mental Health and Wellbeing noting that 13.9% of 4- to 17-year-olds have had a mental health disorder in the past 12 months – of this number, 59.8% had a mild mental disorder, 25.4% had a moderate disorder and 14.7% had a severe disorder (Lawrence et al. 2015).

The response of the World Health Organization to the need for better adolescent health promotion and prevention strategies, including mental health, has been *Global Accelerated Action for the Health of Adolescents (AA-HA!): Guidance to support country implementation*, published in 2017, which provides guidance to policymakers and program managers and highlights the importance of co-production of programs *with* adolescents (World Health Organization 2017).

Historical anecdote 15.1: Young people who experience mental ill health can become leaders

Clifford Beers (1876–1943) was a young person with lived experience who became a pioneer of modern community-based mental health services. When he was 18 years old and studying at Yale University in the United States, Beers' brother was diagnosed with epilepsy. Beers subsequently developed obsessional ideas and anxiety, fearing that he would develop epilepsy himself. He wrote that, 'The more I considered it and him, the more nervous I became and the more nervous, the more convinced that my own breakdown was only a matter of time' (Beers 1908, pp. 7–8). Beers became so unwell that he was admitted several times to mental hospitals. His experiences within mental hospitals of the early 20th century led him to publish a memoir of his experiences titled *A Mind that Found Itself*. He went on to establish America's National Committee for Mental Hygiene, which was later renamed the National Association for Mental Health.

Read more about it: *Beers CW 1908 A mind that found itself: an autobiography. Longmans, Green.*

Developmental issues

There are a range of theories and models covering physical, psychological and cognitive development pertaining to children and young people. Knowledge of these various models can be helpful when working with children and adolescents because they provide us with guidance about what to look for when assessing children and adolescents as well as guide our interactions with them, based on their cognitive or emotional stage of development. For example, knowing that the capacity for abstract thinking does not develop until approximately 12 years of age can help us with the language and concepts we use with younger children. In practice, this means using terms like being 'unhappy' or 'sad' rather than being 'depressed'. Younger children can usually understand unhappy or sad, whereas depression is an abstract concept that they may not understand or relate to.

Physical milestones usually occur within an age range, and knowledge of these normal ranges can alert us to potential problems. For example, most babies learn to walk between 12 and 18 months of age, and a delay in acquiring this skill may indicate a physical or cognitive problem.

Jean Piaget, a Swiss psychologist, identified a number of important milestones in a child's emotional and cognitive development. The first milestone is acquiring a sense of object permanence, which occurs around 9 months of age. The baby comes to realise that things continue to exist even when they are out of sight. This can lead to the baby becoming distressed when their primary caregiver is absent or leaves the room and helps explain why this behaviour begins around the age of 9 months. Between 18 months and 24 months, children develop the capacity for symbolic play and use their imagination in play. This is frequently the time that young children begin to develop their language skills and they can therefore describe what is happening in their play. Language involves using symbols to represent something else, so it is not surprising that these developments occur at around the same time.

Around the age of 7 years children develop an understanding of the conservation of volume. This is a further development of symbolic thinking. For example, if you show a younger child a tall, skinny container and a low, wide container, they will invariably tell you that the tall skinny container contains more liquid. Once they develop conservation of volume, this is no longer the case and the child may experiment with the containers to determine which has the largest volume.

The final stage in Piaget's framework is developing the capacity for abstract thinking at around 12 years of age. Piaget described this as being capable of reasoning not only based on objects but also on the basis of hypotheses or of propositions (Piaget 1962). The capacity for abstract thinking is a sign of sound cognitive development and informs us that the child is developing as expected.

There are other developmental models that will not be discussed here. Piaget's model is probably one of the more useful approaches in mental health work, but it is not the only way to think about developmental issues. Students who have an interest in this area can investigate other possibilities, such as Freud's psychosexual developmental theory, Erikson's psychosocial developmental theory, Bowlby's attachment theory and Bandura's social learning theory.

Knowledge of developmental processes and normal ranges can help us identify any delays in development. Delays can be due to a range of factors including difficulties during the birthing process such as restricted oxygen intake resulting from compression of the umbilical cord, or from exposure to domestic violence or poor caregiving. It is important for all nurses in all clinical settings to identify and delineate the nature of any developmental concerns and make referrals to the most appropriate service.

Critical thinking challenge 15.1

1. Why do nurses (general and specialist) have such a vital role to play in early detection of mental health problems in children and young people?
2. What interventions might nurses (general and specialist) provide?

Mental illness in context

Because mental health issues can affect many aspects of young people's lives, their experiences must be seen in context. It is often the case that the more significant the mental health concern, the greater the possibility of complications in other aspects of their lives. Furthermore, parents and other family members may see these problems as affecting their own lifestyles and activities. While more needs to be understood about the long-term outlook for these young people, it is important for professionals to see the problems in the context of the child's everyday experiences. Help may be needed across a broad range of life issues, including with family functioning, social skills or school problems. While the mental health problem may have caused these difficulties, it is equally important to consider that a life issue may have been the cause *or* a contributing factor in the disorder, and we need to understand the cause to inform prevention strategies (Gunnell et al. 2018). We must take a balanced view so causal factors are not attributed to one area without adequately observing what is happening in other aspects of the young person's life. It may be that the child or adolescent is acting as a 'barometer' for other problems – the young person may be presenting with symptoms that reflect problems in the family or between parents. This may not be recognised initially and may be revealed only after some exploration over time. This is why an important aspect of assessing children and adolescents includes evaluating the family's functioning and coping skills.

Historical anecdote 15.2: Historical labels

In 1856 the French psychiatrist Benedict Morel began describing young people exhibiting signs of mental ill health as experiencing 'dementia praecox' (meaning precocious or early dementia). In 1902 the German psychiatrist Emil Kraepelin (1956–1926) used the term 'dementia praecox' to differentiate psychosis from what he referred to as manic depression (bipolar disorder). Morel and Kraepelin linked 'dementia' with psychotic features because they theorised that the illness was neurologically based, like forms of dementia, and that the clinical pathway led to deterioration and chronicity, similar to dementia. This view was far from optimistic, and the prognosis left minimal hope for the individual's recovery. It is more widely accepted today that it is possible for young people who experience episodes of mental ill health to recover.

Read more about it: *Kendler KS 2018 The development of Kraepelin's mature diagnostic concepts of paranoia and paranoid dementia praecox: a close reading of his textbooks from 1887 to 1899. JAMA Psychiatry 75(12):1280–8.*

Assessment

Assessing the mental health of children and young people can be very complex. Depending on the age of the child, it may not be the young person who identifies a specific problem or seeks assistance. Rather, a referral is often received from an adult (parent, teacher, health worker) presenting their view of the problem, thus providing an interpretation of what they perceive is troubling the child. It is the responsibility of the nurse to then build a therapeutic alliance with all parties involved, ensuring each person feels heard, valued and respected.

In the process of gathering information, an assessment should include not only talking with the child or young person on their own but also asking their consent to talk to others (and explaining the rationale for this), such as their parents, carers, friends and teachers, to gain alternative perspectives. It is helpful to obtain relevant information from several people, given that problems may be interpreted and represented in a variety of ways by others involved in a child's life. Using a biopsychosocial assessment approach can be time-consuming and is often best managed over several short sessions, rather than in one go.

A young person's assessment will follow a similar structure to that undertaken in an adult mental health context; however, some information may require collateral. Having a sound knowledge of expected developmental milestones enables the nurse to differentiate between the responses and developmental challenges of life and the significant psychological problems that may be occurring. Many mental health problems in children and young people may go undetected because signs of the problem are exhibited through their behaviour, physical manifestations or school performance. Exploring the prevalence, persistence, pervasiveness and negative impact of the problem helps appraise and conceptualise its nature and severity so that appropriate interventions can be implemented.

Similarly, gaining an appreciation of the hopes, fears and expectations of each person present – while exploring strengths and protective factors, parenting styles and relationships between family members – can assist in placing the identified problems in context. For instance, issues such as poverty, unemployment, parental substance misuse and cultural isolation can all have a detrimental impact on a child's mental health. Therefore, it is important to collect information that enables the nurse to see the problem through a wider lens so they can work effectively with the child and family (Layard & Hagell 2015). Observation also plays a critical role when assessing children and adolescents. The behaviour and the information provided may not always be congruent. Observing family interactions, non-verbal communication and each person's responses can highlight family dynamics and lead to further understanding of what may be happening for the child within the family or within the child's other social contexts.

Box 15.2 Example of a framework to guide the assessment process

- Presenting concerns
- Family history
- Social history
- Developmental assessment
- Cultural issues
- Psychometric tools
- Mental state assessment
- Observation of interactions
- Risk assessment

Finally, assessing risk is an essential part of any child and adolescent mental health assessment (Mares & Graeff-Martins 2015). In Australia and New Zealand, health professionals are required by law to report any children who they believe are at risk. Mental health nurses therefore have a statutory obligation to report any suspicion of risk to a child or young person with whom they are working. Significant harm or the likelihood of experiencing significant harm from abuse (physical, sexual, emotional, neglect or a combination of all) must be reported. To ensure a unified response, multi-agency collaboration and cohesion is essential in cases where abuse is suspected or disclosed. Risk assessment cannot be achieved through a 'tick box' exercise, since risks concerning children and adolescents are often multifactorial and complex. Risk must be assessed not only from a mental health perspective but also within the caregiving context. Risk factors can include an immediate threat to the child's safety, as in cases of child abuse, or be cumulative, such as a child who is exposed to multiple risk factors such as adversity, neglect, parental illness or domestic violence.

Being sensitive to the presence of child abuse and the impact of the abuse on a child's health and psychological wellbeing is essential in any assessment. The long-term effect of abuse and trauma can have profound consequences in the developing years on brain development, leading to mental health problems, drug and alcohol dependence and associated risk taking.

It can be helpful for a nurse to have a framework from which all aspects of the assessment are completed (see example in Box 15.2). Ultimately, undertaking a comprehensive mental health assessment will enable the mental health nurse to gather the facts and ensure that any decisions made are in the best interests of the child and family.

Services available to children and young people

In many Western countries, specialised input is most often provided by child and adolescent mental health services (CAMHS) or child and youth mental health services (CYMHS). These services have expanded their scope considerably, offering a range of specialist assessment and treatment options. A limitation remains that these services are often found only in main centres. However, smaller populations throughout Australia and New Zealand may have the benefit of eCYMHS, with access to online psychiatric, nursing and allied health input via electronic media generated to smaller populations from main centres.

To offer a comprehensive service to meet the mental health needs of children and adolescents, the focus of service delivery requires a shift from all mental health-related issues being managed by CAMHS to an acceptance that early-onset symptoms can effectively be managed via promotive and preventive strategies. This can be achieved through integration and collaboration between universal services (such as primary health care, education and social and community workers). These professionals, by the nature of their roles, work daily with children and adolescents and are in a prime position to recognise and manage mental health issues early in their development. A range of broad psychosocial strategies, education and general advice can be offered, and more complex mental health issues can be identified and referred to specialist services as required.

This is consistent with the pyramid framework, as advocated by the World Health Organization (2009) (see Fig. 15.1). When planning and organising service delivery, involving people such as nurses working in general practice, rural and remote nurses, teachers, social workers, general practitioners (GPs) and youth workers would reflect the largest tier of the multilayer pyramid (universal informal community care). This tier represents services that are frequently needed and includes interventions that can be provided at a moderately low cost. Nurses working in emergency departments and generalist clinical settings and child and family nurses can provide primary care mental health services (universal and targeted support), while the top tier of the pyramid reflects specialist services that are often expensive and required for only a small percentage of children and young people – for instance, those with moderate to severe and highly complex mental health disorders who require input from specialist health professionals such as mental health nurses (Servili 2015). Nationally in Australia and New Zealand there is active collaboration among the various government and community-based agencies providing care to young people and their families, resulting in considerably less overlap or duplication of services. This has led to various interagency education and training opportunities for workers in the field.

For adolescents in particular, simply providing a traditional outpatient or inpatient service may not be enough. Many teenagers worry about what others would think if they asked for help, while others say they prefer to take care of their own problems, as they struggle with their sense of identity and relationships with adults. A

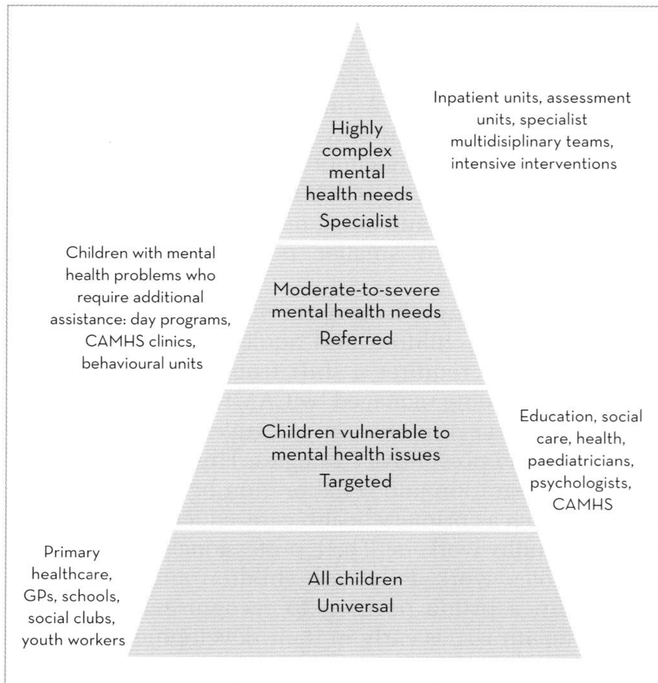

Figure 15.1
A stepped approach to care based on a pyramid framework of healthcare delivery
Adapted from World Health Organization 2009

variety of unhealthy or 'at-risk' behaviours may be present. Despite the National Drug Strategy Household Survey (Australian Institute of Health and Welfare 2017) reporting a decline in the use of tobacco, alcohol and illicit substances in young people, prevalence rates remain fairly high and show a rise in recent methamphetamine users from 22% in 2010 to 50% in 2013 and to 57% in 2016. This highlights the need for more collaboration and more funding for generalised adolescent health services and reach-out programs that can support young people with mild-to-moderate mental health issues.

In some centres in Australia and New Zealand, there are adolescent health centres where no appointment is needed, and teenagers can attend unaccompanied. These centres provide a wide range of services and programs for all health and lifestyle matters. They are often based on a model of primary care promoting early intervention for several health needs and are delivered by a range of multidisciplinary professionals. Such a place in Australia is headspace, a national youth mental health foundation (see www.headspace.org.au), which offers a youth-friendly environment where young people with mental health issues can attend for a range of issues such as general health, mental health, drug and alcohol issues and education or vocational support (Perera et al. 2019; Rickwood et al. 2015). headspace has been so effective in working with young people that a number of primary and tertiary health services have adopted its assessment interview known as HEEADSSS (Home, Education and Employment, Activities, Drugs, Sexuality, Suicide/Depression, Safety) to assist in identifying psychosocial and mental health issues (Hirani et al. 2018).

There is variation between regional services in the types of intervention and treatment available. As with adult services, there are usually a range of walk-in clinics and mobile crisis and support teams, backed up by separate residential units for adolescents and for children – some with programs for families to be admitted in specific circumstances.

The treatment provided also varies from centre to centre, depending on the major problems leading young people to present locally, their age range, the treatment philosophy, theoretical models, expertise available and the living circumstances of the young person and their family. Interventions may include cognitive behaviour therapy, play therapy, psycho-dynamic individual or group work, socialisation and social skills programs, systems-based family therapy, couples therapy, parenting programs or individual therapy for a parent. Sometimes approaches are combined to achieve better outcomes. For example, a child may benefit from cognitive behaviour therapy to help them, while their parents and siblings may benefit from learning positive ways of functioning together. As with adult services, nurses have a range of roles, often developing expertise in various modes of therapy.

The nursing role

Children and adolescents are still developing as individuals, so an intervention while they are young can often have a dramatic positive impact for the rest of their life. Early intervention is often more effective than managing difficulties that have extended into adulthood. With adequate care and a supportive environment, young people can develop resilience – emotionally, psychologically and physically. All nurses have a key role in implementing stepped care arrangements, including services for young people with, or at risk of, mental illness.

Working within a child and adolescent mental health team provides the opportunity to use a wide range of dynamic clinical treatment strategies and therapies. A multidisciplinary team approach is most frequently used. Nurses often play a significant role in various aspects of care, including that of therapist for children, adolescents and families. It is usually expected that a nurse wishing to enter this field will have some years of experience as a mental health nurse and further education, therefore possessing a solid grounding in theory and clinical practice.

Apart from graduate nursing programs, child and adolescent mental health nurses have options available for advanced studies in specialist areas of mental health through postgraduate and master's programs. In addition, nurses can take further training in counselling programs such as family therapy, solution-focused therapy and psychotherapy. Australian child and adolescent mental health services require workers with a high level of knowledge and skills. While Australia does not currently have a set of national competencies relating specifically to nursing in CAMHS, services have adopted guidelines for practice based on the standards of practice developed by the Australian College of Mental Health Nurses (2010). Likewise, some states have developed a competency framework based on those already developed in New Zealand (NSW Ministry of Health 2011; The Werry Centre 2014). These frameworks acknowledge the unique knowledge and skills regarded as fundamental for all professionals working in CAMHS and focus on a number of universal key areas, each with further identified core knowledge and skills to work effectively with children and young people experiencing mental health problems.

Identifying vulnerable children and young people

Parental illness, and specifically mental illness, may have a significant impact on a child's life and mental health. For example, the child may have to take on extra responsibilities, may experience inconsistent parenting or may observe behaviour that is difficult to comprehend, depending on their age. As a result, children of parents who have a mental illness often have social, emotional and psychological needs different from those of children with healthy parents or parents with chronic physical health conditions. Research has even shown that some adult children of parents with mental illness recalled childhood experiences of fear and mistrust, loneliness and isolation that continued into adulthood (Murphy et al. 2015). Over many years the Australian Infant, Child, Adolescent and Family Mental Health Association has campaigned for support for these young people. Since 2001 the Australian Government has provided funds for a project called Children of Parents with a Mental Illness (COPMI) to enable the provision and sharing of resources and support for various groups around Australia working with these families (see www.copmi.net.au).

Other groups of children who may be deemed vulnerable, or at increased risk of developing mental health problems, include: children in care, such as those in foster care or residential care homes, or who are adopted; young offenders; young people with a physical or intellectual disability; young people from culturally diverse backgrounds; homeless children; refugees and asylum seekers; and young people questioning their sexual orientation or gender identity (Australian Health Ministers' Advisory Council 2013). As a nurse it can often be challenging due to the presenting complexity of the problem and the need to work with several agencies, each with a different agenda. It is important that the nurse remains flexible and has clear guidelines for what is expected in their role as an experienced mental health nurse.

Perinatal mental health nursing

Historically, perinatal mental health included only the postpartum stage of childbirth with a focus on the mother's mental health and wellbeing. As more evidence arises, there is a better understanding that both mother and baby require sensitive assessment and the earliest possible intervention to maximise mental wellness for them both. Perinatal mental health encompasses not only the mental health of the mother and the child but also the child–mother relationship, the emotional and psychological wellbeing of other family members and social factors that may impact on the overall health of individuals within the family. Starting from preconception, perinatal mental health includes the antenatal and the postnatal periods, usually until the child is 24 months old. However, Woolhouse et al. (2015) report that a higher number of women experience symptoms related to depression *after* their child has reached 4 years old, compared with the number of women immediately after birth.

Nevertheless, whether a mother has a pre-existing mental health problem or develops a mental health problem in the antenatal or postnatal stage, it can have direct and indirect consequences for the child. Research indicates that mothers experiencing mental distress may not be as sensitive or responsive to their infant's needs and can struggle to complete several activities associated with caring for an infant (Santona et al. 2015). With a strong evidence base demonstrating the importance of secure attachments between a child and their primary caregiver, interactions between a mother experiencing mental illness and her infant can have a detrimental impact on the bonding relationship. Evidence also suggests that the children of mothers who experience longer term illness, such as postnatal depression, may be prone to experiencing developmental delays in areas such as social functioning, language, cognition and behaviour (Goodman 2019).

Recent advances in screening for perinatal mental health issues and a multitude of training courses designed to identify and manage perinatal issues in primary care are now available throughout Australia. Midwives and nurses in all clinical settings need to be aware of mental health during the perinatal period and use these opportunities to identify, assess and refer as necessary. The role of a mental health nurse working in child and adolescent mental health services is to assess and take account of any perinatal mental health issues when undertaking a psychosocial assessment. Part of planning care for a child or young person may involve referring the mother or carer to a more appropriate service to manage their own mental health.

Engaging with children and adolescents

Mental health nurses can become a significant resource for their clients. However, to be able to intervene effectively, the nurse needs to master the art of engaging with children and young people, as individuals and with their parents or carers, in the context of *their* families.

One of the most useful skills a mental health nurse can acquire and refine is the ability to engage clients and establish rapport. Engagement between nurses, young people and their families is fundamental to developing a relationship based on trust. A relationship founded on trust will foster a willingness to work together towards change. This involves communicating in a way that is appropriate within the context of the child's development (The Werry Centre 2014). For example, the communication skills and language used when working with a 5-year-old would differ significantly from those used when working with a 16-year-old. Essentially the nurse is required to master a diverse range of communication skills that not only encourages children and teenagers to listen but also foster effective active listening so that the young person is more likely to communicate in response.

Mental health nurses working with children and adolescents also need to develop and refine the skill of discreet observation of the young person's mood and behaviour, and their interactions with their peers, family, friends and others. Observation of these factors, considered in the broader psychosocial context, will enable the nurse to achieve a more comprehensive understanding of the factors contributing to the current difficulties experienced by the young person and their family.

Ongoing discussion with parents (carers) should clarify which specific factors may be contributing to the person's current problems. With a more specific diagnosis, the nurse and family may then begin the process of exploring solutions (planning), and referral to mental health services may be warranted. Any solutions agreed with the family are best implemented with the family's support and commitment, maximising the probability of positive change. Constant monitoring (evaluation) of behavioural interventions and responses by family members is essential to ensure the mental health team, the young person and their family continue to share a common understanding about managing the problem and a commitment to recovery.

The full participation of young people and their family in their mental health care should not be confined solely to therapeutic outcomes. Organisations have a lot to learn from consumers about planning environments that are sensitive to the needs of young people. 'Family-friendly' environments also need to include processes that respond to the specific needs of younger people, in particular those who are experiencing significant emotional or mental health difficulties.

Engaging young people and families across cultural contexts is key to accurate diagnoses and comprehensive treatment planning. There are implications for the way in which mental health professionals approach assessing clients and families in both Australia and New Zealand. The nurse's understanding of specific cultural practices and beliefs held by clients is imperative to developing trust. Asking for information in such a way that recognises cultural norms will promote the client's confidence in the care provided. Clients are more likely to provide accurate information if they believe the nurse has an understanding of their cultural needs and a genuine respect and commitment to a recovery plan that is culturally sound.

Children

As outlined previously, myriad factors contribute to and affect the mental health of young people. Familial or genetic predisposition to mental illness, the presence of a coexisting medical or neurological problem, developmental problems or growing up in a chaotic or deprived environment are just a few of the considerations of which a beginning mental health nurse should be mindful during assessments of young people and their families. Furthermore, these factors will also affect the direction taken with goal planning and nursing interventions. It should be remembered that the nursing care plan is in fact a recovery plan for the young person and family; therefore, the goals must be achievable, the plan must be collaboratively developed and the strategies must be practical and able to be implemented by the child and parents (with nursing support). If the plan is based on what the nurse can achieve rather than what the family can realistically accomplish, then the medium- to long-term success for recovery may be severely impaired and continuity of care lost. Case study 15.1 and the exploration of the issues discussed illustrates some key concepts.

CASE STUDY 15.1
Adam

A mother takes her four-year-old daughter for an immunisation and mentions to the general practice nurse that she's worried about her 9-year-old son, Adam, who she describes as 'becoming increasingly anxious' and who has developed 'a fixation with tidiness', so much so that it is causing disruption in the family. The family consists of two female siblings, aged 11 and 4, and a father who is an accomplished musician who frequently travels for extended periods performing nationally and internationally. The nurse empathises with the mother and validates her concerns, referring her to the GP and recommending she contacts the community CYMHS. The mother decides to contact CYMHS. The mental health nurse receiving the call assures the mother that her concerns warrant a further assessment by a member of the mental health team, as her child appears to be highly anxious. He is unable to relax and appears to be developing maladaptive behaviours (excessive tidying). Furthermore, his anxiety is having an adverse effect on his relationship with his siblings. The nurse gathers more specific information by phone and explains to the mother that this referral will be discussed at the next team meeting and that she will receive a call within a week regarding an appointment for her, her husband and their son, for further assessment.

DISCUSSION OF CASE STUDY: ADAM

Within the first minutes of a mother's description of her son's problem, the mental health nurse was able to predict a role for the mental health team in assisting this family. The mother was assured that her concerns were well founded. The nurse spent a little more time gathering only the information necessary to discuss the case (assessment) with the clinical team so a plan for a further face-to-face interview could be made. The mother was reassured by the prospect of another appointment (implementation) and felt her initial concerns had been validated. A therapeutic alliance has been initiated between the family and the mental health service.

This early process reflects the beginning of the nurse's role in engaging the family in the therapeutic alliance and emphasises how important each team member's role is in promoting a positive impression on the family (even before meeting them personally). The impression the family gains from an initial phone call can colour their perception of further interactions with the mental health team. Furthermore, the parents' feelings of confidence in the mental health nurse and other team members will most likely have an impact on the confidence that the child and siblings experience. This is important because all family members will be involved in the child's recovery.

The foundation and building of a therapeutic relationship with the young person and the family will usually begin at the time of the initial phone call or face-to-face interview. This interview can be difficult for the young person, who may not perceive that there is a problem and therefore may not fully understand why they are attending an assessment at a mental health service. A skilled mental health nurse will use this opportunity to establish the young person's understanding of their need for an appointment. If the young person seems unsure (or unwilling to concede), they can often be encouraged to describe some difficulties that are occurring at home that they think may have led to their needing this appointment.

It is essential to clarify the child or young person's perception of the problem and their goals for treatment, as well as those of the parents. The nurse's role is to facilitate expression of the difficulties and to make explicit the goal(s) that the client and family have regarding recovery. This is necessary so that all parties (child, family and mental health team) agree on the treatment plan.

Case study 15.2 illustrates these key issues. While a diagnosis such as attention deficit hyperactivity disorder might possibly be indicated in this situation, the case illustrates that it is important to concentrate on the presenting problems and any associated difficulties, rather than giving priority to diagnostic classification. Involving diagnostic controversies can potentially misdirect the focus of care from the individual needs of the child and family.

CASE STUDY 15.2
Tim

Tim is a 6-year-old boy who is attending his first appointment at a community CYMHS, accompanied by his parents. He is the oldest of three children and has a young brother and baby sister. His parents report an escalation in Tim's behaviour just before he turned three: 'It's like he never grew out of the "terrible twos". He just kept on going at a hundred miles an hour,' reported his mother. Tim's father concurred: 'The more limits I set, the worse he gets.' Tim's reply when asked if he knew why he was here was simply: 'I've been naughty.'

DISCUSSION OF CASE STUDY: TIM

A skilled mental health nurse will attempt to clarify these comments using objective language and will eventually identify specific behaviours that the parents regard as priorities for change. The nurse will attempt to match the parents' goals with those of their son.

The nurse's response to Tim's perception that he has been 'naughty' might be: 'Naughty? What do you mean?' The aim for the nurse is to guide Tim to use specific words to tag specific behaviours, and if these match those identified by his parents, a simple goal may be developed to achieve an outcome that is satisfying to both parties. Tim's descriptions of how he sees what's going on may also help the nurse to establish more accurately what the relevant issues might be. Consider this further exchange between Tim and the nurse:

Nurse: Naughty? What does that mean?
Tim: When I run away or squeal.
Nurse: So, you run away?
Tim: My brother ... he's three. He runs away too. When he runs away from Mummy, she chases him.
Nurse: And does your brother squeal?
Tim: No, but when my baby sister squeals, Daddy helps Mummy play with her.

This exchange demonstrates how, through active listening, the nurse has gathered some very specific information about the family dynamics that provides a possible explanation for some of Tim's behaviour. It could be that he is mimicking the behaviours of his younger siblings to receive the same attention from his parents that he perceives his brother and sister receive when they run away or squeal.

Encounters with children and adolescents and their families as illustrated in these case studies demonstrate how the nurse and other team members can engage young people in ongoing treatment, and how treatment will be influenced by further findings. Initiating a sound therapeutic alliance with the child and family is an achievement, although the alliance also requires nurturing.

Generally, a therapeutic alliance is accomplished when respect is paramount in the nurse–client relationship. Like adults, young people respond most positively to being treated with genuine respect. Young people feel respected when they are listened to and given opportunities to make choices and contribute to solving problems. As Roberts et al. (2015) identify, making choices gives the child valuable practice in making decisions, and opportunities for problem solving give them courage to follow things through independently. A commitment by the mental health nurse to facilitating choice and promoting problem-solving opportunities for young people will be further enhanced by a belief in the humanistic idea that all behaviour has meaning. If mental health nurses explore the meaning behind the behaviours we observe, we can plan appropriate strategies to modify behaviour and promote positive change.

Within Australia and New Zealand, CYMHS work with many young people who present in acute emotional distress. Some will internalise their distress and may become withdrawn and depressed. Others may externalise their emotional pain. When this occurs, the child will demonstrate altered behaviours, which may include rigid thinking, compulsive patterns of behaviour, agitation, impulsivity and, in severe cases, aggression. If the nurse has established a therapeutic alliance with the child, the shared trust and respect will provide a foundation for choice-giving and problem solving. An example from practice (case study 15.3) will best illustrate this concept.

CASE STUDY 15.3
Fiona

Fiona is 12 years old and is attending the CYMHS for the first time, accompanied by her mother, with whom she lives. Her younger brother has lived with their father since their parents separated 3 years ago. Fiona's mother is extremely concerned about a gradual change in Fiona's mood over the past 2 years. She has reportedly become angry and unpredictable, a dramatic change from the quiet but confident child she used to be. Her mother describes instances where Fiona will impulsively run from home and engage in risky behaviours such as riding her bike recklessly on their busy street. When met by members of the mental health team, Fiona is at first passive, refusing eye contact, seeming to ignore the conversation between her mother and the nurse and refusing to respond when spoken to directly. Several times during the conversation, however, Fiona interrupts with a hostile comment, countering information provided by her mother.

DISCUSSION OF CASE STUDY: FIONA

Skills required

Even though Fiona is refusing to be involved in the initial assessment, her behaviour and her brief interjections are a valuable source of assessment information. The nurse will document Fiona's behaviour and her comments. In context, this will reflect some family dynamics and give some indication of how Fiona currently feels about life. The challenge for the nurse will be to initially engage Fiona in a shared interest of hers that is non-emotional and therefore less threatening.

Rather than attempting to engage Fiona too early, the nurse wisely chooses to wait for an opportunity. This does not arise until the very end of the initial interview, when the nurse announces that the assessment is almost complete. 'About time', Fiona grumbles, 'I just want to get in the car and listen to my new CD.' The nurse grasps this opportunity:

Nurse: Ah, a new CD ... which group?
Fiona: No one you'd know.
Nurse: Maybe not ... but try me.

To Fiona's surprise, the nurse has recently bought the same CD and although Fiona feigns horror that an adult would even know the band, she cannot completely disguise her admiration.

Nurse: See you in a fortnight then?
Fiona: If I'm not too busy with my music.

Fiona's choice of words ('If I'm not too busy ...') indicates that she is trying to sound uninterested while still leaving her options open.

Approach taken and outcome achieved

Children and adolescents are not always easily engaged. Often the factors contributing to their need for mental health support have affected their ability to trust others; in many cases they have felt let down by adults. The nurse who recognises this will allow time for the young person to engage, initially on their own terms, so the fragile therapeutic alliance can gradually strengthen. Fiona's hostility was ignored; the nurse chose instead to preserve Fiona's fragile sense of dignity. Respecting Fiona's ability to make sound decisions, the nurse did not assume that she would be returning in a fortnight, but rather posed it as a question; this approach was aimed at reassuring Fiona that she had a choice. Her choice to return in a fortnight would demonstrate her courage in recognising that a problem exists and her willingness to explore some supports.

Critical thinking challenge 15.2

1. What might the outcomes have been if the nurse had persisted in asking Fiona questions early in the interview?
2. What assumptions could be made regarding Fiona's need to interrupt while her mother and the nurse were speaking?

Adolescents

When adolescents and their family (carers) present to a healthcare facility, there is an expectation on their part that treatment will achieve the desired outcomes, in terms of the physical, emotional and mental state of the young person. However, it is possible that these outcomes may not be achieved because of many situational factors. One such factor may be the young person's lack of willingness to be part of the referral, assessment and treatment process due to shame, guilt or embarrassment, or to not recognising or acknowledging that a significant problem exists. Mental health nurses providing mental health care for adolescents need to acknowledge that possible influencing factors such as poor insight, resistance to treatment or challenging of authority may be part of normal adolescent behaviour.

Mental health nurses should attempt to form a relationship with the young person through engagement and foster a sense of purpose with the treatment plan for the adolescent. *Engagement* is the process of forming a relationship based on person-centred interactions where there is an ongoing conversation or acknowledgement of a partnership (Dixon et al. 2016). Therefore, an important element of engagement is rapport building, which encompasses not only the formal aspects of mental health care, such as completing a diagnostic interview, but also the social interactions and non-verbal communications that occur. Geldard et al. (2018) state that non-verbal forms of communication may be more significant than verbal interactions when interviewing and engaging young people with mental health problems.

For mental health professionals, language is the key to open communication and creating an environment that can augment engagement. Adolescents may use language and jargon that differs according to their age group or subculture, especially when it comes to 'street lingo'. Adolescents may have a culture that at times seems alien to their parents, caregivers and health professionals. Adolescents and their peer groups may use words and phrases that have a significantly different meaning from that which adults may be accustomed – for example, 'sick', 'bad' or 'gross' may mean 'good'. Health professionals who work with adolescents may need to clarify with the young person what they actually mean by their phrases or words, if the professional does not understand them. This may be particularly relevant when discussing illicit drugs and the street names used for marijuana, amphetamines or hallucinogens.

Understanding language and communicating effectively is integral to engaging with young people and vital to the success of their ongoing treatment. We stated earlier that this chapter does not deal with specific classified conditions but rather the principles of nursing care relating to groupings of disorders. The following section explores the principles of mental health nursing that promote engagement with adolescents with behaviours arising from psychosis, depressive symptoms, social–emotional issues, risk taking and use of technology. Examples of practice situations will highlight some appropriate responses to consider.

Critical thinking challenge 15.3

As a small group exercise, discuss some strategies that nurses can use to foster engagement with an adolescent who is sullen and guarded.

Psychosis and behavioural issues

The terms psychosis and schizophrenia both refer to the same disorder with the same symptoms. Psychosis is the preferred term for use in child and adolescent mental health services and in early intervention services for young people with first-episode presentations. This is due to the negative associations and stigma attached to the term 'schizophrenia', as well as the fact that some people experience an acute and transitory episode of psychosis that does not meet the criteria for a schizophrenia diagnosis.

Psychosis usually emerges in late adolescence or early adulthood, with 80% of people experiencing their first episode of psychosis between the ages of 18 and 30 years (Orygen 2016). There are a small number of adolescents who experience their first episode of psychosis at a younger age, but this is fortunately a rare phenomenon; fortunate, because psychosis is very disruptive to a younger adolescent's developmental trajectory and life in general. Adolescence is a period of rapid development encompassing a range of important tasks such as achieving a sense of individuality and independence, which can be derailed by a psychotic illness. It is also the time when adolescents are engaged in education, and any disruption to this process can have long-term consequences.

Adolescents and young people experience the same symptoms as anyone with a psychotic illness. These symptoms include thought disorder, hallucinations, delusional thinking, poor concentration, lack of energy/motivation and emotional blunting. Not all these symptoms will be present in every person, and it is not uncommon for younger adolescents to present with a limited range of symptoms.

In many cases there is a period of deterioration leading up to the emergence of a fully developed psychotic illness. This is known as the 'prodromal' stage and intervention at this early stage is known to have long-term benefits. It is therefore important for problems to be identified as early as possible to offset the impacts that may occur with untreated psychosis. GPs are often the first port of call when these subtle changes are first recognised, and efforts have been made to educate GPs to recognise these early changes (Orygen 2016).

Treatment for psychosis routinely involves medication. The medication options usually focus on newer atypical antipsychotics such a risperidone and paliperidone. Benzodiazepines such as diazepam or lorazepam may be used in the initial period of treatment while waiting for the antipsychotic medications to take effect. Benzodiazepines can help with agitation and sleep problems and provide a calming effect as an interim measure. Benzodiazepines should not be used long term due to their high potential for dependence. The golden rule when using medication in young people is to start low and go slow. The aim is to find the lowest possible effective dose to help manage the symptoms of psychosis (Orygen 2016). Using the lowest possible effective doses of medication helps to limit the negative impacts of side effects. Young people experience the same side effects as anyone else taking these medications. However, atypical medications such as risperidone and paliperidone have fewer adverse effects than other medications and are less sedating so have fewer negative impacts on the person's ability to function. These medications are less prone to increase appetite, a leading cause of weight gain and subsequent risk of metabolic syndrome. Metabolic syndrome is a group of physical health problems related to weight gain that increase the risk of cardiac problems. Some of the common side effects with these two medications are muscle cramps and joint stiffness. They are also prone to elevate prolactin levels in some people, and this can lead to sexual dysfunction (Stahl 2019). Young people may be embarrassed to discuss this last side effect, so it is important to establish a good therapeutic relationship that supports and encourages open discussion about sensitive topics.

Providing psychoeducation is a key nursing role. This includes information about the effects of the medication (what it is intended to do) and information about side effects and how to manage them. In some cases, where side effects are more troubling, it may be necessary to try a different medication, and it is important to educate patients about the need for these changes. It is especially important to highlight that a change of medication is not a failure of treatment; rather, it is done to find the most effective medication with the least side effects. This approach is driven by the need to maintain hope in the young person, an important aspect of mental health nursing work.

Given the impacts of psychosis on the developmental trajectory of adolescents, psychosocial interventions are also important. Maintaining the young person's connections with their peer group and education has short- and long-term benefits. Some special education facilities for young people with mental health problems are available, and these should be sought out and accessed whenever possible. These facilities provide a more personalised approach and usually have smaller classes with specially trained teachers who have expertise in educating young people with special needs. Where these specialist schools are not available the mental health nurse might work with the school counsellor and classroom teachers to help educate a young person experiencing psychosis. Another option is distance education, which requires considerable support from parents. Mental health nurses may need to provide support to the parents to facilitate this process. Nurses need to know what relevant support services are available in the local area, the referral criteria and how to access these services. Schools often work collaboratively with mental health services, and establishing a positive working relationship with the school has benefits for all concerned. Supporting young people to stay connected with their peer group can require creativity and innovation. Having some knowledge of the young person's interests and activities before developing psychosis provides insight as to what might be effective.

It is also important to work with the families of young people with psychosis. Families are often unaware of what they can do or need to do to support their young person who has psychosis. Ultimately, families provide the lion's share of support for their family members, and supporting them to do this in an effective and helpful way can have significant benefits for both the young person and the family. In addition, it is important to be aware of the effects that a diagnosis of psychosis in their young family member can have on families. They may respond to this with feelings of grief that their child's future potential may be lost or fear about what will happen over time. Family members may also feel helpless in knowing what to do to help their family member achieve their dreams and aspirations and to manage the day-to-day impacts of psychosis. It is important for us to understand how the family reacts to the diagnosis of psychosis so we can support them through this process.

Behavioural issues

Behavioural issues in childhood and adolescence can be complex and difficult to resolve. Generally early intervention is the most effective approach and naturally this requires early identification of behaviours of concern. This might occur in preschools or the early stages of formal education. GPs, paediatricians, child and family nurses, school nurses and nurses working in other primary care settings can also be involved in identifying behavioural problems early.

The causes of behavioural issues in children and adolescents are multifaceted. In some cases, difficult behaviour is a response to exposure to neglect or abuse such as domestic violence or physical, emotional or sexual abuse. Trauma has a significant impact on a young person's capacity to manage their behaviour. Children flourish in consistent, reliable, safe and predictable environments. Some parents, perhaps due to their own experience of poor parenting or other life challenges, have a limited understanding of how best to support children to develop in healthy and adaptive ways. The bonding process between a mother or other primary caregiver and a baby is referred to as 'attachment', and ruptures in this attachment relationship (for example, where a mother is experiencing depression) can create difficulties that manifest as disturbed behaviour as the child develops. The primary task of the attachment relationship is to provide a secure base for the infant from which they can venture out into the world, knowing that they can always return to their safe base. Parents who teach their children emotional regulation provide a language for emotions and help them manage the ups and downs of life. Where parents are not able to support the child to develop these skills, for whatever reason, children can experience greater difficulty regulating their behaviour.

The most effective intervention for problematic behaviours in children and adolescents involves working with the parents or caregivers to support them to develop skills and provide them with strategies to manage difficult behaviours and foster the development of more appropriate behaviours. This is specialised work that is undertaken by a multidisciplinary team, including mental health nurses, who have training in various approaches and techniques. Some interventions can be counterintuitive, which is why training is essential. Success in these therapeutic endeavours takes time and persistence, so developing a positive and supportive relationship with all members of a family is required over the longer term. Supporting a child or young person to more effectively manage their behaviour increases the likelihood that they will succeed in all areas of life, especially their education, family relationships and other social relationships (American Academy of Child and Adolescent Psychiatrists 2007).

The American Academy of Child and Adolescent Psychiatrists (2007, p. 136) provides a brief list of useful interventions that focus on parent management training:

1. Reduce positive reinforcement of disruptive behaviours.
2. Increase reinforcement of prosocial and acceptable behaviour. Positive reinforcement varies widely, but parental attention is predominant. A consequence usually consists of a form of time out or loss of privileges.
3. Apply consequences and/or punishment for disruptive behaviour.
4. Make the parental response predictable, contingent and immediate.

Case study 15.4 looks at a young man experiencing his first episode of psychosis.

CASE STUDY 15.4
David

A 15-year-old boy, David, has been admitted to hospital. He is experiencing a psychotic episode as a result of smoking marijuana for several months. He has been hearing auditory hallucinations (voices telling him he is useless and a nuisance to be around). In the past 6 months there has been a decline in David's academic performance, and he has been isolating himself from his friends and family. Within the past 2 months he has been verbally and physically abusive towards his parents and siblings.

DISCUSSION OF CASE STUDY: DAVID

The presentation of a young person like David experiencing a first episode of psychosis is not uncommon. In considering David's care, the nurse's first priority is to ensure David is physically safe and that those around him also feel safe. When a person's thinking is altered by psychotic phenomena, they may act irrationally as a consequence of feeling fearful and insecure. This may include aggressive behaviour, which is often a response to feeling frightened, threatened or overwhelmed. It is important that the nurse appears calm but confident and offers reassurance and guidance with statements such as, 'David, what you are experiencing must be frightening. You are safe here. We will help you.' Short, clear statements made firmly but quietly and with genuine empathy will be reassuring for David and his family. It is important that it is made clear that, whatever David says or does, he has been heard. At this stage, the nurse should avoid disputing any irrational thoughts David may verbalise. Rather, he should be encouraged to verbalise his confusion and distress. This may assist in diffusing his agitation and may lead to his feeling calmer, thereby reducing the risk of him becoming aggressive.

Another important priority is involving David's family as early as possible, providing them with much-needed support so that they can, in turn, support David. The family will usually be most helpful in providing an accurate history of family health. This will assist in identifying any familial predispositions to mental illness and the nature of onset. This information may help the mental health team to establish the likely severity and prognosis for the illness and organise an individualised treatment plan that will have a higher probability of a positive outcome. Recovery from mental illness demands a high level of support from family, friends and agency staff. The best prognosis and quality of life are achieved when all work collaboratively.

Working with adolescents experiencing psychosis can be extremely challenging. However, where the mental health nurse engages effectively with the young person and can support the client and family through the difficult times towards recovery, it can also be very rewarding work. Once safety has been established and the young person and their family have adjusted to the shock of the initial experience and begun to engage with staff, the medium- to long-term relief of symptoms and psychoeducation towards recovery can begin.

Recovering from psychosis may require a range of interventions including resocialisation through group therapy and individual goal setting that focuses on peer support and re-establishing a social network. Individual goal planning, peer support and group therapy can each promote socially adaptive and acceptable behaviour. Adolescence is a period of personal development involving challenging authority and pushing against the norms of society. The 'normal' adolescent behaviours should not be stifled through treatment but recognised and supported so the young person can return to his or her peer group and family with minimal residual effects of the psychotic episode. One aspect of hospitalisation that can have negative longer term effects is labelling David's condition.

Depression and suicide

Depression and risk of suicide are major concerns in the community, and, while the number of completed suicides of young people appeared to have decreased over the past 20 years, recent data suggests figures are again rising in Western countries, with social media being a cause for concern (Jans et al. 2015). In Australia, considering all causes of death in 2017, suicide accounted for 2% of deaths among males and 1.2% of deaths among females aged 0–14 years. This increased to 36.4% of deaths among males and 32.9% of deaths among females aged 15–19 years and 38.5% of deaths among males and 30.6% of deaths among females aged 20–24 years (Australian Bureau of Statistics 2018). Particularly vulnerable groups at risk include LGBTIQ+ youth (Rivers et al. 2018) and Indigenous Australian youth (Campbell et al. 2016), with a study in the Kimberley region identifying a correlation between death by suicide with the 'wet season', being Indigenous, male and under the age of 25 years (Campbell et al. 2016). In contrast, rates of suicide in pre-pubertal children remain very low. This is possibly due to their lack of understanding of the concept of suicide and that they are less likely to be faced with the risk factors associated with puberty.

The psychological and physical trauma experienced by young people who have attempted suicide may be difficult for everyone to come to terms with, including the resulting fear and grief expressed by their parents/carers. The young person should be reassured that their safety is the treatment team's priority while at the same time providing support to the family. Youth suicide and attempts at self-harm may challenge health professionals and family members to consider their own mortality and the question of why people attempt and complete suicide. It is important that nurses develop skills that enable them to feel comfortable addressing these issues directly with the young person and their family – this is particularly essential for nurses working in clinical areas where contact with young people who have attempted suicide is more common (nurses working in emergency departments, nurses working in rural and remote medicine, mental health nurses working in acute care teams or CYMHS).

Engaging with adolescents who are depressed or suicidal can be extremely difficult due to their tendency towards socially withdrawn and isolative behaviour, or due to cognitive impairment. Nurses can engage with adolescents through routine nursing care, social interactions, groups and individual therapy. It is often a nurse who spends long hours with the young person and is present with them as their mood shifts throughout the day who may be alerted to a subtle increase in risk to the young person's emotional or physical safety. A nurse's ability to reassure young people of their availability as needed helps young people feel free to discuss issues with the nurse when the time seems most appropriate for them.

An issue that can be confusing for nurses is that at times adolescents who are clinically depressed may present with aggressive traits or behaviours. Some adolescents are not able to communicate their emotions verbally. As a result, their only means of expressing distress may be through verbal or physical aggression, towards themselves or others. Getting involved in physical activity, sport, music or art may help engagement. Sharing the young person's physical space and activities may help in forging a therapeutic alliance. Using diversional activities can enable mental health nurses to further engage the young person and progress the therapeutic relationship. Establishing a confidante may be the turning point in the young person's treatment.

Case study 15.5 looks at 14-year-old girl who is self-harming.

CASE STUDY 15.5
Julia

Julia is a 14-year-old who, over the past year, has become increasingly withdrawn from her peer group. She was previously an A-grade student in a select school, but over the past 4 months her school grades have dropped noticeably and she is not completing her homework. She no longer has an interest in playing netball or attending her athletics club. Julia's mother says that Julia has been aggressive towards her and has been harming herself by cutting her wrists with any sharp object available. Julia's GP prescribed antidepressant medication 6 weeks before admission, but there has been minimal change in her mental state.

DISCUSSION OF CASE STUDY: JULIA

Julia requires intensive therapy, which may include cognitive behaviour therapy, family therapy, individual psychotherapy and a review of her medication. Psychosocial issues also need to be considered during Julia's treatment. This may include exploring school issues, as well as whether there is any risk of Julia having been physically, emotionally or sexually abused. Also, there may have been significant losses that have contributed to her depression.

In assisting young people like Julia, the mental health nurse will need to establish rapport and maintain engagement. It will be important to gain the client's confidence from the initial meeting because there will be many sensitive issues to address. Adolescents seeking help from adults will not always commit time for a therapeutic relationship to grow if they doubt in any way the sincerity of the person in whom they are confiding.

In some instances, the action of inflicting harm upon oneself can provide a sense of relief from severe emotional distress and psychic pain. It is therefore essential that the nurse recognises this possibility and, while working with the young person, makes every effort for them to feel respected and not judged on the behaviour that has led to them seeking help. Medical care, such as attention to a wound, should be addressed discreetly and professionally. The key aspect of providing care for the young person is establishing their current level of safety and working with them on how this can best be achieved. It will be helpful to ensure the young person has adequate support networks so they can strengthen these connections with a view to obtaining help in more adaptive ways in the future.

Critical thinking challenge 15.4

List the potential barriers to establishing a therapeutic alliance with Julia.

Self-harm and young people

Self-harm refers to a specific set of behaviours, but the term is used somewhat loosely to cover a wider range of issues including suicidal behaviour and thinking. In this section self-harm refers specifically to intentional self-injury or poisoning that does not have suicidal intent. This does not mean that self-harm is never associated with suicidal thinking or behaviour, but it is important to make a clear distinction between self-harm without suicidal intent and self-harm in the context of suicidal thinking (Hungerford et al. 2018). The reasons for this distinction are concerned with the different causes and interventions that are needed to manage non-suicidal self-harm compared with suicidal behaviour and thinking. It is important to bear in mind that self-harm is an expression of personal distress, not an illness, and there are many varied reasons for a person to harm her or himself (NICE 2004).

Self-harming is reasonably common, with a prevalence rate of 371.4 per 100,000 of the population among females aged 15–19 years. The highest rate for males, at 163.4 per 100,000, occurs in the 30–34-year age group (Hungerford et. al. 2018). Overall lifetime prevalence is 16.9%, with a mean starting age of 13. The most frequent reasons for self-harm is to achieve relief from thoughts or feelings, and the most frequent self-harming behaviour is cutting (American Academy of Child and Adolescent Psychiatrists 2018), although a wide variety of self-harming behaviours are seen in practice. Young people who self-harm commonly present to general practice or hospital emergency departments to have their injuries attended to. Frequently, they are brought in or sent to hospital by parents, teachers or concerned friends.

Self-harm is used as a coping mechanism to manage feelings of distress arising from a variety of sources including abuse and trauma. In some cases it becomes a fashion among a group of adolescent peers and is done in an effort to fit in with a peer group. It is therefore important when assessing young people who self-harm to understand the motivations for their self-harming behaviour. Where a history of abuse or trauma is revealed as the underlying cause it is important to gain an understanding of the nature and extent of this issue. This can be difficult due to the high levels of shame and embarrassment that accompany the experience of abuse and trauma. An underlying mental illness such as anxiety, depression or psychosis may also contribute to self-harming behaviour, and it is helpful for this to be identified as part of any assessment of a person who engages in self-harm (Hungerford et. al. 2018).

Critical thinking challenge 15.5

Either individually or in a group, have a brainstorming session and list all the skills that a child and youth mental health nurse would require. Subdivide these into skills that you think may be specific to either a community mental health nurse or a mental health nurse working in an inpatient setting.

Interventions

It is important for all members of the healthcare team to treat people who self-harm with respect and courtesy, using a non-judgemental, non-critical approach. This includes nurses working in triage, assessment and treatment, as well as nurses conducting mental health assessments. People who self-harm are frequently ashamed of their behaviour and fear judgement and discrimination from others due to a lack of understanding about self-harming behaviour. Adopting a stance of genuine curiosity and acceptance can have powerful therapeutic effects.

Immediate interventions for self-harm need to focus on managing any injuries that have occurred. This may involve stitches, dressings or managing intentional poisoning. Once the person's physical healthcare needs have been addressed it is usual for mental health staff to conduct an assessment. This should be conducted as soon as possible and can be done before physical health care has been completed, if it is safe to do so. All staff who have contact with people who self-harm need to adopt an accepting, respectful, non-critical approach. Remembering that people who self-harm are managing their distress in the only way they know how can help with this process. Those who self-harm, particularly those who have been subject to abuse or trauma, are usually hypersensitive to the reactions of the people around them so it is important to maintain a positive therapeutic stance. This is a particularly important strategy because people who self-harm can be seen in a negative light by some staff, possibly due to lack of understanding about the levels of distress these people experience and the apparently ineffective methods used to manage this distress.

The aim of assessment with people who self-harm is to gain an understanding of the extent and frequency of their behaviours. It is also important to gain an understanding of the motivations for self-harming behaviour. This can help us work with the person to develop interventions that will address the underlying problems.

Some people who self-harm find it extremely difficult to stop their behaviours for a range of reasons including ongoing exposure to trauma and abuse. In such situations, identifying harm-reduction strategies, accepting that self-harm will most likely continue into the foreseeable future, should be the focus. Harm reduction involves working with the person to find less harmful ways to manage their distress and thereby minimise the damage that may result from self-harming behaviour. This can be something as simple as getting the person to attach a rubber band to their wrist and to flick the rubber band when they feel the need to self-harm. The pain from the rubber band mimics the pain from cutting and can serve the same purpose as cutting. In the longer term, various psychological and talking therapies can be helpful for people who self-harm. This includes cognitive behaviour therapy and dialectical behaviour therapy. These therapies are delivered by suitably trained and qualified practitioners including mental health nurses (NICE 2011).

As with all areas of work with children and adolescents, working with family or carers (wherever possible and appropriate) is an important part of interventions for self-harm. Helping parents and caregivers gain an understanding of self-harming behaviour can reduce interpersonal conflicts within the family. Working to help family members develop strategies to support their young family member can also be beneficial. Knowing about self-harming behaviours and developing ways to provide support and care to their young family member and being open to talking about the issues can help ameliorate the distress and difficulties resulting from self-harm.

Risk taking and young people

Some problematic or risk-taking behaviours among adolescents and young people are often seen to be part of normal development and the transition from adolescence to adulthood. Problematic or risky behaviours can take a number of forms including tobacco use, binge drinking, cannabis or other drug use, reckless driving (e.g. texting while behind the wheel) and risky sexual activity. The adolescent brain is still maturing during adolescence, and young people are strongly influenced by peers in their decision making, which leads to increased impulsivity and risky behaviours in an attempt to avoid peer exclusion. There also appears to be a neurobiological link and correlations between certain personality factors and risk taking in youth, and these include greater levels of risk tolerance, sensation, thrill seeking and impulsivity (Nagel 2019). For some young people engaging in risk taking is experimental and forms part of their search for identity and values, social and financial independence, and peer networks (Sanci et al. 2018). However, in Australia Dillon (2019) has identified some concerning trends with an increase in the use of cannabis, normalisation of ecstasy/MDMA and use of nitrous oxide ('nangs') among school-aged young people, with some believing that these substances are less harmful than alcohol. Yet for around one in four adolescents, risk taking can affect their mental and physical wellbeing (Sanci et al. 2018) and may be a maladaptive coping strategy for young people who are already experiencing poor mental health.

Education and role-modelling within the home, school and community is crucial in teaching young people how to act in a socially responsible way. As a clinician, early detection is important. Take any opportunity that presents to talk with young people about risk-taking behaviours. Young people may be reluctant to disclose and access healthcare services but value the advice of clinicians (Sanci et al. 2018). Some of the barriers for young people in accessing healthcare services are listed in Box 15.3. Building resilience is key and using the HEEADSSS health assessment (Box 15.4) supports a clinician to explore protective factors that the young person already has in their lives and ways to strengthen these while respecting choices and decisions. Bear in mind, that while peers may be a risk factor, in some cases they may also be the person who take steps or intervenes to prevent harm (Centre for Accident Research & Road Safety Queensland 2014) so greater knowledge of peers about the potential risks of behaviours can be empowering.

Box 15.3 Barriers for adolescents accessing healthcare services

The 5 Cs:

- **Cost** of care
- **Confidentiality** – fear of a lack thereof
- **Compassion** – lack of non-judgemental clinicians with sensitivity to developmental stage
- **Clinical skill** – poor communication by clinician (e.g. use of jargon) and low evidence-based management of common problems such as depression and anxiety or requests for effective contraception
- **Convenience** – difficulty getting a timely appointment, inflexible appointment systems, waiting times, inadequate transport options, restrictions on when can make time to attend care independently

and the D:

- **Developmental issues** – embarrassment, poor self-identified needs, low knowledge of services, little experience with healthcare systems and expressing needs, low health literacy

Reproduced with permission from The Royal Australian College of General Practitioners from: Sanci L, Webb M, Hocking J. Risk-taking behaviour in adolescents. Aust J Gen Pract 2018;47(12):829–34. Available at www1.racgp.org.au/ajgp/2018/december/risk-taking-behaviour-in-adolescents

Box 15.4 HEEADSSS assessment

- **H**ome environment
- **E**ducation and employment
- **E**ating and exercise
- Peer-related **A**ctivities
- **D**rugs, tobacco and alcohol
- **S**ex and sexuality
- **S**uicide, depression and other mental health issues
- **S**afety from injury, violence, abuse, and safety precautions to reduce sun damage and vaccine preventable infections

Klein DA, Goldenring JM, Adelman WP. Probing for scars: How to ask the essential questions. Contemporary Pediatrics 2014;31(1):16–28

Technology and young people

Children and young people are spending more and more time online or connected to devices. Nine out of 10 Australian teenagers aged 14–17 years have a mobile phone, and nearly all have a smartphone (Roy Morgan 2016). There are benefits to the social connectedness that technology and social media affords, and there are also risks. Cyberbullying is a real risk and can be the source of emotional disturbances and substance use; it can lead to self-harm and thoughts of suicide in children and young people (Kids Helpline 2019). Cyberbullying is when technology is used in a negative and unhealthy way and can include sending or sharing hurtful, embarrassing or abusive emails/messages, humiliating others online through videos or posting of images, spreading rumours online, excluding others or threatening others, making people feel afraid (Kids Helpline 2019). One in five Australian children aged 8–17 years has reported cyberbullying over a 12-month period (Katz et al. 2014). The potential danger of cyberbullying is that the reach is much greater because of the internet, technology and mobile phones, which provide access to world-wide communication options such as text, email and social media such as Snapchat, Instagram and Facebook. There is also greater anonymity for the perpetrator and difficulty in removing statements or images once shared publicly because we leave our 'digital footprints' (Kids Helpline 2019).

Family members may notice if their child or young person is affected by cyberbullying. Signs can include greater isolation from peers or social activities, trouble sleeping, complaints of somatic symptoms, poor school performance, seeming unhappy or stressed after being on their mobile phone or computer, or receiving more messages than usual by text or on social media. Health professionals should be aware of the potential mental health risks associated with cyberbullying and how social support from school and family can be a protective mechanism (Beyond Blue 2019). Family can be instrumental in encouraging the young person to talk openly about what is happening and their feelings or, alternatively, helping them find someone safe to talk to such as a health professional or accessing counselling supports such as the Kids Helpline, eheadspace or Lifeline. Family members, school staff and health professionals can also help the young person to develop a plan or steps to respond and cope with the bullying. Steps can include not responding and blocking the bully in privacy settings, collecting evidence and reporting the abuse to the service or social media outlet for removal of material and, depending on the severity of the offence, reporting it to an e-safety agency such as the Office of the eSafety Commissioner in Australia or law enforcement (eSafety Commissioner 2019).

With the rise in the need to be 'connected', there has also been a rise in young people's use of social media with the emergence of platforms such as Facebook (2004), Twitter (2006), Instagram (2010) and Snapchat (2011). Gunnell et al. (2018, p. 1) explains that 'social media use may result in less face to face communication, overdependency on being "liked" for social validation (particularly for girls), and pressure to keep up with discussions 24 hours a day, leading to poor sleep'. 'Fear of missing out' has come to the fore among young people who feel the need to be continually connected with what others may be doing to avoid missing out, having significant effects on their mental wellbeing (Stephen & Edmonds 2018). Similarly, problem gaming, particularly for boys, may be a symptom of factors such being lonely or feeling anxious or depressed. And while there is debate about whether it should be classified as a disorder, the amount of time a young person spends gaming can have significant negative effects on daily life (relationships, school or work, health and wellbeing) (Orlando 2019).

Greater access to the online environment and technology also means young people are exposed to pornography. Research shows that nearly half of children 9–16 years of age experience regular exposure to sexual images, and young males are more likely to seek out pornography and do so frequently. The impact of this exposure can increase sexual behaviour and risk taking in teenagers, with pornography associated with unsafe sexual health practices such as multiple partners and not using condoms because they don't see this as 'normal', increasing risk for unplanned pregnancies and sexually transmitted infections (Quadara et al. 2017).

Taking this all into account, nurses should support recommendations for appropriate screen time, encouraging 8–12 hours of sleep and 1 hour of exercise each day as a priority over screen time. Nurses can also support families with setting screen time guidelines and family media agreements to help young people 'stay safe', 'think first' (before posting), 'stay balanced' and 'communicate openly'. An example of an agreement can be found on the Common Sense Media website: https://www.commonsensemedia.org/family-media-agreement.

Family work

Nurses working with children and adolescents experiencing mental health issues should be aware that it is best that this client group should, if possible and appropriate, not be seen, assessed or treated in isolation. Ideally, nurses working with this client group should incorporate all members of the family who have a significant role within the household. This ensures the 'identified consumer' of CAMHS is not perceived to be the family scapegoat. A family scapegoat is used to divert attention away from other problems that may exist in a family such as difficulties in the parental relationships. It is also the case that children and adolescents live within and depend on their families for sustenance and emotional support, and families need to be involved in helping their young person manage whatever difficulties they face. At times this may involve changes in the way the family operates in terms of support and discipline. Therefore, a major component of CAMHS nursing is involving the family in treatment through family work. In recent times there has been a shift in focus towards family-centred mental health nursing, which includes family-based assessments and treatments, spreading the attention across the whole family rather than focusing on the identified client. Family work is based on the principles of family therapy, which requires a specific way of working and requires specialist training.

In some cases, family work is contraindicated. This applies where there is violence or physical abuse in a family or where there is a suspicion of sexual abuse. Engaging all members of the family in therapeutic work can have negative consequences for the young person because they may be held responsible for exposing the family to outside scrutiny.

Family therapy has been constantly evolving since its inception in the middle of the 20th century. Traditionally, it has focused on the identified problems with the child or adolescent and how the family has dealt with these issues from a particular theoretical perspective. There is a wide variety of theoretical frameworks operating in the family therapy space, and family therapists usually adhere to the framework in which they are trained. Family therapy works within the following principles:

- Problems in families are best understood and treated from a circular rather than a linear perspective. A linear perspective uses a straightforward cause-and-effect relationship, whereas a circular approach considers all contributing factors, some of which may not seem, on the surface, to be directly related to the issues at hand. For example, difficulties in the parental relationship may be played out through relationships with the children, particularly where one child is favoured above others by one of the parents.
- Families experiencing problems need to be supported to develop their own problem-solving abilities.
- The ability of family members to change depends on their ability to alter their perception of the problem.
- A family's understanding of problems does not itself lead to changes in behaviour.
- A therapeutic context for change must be created for families.
- Problems or symptoms may serve a positive family function.
- Outcomes are more positive if problems are treated from an eco-systemic perspective (Dallos & Draper 2010).

From these key aspects of family involvement, nurses can formulate their own methods of working with families that best suit their clinical environment. Undertaking family work can be both challenging and rewarding. It is recommended that nurses involved in such work or working in child and adolescent teams undertake specialist training and engage in ongoing clinical supervision to ensure that optimal patient/family–nurse relationships are maintained and that the family achieves their desired outcomes.

Working with families is discussed in more detail in Chapter 5.

Critical thinking challenge 15.6

Imagine you are contacting a health service about worries and concerns you have for a family member. What nursing attributes and skills would you find reassuring during the first phone contact?

Confidentiality

An important issue for young people is being able to understand how the information shared during interactions with team members is documented and knowing who has access to these records. It is important to them that their need for confidentiality be maintained; however, there are constraints on the confidentiality available to children and adolescents. One such constraint is the presence of risk factors. The young person must know that nurses and their colleagues are bound to share information that has a direct effect on their safety or the safety of others. The age of the young person is another issue we need to consider. There is no statute law covering confidentiality or consent and, as such, case law (see Chapter 8) and health service policy should guide action in this area. When working with families in the child and adolescent sphere it is unwise to promise complete confidentiality when working with young people. For young people aged 14 years or older it is generally wise to let them know that information may be shared with others and that this will be discussed and negotiated with the young person before this is done. Exceptions to this process should also be discussed in the early stages of the therapeutic relationship. The exceptions are generally related to issues of safety such as the emergence of suicidal thinking, the young person engaging in dangerous behaviours like drug taking or revelations about abuse. It is not necessary to list every possible exception. A general statement about issues of concern or safety is usually enough. If the young person is forewarned that there are exceptions to confidentiality, this can lead to a more open and productive relationship.

Interviews with adolescents should not be restricted to the formality of interview rooms. So long as safety can be assured, some adolescents may prefer to be interviewed in a more public place such as a courtyard. Flexibility (and not a small dose of ingenuity!) is the key to providing a quality service that will encourage young people to return when needed.

Psychoeducation

As stated previously, having to take regular medication can be a major issue for adolescents, regardless of their condition. Many young people do not want to be different from their peer group. This may include not wanting to be seen as being different by needing to take tablets. Through psychoeducation, the rationale for taking medication should be explained and adverse effects discussed, together with how to reduce any potential complications of medication therapy. Problem solving with the young person about ways to discreetly include taking the prescribed medication in their daily lifestyle will be of benefit. The risk of taking non-prescribed medications and taking medications in addition to illegal substances and alcohol should also be highlighted. This can be achieved by maximising therapeutic interventions. In adolescent mental health, engagement through developing rapport and trust are key elements to achieving change. Without these elements, minimal change might be achieved.

Legal issues

Nurses caring for young people admitted to mental health services often have to deal with legal issues relating to duty of care, child protection and mental health legislation. In the developed world, children and younger adolescents (usually aged 13 years or under) must have a parent's or guardian's consent to seek treatment for any form of medical intervention, including mental health assessments and treatment. Young people in Australia aged 14 years or older can give their own consent to receive medical or nursing treatment, as long as their parents are aware and the health professionals believe that the young person is competent to give consent.

The ability for young people to consent to medical treatment or seek medical consultations is referred to as 'Gillick competence' (*Gillick v. West Norfolk and Wisbech Area Health Authority 1986*). Medical and nursing staff may question whether the young person is 'Gillick competent' or has the cognitive ability to make an informed judgement to give their own consent for treatment. The legal precedent is the case where a parent took a local health authority to court after one of her children received treatment from a GP without her consent. This case has had a major impact on the provision of paediatric health care and, consequently, health workers must consider each child's competence on a case-by-case basis, assessing both the competence and the maturity of the child (Hein et al. 2015).

In mental health, as with general health care, consent could be challenged by parents and doctors; however, to ensure the safety and wellbeing of young people, mental health legislation provides strong guidelines and rights of appeal. Mental health nurses who treat young people aged under 16 years should be aware that it is unethical and legally unsafe to engage a young person in treatment without informing their parent(s). Healthcare agencies and inpatient units tend to have specific protocols and policies to address this issue.

The legal process by which young people can be admitted involuntarily to mental health agencies is similar to that for adult patients. This ensures legal processes and due process are followed regarding human rights, issues of liberty and protecting the rights of others. It is always preferable that young people are admitted voluntarily. However, if the safety of an adolescent is at risk and they are unable to consent to voluntary treatment, the relevant mental health Act can be invoked. Younger people, aged 13 or under, are usually regarded as voluntary if their parents have provided consent. If a young person is aged 14 or 15 it is beneficial, if possible, to gain their consent to treatment, as well as a parent's consent.

The other main legal issues that need to be observed in child and adolescent mental health are child protection and statutory orders regarding custody. Nurses are mandatory reporters under child protection legislation, and all nurses need to be familiar with the legislation in their jurisdiction. New Zealand and the states and territories of Australia have their own legislation governing child protection and guardianship. However, the overriding principles are those of the World Health Organization and the United Nations Convention on the Rights of the Child (Parliament of the Commonwealth of Australia Joint Standing Committee on Treaties 1998). In theory, all children and adolescents have legal rights to education, health and wellbeing.

NURSE'S STORY 15.1

Kristin Henderson

As an experienced mental health nurse, I'd regarded myself as a spontaneous, reflective clinician, confident that my interactions with patients were at all times respectful, helpful and kind. I was taken by surprise, then, when I began working with young people in an inpatient mental health setting – surprised that I now felt hesitant and doubtful about how to respond. What was appropriate? What would be a better response? My confidence and spontaneity had given way to feeling stilted and unsure ... until a defining moment when I realised that I should open my senses to cues within myself and from others, taking time to reflect upon what I was seeing in myself. This could deepen my understanding of how others see themselves. This is my story ...

With his bath finished and his pyjamas on, 8-year-old Cobey and I stand in front of the full-length mirror looking straight at ourselves, occasionally glancing across at each other's reflection, then back to our own. As we look at our reflections, I wonder what we are *really seeing*.

I see myself: casually dressed, complete and unchanging ... oh, and looking a wee bit tired! I suspect that Cobey, like me, sees an image of himself, but I can only speculate what self-image that might be ...

I kneel down beside Cobey to try to observe his reflection as he might be seeing it. I note a small crack in the glass near where Cobey is standing. The mirror has been damaged, but because of the safety component of the glass, it has not shattered but simply absorbed the knock, leaving three fractures darting out from the one stress point. As I had anticipated, his image is disjointed, and the symbolic implications momentarily tug at me.

'What do you see?' I ask quietly.

No answer. He continues looking into the broken mirror. He is observing fragmented self – lots of small pieces, together, but not quite. He moves bodily up and down and sideways, all the time trying to piece together his reflection in a harmonious union. But it is not to be – whichever position he views himself from, he is in several pieces, a fragmented whole.

'I'm in pieces ... nothing fits together properly,' he eventually says, giggling. Then for a few more minutes he moves about, trying to find where he might place himself so that the pieces of him do come together, as they should. In a short while, in frustration, he curses the mirror and leaves the room. I stand stunned. Cobey's complex and distressing childhood history symbolically laid bare before the mirror. So much about us both, reflected in this brief encounter.

Chapter summary

This chapter has highlighted knowledge and skills that a beginning nurse requires when working for the first time with children and adolescents in the mental health field. It has focused primarily on engagement – establishing a therapeutic relationship and forging a therapeutic alliance. Nurses must first master strategies for engaging young people and their families before more advanced skills in mental health nursing can be consolidated effectively. Engaging young people and families early and developing a therapeutic relationship will enhance the quality of assessment information clients provide. Furthermore, a sense of trust shared between parties will promote commitment to a shared treatment plan created in partnership between the young person, their parents and the mental health team.

The case studies in this chapter have sought to reinforce the importance of engagement and working in partnerships. Demonstrating empathy and performing with absolute sincerity are important factors in caring for children and adolescents. It is important that young people feel that they are the priority for the nurse at this particular time.

EXERCISES FOR CLASS ENGAGEMENT

1. Contact your nearest CYMHS and ask for information on the services available to children and young people. Share this information with your group.
   - Are these services proactive and responsive?
   - Does the service actively promote early intervention?
2. Contact a nurse working in a community setting and another from an inpatient unit and ask them to speak to your group about their roles. Note any differences between the mental health nursing of young people in the community and that of young people in an inpatient setting.
3. In small groups, nominate one person to act as a mental health nurse and another to play the role of a sullen, guarded adolescent. Remaining group members are to observe and document the difficulties presented in establishing rapport.
4. Contact a child and youth mental health agency or community youth shelter and arrange to speak with a person who has experience with depressed or suicidal youth. Then clarify your responses to Critical thinking challenge 15.5.
5. Seek out the mental health and child protection Acts applicable in your state, territory or region. Summarise key points in applying these to establishing safety for young people. Share your findings.

Useful websites

Children of Parents with a Mental Illness (COPMI): http://www.copmi.net.au/
Headspace: https://headspace.org.au/
Kidshelpline: https://www.kidshelpline.com.au/

References

Achenbach, T.M., Ndetei, D.M., 2015. Clinical models for child and adolescent behavioral, emotional, and social problems. In: Rey, J.M. (Ed.), IACAPAP E-Textbook of Child and Adolescent Mental Health. International Association for Child and Adolescent Psychiatry and Allied Professions, Geneva.

American Academy of Child and Adolescent Psychiatrists, 2018. Prevalence and characteristics of self-harm in adolescents: meta-analyses of community-based studies 1990–2015. J. Am. Acad. Child Adolesc. Psychiatr. 57 (10), 733–741.

American Academy of Child and Adolescent Psychiatrists, 2007. Practice parameter for the assessment and treatment of children and adolescents with oppositional defiant disorder. J. Am. Acad. Child Adolesc. Psychiatry 46 (1), 126–141.

American Psychiatric Association, 2013. Diagnostic and Statistical Manual of Mental Disorders, fifth ed. APA, Washington, DC.

Australian Bureau of Statistics, 2018. Causes of death, Australia 2017. Catalogue 3303.0. Commonwealth of Australia, Canberra.

Australian College of Mental Health Nurses, 2010. Standards of practice in mental health nursing. Available: http://www.acmhn.org/publications/standards-of-practice.

Australian Health Ministers' Advisory Council, 2013. A national framework for recovery-oriented mental health services: Guide for practitioners and providers. Commonwealth of Australia, Canberra.

Australian Institute of Health and Welfare, 2017. National Drug Strategy Household Survey 2016: Detailed findings 2017. Drug Statistics Series No. 31. Cat. no. PHE 214. AIHW, Canberra.

Australian Institute of Health and Welfare, 2011. Young Australians: their health and wellbeing 2011. Cat. no. PHE 140 Canberra: AIHW.

Beers, C.W., 1908. A Mind That Found Itself: An Autobiography. Longmans, Green, New York.

Beyond Blue, 2019. Bullying and cyberbullying. Available: https://healthyfamilies.beyondblue.org.au/age-13/raising-resilient-young-people/bullying-an d-cyberbullying.

Campbell, A., Chapman, M., McHugh, C., et al., 2016. Rising Indigenous suicide rates in Kimberley and implications for suicide prevention. Australas. Psychiatry 24 (6), 561–564.

Centre for Accident Research & Road Safety – Queensland, 2014. Adolescent Risk-Taking. Queensland University of Technology, Brisbane.

Dallos, R., Draper, R., 2010. An Introduction to Family Therapy: Systemic Theory and Practice, third ed. McGraw-Hill Education, Maidenhead.

Dillon, P., 2019. Teenagers, alcohol and other drugs 2019: What's happening, what's out there and how much influence do parents really have? Available: http://darta.net.au/wordpress-content/uploads/2019/04/WHATS_HAPPENING_2019.pdf.

Dixon, L.B., Holoshitz, Y., Nossel, I., 2016. Treatment engagement of individuals experiencing mental illness: review and update. World Psychiatry 15 (1), 13–20.

Erskine, H.E., Moffitt, T.E., Copeland, W.E., et al., 2015. A heavy burden on young minds: the global burden of mental and substance use disorders in children and youth. Psychol. Med. 45 (7), 1551–1563.

eSafety Commissioner, 2019. Cyberbullying. Available: https://www.esafety.gov.au/esafety-information/esafety-issues/cyberbullying.

Geldard, K., Geldard, D., Foo, R.Y., 2018. Counselling Children: A Practical Introduction, fifth ed. Sage, London.

Goodman, J.H., 2019. Perinatal depression and infant mental health. Arch. Psychiatr. Nurs. 33 (3), 217–224.

Gore, F.M., Bloem, P.J.N., Patton, G.C., et al., 2011. Global burden of disease in young people aged 10–24 years: a systematic analysis. Lancet 377, 2093–2102.

Gunnell, D., Kidger, J., Elvidge, H., 2018. Adolescent mental health in crisis. BMJ 361, k2608.

Hein, I.M., Troost, P.W., Broersma, A., et al., 2015. Why is it hard to make progress in assessing children's decision-making competence? BMC Med. Ethics 16, 1.

Hirani, K., Cherian, S., Mutch, R., et al., 2018. Identification of health risk behaviours among adolescent refugees resettling in Western Australia. Arch. Dis. Child. 103, 240–246.

Hungerford, C., Hodgson, D., Bostwick, R., et al., 2018. Mental Health Care, third ed. John Wiley, Milton.

Jans, T., Taneli, Y., Warnke, A., 2015. Suicide and self-harming behaviour. In: Rey, J.M. (Ed.), IACAPAP E-Textbook of Child and Adolescent Mental Health. International Association for Child and Adolescent Psychiatry and Allied Professions, Geneva.

Katz, I., Keeley, M., Spears, B., et al., 2014. Research on youth exposure to, and management of, cyberbullying incidents in Australia: Synthesis report (SPRC Report 16/2014). Sydney, Social Policy Research Centre, UNSW, Sydney.

Kendler, K.S., 2018. The development of Kraepelin's mature diagnostic concepts of paranoia and paranoid dementia praecox: a close reading of his textbooks from 1887 to 1899. JAMA Psychiatry 75 (12), 1280–1288.

Kids Helpline, 2019. Cyberbullying. Available: https://kidshelpline.com.au/teens/issues/cyberbullying.

Lawrence, D., Johnson, S., Hafekost, J., et al., 2015. The mental health of children and adolescents. Report on the second Australian Child and Adolescent Survey of Mental Health and Wellbeing. Department of Health. Canberra.

Layard, R., Hagell, A., 2015. Healthy young minds: transforming the mental health of children. Report of the WISH Mental Health and Wellbeing in Children Forum, World Innovation Summit in Health, Qatar.

Mares, S., Graeff-Martins, A.S., 2015. The clinical assessment of infants, preschoolers and their families. In: Rey, J.M. (Ed.), IACAPAP E-Textbook of Child and Adolescent Mental Health. International Association for Child and Adolescent Psychiatry and Allied Professions, Geneva.

Morris, J., Belfer, M., Daniels, A., et al., 2011. Treated prevalence of and mental health services received by children and adolescents in 42 low-and-middle-income countries. J. Child Psychol. Psychiatry 52, 1239–1246.

Murphy, G., Peters, K., Wilkes, L., et al., 2015. Childhood parental mental illness: living with fear and mistrust. Issues Ment. Health Nurs. 36, 294–299.

Nagel, M.C., 2019. The neurobiology of risk taking and impulsivity. Encycl. Child Adolesc. Dev. doi:10.1002/9781119171492.

Naghavi, M., 2019. Global, regional, and national burden of suicide mortality 1990 to 2016: systematic analysis for the Global Burden of Disease Study 2016. BMJ 316, 194.

NICE, 2011. Self-harm in over 8s: long term management. National Institute for Health and Care Excellence. Accessed at: nice.org.uk/guidance/cg133.

NICE, 2004. Self-harm in over 8s: short term management and prevention of recurrence. National Institute for Health and Care Excellence. Accessed at: nice.org.uk/guidance/cg16.

NSW Ministry of Health, 2011. NSW Child and Adolescent Mental Health Services (CAMHS) Competency framework. NSW Government, Sydney.

Orlando, J., 2019. How to know if your child is addicted to video games and what to do about it. The Conversation. Available: http://theconversation.com/how-to-know-if-your-child-is-addicted-to-video-games-and-what-to-do-about-it-118038.

Orygen. The National Centre for Excellence in Youth Mental Health, 2016. Australian Clinical Guidelines for Early Psychosis, second ed. Orygen Youth Health, Melbourne.

Parliament of the Commonwealth of Australia Joint Standing Committee on Treaties, 1998. United Nations Convention on the Rights of the Child, 17th report. Commonwealth of Australia, Canberra.

Perera, S., Hetrick, S., Cotton, S., et al., 2019. Awareness of headspace youth mental health service centres across Australian communities between 2008 and 2015. J. Ment. Health. doi:10.1080/09638237.2019.1630718.

Piaget, J., 1962. The stages of the intellectual development of the child. Bull. Menninger Clin. 26 (3), 120–128.

Quadara, A., El-Murr, A., Latham, J., 2017. The Effects of Pornography on Children and Young People: An Evidence Scan. Australian Institute of Family Studies, Melbourne.

Rey, J.M., Bella-Awusah, T.T., Jing, L., 2015. Depression in children and adolescents. In: Rey, J.M. (Ed.), IACAPAP E-Textbook of Child and Adolescent Mental Health. International Association for Child and Adolescent Psychiatry and Allied Professions, Geneva.

Rickwood, D.J., Telford, N.R., Mazzer, K.R., et al., 2015. The services provided to young people through the headspace centres across Australia. Med. J. Aust. 202 (10), 533–536.

Rivers, I., Gonzalez, C., Nodin, N., et al., 2018. LGBT people and suicidality in youth: a qualitative study of perceptions of risk and protective circumstances. Soc. Sci. Med. 212, 1–8.

Roberts, J., Fenton, G., Barnard, M., 2015. Developing effective therapeutic relationships with children, young people and their families. Nurs. Child. Young People 27 (4), 30–35.

Roy Morgan, 2016. 9 in 10 Aussie teens now have a mobile (and most are already on to their second or subsequent handset). Press Release Finding No. 6929. Australia. Available: http://www.roymorgan.com/findings/6929-australian-teenagers-and-their-mobile-phones-june-2016-201608220922.

Sanci, L., Webb, M., Hocking, J., 2018. Risk-taking behaviour in adolescents. Aust. J. Gen. Pract. 47, 829–834.

Santona, A., Tagini, A., Sarracino, D., et al., 2015. Maternal depression and attachment: the evaluation of mother–child interactions during feeding practice. Front. Psychol. 6, 1235. http://doi.org/10.3389/fpsyg.2015.01235.

Sawyer, M.G., Miller-Lewis, L.R., Clark, J.J., 2007. The mental health of 13–17-year-olds in Australia: findings from the National Survey of Mental Health and Wellbeing. J. Youth Adolesc. 36, 185–194.

Servili, C., 2015. Organizing and delivering services for child and adolescent mental health. In: Rey, J.M. (Ed.), IACAPAP E-Textbook of Child and Adolescent Mental Health. International Association for Child and Adolescent Psychiatry and Allied Professions, Geneva.

Stahl, S.M., 2019. Stahl's Prescribing Guide: Children and Adolescents. Cambridge University Press, Cambridge.

Stephen, R., Edmonds, R., 2018. Briefing 53: Social Media, Young People and Mental Health. Centre for Mental Health, London.

The Werry Centre, 2014. Real Skills Plus ICAMH/AOD: A Competency Framework for the Infant, Child and Youth Mental Health and Alcohol and Other Drug Workforce. The Werry Centre, Auckland.

Thompson, M., Hooper, C., Laver-Bradbury, C., et al., 2012. Child and Adolescent Mental Health Theory and Practice, second ed. Hodder Arnold, UK.

Woolhouse, H., Gartland, D., Mensah, F., et al., 2015. Maternal depression from early pregnancy to 4 years postpartum in a prospective pregnancy cohort study: implications for primary health care. BJOG 122 (3), 312–321.

World Health Organization, 2019. Coming of age: adolescent health. Available: https://www.who.int/health-topics/adolescents/coming-of-age-adolescent-health.

World Health Organization, 2018. Adolescent mental health. Available: https://www.who.int/news-room/fact-sheets/detail/adolescent-mental-health.

World Health Organization, 2017. Global accelerated action for the health of adolescents (AA-HA!): guidance to support country Implementation. Available: https://www.who.int/maternal_child_adolescent/topics/adolescence/framework-accelerated-action/en/.

World Health Organization, 2014. Health for the World's Adolescents: A Second Chance in the Second Decade. WHO, Geneva.

World Health Organization, 2009. Improving health systems and services for mental health. Available: http://whqlibdoc.who.int/publications/2009/9789241598774_eng.pdf.

CHAPTER 16

Mental disorders of older age

Melissa Robinson-Reilly and Peta Marks

KEY POINTS

- People are living longer and, as populations age, understanding the mental disorders and needs of older people, and considering the factors that impede care such as ageism, stereotyping and stigma is important.
- Throughout life's trajectory changes which influence and impact on a person as they age should be considered.
- Functional deterioration is a normal part of ageing and, although mental illness may increase with age, not all older age will require health and social support.
- Nursing management of mental illness in older people should include listening to the individual, encouraging an active and healthy lifestyle, and cultivating an interactive therapeutic nurse–patient relationship.
- Nurses' attitudes are important in influencing the delivery of care to older people. In assessing an older person, avoid making ageist assumptions such as assuming that dementia is the cause of changes in behaviour and activity.
- Mental health disorders in old age include depression, anxiety, delirium, dementia and schizophrenia. Substance misuse is also an issue. The most common disorders are depression and anxiety.

KEY TERMS

- Ageing
- Ageism
- Alzheimer's disease
- Anxiety
- Cognitive assessment tools
- Delirium
- Dementia
- Depression
- Indigenous Australians
- LGBTIQ+ (lesbian, gay, bisexual, transgender, intersex or queer/questioning)
- Mental disorders
- Schizophrenia
- Stepped care
- Substance misuse
- Suicide

LEARNING OUTCOMES

The material in this chapter will assist you to:

- understand the difference in ageing for young-old to old-old people
- develop knowledge to help identify risks and respond in context to older aged people
- identify life trajectory changes that can contribute to new or established mental disorders
- apply new knowledge and support strategies in caring for older aged people with depression, anxiety, substance misuse, delirium, dementia, schizophrenia and suicide risk
- support consumers to improve mental health in older age.

Introduction

Ageing brings with it many life-changing events. Older aged people (65 years or older) have lifelong experiences and some have pre-existing health disorders. With this in mind it is important to have an understanding of the changes that occur in ageing including physical changes and mental disorders that can coincide with, and impact on, health care.

This chapter presents an insight into the mental disorders that are common in older people. The principles underlying nursing diagnosis, assessment and management are explored. Strategies to promote mental health and reduce negative attitudes to enhance the quality of care for older aged people as consumers of mental health care are discussed.

Demography of ageing

Older age is categorised into three broad groups: young-old (65–74 years), middle-old (75–84 years) and old(est)-old (85+ years). Age does not always reflect a person's abilities or capabilities, and some older aged people may not identify with being old or with their living age. Older aged people may feel discriminated against because of their chronological age, which to them may be simply a number. This in itself leads to anxiety and stress and missed opportunities for seeking support and a positive mental health outcome (Lyons et al. 2018).

The Australian Institute of Health and Welfare (AIHW) reports that in 2017 one in seven Australians were aged 65 years or older (AIHW 2018a), with more than half of older people (57% or 2.2 million) aged 65–74, one-third aged 75–84 (30% or 1.2 million) and 13% aged 85 or older (497,000). By 2047 it is projected there will be just under 3.4 million people aged 65–74 in Australia, people aged 75–84 will account for 35% (2.6 million) of the population and one in five older people will be aged 85 or older (20% or 1.5 million) (Australian Bureau of Statistics 2017). The proportion of older adults in New Zealand is similar, with more than 15% of the population aged over 65 years (Statistics New Zealand 2018) and average life expectancy increasing, with the number of New Zealanders aged 65 years or older expected to grow by nearly 40% over the next decade (Te Pou o te Whakaaro Nui 2019). Older populations are increasingly diverse across cultural background and ethnicity, religious and spiritual beliefs, gender identity, relationships and sexuality (older adults who identify as lesbian, gay, bisexual, transgender, intersex or queer/questioning (LGBTIQ+)).

There are relatively few older people in the Australian Indigenous population, reflecting the life expectancy gap between Indigenous and non-Indigenous Australians and the lower proportion of Indigenous people aged 65 years or older. This reflects the generally poorer health of Indigenous Australians compared with other Australians (AIHW 2018a). In New Zealand's 2018 census, the proportion of the population aged over 65 years grew to 15% and included 6% older Māori (Statistics New Zealand 2018). Both New Zealand Māori and Australian Indigenous populations have poor health as they age as a result of the compounded negative effects of intergenerational disadvantage and a lower life expectancy than the non-Māori and non-Aboriginal populations (Te Pou o te Whakaaro Nui 2019).

Although ageing is not necessarily synonymous with illness or frailty it does correlate with disability and impairment as chronic conditions and multimorbidity become more common in older adults (Beard et al. 2016; Prince et al. 2015). In 2013 the World Health Organization (WHO) reported that more than 20% of older adults had a mental or neurological disorder, with the most common disorder diagnoses in this age group being dementia and depression. WHO (2013) also reported that anxiety disorders were found in 3.8% of the older population, as well as low levels of substance misuse (1%). In particular, risk factors for depression – such as loss and grief, social isolation and loneliness, medical illness and disability, changes in socioeconomic status related to retirement and being a caregiver – are more common in older age. The predicted increase in the older population is therefore expected to multiply the numbers of adults with mental illness (WHO 2013).

It is difficult to have a firm sense of how many older people have a mental illness because prevalence figures vary considerably according to the populations surveyed and the methodologies used (Volkert et al. 2012). In addition, there are also a number of negative stereotypical perceptions of age and older people that may inhibit the diagnosis and treatment of physical and mental illness. 'Ageism' was a broad term introduced in the late 1960s by Dr Robert Butler in response to the dismissive attitude towards older people in America (Butler 1969). However, the term 'ageism' marginalises older aged people and can have a negative impact on their health and wellbeing (WHO 2016). In older people, ageism and stigma are deemed a consequence of losing or gradually losing independence, whether it be physical or functional, and results in tactless stereotyping. Although ageism is experienced almost universally by older people, younger people have also reported having ageist views reciprocated against them (Wilson 2019). Ageist views may affect the recorded prevalence rates of mental illness in the older population through misdiagnosis or unwillingness to diagnose individuals because their experiences are stereotyped as being related to age. Ageism can also influence assessment and treatment – for example, where conclusions are drawn too quickly about what the person is experiencing and why, or where treatment is withheld due to perceived value and the person's age. Self-stigma around ageing may also influence health literacy, help-seeking and health outcome.

The AIHW (2018a) states that health literacy can influence how much and how effectively a person manages their health. Health literacy has two major components: individual health literacy is about a person's ability to access, understand and apply health information; and the health literacy environment describes the infrastructure, people, policies and relationships of the healthcare system (AIHW 2018a). Health literacy in older aged people is associated with cognitive function and the ability to access information and the capacity to support adherence to interventions and management of mental disorders (Chesser et al. 2016). Low levels of health literacy are associated with undesirable outcomes such as premature death among older people. An Australian survey compared subgroups based on age, gender, Indigenous status and previous service access or experience of mental illness. Cost, stigma and mental health literacy were found to be prominent barriers to help-seeking (Coates et al. 2018).

Screening and assessment of older people

The world is full of active and healthy older people, and most older people do not require additional health and social support. How each person ages is individual and unique. Some of these characteristic changes are noticeable, such as the extrinsic effects on the skin, thinning of hair and stature, but many are not. Physiologically, there are bodily organ changes that occur as a result of ageing – for example, the motility of the gastrointestinal tract decreases, which may affect medication absorption and contribute to constipation. There are also organ changes that may affect cognition and bring about vascular changes, hypertension and diabetes (Koppara et al. 2015; Yohannes et al. 2017).

There are several theories about ageing:

- It occurs as the result of pre-programmed switching on and off of certain genes.
- It is the result of normal 'wear and tear' or a biological deteriorative process.
- It is an environmental process due to the links between chronic inflammation, DNA damage and metabolic factors influenced by diet (Bektas et al. 2018).

Whatever theory you support, the life changes that can occur in older people – including physical illness and chronic disease, as well as emotional, financial and social factors – may contribute to developing new mental health issues or exacerbate pre-existing mental illness.

Isolation:
social
financial
retirement
Illness:
chronic
mental disorder
altered function
Death:
spouse/partner
friends
family
self
Vulnerability:
physical changes
cognitive
changes
disability
Loss of
independance:
residential care
Sensory changes:
deafness, sight,
taste, touch,
smell
Factors that
affect older
age

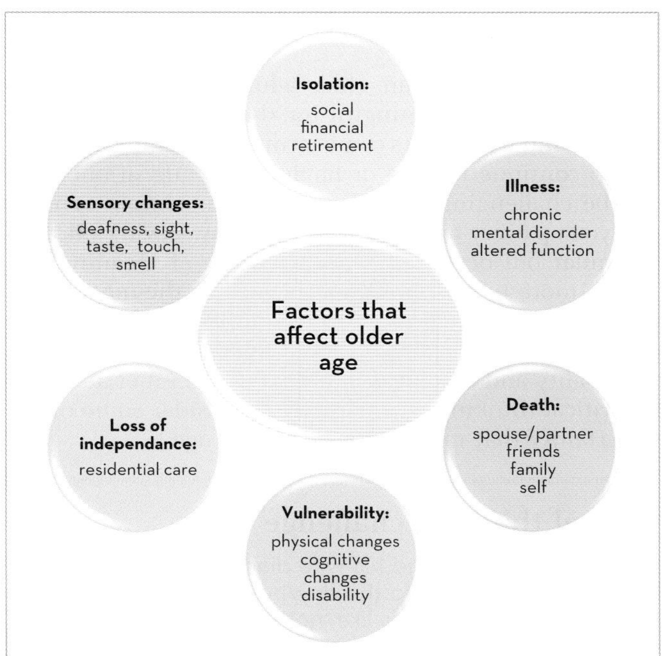

Figure 16.1
Experiential impacts in ageing

Biopsychosocial factors and life-stage transition

Biopsychosocial factors and life-stage transition points (e.g. retirement, death of a spouse, outliving friends or children (Fig. 16.1)) can interact and lead to changes in a person's physical and mental health. For example, a person's physical activity level may alter, given changes in motivation as the result of a bereavement, a chronic disease, pain or increasing frailty (or a combination of these). As a consequence of a more sedentary lifestyle, a person may be more predisposed to obesity, though diet and poor oral health can also contribute, particularly if nutrition becomes poorer as the result of selecting convenience meals or making food choices based on cost. Social withdrawal, loss of social engagement, social isolation and increased loneliness may also occur and are profound risk factors for depression. Loneliness in the general population is a determinant of mental health and increases in older age (Beutel et al. 2017) – feeling of emptiness, even when surrounded by other people, often go hand in hand with feelings of failure. In this context negativity then outweighs positive emotions, which can lead to depression and poorer physical and mental health (Zhao et al. 2018).

Ageing and becoming older can also affect a person's independence. Living arrangements can change from being a homeowner, transitioning to retirement lifestyle accommodation, and to requiring supportive care in a residential aged care facility. These life-stage changes can impact on a person's independence, sense of self and mental health. Older adults who live in residential aged care are particularly vulnerable to developing mental illness, where the experience of loneliness is up to four times higher than for those living in the community (Anderson et al. 2017). Furthermore, older adults who are institutionalised face a number of changes to their normal routine and they often struggle to adjust to living in an environment where there are a lot of people, noises and routines that seem strange. Such factors, including limited nurse–patient interaction, increases vulnerability to mental illness (Haugan et al. 2013).

When assessing an older adult, it is important to identify what is meaningful for them, what gives them purpose and what offers connectedness. Meaning is crucial, but to continue finding or having meaning in one's life can be challenging. Meaning can be as simple as what gets you up every morning to start the day. Having 'purpose' is similar but describes a deeper sense of meaning and relates more to existential issues such as the meaning of life. While meaning and purpose impact on how we are connected, the idea of 'connectedness' also includes spirituality and closeness to others (Drageset et al. 2017). In Critical thinking challenge 16.1, consider some of the uncertainty that may develop in older age.

Critical thinking challenge 16.1

Paul is 88 years old and his wife died 2 years ago, yet he could tell you exactly to the day/hour/minute how long it has been. He uses words like 'nothingness', 'hatred', 'anger' and 'emptiness' when he is talking about life and feels he is now a nuisance to all. He also feels worn out and disappointed that he too has not yet died.

From this short scenario, consider where meaning, purpose and connectedness is evident (or not). What more would you want to know about Paul?

When communicating with an older age person allow extra time, use simple sentences and do not rush. It is important for nurses to remember the person may be experiencing sensory or cognitive impairment, or both. Sight, hearing and memory may be affected. Avoid speaking in an environment filled with distractions and sit opposite to enable eye contact. Always listen and give the person time to respond or to ask you questions. To know if you have been understood you can summarise the discussion. Help the person to focus on activities that may enable meaning, purpose and connectedness.

Chronic disease and mental health

Ageing is a risk factor for developing chronic disease. Evidence also aligns chronic disease as a risk factor for, or contributing factor of, mental disorder, specifically: coronary heart disease, respiratory disease (asthma and chronic obstructive pulmonary disease), stroke, type 2 diabetes, chronic kidney disease, arthritis, osteoporosis, cancer and depression (Scott et al. 2016). Other modifiable risk factors include smoking and illicit drug and alcohol misuse.

It is important for nurses to be aware of the interrelationship between mental health and chronic disease; a person's health outcomes are better when their mental health is addressed, and worse when it is not. The following list outlines some of the mental health impacts of chronic disease:

- Chronic heart failure has been linked to depression, and symptoms for the two overlap – for example, low energy, fatigue, sleep disturbance, weight loss or gain, decreased attention and memory impairment (Liguori et al. 2018). Neurotransmitters or neurohormonal dysfunction contribute to the onset and worsening of the symptoms related to depression. The implication of cortisol, which is a steroid hormone, is released at times of stress, and this can exacerbate cardiac conditions and subsequently bring out depressive symptoms.
- Respiratory dysfunction can lead to, or exist with, other comorbidities and loss of physical function. Respiratory disease, asthma and chronic obstructive pulmonary disease can also affect longevity. Cognitive impairment is common in people with chronic obstructive pulmonary disease due to poorer physical fitness and the ability to manage own care (Yohannes et al. 2017).
- Neurological injury can lead to depression and a significantly increased risk of mortality given the functional disability incurred. More than 30% of stroke survivors will develop depression in the first 6 months following the stroke (Volz et al. 2016). The functional decline resulting from this life-threatening event can also bring about anxiety.
- Late-onset type 2 diabetes also has implications for depression. People who are well and manage their diabetes are at lesser risk. Diabetes is a factor in increasing mortality and functional impairment due to episodes of hypoglycaemia that effects microvascular changes. These changes can lead to cardiac events. Prolonged hypoglycaemia may increase the risk of dementia and is a significant risk in altered cognition (Meneilly et al. 2018). As a preventative strategy, guidelines suggest that an older person's glycaemic level should be slightly higher than in people with younger onset diabetes (The Royal Australian College of General Practitioners 2016).
- Chronic kidney disease and end-stage renal disease, which requires renal replacement therapy such as haemodialysis, is linked to risk factors such as smoking, obesity and diabetes and is common among people with mental illness compared with the general population (Iwagami et al. 2018). The risk factors and treatment for mental disorders may influence the risk of chronic kidney disease, although increasing age is a predominant feature (Iwagami et al. 2018). International research has identified that using antipsychotics and medication such as lithium are risk factors for nephrotoxicity (Iwagami et al. 2018). A decreased level of kidney function and renal impairment is also associated with cardiac disease and often leads to premature death (Ramesh et al. 2016). Careful monitoring of kidney function, blood glucose and cholesterol is important for early management.
- Arthritis, osteoarthritis, osteoporosis and pain are common and debilitating in older aged people. Onset

can occur in early to mid-life and becomes more severe in later years. Commonly, joints, hips, knee(s) and hands are most affected. Chronic pain is also associated with depression – daily life is challenged by limited mobility and physical function, compounded by pharmacotherapy to relieve pain (de Koning et al. 2018).
- Cancer is well evidenced to affect cognition, mental and physical health. In older aged people, this can be a subjective experience and there are many physical and psychological factors that can lead to mental disorders. Cancer is often considered a chronic disease and can be emotionally disabling. Cognitive dysfunction is associated with end of life (Kurita et al. 2018).

Screening and observation

The main reasons for assessing older people are:
- to obtain a baseline assessment of function – this can assist in avoiding unrealistic goals
- to demonstrate positive changes to clients and to gather evidence for relatives, nurses and other health professionals
- for selection purposes (e.g. in research) to ensure that groups of people are of similar levels
- to evaluate a new approach, treatment program or service
- for legal purposes (e.g. complications following a head injury)
- to assist with diagnosis, treatment planning and expectations about prognosis.

Most of the time nurses are involved in obtaining a baseline assessment of function and assisting with diagnosis and determining the factors relevant to prognosis. Cognitive assessment should be included in any evaluation of older adults. When a client is experiencing psychological distress, there may be little time to conduct a full assessment. Using observation skills and a brief assessment of the client's cognitive functioning via the Mini-Mental State Examination (MMSE) (Folstein et al. 1975) provides valuable baseline data on which to base subsequent observations and care. Cognitive changes can affect memory and retention, orientation to place and time and the ability to complete simple and complex tasks through executive functioning.

When making a diagnosis of mental illness, cultural concepts related to physical and mental wellbeing must be considered. The MMSE, which must be purchased to use (https://www.parinc.com/Products/Pkey/237), is available in a number of different language versions that take into consideration an individual's educational attainment and culture. The consequence of using the standard MMSE in groups that differ on cultural and linguistic grounds is the potential to attribute low scores to pathological processes rather than to other factors such as education level, literacy and cultural differences in cognitive and perceptual information processing. The Rowland Universal Dementia Assessment Scale (RUDAS) is a short cognitive screening instrument designed to minimise the effects of cultural learning and language diversity (Storey et al. 2004). The RUDAS is freely available and the instrument and guide can be found at www.health.qld.gov.au/tpch/html/rudas.asp.

When screening older people, use instruments that consider the attributes of older people as well as reporting other conditions. For example, the Cornell Scale for Depression in Dementia is useful for identifying depression in older people with dementia (Snowdon 2010). In addition, the Mini-Cog is a short screening tool that combines the clock drawing test and three-word recall. While some studies report the superior screening properties of the Mini-Cog compared with the MMSE (Borson et al. 2005; Milian et al. 2012), others report similar screening results (Borson et al. 2003; Dougherty et al. 2010). The Mini-Cog assessment and instructions are freely available via https://mini-cog.com/.

For older people 'with complex comorbidities, multimorbidity, frailty, or polypharmacy, a comprehensive geriatric assessment should be performed' (Kok & Reynolds 2017).

Obtaining a health history and nursing assessment

The determinants of health are grouped into four categories:
- physical environment – housing
- social environment – education, employment, relationships
- economic environment – income
- individual environment – sex, physical or mental determinants (WHO 2016).

Pay attention to each of these determinants when obtaining a health history in older aged people, particularly where the person has comorbidities and a mental disorder, to ensure you identify all the issues that may inform nursing care and management (Talley & Jones 2018). A methodical approach to history taking is necessary because older aged people tend to under-report symptoms and problems. Building a rapport will foster trust. Remember not to use terms of endearment, which can feel patronising. Use the person's name. Wherever possible, have a carer or relative present to assist in gathering collateral information.

Establish what is the presenting issue and obtain an in-depth history. Asking about a person's social history and the physical environment where they live can help to flag any difficulties or habits that may be influencing their symptoms or impacting on their activities of daily living. Follow through with a review of body systems. This can be modified to reduce the burden of answering questions, which may have already been asked on many occasions, to specific areas such as mobility and falls, elimination, diet, vision and hearing. Ask about current medications, why the person is taking them and whether they adhere to what has been prescribed. You may also have access to previous health records and you can check medications with the person's general practitioner or prescriber if you are unsure.

A dementia assessment is only appropriate if suspected. Complete Critical thinking challenge 16.2 before moving onto the next section, where specific assessment tools are discussed.

Critical thinking challenge 16.2

List the specific areas you have observed a medical or nursing colleague perform in a health history assessment for an older age person. What did you notice is different from a younger person's assessment?

Cognitive assessment tools

Assessment tools are often used to assist in care strategies and are well validated globally to the general population. Though in a recent Australian study involving Aboriginal and Torres Strait Islander peoples, the findings suggested considering the efficacy of alternative assessment tools for visual and motor impairment, and people with lower education levels (Lavrencic et al. 2018). Culturally specific adaptions, such as 'logical memory' support the use of stories for memory assessment in this cohort (Lavrencic et al. 2018). Logical memory involves being told a story and asking the person to recall it 30 minutes later.

The most commonly used validated cognitive assessment tools are:

- the Standardised Mini Mental-State Examination (Molloy & Standish 1997)
- the Abbreviated Mental Test Score (Hodkinson 1972)
- the Clock Drawing Test (Rakusa et al. 2018)
- the Addenbrooke's Cognitive Examination – Revised (Beishon et al. 2019).

Tools developed for use with people from culturally diverse backgrounds are:

- Mini-Cog (Seitz et al. 2018)
- Rowland Universal Dementia Assessment Scale (Komalasari et al. 2019)
- Kimberley Indigenous Cognitive Assessment short form (LoGiudice et al. 2010).

Other tools to consider for older aged people include the following:

- The Cornell Scale for Depression in Dementia is designed for people with dementia (Alexopoulos et al. 1988). It comprises both an informant and patient interview. Many patient interview items can be completed by simply observing the patient. About 20 per cent of people with dementia have moderate or severe depression; both conditions need to be addressed if present (de Koning et al. 2018).
- The Geriatric Depression Scale short form (GDS-15 or GDS 5/15) is used for cognitively intact people (Sheikh & Yesavage 1986).
- The UCLA Loneliness Scale is used if it is suspected the person is experiencing loneliness. It is a set of three questions currently recommended in the International Consortium for Health Outcome Measures (Akpan et al. 2018).

Given the variety of validated tools available, complete the Critical thinking challenge 16.3.

Critical thinking challenge 16.3

Choose a tool and try it on yourself and then a friend. How was the experience for you? Discuss the experience with your friend and comment on how useful the tool was.

Mental health disorders in older age

Although a number of conditions, including anxiety disorders, depression, suicide, substance misuse, delirium, dementia and schizophrenia, fall within the context of mental illness in old age, they do not occur *because* of ageing. Approximately 15% of people aged 60 or older experience a mental disorder (Kenbubpha et al. 2019).

All psychological symptoms should be assessed in the context of medical or cognitive impairments to ensure the most appropriate treatment is provided; pharmacological treatment is complex (Crocco et al. 2017). Often differential symptom presentation can be difficult because survey criteria specifically for older aged people (e.g. 'fear of burden on family') is not included (Balsamo et al. 2018). Older people may fear situations or objects, experience memory impairment or confusion, and their symptoms may coexist with another mental illness such as depression and dementia (Balsamo et al. 2018).

Common mental health disorders are explored in the following sections with relation to older people and also in separate chapters devoted to the relevant disorder.

Anxiety disorders

Anxiety disorders are one of the most common mental disorders experienced by older adults and are highly comorbid with depression, substance use disorder and sleep disorder (Hellwig & Domschke 2019). They can continue through life from an early onset, or can manifest later in life, but are often under-recognised, perhaps in part because older adults have lower mental health literacy around anxiety than younger people (Beaunoyer et al. 2019). A presentation of anxiety in older people is similar to that in younger people. However, as with depression, diagnosis is complicated by the tendency of older adults to focus on physical rather than psychological illness and by sensory deficits, medical comorbidities and cognitive impairment (Creighton et al. 2018). The most common anxiety disorders in older adults are generalised anxiety disorder and phobias. Anxiety disorder is associated with a high number of somatic medications, a high number of chronic illnesses (Zhang et al. 2015) and an increased risk for cognitive impairment and dementia in the community (Gulpers et al. 2016).

There is insufficient research examining the aetiology of anxiety disorders in older adults. However, evidence suggests that while risk factors are similar to those for depression, social factors such as low affective support during childhood, negative parenting and experiencing negative life events are uniquely associated with anxiety (Zhang et al. 2015). Women are more likely to experience anxiety than men, and residents of residential aged care facilities are at high risk for developing an anxiety disorder (Creighton et al. 2018). Discrimination experienced by older people in the LGBTIQ+ community has been considered a factor for anxiety in disclosing sexual orientation and gender identity, with 34% hiding their sexuality when seeking health care (Australian Human Rights Commission 2015).

Comorbidity is common and affects treatment and outcome. Comorbid anxiety disorder in clients with major depression lowers the rate of recovery and is also associated with a higher rate of cognitive decline and suicide (Santini et al. 2015). The presence of anxiety symptoms decreases the efficacy of depression treatment and, although treatment for depression may reduce anxiety, this is not always the case, with anxiety symptoms persisting despite the resolution of other depressive symptoms (van der Veen et al. 2015). Those experiencing a cognitive disorder and behaviour problems often have a more rapid functional loss when they also present with anxiety symptoms (Crocco et al. 2017).

Given that anxiety is so frequently under-diagnosed, awareness of how anxiety presents and routine screening in older adults is an important nursing role – regardless of the clinical setting. Talking and building a rapport that is therapeutic can help to identify anxiety and enables early intervention, treatment and referral as appropriate. Treatment strategies involve individual planning with the person and may require modifications in lifestyle and addressing psychosocial stressors. Depending on the severity of the illness, the comorbidities and the clinical setting, nurses can assess the capacity of the older age person to engage with different types of therapy and support skill development (e.g. mindfulness and breathing techniques, online self-help). The Royal Australian and New Zealand College of Psychiatrists' clinical practice guidelines recommend cognitive behaviour therapy (CBT), either face-to-face or digital, as first-line management (Andrews et al. 2018). Digital CBT, whether via a computer, hand-held device or mobile phone, has been shown to be effective even in people with mild cognitive impairment (Andrews et al. 2018). CBT is also an effective treatment for anxiety disorders where the patient's focus is on catastrophic thinking and where they use patterns of behaviour that reinforce their anxiety (Wilkinson 2013). Pharmacotherapy choices, namely selective serotonin reuptake inhibitors (SSRIs) and serotonin norepinephrine reuptake inhibitors (SNRIs), depend on the triggers of the anxiety and should be reviewed every 4–6 weeks (Andrews et al. 2018; Crocco et al. 2017).

The three Ds: depression, delirium and dementia

Depression is not unique to older age and it can manifest untreated for many years at different times in a person's life. Delirium and dementia are also not necessarily age-related and can occur in younger people. However, because depression, delirium and dementia are common in older adults and are frequently confused, it is important to understand the differences and similarities. Keep in mind that an older age person may present with more than one of these disorders and the symptoms may overlap as shown in Table 16. 1.

TABLE 16.1 Comparison of dementia, delirium and depression

FEATURES	DEMENTIA	DELIRIUM	DEPRESSION
Onset and duration	Slow deterioration over time - months to years	Sudden onset - hours or days	Mood change over 2 weeks and may coincide with a life event or change such as the death of a loved one
Course	Slow and progressive cognitive decline; non-reversible	Sudden, short and fluctuating; reversible underlying cause	Diurnal fluctuations - can be worse of a morning or evening; reversible with treatment
Signs and symptoms	Wandering, agitation, sleep disturbance, fluctuations in behaviour during the day, generally alert, depression may be present, difficulty with word recall	Restless and uneasy, with fluctuations in agitation, restlessness and hallucinations, impaired attention, mood changes from anger, tearful outbursts and fear, disorganised thinking	Withdrawn, apathetic, feelings of hopelessness and alert, though attention fluctuates with mood; appetite may be increased or diminished

DEPRESSION

There is a common perception that older people become depressed as a part of the normal ageing process. This is not so, but older people are vulnerable to developing a depressive illness because of age-related biochemical changes and psychological factors.

Depression is one of the most common remediable mental disorders in older people (Laborde-Lahoz et al. 2014). In some older adults it has been found to be associated with vascular brain changes; however, 'the causal relationship between brain changes, related lesions, and late life depression remains controversial' (Aizenstein et al. 2016, p. 1). There is also a lack of clarity around the interrelationship between depression, cognitive decline and dementia, with some reporting depression as a dementia risk factor and others naming depression as a consequence of cognitive decline. Others still have theorised that depression and cognitive decline might both be the result of underlying neurodegenerative processes (Kaup et al. 2016). To make this distinction even more difficult, depression often coexists with dementia. Furthermore, diagnosis may be hindered if the person also has a physical illness, which leads health professionals to believe that the person's depressive symptoms are understandable given their physical status – depression is frequently associated with many common medical conditions found in later life such as stroke, cancer, myocardial infarction, diabetes, rheumatoid arthritis and Parkinson's disease (Julien et al. 2016).

As described above, significant life changes that are associated with growing older can also place older people at risk of depression. It is suggested that lower social support and even hospitalisation can be factors in developing distress that can lead to depression (Liguori et al. 2018). Prevalence increases for people aged 85 years or older, those who are hospitalised and those in living in residential aged care facilities. Factors associated with depression include female gender, poor education, early trauma, chronic somatic illness, cognitive impairment, stressful life events (e.g. bereavement), medications, a decrease in activity and losses related to physical illness, financial security, accommodation and independence (Kok & Reynolds 2017).

Presentation

Although older people may exhibit the cardinal features of depression such as low mood and loss of interest, they often attribute these feelings to their physical condition; this will then be the focus of the presentation rather than an acknowledgement of feeling depressed. Complaints might include fatigue, weight loss, pain, problems with self-care, memory concerns or unexplained medical symptoms (Hegeman et al. 2015; Kok & Reynolds 2017).

Depression and dementia share common features such as poor concentration, low mood and social isolation and may both present with psychomotor slowing, apathy, impaired memory, fatigue, sleep disturbance and poor concentration. Distinguishing between grief and depression can also be difficult, since they also share many symptoms. Grief, however, tends to fluctuate, with the person experiencing good and bad days, whereas feelings of emptiness and despair are constant in a person with depression.

Screening and assessment

Initiating a conversation with an older age person about their mood is a good starting point to identifying depression and ensuring appropriate care and treatment are implemented. In evaluating symptoms of depression, the person's context is important; remember that concurrent diagnoses contribute to (and complicate) the clinical picture. Interviewing the person's family or carer can both corroborate the person's history and substantiate a professional assessment, as well as gather additional information to assist in the assessment. Family or a carer will commonly report changes that the person has not recognised such as social withdrawal, irritability, avoiding family and friends, poor hygiene and memory change. Losses such as status, income and bereavement can contribute to feelings of dejection.

Undiagnosed and untreated depression places the person at risk of mental suffering, poor physical health, social isolation and suicide. Screening for depression should be undertaken for people who are recently bereaved and, in particular, when they have unusual symptoms such as marked functional impairment, mood-congruent delusions and psychomotor retardation. It is important to note that older people may use different language to describe their depressed mood. For example, rather than describing sadness they may talk about 'their nerves'.

The Geriatric Depression Scale (short form) (Box 16.1) is an age-specific screening tool for use in those who are cognitively intact (Sheikh & Yesavage 1986; Yesavage et al. 1983). There is also a longer version of 30 items, though it does not measure physical symptoms. The GDS is available in many languages (see https://web.stanford.edu/-yesavage/GDS.html).

The Patient Health Questionnaire or PHQ9 (Spitzer et al. 1994) is another simple screening tool that may help identify depression. In particular there are three questions that ask directly if there is a loss of mood or sense of hopelessness, a lack of interest and thoughts of death.

The possibility of a depressive illness should also be considered in older people if they develop anxiety or cognitive impairment (depression is common in people with mild cognitive impairment (Ismail et al. 2017)). Up to 40% of people with dementia may also experience depression (Kitching 2015). To assist with the diagnosis of depression:

- Check for the presence of depressive symptoms using a screening instrument for this age group, such as the GDS, but note that the reliability of the GDS is reduced when clients have cognitive impairment. Remember

Box 16.1 Geriatric Depression Scale (short form)

A series of yes and no questions, with the answer in bold equalling one point.

1.	Are you basically satisfied with your life?	**No**
2.	Have you dropped many of your activities or interests?	**Yes**
3.	Do you feel that your life is empty?	**Yes**
4.	Do you often get bored?	**Yes**
5.	Are you in good spirits most of the time?	**No**
6.	Are you afraid that something bad is going to happen to you?	**Yes**
7.	Do you feel happy most of the time?	**No**
8.	Do you feel helpless?	**Yes**
9.	Do you prefer to stay at home, rather than go out and do things?	**Yes**
10.	Do you feel that you have more problems with memory than most?	**Yes**
11.	Do you think it is wonderful to be alive now?	**No**
12.	Do you feel pretty worthless the way you are now?	**Yes**
13.	Do you feel full of energy?	**No**
14.	Do you feel that your situation is hopeless?	**Yes**
15.	Do you think that most people are better off then you are?	**Yes**

When a score of more than five is indicated, a more thorough clinical investigation should be undertaken.

This short version has been adapted by many organisations.

Source: Yesavage 1988

that people can experience depression, a physical disorder and/or dementia all at the same time. Do not assume that symptoms can be easily related to the person's life circumstances or their age.

- Where clients have significant cognitive impairment the Cornell Scale for Depression in Dementia (CSDD) should be used. The CSDD is a screening tool and is not diagnostic. The nurse will interview the client's caregiver on the 19 items of the scale. The caregiver then reports their observations based on the previous week. The nurse then briefly interviews the client. The tool is useful if aiming to evaluate the effect of therapy. Permission must be sought to use the CSDD.

Treating depression in older people

The most effective treatment for depression is early intervention. Nurses are often in the unique position of being able to identify behaviour changes and specific symptoms early or at onset because they have more contact with clients in hospital and community settings. Documenting what you have observed clearly in the person's medical record and escalating a referral for further assessment and treatment by health professionals who are skilled and educated in the care and management of older people with mental illness is essential (Haugan et al. 2013).

Nurses can support people to engage in regular exercise, which has been identified as effective for improving physical and mental health in older adults with mental illness, particularly for those who are experiencing depression (Chen et al. 2018). Mental health nurses provide psychotherapeutic support and interpersonal psychotherapy to enable clients to problem solve and to talk about their feelings. Psychotherapy is recommended for older adults experiencing mild to moderately severe depression and is as effective as antidepressants (Kok & Reynolds 2017). Acceptance and commitment therapy, cognitive therapy, CBT, mindfulness-based cognitive therapy, compassion-focused therapy, group therapy and counselling are useful, especially when the depressive illness is loss-related. CBT is the best studied and has been reported as an effective treatment for depression in older people (Jayasekara et al. 2015), but whether it is effective in very old people aged 75 years or older is unclear (Kok & Reynolds 2017). Mindfulness-based cognitive therapy is a meditation-based intervention that has been reported as a promising and cost-effective treatment for older adults with depression and anxiety (Foulk et al. 2014).

Although pharmacological treatment is often effective in treating depression, adverse events due to medical comorbidities and medication interactions can be problematic in older people. Some medications can induce or worsen depressive symptoms (Kok & Reynolds 2017). It is crucial that the introduction (and discontinuation) of antidepressants are titrated (and tapered) gradually to ensure the drug is tolerated (and to ensure relapse or recurrence does not occur). Problems with polypharmacy can be minimised through a tool such as the Screening Tool of Older Persons Prescriptions and Screening Tool to Alert doctors to Right Treatment (STOPP/START) that supports prescribing doctors to make appropriate medication prescriptions and avoid undertreatment (Kok & Reynolds 2017). In older clients with severe depression associated with dementia, evidence does not support using antidepressant medication (Kok & Reynolds 2017) and prognosis is poor. Electroconvulsive therapy may also be prescribed for older adults with depression and be used alone or in conjunction with psychosocial therapies.

See the 'Useful websites' list at the end of the chapter for more information and fact sheets on depression.

DELIRIUM

Delirium (or acute confusion) is a serious acute reversible medical condition whereby a person's mental ability is affected (an acute decline in consciousness and cognition). It develops over a short period of time (usually within hours or days) and symptoms tend to fluctuate throughout the day. It is a common condition in older people who are hospitalised (prevalence up to 56% (Lee et al. 2017), but it can also occur in older people in the community. Delirium is potentially preventable in up to two-thirds of hospitalised patients and is often treatable; however, it is associated with an increased risk of death, institutionalisation and dementia (Lee et al. 2017). Delirium causes distress for the person, their family and treating healthcare providers. Addressing delirium includes predicting, preventing, diagnosing and treating older people who are affected (Lee et al. 2017).

Older aged people are at risk of developing delirium if they:

- are acutely unwell or have a chronic illness
- have a pre-existing diagnosis of dementia or depression
- are 70 years of age or older
- have sensory impairment such as poor eyesight
- are taking multiple medications
- are in drug withdrawal, including from alcohol
- are undergoing a surgical procedure requiring general anaesthetic (e.g. hip fracture) (Lee et al. 2017).

The causes of delirium can include physical illness, urinary tract infection, constipation, dehydration, pain, polypharmacy, excessive alcohol consumption and abruptly withdrawing from alcohol or medications. Presenting symptoms can vary and are often masked by comorbid symptoms of other diseases. Symptoms include confusion and forgetfulness, inattention, unusual behaviour, agitation or withdrawn behaviour, night wakening and day sleeping, exhibiting fear or upset, mood change, hallucinations and incontinence (Lee et al. 2017). It is imperative to determine the causal factors and treat the underlying problem if possible. Taking a comprehensive history in consultation with the family and including medical, physical, cognitive, social and behavioural function will help identify the underlying condition and inform interventions to reverse delirium.

The approach to delirium

The Confusion Assessment Method is a tool developed for non-psychiatrically trained clinicians and researchers (Inouye et al. 1990). This tool is available in a short form, which has four items commonly used for screening and a long form, which has 10 items for diagnostic confirmation, subtyping and research (Inouye 2018). To support a diagnosis of delirium, there must be evidence of an acute onset and fluctuating changes in the person's condition. The presence of inattention, with either disorganised thought processes or an altered level of consciousness, is required.

Although there is no specific pathology test for diagnosing delirium, there are studies that suggest an association with raised inflammatory markers C-reactive protein and interlukein-6 (Inouye 2018).

Prior to an older person undergoing surgery it is important that the nurse assesses the person to ensure any changes in behaviour following surgery can be detected and early intervention given. There are two established risk factors for older people undergoing surgery: previous alcohol/drug abuse and prolonged operating time under a general anaesthetic. Evidence supports a preventive approach including all staff being aware of delirium risk factors, reductions in the use of medications that increase risk and delirium-friendly post-surgery medication orders, addressing constipation and other known risk factors, and attending to sensory impairment and individual complications (Freter et al. 2016). Managing delirium includes supportive therapy and pharmacological management. Supportive therapy that nurses can offer includes ensuring patient safety, attention to fluid and nutrition and reorientation (e.g. memory cues including calendars, clocks and photographs of family and pets).

DEMENTIA

Prevalence

There are more than 100 diseases, including brain injury or trauma, that can cause dementia, but it is not a normal part of ageing. However, as the prevalence of dementia increases exponentially with age, the number of people with dementia is increasing in Australia and New Zealand because more people are living longer. In 2019 an estimated 447,115 Australians were living with dementia, with 43% being over the age of 85 years and 52% living in a residential aged care facility (AIHW 2018a; Dementia Australia 2018). The number of people diagnosed with young-onset dementia (before the age of 65) is also increasing, with approximately 27,247 people affected, including people as young as 30 years of age (Dementia Australia 2018). Dementia is the second leading cause of death in Australia and the leading cause of death in women (Australian Bureau of Statistics 2018). In Aboriginal and Torres Strait Islander people aged over 65 years, dementia is three times higher than the wider Australian older age population (AIHW 2018a; Radford et al. 2015). The New Zealand estimates are similar – in 2016, the prevalence estimate of dementia in New Zealand was 62,287 people (Deloitte Economics 2017) – a 29% increase since the 2011 estimate of 48,182 in 2011. This number is also predicted to increase to 170,212 (2.9% of the population) by 2050 (Deloitte Economics 2017).

In the early stages of dementia, people usually live in the community, while people with higher levels of cognitive loss are often accommodated in residential aged care facilities. Approximately one in five people experiencing dementia will also experience depression, but it is often underdiagnosed in this population (Gaugler et al. 2014).

'Dementia' is the common umbrella term used for Alzheimer's disease, vascular dementia and Lewy body dementia and is the single greatest cause of disability in older Australians (AIHW 2018a). Other types of dementia are frontotemporal lobe, alcohol-related dementia, Down syndrome and HIV-associated dementia. Another term for dementia is 'neurocognitive disorder' and, while this refers to the type (mild, major) and includes many subtypes, for the purpose of this section dementia will be referred to in this context.

Clinical features

Older aged people with dementia experience cognitive decline/impairment, behavioural and/or psychological symptoms. Cognitive impairment can also result in the person displaying problems that may be identified by care staff as being challenging to manage. Behaviours of aggression and agitation are easily recognised and include, for example, an increase in disorientation, restlessness, agitation, anxiety and behavioural problems occurring in the late afternoon, evening or at night termed 'sundowning' (Khachiyants et al. 2011). This increase in disorientation has variously been attributed to diurnal variations in hormones and light, as well as to fatigue and a search for familiar surroundings in which to rest. However, in some people this pattern is reversed – they are more disoriented in the morning. Apathy and depression are often misinterpreted and underdiagnosed. Excluding other causes for the fluctuations in behaviour such as pain or infection should be considered. Memory loss may be misconstrued as a psychosis event. This can lead to inappropriate prescribing of antipsychotics that elevate the risk of fall and injury and should only be used when behavioural interventions have failed (Macfarlane & O'Connor 2016).

Assessing the following cognitive domains help to establish the presence of dementia and determine severity:

- complex attention – includes sustained attention, divided attention, selective attention and information processing speed
- executive function – includes planning, decision making, working memory, responding to feedback, inhibition and mental flexibility
- learning and memory – includes free recall, cued recall, recognition memory, semantic and autobiographical long-term memory and implicit learning
- language – includes object naming, word finding, fluency, grammar and syntax and receptive language
- perceptual-motor function – includes visual perception, visio-constructional reasoning and perceptual-motor coordination
- social cognition – includes recognition of emotions, theory of mind and insight.

Nursing management of people with dementia

Nurses can support the person with dementia to manage their feelings and thoughts, to deal with their stresses, to link them to their community (including a safe environment) and to support the individual and family to build resilience. A person-centred approach to care aims to understand the person and seeks to engage with and respond appropriately to their individual situation.

Distraction, redirection, reassurance and reorientation form the core behavioural interventions. Observe for triggers that pre-empt behavioural symptoms – an individualised care plan should identify and address the person's triggers and behaviours (Macfarlane & O'Connor 2016). People with dementia are often highly responsive to the environment they find themselves in. Therefore, wherever possible, the environment needs to be made safe and familiar, with objects that have meaning for the person (e.g. family photographs). Avoid unnecessary changes to routines.

Given the challenging behaviours, medical practitioners often prescribe pharmacotherapy that should be reviewed and reduced after 2–3 months, then stopped once the behaviour is resolved (Lavan et al. 2016). Drug therapy should only be used when simple behavioural interventions have failed. However, not all people with dementia have behavioural problems as Stephen's story presents.

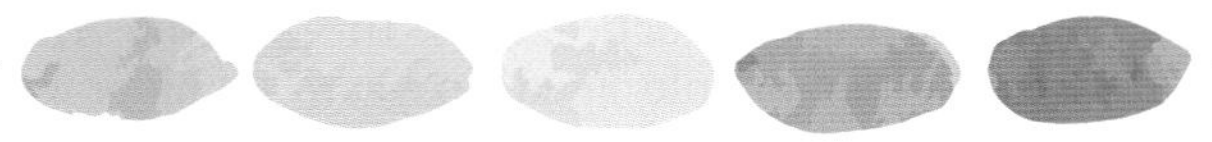

NURSE'S STORY 16.1

Stephen

As a newly qualified registered nurse commencing in aged care, I had not considered that LGBTIQ+ issues would have to be considered. It came to my attention with the admission of Alex (61 years), who was brought to the facility by his partner, James. James reported that Alex had been displaying strange behaviours for the past two years. He had been an architect in a small local company, and one of the senior partners had contacted James with concerns about his quality of work, which was deteriorating. James had also noted that Alex was becoming increasingly dependent on him in decision making. At this point James took Alex to see his general practitioner and was diagnosed with early dementia and referred to an aged care assessment team (ACAT). ACAT arranged home help to assist James in his care of Alex. The intimacy James and Alex shared in their relationship was also challenged. In the aged care facility, Alex experienced loneliness, new surroundings and the absence of his lifelong partner. The ACAT occupational therapist introduced Alex to art therapy. Initially this was enjoyed, but Alex thought the people who were there were odd, and this was getting him down. He thought of them as unfamiliar and 'old'. Alex's niece mentioned to James that she had met some of his old acquaintances at a community centre, which prompted connecting with their old network of friends and the social life they both had led. Some of his friends attended social functions at the aged care facility, which were very colourful and joyful. It was a different experience for the staff being exposed to the theatrical lifestyle of Alex' circle of friends. They noticed the change in Alex as a resident and his increased acceptance and engagement with the other residents.

Non-pharmacological principles for dementia care include safe environments that are familiar, using cues to assist the individual, such as routines, and using familiar repetitive activities. This may be in the form of music, art, household chores or having personal belongings that connect to their past. Stimulate activity engagement with pets or sensory stimulation (Scales et al. 2018).

To recap, depression, delirium and dementia may present with similar features. Table 16.1 provides an overview of the onset and duration, course, activity, alertness, attention mood and thinking pattern.

Substance use and misuse

Substance use and misuse is a problem within the older age population (Rao & Roche 2017). In 2018 the AIHW reported that older people aged 70 years or older were more likely to exceed lifetime risks and alcohol-related harm, with alcohol consumption more than 5 days per week (AIHW 2018b). The 2016 National Drug Strategy House Survey reported an increase in the proportion of older Australians using illicit drugs, indicating that there is now an ageing cohort of drug users (AIHW 2017). In 2016–17 the principal drugs of concern for those aged over 50 years old were alcohol (66%), followed by 9% for cannabis, 7% for amphetamines and 5% for heroin (AIHW 2018b). Problematic use is clearly under-reported, with drug use prevalence occurring in baby boomers and post baby boomers (Carew & Comiskey 2018). As previously discussed, physical health changes associated with ageing may also affect the body's metabolism of these substances.

Likely triggers for substance use and misuse in older age is often associated with tolerance to previously used substances, although life-changing events, as well as planned and unplanned stressors, have a significant influence. These may occur at retirement and as a result of unforeseen financial strain, death of a spouse, chronic illness both physical and mental, family disputes/estrangement, sleep disturbances or change of living arrangements.

Often referred to as a soft drug, cannabis use in older Australians is increasing given the contemporary influence of medicinal cannabinoids (Kostadinov & Roche 2017). Opioid use for chronic pain is also not without risks. Pain is diverse, with chronic comorbidities. Benzodiazepines prescribed for sleep deprivation are among the most frequently prescribed drugs for older people (Musich et al. 2019). This in itself is problematic because benzodiazepines are highly addictive and increase the risk of falls. Symptoms of substance misuse can also be masked by symptoms of chronic illness such as diabetes, or even depression and dementia. Review the possible symptoms in Critical thinking challenge 16.4.

Critical thinking challenge 16.4

Signs and symptoms of drug use can be both behavioural and physical. Substances manifest with many overlapping symptoms with chronic illness. Access the following NARCONON web link and review the listed signs and symptoms. Which do you believe may be misinterpreted as a chronic illness?

https://www.narconon.org/drug-abuse/signs-symptoms-of-drug-abuse.html

During hospitalisation there is an opportunity to identify substance use during the nursing assessment. Ascertaining the substance to be addressed is the primary goal. And ask for specifics. Rather than asking someone whether they drink alcohol, ask: 'How much alcohol do you drink per day?' If they say 'not much' or 'I only drink socially', ask them to tell you exactly how much alcohol this involves. Older clients may relate that they do not drink 'much' but may be unaware of the guidelines and consider their intake to be less harmful than it is (see also Chapter 11 for more information). Given the complexity of older age care, targeted age-appropriate interventions should be implemented (Kostadinov & Roche 2017; Musich et al. 2019). Meeting the individual needs of an older age person can be complex because withdrawal symptoms may be delayed, so ongoing nursing observation and assessment is required. Providing social and emotional support requires an interdisciplinary team approach. Escalation of care should be considered during detoxification.

Schizophrenia

Psychosis usually onsets in the early 20s; however, in 15–20% of those with a diagnosis of schizophrenia, symptoms appear in middle to later life (Cohen 2018). Precise age onset is difficult to determine given it may be based on the person's age when clinically assessed, but it is estimated 17% of the general older age have mild cognitive impairment (Cohen 2018). Older-onset schizophrenia is more likely in women given physiological changes, such as oestrogen depletion after menopause, which is thought to affect neuron function and decrease cognition (Cai & Huang 2018). In older aged people, paranoia is common and not necessarily due to cognitive changes.

As with other mental health disorders in old age, assessment is complicated by comorbidity, and stigma is also an issue. There is also a relationship between schizophrenia and risk of dementia, specifically in women, which is associated with loneliness, and women being more prone to mood swings, insomnia, irritability, anxiety and depression (Cai & Huang 2018). If we consider the symptoms of schizophrenia in the older aged (65 years or older), there are common features with dementia, though dementia is characterised by a progressive loss of cognition and function.

In older people, psychosis in schizophrenia is often associated with brain abnormalities such as stroke, tumours and trauma, with marked neuropsychological impairment (Cai & Huang 2018). Behaviours can be challenging to manage, and determining the underlying factors is crucial.

Historical anecdote 16.1: Basket cases and Bedlam!

After St Marys of Bethlehem was established in 1247 the monks there became known as 'basket men' for their habit of carrying baskets to collect and distribute food and alms for the sick – this led to our modern stigmatising term 'basket case'. By 1377 St Marys had become known as 'Bethlem', which local townspeople vulgarised to 'Bedlam'. The modern-day term 'bedlam', meaning uproar and confusion, is derived from the asylum's name. Like many asylums of the Middle Ages, Bedlam was overcrowded and maladministered. A dehumanising practice developed in the mid-1700s when, for the price of a penny, a visitor could spend what was advertised as a 'very amusing' afternoon touring the facility observing the 'old loonies'. During visits, people were provided with a glimpse of the horrific, yet socially acceptable, treatment of people in grisly living conditions receiving bizarre painful, dehumanising treatments.

Read more about it: *Clarke BFL 1975 Mental disorder in earlier Britain: exploratory studies. University of Wales Press, Cardiff*

Historical anecdote 16.2: Treatment or neglect?

History teaches that treatment of mental illness has been used to justify healthcare and nursing negligence. During the 1960s and 1970s, a program referred to as 'deep sleep therapy' was practised (in combination with electroconvulsive therapy) by Dr Harry Bailey in at Chelmsford Private Hospital in Sydney. Deep sleep therapy involved long periods of barbiturate-induced unconsciousness. It was prescribed for conditions ranging from schizophrenia and depression and addiction. Twenty-six patients died due to the therapy during the 1960s and 1970s. After the failure of medical agencies to investigate or address complaints, a series of newspaper articles in the early 1980s in the *Sydney Morning Herald* and television coverage exposed the abuses at the hospital.

Read more about it: *Walton M 2013 Deep sleep therapy and Chelmsford Private Hospital: have we learnt anything? Australasian Psychiatry, 21(3): 206–12*

In people with Alzheimer's and psychosis related to schizophrenia (rather than to dementia), remission is common. Management should be collaborative, with clinical symptom management and involving the older age person in addressing any concerns affecting their daily life. CBT and social skills training are useful strategies. Social contact and education of caregivers can reduce associated anxiety and normalise the person's environment.

The use of second-generation antipsychotics has increased even though the side effects risk serious harm in older age (Kjosavik et al. 2017). The duration of use should be monitored and limited in older people.

Suicide

Older aged people have a significantly higher rate of death by suicide in Australia than the younger population. In 2017, there were 3,128 suicide deaths in people over the age of 60 years and 39.3 per 100,000 in males aged 85 years and older (Australian Bureau of Statistics 2017). In New Zealand, the rate of suicide in people aged over 65 years is significantly lower. However, across all age groups, men and Māori were highly represented in the figures, with 457 men dying by suicide in 2016–17, a rate of 19.36 per 100,000, up from 409 and 17.71 per 100,000 the previous year. The number of Māori who died by suicide, not age specific, in 2016–17 was 130 and 21.73 per 100,000 (Statistics New Zealand 2018).

Risk factors for suicide in older people

Older aged people may be vulnerable to suicide, particularly where there is an increase in the complexity of lifelong stressors. Significant issues may enhance feelings of loss: being or becoming a widow/widower; bereavement and becoming socially isolated; feeling a lack of social support; or being lonely or alone. Other risks include cognitive impairment or decline, whether from a physical or neurodegenerative cause. Chronic illness, physical/psychological pain, substance use/misuse and mental health disorders are also key risk considerations, as are previous suicide attempts. Depression and dementia, stroke and a new or existing diagnosis of a life-limiting disease such as cancer may contribute to suicidal ideation due to loss of physical and cognitive function (Ahmedani et al. 2017). Unmistakably, suicide risk is linked to poor physical health. In an American study, 17 physical health conditions were associated with increased suicide in older people (Ahmedani et al. 2017).

Building an awareness of these risks places nurses in a position to be more involved in mental health promotion and early intervention focused on preventing suicidal behaviours in older aged people. Like anyone who says they are experiencing suicidal thoughts, an older age person who talks about suicide must be taken very seriously – never assume that because someone is an older person and hospitalised, or accessing aged care services or living in a residential aged care facility, that they are not capable of a suicide attempt. The person offering information about their intended suicide, identifying how, when and by what means, will enable the level of risk to be assessed (see Chapter 7 for risk assessment).

A suicide intent may not always be obvious, as Peter's story shows.

NURSE'S STORY 16.2

Peter

I had been allocated an older male client, Bill, who had been bounced around to different organisations before securing funding with the non-government organisation I was working at. Because of Bill's circumstances (socioeconomic, health and age), he qualified for several care packages. So, two community support workers were allocated to work with him across the week for nominal hours. I visited Bill in the first week and began to establish a relationship with him. My co-worker was on sick leave, so my 1-hour visit was the only support Bill had received for the first week. In the second week, Bill received support from both packages (total of 3 hours). During this visit, I noted Bill to be comfortable to verbalise that he was feeling unsure about his future, though we spoke of his long-term goals. In his younger years he had been interested in studying computing at TAFE, so he agreed that in our next visit we would focus on short-term achievable goals. Two days after this visit, he committed suicide.

I had mixed emotions about this. I had a duty of care to Bill. Did I miss something? Were there signs that I should have picked up? Am I qualified enough to be dealing with these types of people? I became angry – the system had let Bill down. Why had he been bounced around? Would the outcome have changed with a more consistent approach to his care? I even questioned if this reflected on my capacity to manage people with mental health disorders as a community support worker. To rationalise this I tried to weigh up how much I could really achieve in such a short time with him. We had a total of 2 hours together.

Suicide prevention is based on the overall burden of physical disease (Ahmedani et al. 2017). One approach to restoring recovery is through a chronic care model. The chronic care model, developed by Dr Edward Wagner (2014), is based on organisational and patient–provider relationships, which aims to address the management of long-term conditions that may result in depression and potentially lead to suicide ideation (Conejero et al. 2018). It is also suggested that suicide risk assessment should be part of the older age assessment (van Orden & Deming 2018).

Health and stress factors increase the complexity of the explanatory model for suicide in older age (Conejero et al. 2018). Psychological pain and somatic distress have been implicated in people who have had lifelong suicide ideation (Conejero et al. 2018). In Jill's story, she shares her experience with the suicide of her friend.

CONSUMER'S STORY 16.1

Jill

I had what I thought was an honest and strong relationship with Margaret. I was introduced to her at a stroke support group meeting, and she was a lot older than me. We had consistently communicated for around 9 months. She shared with me on different occasions when she was feeling anxious about being alone with her thoughts for too long. She would say things like: 'Make sure you are coming on Thursday – I know I'll need to see someone by then'.

Coming from a rural community originally, we had long-term plans to visit her family home because her much older brother, Jim, I think he was 82 years old, was still living there. The chosen weekend was approaching and despite me noticing a decline in her mood, Margaret insisted that she would be alright and that this would be good for her. She called it her 'out'. I contacted her brother and, without breaking Margaret's confidence, I indicated that she was not well and hoped Jim could keep an eye on her. The drive was uneventful, and she seemed happy to see her home and her brother. After her first night with Jim, she committed suicide on the property.

Working with older people and responding appropriately to early cues is a proactive approach. Assessment for depression, if not already an underlying mental disorder, can be an effective strategy, and providing timely therapeutic management may help. Interventions to prevent experiences of loneliness, hopelessness and isolation can be explored by nurses working in primary care and community settings with older people, as well as by those working in aged care and residential aged care services. Monitoring and reviewing current care strategies for effectiveness and escalating care to the appropriate mental health or crisis intervention service when it is required is vital.

Be mindful that it is important to engage in self-care when working with people who are expressing suicidal thoughts, attempting suicide or dying by a catastrophic event like suicide (see Chapter 6).

Nursing management of older people

Health professionals, as well as the public, often have negative attitudes towards ageing and poor attitudes to and tolerance of mental illness. Stereotypical images of older people and ageist beliefs can affect the quality of nursing care and therefore on a person's health outcomes (Rush et al. 2017). For nurses, an important aspect of managing older people is reflecting on your own attitudes and biases, and how these might affect care.

Several nursing interventions are known to assist older people:

- Listen to the person in an active way; in particular, try to notice the feelings and emotions behind the words.
- Encourage older people to participate in physical and social activities that invite them to focus on aspects of their life apart from illness.
- Assist older people to understand disease processes, how to take medications and to maintain a physically and mentally active lifestyle.
- Help older people to find coping strategies to assist them with any losses such as a decline in health or financial status or bereavement.
- Support the person to work through the pain of grief and to adjust to an environment where the deceased is no longer available.
- Identify informal supports such as social networks and support services.

Use a person-centred care approach – develop a collaborative and respectful partnership with the person and respect the contribution that the older person can bring. This approach requires the nurse to get to know the person – their needs, preferences and life history – and to empower them by encouraging them to be involved in the decisions that affect their health and wellbeing as much as possible. Providing flexible and accessible services that respond to the individual's needs is vital.

Nurses can assist older people in maintaining function by ensuring they have small, frequent meals, are well hydrated and maintain bowel function through a high-fibre diet, hydration and exercise. Clients should be encouraged to mobilise and be independent, and nurses should ensure they have undisturbed rest and relaxation. Other therapies that older people may find therapeutic include listening to music they enjoy, hand and back massage and pet therapy (Moyle 2014). Massage, for example, can induce a calming sensation that may reduce anxiety (Moyle et al. 2013a). In addition, companion robots such as animal robots have also been reported to reduce agitation and improve quality of life, in particular for older people with non-communicable disease (Moyle et al. 2013b).

These interventions are generalised and so it is important to evaluate care processes regularly to ensure the interventions are appropriate for the situation. As previously highlighted, it is also imperative that health professionals consider the person's culture, as decisions about care may be affected by cultural differences. For example, institutional care for family members is not an accepted way of providing care in some cultures. People from non-English-speaking populations often present at later stages of mental illness due to low levels of English proficiency or unfamiliarity with mental health services. People who come to Australia and New Zealand as refugees or asylum seekers have frequently experienced extreme hardship and trauma in their country of origin and/or in their migration journey. The effects of displacement and trauma place them at high risk of developing post-traumatic stress disorders and depression, but the stigma associated with mental-health–related conditions can affect a person's desire to seek help (Procter 2016). (See Chapter 3 for more information about trauma, crisis, loss and grief.)

When mental health nurses are providing psychological therapy, they will need to consider the needs of the individual and the underlying conditions or circumstance. For example, CBT has demonstrated social wellbeing along with lower levels of depression; fewer physical symptoms and sleep complaints have also been evidenced (Friedman et al. 2017). CBT could be used to help address fears of falling and lead to adaptive behaviours such as exercising regularly (Liu et al. 2018). Not all older aged people will be able to participate in psychological therapy given the level of their cognitive or sensory impairment, but given the complexities associated with the use of medicines in older people, wherever possible, non-pharmacological treatments should be used.

Polypharmacy for older age and medication safety

Polypharmacy in older aged people can be complex and not without risks (Wallis et al. 2018). Risks such as inappropriate prescribing, medication omission and adverse reactions due to interactions of drug groups is of a concern. Adjunct to this is a possible acute illness and admission to hospital, multiple prescribers, and inaccurate/incomplete medical records. There is also the issue of older aged people memory recall on which medications they are taking. Confusion over generic names versus trade names and over-the-counter medications may contribute to pharmacy errors at point of care. Non-adherence to prescribed regimes is another problem and may be related to memory or an issue such as being unable to pay for the number of scripts that have been issued. The provision of verbal and written drug information may allay some of these issues.

Prescribing in this context requires sound knowledge of ageing physiology, geriatric medicine and pharmacotherapy to reduce potential error (Lennox et al. 2019). Physiological changes, chronic illness and even malnutrition affect drug pharmacokinetics and pharmacodynamics (Lavan et al. 2016). In particular, absorption, distribution, metabolism and excretion (Australian Medicines Handbook 2019; Lavan et al. 2016). As previously discussed, physical ageing, especially renal function, and chronic co-morbidities, can impact on sensitivity to specific drugs and may contribute to the person's presenting symptoms. Take the time to ponder Critical thinking challenge 16.5.

Critical thinking challenge 16.5

It is important to consider polypharmacy as up to 40% of people over the age of 60 may take five or more different medications. How should prescribing in older age be approached to prevent adverse effects?

The role of antipsychotics and antidepressants to manage symptoms in older aged people requires special consideration. Quetiapine is the most prescribed antipsychotic (Kjosavik et al. 2017). Using antipsychotics can increase the risk of stroke and death when beginning treatment. It is recommended to use lower starting doses of any medication and gradually titrate to reduce side effects and to limit the period of use (Australian Medicines Handbook 2019). Although in Australia there has been a reduction in prescribing frequency, there has been an increase in 'prn' prescribing (Westbury et al. 2018). In an Australian study, off-label prescribing of antipsychotics occurred in 63% of people over 75 years of age with dementia for behavioural and psychological symptoms (Kjosavik et al. 2017). Yet, antipsychotic use can worsen behavioural and psychological symptoms of dementia (Westaway et al. 2018).

Note the following precautions for antipsychotics that are used in acute and chronic psychoses:

- respiratory failure or respiratory depression – exacerbated by alcohol use
- hyperthyroidism – check thyroid function routinely
- hypo/hyperthermia – may lead to shock
- gastrointestinal obstruction, urinary retention, myasthenia gravis – may be exacerbated by anticholinergic effects
- diabetes – may have raised glycaemic levels
- neurological effects – can aggravate Parkinson's or tremors, cognitive deterioration in Lewy body dementia, risk of seizures
- cardiovascular effects – risk of arrhythmias and prolonged Q-T intervals
- use of antipsychotics in older people – associated with increased risk of stroke (Australian Medicines Handbook 2019).

Given the ongoing dialogue within the literature, antidepressants, SSRIs and SNRIs are most suited to managing specific mental health disorders in older age (Andrews et al. 2018). Side effects should be monitored and observation for any metabolic effects (Australian Medicines Handbook 2019). Both SSRIs and SNRIs have a risk of serotonin toxicity and require tapering of the dose over at least 4 weeks to prevent withdrawal effects. Common adverse effects include gastrointestinal upset, nausea, diarrhoea, agitation, insomnia/drowsiness, decreased libido, myalgia and rash (Australian Medicines Handbook 2019). Blood pressure and sodium levels (risk of hyponatraemia) should be monitored, with a baseline measurement taken before treatment.

To recap, providing older aged people with information about their medications and associated effects is crucial. Any new medication should be started at a low dose to monitor effect. It is also preferable to only begin one new treatment at a time to enable any side effects to be identified. Critical thinking challenge 16.6 provides an opportunity for you to review pharmacology.

Critical thinking challenge 16.6

Complete the following table to consolidate your learning about pharmacology in the following mental health disorders. Complete the missing information and provide the precautions, adverse effects and any practice point pertaining to older aged people.

MENTAL HEALTH DISORDER	DRUG GROUP	PRECAUTION	ADVERSE EFFECTS	PRACTICE POINT FOR OLDER PEOPLE
Depression	Antidepressant			
Dementia	Benzodiazepine			
Anxiety	SSRI			
Schizophrenia	Antipsychotic			

Chapter summary

Healthy ageing involves more than promoting good mental and physical health. It includes social and emotional wellbeing; nurses can support older people to maintain social connections and regular engagement with supports and community. As people age they experience psychosocial factors such as bereavement as well as loss of physical and mental functioning. This may place them at risk of mental disorders and, in particular, depression or anxiety, which are both common and treatable. However, mental disorders are not a normal part of ageing, and clients require adequate assessment and diagnosis to ensure their symptoms are not related to other issues such as adverse effects of medications or underlying physical disease. The diagnosis and treatment of mental disorders in older adults can be complex and are complicated by the presence of comorbid conditions. Negative stereotypical ageist assumptions are also problematic.

Nurses have an important role to play with older people experiencing mental disorders. Establishing a therapeutic relationship provides the opportunity for nurses to recognise the symptoms of mental illness and to suggest/provide/refer for further assessment and treatment as required. The knowledge that older people have a high risk of suicide means it is imperative that they are assessed and treated appropriately and effectively. Skills in establishing a therapeutic relationship, and in using psychotherapeutic support such as CBT, can assist older people to address the impacts of grief and bereavement, role disputes and transitions, or interpersonal issues, and can, along with pharmacotherapy and at times electroconvulsive therapy, improve older people's quality of life.

Useful websites

Australian and New Zealand Society for Geriatric Medicine: http://www.anzsgm.org/
Australasian Delirium Association: https://www.delirium.org.au/
Beyond Blue: https://www.beyondblue.org.au/
Black Dog Institute: https://www.blackdoginstitute.org.au/clinical-resources/depression
Capital Health Network: https://www.chnact.org.au/mental-health-programs-hp
Dementia Australia: https://www.dementia.org.au/
Dementia Training Australia: https://www.dta.com.au/
Department of Health: http://www.health.gov.au/internet/publications/publishing.nsf/Content/mental-pubs-p-mono-toc~mental-pubs-p-mono-pop~mental-pubs-p-mono-pop-old
Head to Health – Australian Government: https://headtohealth.gov.au/supporting-someone-else/supporting/aged-and-elderly
Health Direct: https://www.healthdirect.gov.au/older-people-and-mental-health
HELP: https://www.hospitalelderlifeprogram.org/about/
Khan Academy: https://www.khanacademy.org/science/health-and-medicine/mental-health/dementia-delirium-alzheimers/v/what-is-delirium
Mental Health Commission of NSW: https://nswmentalhealthcommission.com.au/mental-health-and/older-people
NARI: https://www.nari.net.au/research/current-projects/mental-health
Narconon Drug Rehab and Drug Education Centre: https://www.narconon.org/drug-rehab/centers/narconon-melbourne-australia.html
National Depression Initiative: www.depression.org.nz
New Zealand suicide prevention: www.mentalhealth.org.nz/suicideprevention
SANE Australia: https://www.sane.org/images/PDFs/GrowingOlderStayingWell.pdf
World Health Organisation: https://www.who.int/mental_health/en/

References

Ahmedani, B.K., Peterson, E.L., Hu, Y., Rossom, R.C., Lynch, F., Lu, C.Y., et al. 2017. Major physical health conditions and risk of suicide. Am. J. Prev. Med., 53 (3), pp.308–315.
Aizenstein, H.J., Baskys, A., Boldrini, M., et al., 2016. Vascular depression consensus report – a critical update. BMC Med. 14, 161.
Akpan, A., Roberts, C., Bandeen-Roche, K., et al., 2018. Standard set of health outcome measures for older persons. BMC Geriatr. 18 (1), 36.
Alexopoulos, G.S., Abrams, R.C., Young, R.C., et al., 1988. Cornell scale for depression in dementia. Biol. Psychiatry 23 (3), 271–284.
Anderson, J., Deravin-Malone, L., Croxon, L., 2017. A review of aged care provision in multipurpose services (MPS). Aust. Nurs. Midwifery J. 24 (7), 34.
Andrews, G., Bell, C., Boyce, P., et al., 2018. Royal Australian and New Zealand College of Psychiatrists clinical practice guidelines for the treatment of panic disorder, social anxiety disorder and generalised anxiety disorder. Aust. N. Z. J. Psychiatry 52 (12), 1109–1172.
Australian Bureau of Statistics, 2018. National Health Survey: first results 2017-2018. Available from: http://www.abs.gov.au/ausstats/abs@.nsf/mf/4364.0.55.001.
Australian Bureau of Statistics, 2017. Australian Demographic Statistics, Jun 2016. ABS cat. no. 3101.0. Canberra: ABS.
Australian Human Rights Commission (AHRC), 2015. Resilient individuals: sexual orientation, gender identity & intersex rights 2015. Sydney: AHRC.
Australian Institute of Health and Welfare (AIHW), 2018a. Older Australia at a glance. Canberra: AIHW.
Australian Institute of Health and Welfare (AIHW), 2018b. Alcohol and other drug treatment services in Australia 2016–17. Drug treatment services series no. 31. Cat. no. HSE 207. Canberra: AIHW.
Australian Institute of Health and Welfare (AIHW), 2017. National Drug Strategy Household Survey 2016: detailed findings. Drug statistics series no. 31. Cat. no. PHE 214. Canberra: AIHW.
Australian Medicines Handbook, 2019. Australian Medicines Handbook. Online. https://amhonline.amh.net.au/.
Balsamo, M., Cataldi, F., Carlucci, L., et al., 2018. Assessment of anxiety in older adults: a review of self-report measures. Clin. Interv. Aging 13, 573.
Beard, J.R., Officer, A.L., de Carvalho, I.A., et al., 2016. The World report on ageing and health: a policy framework for healthy ageing. Lancet 387 (10033), 2145–2154.
Beaunoyer, E., Landreville, P., Carmichael, P.H., 2019. Older adults' knowledge of anxiety disorders. J. Gerontol. B Psychol. Sci. Soc. Sci. 74 (5), 806–814.
Beishon, L.C., Batterham, A.P., Quinn, T.J., et al., 2019. Addenbrooke's Cognitive Examination III (ACE-III) and mini-ACE for the detection of dementia and mild cognitive impairment. Cochrane Database Syst. Rev. (12), CD013282, doi:10.1002/14651858.
Bektas, A., Schurman, S.H., Sen, R., et al., 2018. Aging, inflammation and the environment. Exp. Gerontol. 105, 10–18.
Beutel, M.E., Klein, E.M., Brähler, E., et al., 2017. Loneliness in the general population: prevalence, determinants and relations to mental health. BMC Psychiatry 17 (1), 97.
Borson, S., Scanlan, J.M., Watanabe, J., et al., 2005. Simplifying detection of cognitive impairment: comparison of the Mini-Cog and Mini-Mental State Examination in a multiethnic sample. J. Am. Geriatr. Soc. 53, 871–874.
Borson, S., Scanlan, J.M., Chen, P., et al., 2003. The Mini-Cog as a screen for dementia: validation in a population-based sample. J. Am. Geriatr. Soc. 51, 1451–1454.
Butler, R.N., 1969. Age-ism: another form of bigotry. Gerontologist 9 (4 Pt 1), 243–246.

Cai, L., Huang, J., 2018. Schizophrenia and risk of dementia: a meta-analysis study. Neuropsychiatr. Dis. Treat. 14, 2047.

Carew, A.M., Comiskey, C., 2018. Treatment for opioid use and outcomes in older adults: a systematic literature review. Drug Alcohol Depend. 182, 48–57.

Chen, L.J., Ku, P.W., Fox, K.R., 2018. Exercise for older people with mental illness. In: Stubbs, B., Rosenbaum, S. (Eds.), Exercise-Based Interventions for Mental Illness: Physical Activity as Part of Clinical Treatment. Academic Press, Cambridge, (Chapter 7).

Chesser, A.K., Keene Woods, N., Smothers, K., et al., 2016. Health literacy and older adults: a systematic review. Gerontol. Geriatr. Med. 2, 2333721416630492. doi:10.1177/2333721416630492.

Clarke, B.F.L., 1975. Mental Disorder in Earlier Britain: Exploratory Studies. University of Wales Press, Cardiff.

Coates, D., Saleeba, C., Howe, D., 2018. Mental health attitudes and beliefs in a community sample on the central coast in Australia: barriers to help seeking. Community Ment. Health J. 55 (3), 1–11.

Cohen, C.I., 2018. Very late-onset schizophrenia-like psychosis: positive findings but questions remain unanswered. Lancet Psychiatry 5 (7), 528–529.

Conejero, I., Olié, E., Courtet, P., et al., 2018. Suicide in older adults: current perspectives. Clin. Interv. Aging 13, 691.

Creighton, A., Davidson, T., Kissane, D., 2018. The assessment of anxiety in aged care residents: a systematic review of the psychometric properties of commonly used measures. Int. Psychogeriatr. 30 (7), 967–979.

Crocco, E.A., Jaramillo, S., Cruz-Ortiz, C., et al., 2017. Pharmacological management of anxiety disorders in the elderly. Curr. Treat. Options Psychiatry 4 (1), 33–46.

de Koning, E.J., Timmermans, E.J., van Schoor, N.M., et al., 2018. Within-person pain variability and mental health in older adults with osteoarthritis: an analysis across 6 European cohorts. J. Pain 19 (6), 690–698.

Deloitte Economics, 2017. Dementia Economic Impact Report 2016. Alzheimers New Zealand. https://www.alzheimers.org.nz/getmedia/79f7fd09-93fe-43b0-a837-771027bb23c0/Economic-Impacts-of-Dementia-2017.pdf.

Dementia Australia, 2018. Dementia Prevalence Data 2018-2058, commissioned research undertaken by NATSEM, University of Canberra, Canberra.

Dougherty, J.H., Cannon, R., Nicholas, C.R.N., et al., 2010. The computerized self-test (CST): an interactive, internet accessible cognitive screening test for dementia. J. Alzheimers Dis. 20, 185–195.

Drageset, J., Haugan, G., Tranvåg, O., 2017. Crucial aspects promoting meaning and purpose in life: perceptions of nursing home residents. BMC Geriatr. 17 (1), 254.

Folstein, M.F., Folstein, S.E., McHugh, P.R., 1975. Mini-Mental State: a practical method for grading the state of patients for the clinician. J. Psychiatr. Res. 12, 189–198.

Foulk, M.A., Ingersoll-Dayton, B., Kavangh, J., et al., 2014. Mindfulness-based cognitive therapy with older adults: an exploratory study. J. Gerontol. Soc. Work 57, 498–520.

Freter, S., Dunbar, M., Koller, K., et al., 2016. Prevalence and characteristics of pre-operative delirium in hip fracture patients. Gerontology 62, 396–400.

Friedman, E.M., Ruini, C., Foy, R., et al., 2017. Lighten UP! A community-based group intervention to promote psychological well-being in older adults. Aging Ment. Health 21 (2), 199–205.

Gaugler, J.E., Mittelman, M.S., Hepburn, K., et al., 2014. Identifying at-risk dementia caregivers following institutionalization. J. Appl. Gerontol. 33 (5), 624–646.

Gulpers, B., Ramakers, I., Hamel, R., et al., 2016. Anxiety as a predictor for cognitive decline and dementia: a systematic review and meta-analysis. Am. J. Geriatr. Psychiatry 24 (10), 823–842.

Haugan, G., Innstrand, S.T., Moksnes, U.K., 2013. The effect of nurse-patient interaction on anxiety and depression in cognitively intact nursing home patients. J. Clin. Nurs. 22 (15–16), 2192–2205.

Hegeman, J.M., de Waal, M.W., Comijis, H.C., et al., 2015. Depression in later life: a more somatic presentation? J. Affect. Disord. 170, 196–202.

Hellwig, S., Domschke, K., 2019. Anxiety in late life: an update on pathomechanisms. Gerontology, 65 (5), 465–473.

Hodkinson, H.M., 1972. Evaluation of a mental test score for assessment of mental impairment in the elderly. Age. Ageing 1 (4), 233–238.

Inouye, S.K., 2018. Delirium – a framework to improve acute care for older persons. J. Am. Geriatr. Soc. 66 (3), 446–451.

Inouye, S.K., van Dyck, C.H., Alessi, C.A., et al., 1990. Clarifying confusion: the confusion assessment method: a new method for detection of delirium. Ann. Intern. Med. 113 (12), 941–948.

Ismail, Z., Elbayoumi, H., Fischer, C.E., et al., 2017. Prevalence of depression in patients with mild cognitive impairment: a systematic review and meta-analysis. JAMA Psychiatry 74 (1), 58–67.

Iwagami, M., Mansfield, K.E., Hays, J.F., et al., 2018. Severe mental illness and chronic kidney disease: a cross-sectional study in the United Kingdom. Clin. Epidemiol. 10, 421.

Jayasekara, R., Procter, N., Harrison, J., et al., 2015. Cognitive behavioural therapy for older adults with depression: a review. J. Ment. Health 24, 168–171.

Julien, C.L., Rimes, K.A., Brown, R.G., 2016. Rumination and behavioural factors in Parkinson's disease depression. J. Psychosom. Res. 82, 48–53.

Kaup, A.R., Byers, A.L., Falvey, C., 2016. Trajectories of depressive symptoms in older adults and risk of dementia. JAMA Psychiatry 73 (5), 525–531.

Kenbubpha, K., Higgins, I., Wilson, A., et al., 2019. Psychogeriatrics, testing psychometric properties of a new instrument 'Promoting Active Ageing in Older People with Mental Disorders Scale' from a cross-sectional study. Psychogeriatrics 19 (4), 370–383.

Khachiyants, N., Trinkle, D., Son, S.J., et al., 2011. Sundown syndrome in persons with dementia: an update. Psychiatry Investig. 8, 275–287.

Kitching, D., 2015. Depression in dementia. Aust. Prescr. 38, 209–211.

Kjosavik, S.R., Gillam, M.H., Roughead, E.E., 2017. Average duration of treatment with antipsychotics among concession card holders in Australia. Aust. N. Z. J. Psychiatry 51 (7), 719–726.

Kok, R.M., Reynolds, C.F., 2017. Management of depression in older adults: a review. JAMA 317 (20), 2114–2122.

Komalasari, R., Chang, H.C., Traynor, V., 2019. A review of the Rowland Universal Dementia Assessment Scale. Dementia 18 (7–8), 3143–3158.

Koppara, A., Wagner, M., Lange, C., et al., 2015. Cognitive performance before and after the onset of subjective cognitive decline in old age. Alzheimers Dement. (Amst.) 1 (2), 194–205.

Kostadinov, V., Roche, A., 2017. Bongs and baby boomers: trends in cannabis use among older Australians. Australas. J. Ageing 36 (1), 56–59.

Kurita, K., Reid, M.C., Siegler, E.L., et al., 2018. Associations between mild cognitive dysfunction and end-of-life outcomes in patients with advanced cancer. J. Palliat. Med. 21 (4), 536–540.

Laborde-Lahoz, P., El-Gabalawy, R., Kinley, J., et al., 2014. Subsyndromal depression among older adults in the USA: prevalence, comorbidity, and risk for new-onset psychiatric disorders in late life. Int. J. Geriatr. Psychiatry 30 (7), 677–685.

Lavan, A.H., Gallagher, P.F., O'Mahony, D., 2016. Methods to reduce prescribing errors in elderly patients with multimorbidity. Clin. Interv. Aging 11, 857.

Lavrencic, L.M., Richardson, C., Harrison, S.L., et al., 2018. Is there a linke between cognitive reserve and cognitive function in the oldest-old? J. Gerontol. A Biol. Sci. Med. Sci. 73 (4), 499–505.

Lee, M., Kim, T., Ahn, S., et al., 2017. Effectiveness of antipsychotics on delirium in elderly patients. J. Psychiatry 20, 4.

Lennox, A., Braaf, S., Smit, D.V., et al., 2019. Caring for older patients in the emergency department: health professionals' perspectives from Australia – the Safe Elderly Emergency Discharge project. Emerg. Med. Australas. 31 (1), 83–89.

Liguori, I., Russo, G., Curcio, F., et al., 2018. Depression and chronic heart failure in the elderly: an intriguing relationship. J. Geriatr. Cardiol. 15 (6), 451.

Liu, T.W., Ng, G.Y., Chung, R.C., et al., 2018. Cognitive behavioural therapy for fear of falling and balance among older people: a systematic review and meta-analysis. Age. Ageing 47 (4), 520–527.

LoGiudice, D., Strivens, E., Smith, K., et al., 2010. The KICA screen: the psychometric properties of a shortened version of the KICA (Kimberley Indigenous Cognitive Assessment). Australas. J. Ageing 30, 215–219. https://doi.org/10.1111/j.1741-6612.2010.00486.x.

Lyons, A., Alba, B., Heywood, W., et al., 2018. Experiences of ageism and the mental health of older adults. Aging Ment. Health 22 (11), 1456–1464.

Macfarlane, S., O'Connor, D., 2016. Managing behavioural and psychological symptoms in dementia. Aust. Prescr. 39 (4), 123–125.

Meneilly, G.S., Knip, A., Miller, D.B., et al., 2018. Diabetes in older people. Can. J. Diabetes 42, S283–S295.

Milian, M., Leiherr, A.M., Straten, G., et al., 2012. The Mini-Cog versus the Mini-Mental State Examination and the Clock Drawing Test in daily clinical practice: screening and value in a German memory clinical. Int. Psychogeriatr. 24 (5), 766–774.

Molloy, D.W., Standish, T.I., 1997. A guide to the standardized Mini-Mental State Examination. Int. Psychogeriatr. 9 (S1), 87–94.

Moyle, W., 2014. Evidence-based nursing interventions: fostering quality of life. In: Moyle, W., Parker, D., Bramble, M. (Eds.), Care of Older Adults: A Strengths-Based Approach. Cambridge University Press, Sydney.

Moyle, W., Cooke, M., Beattie, E., et al., 2013a. Foot massage versus quiet presence on agitation and mood in people with dementia: a randomized controlled trial. Int. J. Nurs. Stud. 51, 856–864.

Moyle, W., Cooke, M., Beattie, E., et al., 2013b. Exploring the effect of companion robots on emotional expression in older people with dementia: a pilot RCT. J. Gerontol. Nurs. 39, 46–53.

Musich, S., Wang, S.S., Slindee, L., et al., 2019. Prevalence and characteristics associated with high dose opioid users among older adults. Geriatr. Nurs. (Minneap) 40 (1), 31–36.

Prince, M.J., Wu, F., Guo, Y., et al., 2015. The burden of disease in older people and implications for healthy policy and practice. Lancet 385 (9967), 549–562.

Procter, N.G., 2016. Person-centred care for people of refugee background. J. Pharm. Pract. Res. https://doi.org/10.1002/jppr.1222.

Radford, K., Mack, H.A., Draper, B., et al., 2015. Prevalence of dementia in urban and regional Aboriginal Australians. Alzheimers Dement. 11, 271–279.

Rakusa, M., Jensterle, J., Mlakar, J., 2018. Clock drawing test: a simple scoring system for the accurate screening of cognitive impairment in patients with mild cognitive impairment and dementia. Dement. Geriatr. Cogn. Disord. 45 (5–6), 326–334.

Ramesh, S., Zalucky, A., Hemmelgarn, B.R., et al., 2016. Incidence of sudden cardiac death in adults with end-stage renal disease: a systematic review and meta-analysis. BMC Nephrol. 17 (1), 78.

Rao, R., Roche, A., 2017. Substance misuse in older people. BMJ 2017, 358. https://doi.org/10.1136/bmj.j3885.

Rush, K.L., Hickey, S., Epp, S., et al., 2017. Nurses' attitudes towards older people care: an integrative review. J. Clin. Nurs. 26 (23–24), 4105–4116.

Santini, Z.I., Koyanagi, A., Tyrovolas, S., et al., 2015. The association of relationship quality and social networks with depression, anxiety, and suicidal ideation among older married adults: findings from a cross-sectional analysis of the Irish Longitudinal Study on Ageing (TILDA). J. Affect. Disord. 179, 134–141.

Scales, K., Zimmerman, S., Miller, S.J., 2018. Evidence-based nonpharmacological practices to address

behavioral and psychological symptoms of dementia. Gerontologist 58 (Suppl. 1), S88–S102.
Scott, K.M., Lim, C., Al-Hamzawi, A., et al., 2016. Association of mental disorders with subsequent chronic physical conditions: world mental health surveys from 17 countries. JAMA Psychiatry 73 (2), 150–158.
Seitz, D.P., Chan, C.C., Newton, H.T., et al., 2018. Mini-Cog for the diagnosis of Alzheimer's disease dementia and other dementias within a primary care setting. Cochrane Database Syst. Rev. (2), CD011415, doi:10.1002/14651858.CD011415.pub2.
Sheikh, J.I., Yesavage, J.A., 1986. Geriatric Depression Scale (GDS): recent evidence and development of a shorter version. Clin. Gerontol. 5 (1–2), 165–173.
Snowdon, J., 2010. Depression in nursing homes. Int. Psychogeriatr. 22 (7), 1143–1148.
Spitzer, R.L., Williams, J.B.W., Kroenke, K., et al., 1994. Utility of a new procedure for diagnosing mental disorders in primary care: the PRIME-MD 1000 study. JAMA 272, 1749–1756.
Statistics New Zealand, 2018. Projections Produced by Statistics New Zealand According to Assumptions Specified by the Ministry of Health – 2018 Update. Ministry of Health, Wellington.
Storey, J., Rowland, J., Basic, D., et al., 2004. The Rowland Universal Dementia Assessment Scale (RUDAS): a multicultural cognitive assessment scale. Int. Psychogeriatr. 16 (1), 13–31.
Talley, N.J., Jones, S., 2018. Clinical Examination: A Guide to Specialty Examinations, vol. 2, eighth ed. Elsevier, Sydney, pp. 826–833.
Te Pou o te Whakaaro Nui, 2019. Working with older people: Mental health and addiction workforce development priorities. Auckland: Te Pou o te Whakaaro Nui.
The Royal Australian College of General Practitioners, 2016. General practice management of type 2 diabetes: 2016–18. East Melbourne: RACGP.
van der Veen, D.C., van Zelst, W.H., Schoevers, R.A., et al., 2015. Comorbid anxiety disorders in late-life depression: results of a cohort study. Int. Psychogeriatr. 27, 1157–1165.
van Orden, K., Deming, C., 2018. Late-life suicide prevention strategies: current status and future directions. Curr. Opin. Psychol. 22, 79–83.
Volkert, J., Schulz, H., Härter, M., et al., 2012. The prevalence of mental disorders in older people in Western countries – a meta-analysis. Ageing Res. Rev. 12 (1), 339–353.
Volz, M., Möbus, J., Letsch, C., et al., 2016. The influence of early depressive symptoms, social support and decreasing self-efficacy on depression 6 months post-stroke. J. Affect. Disord. 206, 252–255.
Wagner, E., 2014. The chronic care model and integrated care. [Video file]. Available from https://www.youtube.com/watch?v=K-z6HjRkKSc.
Wallis, K.A., Elley, C.R., Lee, A., et al., 2018. Safer Prescribing and Care for the Elderly (SPACE): protocol of a cluster randomized controlled trial in primary care. JMIR Res. Protoc. 7 (4).
Walton, M., 2013. Deep sleep therapy and Chelmsford Private Hospital: have we learnt anything? Australas. Psychiatry 21 (3), 206–212.
Westaway, K., Sluggett, J., Alderman, C., et al., 2018. The extent of antipsychotic use in Australian residential aged care facilities and interventions shown to be effective in reducing antipsychotic use: a literature review. Dementia doi:10.1177/1471301218795792. [Epub ahead of print]; 1471301218795792.
Westbury, J., Gee, P., Ling, T., et al., 2018. More action needed: psychotropic prescribing in Australian residential aged care. Aust. N. Z. J. Psychiatry 53 (2), 136–147.
Wilkinson, P., 2013. Cognitive behavioural therapy with older people. Maturitas 76 (1), 5–9.
Wilson, D.M., 2019. Where are we now in relation to determining the prevalence of ageism in this era of escalating population ageing? Ageing Res. Rev. 51, 78–84.
World Health Organization, 2016. Health Impact Assessment (HIA) – The Determinants of Health [Internet]. WHO, Geneva. Available from: http://www.who.int/hia/evidence/doh/en/.
World Health Organization, 2013. Mental Health Action Plan 2013–2020. WHO, Geneva. Available from: https://www.who.int/mental_health/publications/action_plan/en/.
Yesavage, J.A., Brink, T.L., Rose, T.L., 1983. Development and validation of a geriatric depression rating scale: a preliminary report. J. Psychiatr. Res. 17, 27.
Yohannes, A.M., Chen, W., Moga, A.M., et al., 2017. Cognitive impairment in chronic obstructive pulmonary disease and chronic heart failure: a systematic review and meta-analysis of observational studies. J. Am. Med. Dir. Assoc. 18 (5), 451-e1.
Zhang, X., Norton, J., Carriere, I., et al., 2015. Generalized anxiety in community-dwelling elderly: prevalence and clinical characteristics. J. Affect. Disord. 172, 24–29.
Zhao, X., Zhang, D., Wu, M., et al., 2018. Loneliness and depression symptoms among the elderly in nursing homes: a moderated mediation model of resilience and social support. Psychiatry Res. 268, 143–151.

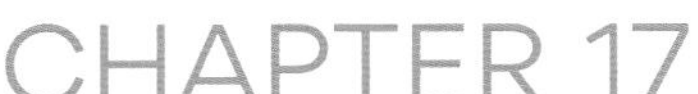

Autism and intellectual disability

Andrew Cashin

KEY POINTS

- Person-centred care necessitates a conscious effort to understand how the person at the centre of care thinks and processes information.
- Autism encompasses a different style of thinking and information processing to that experienced by neurotypical thinkers.
- Intellectual disability relates to the volume of information that can be handled at any one time, the speed of processing this information and the associated functional impairment.
- Assessment and intervention needs to be adjusted to be meaningful for people with autism spectrum disorder and intellectual disability.

KEY TERMS

- Ability versus disability
- Autism and intellectual
- Diagnosis and difference
- Neurotypical thinking
- Nursing and difference
- Information processing

LEARNING OUTCOMES

The material in this chapter will assist you to:

- understand the thinking and information-processing styles that characterise autism spectrum disorder and intellectual disability
- distinguish between neurotypical thinking and the differences experienced by those with autism spectrum disorder and intellectual disability
- identify what is meant by diagnostic overshadowing and appreciate the impact of this phenomena on health outcomes for people with disability
- design adjustments to mental health nursing interventions to be used with people with autism spectrum disorder and intellectual disability to promote better and more equitable health outcomes.

Introduction

Understanding how people think and process information is essential for mental health nurses. This understanding includes what are transitory changes in thinking related to the symptoms of a mental illness, such as that experienced in psychosis, and what are permanent traits that result from a developmental process. This chapter contains essential knowledge to progress the development of this understanding.

Person-first language will be used in this chapter in full acknowledgement that it is understood that people are not defined by an illness or disability. This approach is consistent with person-centred nursing, a concept embedded in nursing standards in Australia and New Zealand (Cashin et al. 2017, Nursing Council of New Zealand 2016). However, it is acknowledged that, in the context of autism, this use of language is contested by proponents of identity-based language. In the case of identity-based language it is conceptualised that a trait may define who a person is. If we were to adopt identity-based language, as an example, in place of referring to a person with autism, we would refer to the person as autistic. In practice it is important as part of person-centred care to identify how the person you are working with understands what is going on for them and to identify if they have a preference of identifying language and what it is (Shakes & Cashin 2018).

Autism and intellectual disability are conceptualised as spectrums. For autism this is represented in the diagnostic nomenclature of autism spectrum disorder (ASD). For intellectual disability the spectrum is signified in the diagnostic nomenclature of the level of disability that ranges from mild to severe. The diagnostic classifications in both the *Diagnostic and Statistical Manual of Mental Disorders,* 5th edition (DSM-5) (American Psychiatric Association 2013) and the *International Classifications of Disease* (ICD) will be explored in the discussion of the types of disorder.

Autism represents a fundamental difference in thinking and information processing that results from a developmental process. In the world there are two recognised styles of thinking and information processing. One is autism, and the second, far more common style, is typical thinking (Cashin & Barker 2009). The term used to describe those with a typical thinking style is commonly accepted to be 'neurotypical'. Thinking differences that underpin behaviours recognised as difference in people with ASD include impaired abstraction (the ability to recognise like and similar as opposed to concrete black and white), impaired linguistic processing with a relative strength in visual processing and impaired theory of mind (the awareness that people all have minds and these minds are particular to individuals with the ability to put oneself figuratively in another person's shoes and guess what they are thinking and feeling) (Cashin et al. 2012). The impact of these differences is significant and tends to compound, resulting in a lack of formation of a unified base of knowledge about the world, a central characteristic of neurotypical thinking. While thinking changes are a frequent symptom of mental illness, they are often transitory in the form of psychotic phenomena. At times people become stuck in such thinking patterns for long periods and people refer to such things as fixed thinking or chronicity; however, these changes became superimposed on what was originally a typical thinking style.

At this point an astute reader may wonder about the negative or deficit symptoms of schizophrenia. Negative symptoms commonly include decreased emotional expression and decreased abstraction. Similar to that experienced in ASD, there is often impaired theory of mind and executive functioning (Nylander et al. 2008). Such an example brings to our attention that boundaries between disorders are artificial constructions as we attempt to linguistically construct our world and demarcate understanding (Cashin 2016). Boundaries are fluid and will change as our understanding of the brain and genetics improve.

In contrast to ASD, intellectual disability does not represent a different thinking style but rather a difference in the speed of processing within a person's thinking style and a difference in the volume of information that can be handled at any point in time. While intellectual disability is comorbidly experienced in a larger proportion of people who also have ASD, as compared to neurotypical thinkers, overall it is still experienced by the minority in that population (Cashin & Yorke 2016).

With the incidence of approximately 1% of the population having ASD and approximately 1% overall having an intellectual disability (American Psychiatric Association 2013), all nurses will at some time care for someone with these disabilities, even in generalist services. Working with people with ASD and with people with intellectual disability is a specialty area of practice. An emerging and even more specialised area of practice is work in specialty services that support care for people with ASD and/or intellectual disability and comorbid mental illness. These services do not yet exist in a way to meet the required demand and are not evenly geographically spread.

Types of disorder

Autism spectrum disorder

ASD is the current diagnostic entity for autism and encompasses the diagnoses previously used colloquially and in the DSM and ICD. The diagnostic entities used in versions of the DSM up to DSM-5 of autistic disorder, Asperger's disorder and pervasive developmental disorder not otherwise specified have now been encompassed by the term 'autism spectrum disorder'. In the ICD, atypical autism was used as an equivalent descriptor to pervasive development disorder not otherwise specified that appeared in the DSM. Both terms were frequently employed to denote a sub-threshold diagnosis and less frequently to diagnose someone where symptoms were not recognised until later in life.

High-functioning autism was never a DSM diagnosis but a colloquial term at times employed by people to signify ASD without a comorbid intellectual disability. At an earlier phase of understanding autism, some people used it to denote ASD without impairment of speech (note this is the function of speech not a judgement on communication). While some people still use this term, it is incorrect. To correctly describe the comorbid presence of intellectual disability or language impairment it should be stated as a comorbidity and the level and type of disability described.

The multitude of terms that have now been collapsed into recognising the spectrum nature of ASD evolved based on the neurotypical thinking trait of needing to name things, followed by the need to define the level or to answer the question of how much of the thing is present. In terms of disability this often takes the form of a quest to determine if the disability is mild, moderate or severe. In ASD, severity levels have been incorporated into the DSM-5 to accommodate this need. However, there are caveats around the levels based on full acknowledgement that the frequency and intensity of the characteristic behaviours of ASD will fluctuate based on mediating factors such as anxiety; that is, severity levels are not consistent for a person and will go up and down depending on context. A person with ASD in a very social and unfamiliar environment, as an example, would potentially meet the criteria for a higher severity rating than when in a more familiar and less socially demanding space. Hence transition periods often see a sustained, albeit not permanent, increase in severity ratings.

The ICD 11 and DSM-5 classifications have converged and are more closely aligned than ever before. Both classifications conceptualise autism as based on a dyad of impairment. The two underpinning domains are impaired social communication and the presence of restrictive and repetitive interests, activities and behaviours. This dyad replaces the earlier triad of impairment that underpinned classification symptoms. Previously autism was conceptualised as being underpinned by impairment in the domains of communication, social skills and behavioural flexibility. It became clear that the separation of communication and social skills was redundant and so the two areas were collapsed into 'impaired social communication'.

The DSM-5 diagnostic criteria is presented in Box 17.1.

ASD is a behavioural diagnosis as can be seen from the criteria used to diagnose it. There are no physical tests that can be used to diagnose or confirm the diagnosis of ASD. The behaviours, it has come to be recognised, are the outward expression of difference in thinking and information processing. Just like the previously conceptualised triad of behavioural impairment, there is a triad of thinking impairments or difference represented by the diagnosis of ASD. These impairments are impaired abstraction, impaired theory of mind and impaired linguistic processing (having a relative strength in visual processing). Understanding these differences are key to successfully working with a person with autism. This includes work at the assessment phase and the intervention/support phase. The thinking differences will be discussed further under the heading signs and symptoms.

Intellectual disability

Intellectual disability (intellectual developmental disorder) is the diagnostic nomenclature used in the DSM-5 (American Psychiatric Association 2013). The ICD 11 uses the term 'disorders of intellectual development', a shift from mental retardation, the terminology used in earlier editions (Girimaji & Pradeep 2018). The shifting terminology again reflects evolution in understanding difference and in this case the developmental aspect of intellectual development.

In Australia and New Zealand, the terminology 'intellectual disability' is commonly used. In the United States 'developmental disability' is most commonly used, and in the United Kingdom 'learning disability' is the preferred nomenclature (Burghardt 2018). Just as 'mental retardation' is now exiting as a term from the diagnostic vernacular, earlier nomenclature used terms such as 'idiocy', 'mental deficiency', 'moron' and 'imbecile' that are now out of use. When reflecting on community attitudes to intellectual disability it is important to note that these terms have been incorporated as slurs in everyday language use. One point of accessible self-reflection is to consider whether and when you use these terms, and whether it reflects a position on individual value of people with intellectual disability?

In both the DSM and ICD intelligence or intellect is now represented as more than that which can be represented by an intelligence quotient (IQ) test alone. Intelligence includes the capability to demonstrate functioning through adaptive behaviour (Girimaji & Pradeep 2018). This situates clinical assessment as an important element of the diagnostic practice alongside the use of standardised tests. Intellectual disability is a disorder therefore in which deficits are assessed to occur through IQ testing and assessment of adaptive functioning across the domains of conceptual, social and practical application (DSM-5).

Intellectual disability is the opposite to ASD in our evolution of understanding. In intellectual disability the original focus was thinking alone, and this has now extended to the acceptance of the need to look at behaviours in the form of adaptive functioning. In ASD the understanding first evolved in understanding the triad of impaired behaviours and then moved to the underlying thinking and information processing differences. For the DSM-5 diagnostic criteria see Box 17.2.

Box 17.1 Autism spectrum disorder diagnostic criteria 299.00 (F84.0)

Persistent deficits in social communication and social interaction across multiple contexts, as manifested by all the following, currently or by history (examples are illustrative, not exhaustive):

- deficits in social–emotional reciprocity, ranging, for example, from abnormal social approach and failure of normal back-and-forth conversation, to reduced sharing of interests, emotions or affect, to failure to initiate or respond to social interactions
- deficits in non-verbal communicative behaviours used for social interaction, ranging, for example, from poorly integrated verbal and non-verbal communication, to abnormalities in eye contact and body language or deficits in understanding and use of gestures, to a total lack of facial expressions and non-verbal communication
- deficits in developing, maintaining, and understanding relationships, ranging, for example, from difficulties adjusting behaviour to suit various social contexts; to difficulties in sharing imaginative play or in making friends; to absence of interest in peers.

SPECIFY CURRENT SEVERITY:

Severity is based on social communication impairments and restricted, repetitive patterns of behaviour.

Restricted, repetitive patterns of behaviour, interests, or activities, as manifested by at least two of the following, currently or by history (examples are illustrative, not exhaustive:

- stereotyped or repetitive motor movements, use of objects or speech (e.g. simple motor stereotypies, lining up toys or flipping objects, echolalia, idiosyncratic phrases)
- insistence on sameness, inflexible adherence to routines, or ritualised patterns of verbal or non-verbal behaviour (e.g. extreme distress at small changes, difficulties with transitions, rigid thinking patterns, greeting rituals, need to take the same route or eat the same food every day)
- highly restricted, fixated interests that are abnormal in intensity or focus (e.g. strong attachment to or preoccupation with unusual objects, excessively circumscribed or perseverative interests)
- hyper- or hyporeactivity to sensory input or unusual interest in sensory aspects of the environment (e.g. apparent indifference to pain/temperature, adverse response to specific sounds or textures, excessive smelling or touching of objects, visual fascination with lights or movement).

SPECIFY CURRENT SEVERITY:

Severity is based on social communication impairments and restricted, repetitive patterns of behaviour.

Symptoms must be present in the early developmental period (but may not become fully manifest until social demands exceed limited capacities or may be masked by learned strategies in later life).

Symptoms cause clinically significant impairment in social, occupational or other important areas of current functioning.

These disturbances are not better explained by intellectual disability (intellectual developmental disorder) or global developmental delay. Intellectual disability and ASD frequently co-occur; to make comorbid diagnoses of ASD and intellectual disability, social communication should be below that expected for general developmental level.

Note: Individuals with a well-established DSM-IV diagnosis of autistic disorder, Asperger's disorder or pervasive developmental disorder not otherwise specified should be given the diagnosis of ASD. Individuals who have marked deficits in social communication, but whose symptoms do not otherwise meet criteria for ASD, should be evaluated for social (pragmatic) communication disorder.

Specify if:

- with or without accompanying intellectual impairment
- with or without accompanying language impairment
- associated with a known medical or genetic condition or environmental factor
- associated with another neurodevelopmental, mental or behavioural disorder
- with catatonia (refer to the criteria for catatonia associated with another mental disorder, pp. 119–120 of DSM-5, for the definition).

Adapted from American Psychiatric Association 2013

Historical anecdote 17.1: Autism

The term autism can be traced back to the work of Eugene Bleuler, who as early as 1910 described autism as a symptom of schizophrenia involving an inability to distinguish internal fantasy from reality. Later in 1943 American child psychiatrist Leo Kanner described autism in children as being distinguished by an inability to relate self towards other people and the world from the beginning of life he described an 'extreme autistic aloneness that whenever possible disregards, ignores, shuts out anything that comes to the child from the outside' (Kanner 1943). In 1944, and with no knowledge from Kanner's work, paediatrician Hans Asperger published a paper describing similar types of children in Vienna. He observed children who had high intelligence and creativity but often experienced learning difficulties. They would habitually avoid eye contact and did not speak in a way that was attuned to their listener but aimed into the distance. Initially unacclaimed, Asperger's work later become well known and lead to the naming of the condition known as Asperger's syndrome. The name of this disorder has been challenged in recent times due to the unearthing of historical documents that revealed Hans Asperger was heavily involved in Nazi eugenics. Further to this, and with greater understanding, it has become clear that the main distinguishing factor between what came to be seen as autistic disorder and Asperger's disorder was the presence of comorbid intellectual disability and both disorders referred to the same thing, so the terms have been collapsed into ASD.

Read more about it: *Feinstein A 2011 A history of autism: conversations with the pioneers.John Wiley & Sons, West Sussex*

Box 17.2 Diagnostic criteria

Intellectual disability (intellectual developmental disorder) is a disorder with onset during the developmental period that includes both intellectual and adaptive functioning deficits in conceptual, social and practical domains. The following three criteria must be met:

- deficits in intellectual functions, such as reasoning, problem solving, planning, abstract thinking, judgement, academic learning and learning from experience, confirmed by both clinical assessment and individualised, standardised intelligence testing
- deficits in adaptive functioning that result in failure to meet developmental and sociocultural standards for personal independence and social responsibility (without ongoing support, the adaptive deficits limit functioning in one or more activities of daily life, such as communication, social participation or independent living, across multiple environments such as home, school, work and community)
- onset of intellectual and adaptive deficits during the developmental period.

Note: The diagnostic term 'intellectual disability' is the equivalent term for the ICD-11 diagnosis of 'intellectual developmental disorders'. Although the term 'intellectual disability' is used throughout this manual, both terms are used in the title to clarify relationships with other classification systems. Moreover, a federal statute in the United States (Public Law 111-256, Rosa's Law) replaces the term 'mental retardation' with 'intellectual disability', and research journals use the term 'intellectual disability'. Thus, 'intellectual disability' is the term in common use by medical, educational and other professions and by the lay public and advocacy groups.

Specify current severity:

- 317 (F70) Mild
- 318.0 (F71) Moderate
- 318.1 (F72) Severe
- 318.2 (F73) Profound.

The various levels of severity are defined based on adaptive functioning and not IQ scores because it is adaptive functioning that determines the level of supports required. Moreover, IQ measures are less valid in the lower end of the IQ range.

NURSE'S STORY 17.1

Toby

Michael, aged 25 years, had his first mental health admission when he was 15 years old. The admission was linked to concerns about anxiety and that he had been physically harassing girls at his high school. In addition to having an anxiety disorder diagnosed, a psychometric evaluation revealed that Michael had an intellectual disability. Due to a long history of preadmission difficulties at school he was subsequently transferred to a special needs high school. Despite the best efforts of his teachers, whenever he became excited during his senior years at high school Michael had a tendency to get into trouble because he would stand very close to females and sometimes touch them inappropriately, becoming demanding and irritable when told to provide space. Female teachers and students were warned that he was potentially dangerous and that they should not get too close to him. A common term used to describe Michael's behaviour was 'predatory'. Because of this he experienced very little physical human contact and did not get to attend school excursions or co-ed events unless there were male staff members present. After finishing high school aged 18, Michael started on a Disability Support Pension and became increasingly socially isolated. He spent all his time with his mother at home, who also had an intellectual disability, where they engaged in hoarding behaviour, collecting rubbish from their local neighbourhood and storing it at home.

My work with Michael began following complaints to the local council about his family's hoarding behaviour. After a general practitioner review, I began providing regular consultations with Michael, which were often also attended by his mother as a support person. Following a full case review of his history of care, what came to light was that although he was constantly told his behaviour was inappropriate during high school, the school had made little headway in helping Michael to understand what 'appropriate behaviour' was. The focus of my treatment from that point on was exploring Michael's interpretation of his world, understanding it from a developmental perspective in that Michael had not really advanced past junior 'adolescent type' behaviour in the way he related to females and how he interpreted personal space.

When alone with his mother and engaged in routine, his anxiety remained low and his behaviour was relatively predictable. But if he visited a shopping centre or used public transport his mood could quickly become elevated and he then tended to start invading the personal space of nearby females. My work with him had a strong educational flavour, using graded exposure to teach about personal space and about what was acceptable and non-acceptable social behaviour in public spaces (e.g. shaking hands, not hugging or touching others unless they gave him permission). This was combined with work to promote recognition of contexts in which his anxiety was his high and symptoms that suggest anxiety levels are rising. Although it took a couple of years of regular consultations, with repetition, which was helpfully supported and reinforced by his mother, Michael eventually learned the concept of personal boundaries. He became very proud of himself, enjoying the positive responses he got from people. He became better at regulating his behaviour in unpredictable and anxiety-provoking environments. Michael's mother has since passed away and he now lives in a group home where he receives daily support and works on a production line at a local factory. I have seen him a couple of times since our meetings ended and on each occasion he proudly shook my hand.

Prevalence

The prevalence of ASD globally in the general population is reported to be 1% in children and adult populations (American Psychiatric Association 2013). Reported prevalence rates in studies vary greatly depending on whether the study is retrospective or prospective in design.

Prevalence of intellectual disability in the general population is approximately 1%, with the percentage varying by age and severity rating (American Psychiatric Association 2013).

The prevalence of people with ASD having comorbid intellectual disability is estimated to range from 20% (Croen et al. 2015) to 40% (Van Naarden Braun et al. 2015). The variance is based, as in the studies determining prevalence, on the design of the studies.

Contributing factors

AUTISM SPECTRUM DISORDER

Causation of ASD has been discussed from a variety of viewpoints across time. We have come to know more clearly what does not cause ASD through the process than to understanding the cause.

Parenting as a causative factor was an early point of consideration progressing from Leo Kanner's observation of a cold and uncaring parenting style in the sample he reported on, to the coining of the term 'refrigerator mother' by Bruno Bettleheim (Bettleheim 1990; Kanner 1943). Bettleheim based his theory on the observation that children with autism shared many characteristics with prisoners he had observed in World War II concentration camps. These factors he attributed to the guards' cold and uncaring behaviours in the camps and projected this onto parental behaviours in the context of parenting children with autism. This psychogenic theory eventually dissipated, as research demonstrated no relationship between parenting style and causation of ASD.

There was a long debate on the link with the measles, mumps rubella vaccination and the role of the preservative thimerosal in the vaccine; however, this has not been supported by any evidence despite several large-scale commissions to examine it. The early work of the scientist who proposed this link has now been discredited and withdrawn.

The notion of neurodiversity has been put forward to challenge the logic of the idea of searching for causation. The neurodiversity movement promotes the concept that ASD is not a pathology with a cause but part of the diversity of humanity (Shakes & Cashin 2018). This discourse, while making some strong points, does suffer from an internal inconsistency in that an entitlement for support is championed, yet parallels are drawn with previous social movements related to race, colour and sexual preference, areas of obvious diversity that are not conceptualised as including the need for support in adaptive functioning and comprehension.

The emergence of the strong suspicion of genetic difference, represented by partial dislocation identified on many genes in people with ASD, and the heritability of ASD in that prevalence is higher among biological siblings than the general population, supported suspicions that ASD as a developmental disorder developed in utero and was present at birth as part of the different way of thinking and processing information. As early as 2001 changes had been identified in people with ASD on all chromosomes excepting 14 and 20 (Committee on Children with Disabilities 2001). There is increased prevalence of ASD in groups of people with other genetic conditions, suggesting some shared liability. At this point we are left without known causation of ASD. There is a strong suspicion that ASD as a spectrum disorder is heterogeneous by nature and, as technology develops, what we now cluster under the umbrella of ASD may have different causative trajectories.

INTELLECTUAL DISABILITY

Prenatal, perinatal and postnatal factors have been associated with developing intellectual disability (American Psychiatric Association 2013). Examples of prenatal factors that affect development include genetic syndromes, environmental factors (e.g. toxins and maternal alcohol consumption), maternal illness (e.g. blood-borne viruses and placental disorders) and structural differences/ abnormality in the physical development of the brain. Examples of perinatal factors include delivery-related incidents and development of acute inflammation of the brain. Postnatal factors may include a wide variety of traumas originating from physical injury, infections, syndromes and situations that impair oxygen supply in the brain (American Psychiatric Association 2013).

In addition to the examples described above, extreme social deprivation has been associated with developing intellectual disability. While the potential causes are many, it must be emphasised that in many cases no cause can be identified.

The experience of inclusion and exclusion

One unifying element in the discourse related to the experience of both ASD and intellectual disability is that of inclusion and a sense of community belonging (Robinson 2013). Society could be described 'a large group of people who live together in an organized way, making decisions about how to do things and sharing the work that needs to be done' (Cambridge English Dictionary 2020). Around the world, societies are mediated by a complex mix of implicit and explicit rules as elements of governance. The rules determine what is acceptable both in behavioural performance of societal tasks and routines and also in the process of social mediation.

Belonging in society is determined through participating in activities designed to promote thriving. Participation is predicated on the ability to comprehend both the explicit and implicit rules and to participate in the social mediation. While often taken for granted, the underpinning abilities required to meet these demands are many and complex.

In ASD the core features of impaired social communication and impaired behavioural flexibility, manifested as restrictive and repetitive behaviour, represent challenges. The abilities of those with ASD in many cases do not align with those complex abilities identified and needed for active participation, and so the deficit in the required abilities, by definition, become a disability.

The challenge in intellectual disability is that of being able to handle the volumes of information needed to navigate participation and to have the necessary processing speed to manage the information in a timely manner. The social mediation occurs in real time and requires a multitude of on-the-spot decisions.

Signs and symptoms

It is useful to discuss the signs and symptoms of ASD and intellectual disability to understand how they shape the requirements needed for adjustments in the mental health assessment and in intervention strategies. Developing capability in assessing the mental health of people with ASD and intellectual disability is essential for mental health nurses, as not only do people with ASD and intellectual disability each represent approximately 1% of the population (American Psychiatric Association 2013) but, as population groups, they both have a disproportionate prevalence of mental ill health and mental illness.

Autism spectrum disorder

Earlier in the chapter the behavioural dyad of impairment and the underpinning thinking and information-processing triad of impairment was discussed. In this section the signs and symptoms as manifested in thinking and information processing, and the subsequent behaviour, will be unpacked further. These differences are the characteristic signs and symptoms of ASD.

The thinking and information-processing impairments of ASD are inherent traits. As we discovered in the historical evolution of our understanding of ASD, and our passage through psychogenic theory in which parenting was the focus, we have come to know that the traits are not learned, and that a new way of thinking cannot be taught. They are gifts, as in the great gift of abstraction, first identified by Aristotle. The differences are most likely linked to genetically mediated differences that affect brain structure and function, although these differences have not yet been conclusively identified. The differences in thinking and information processing are impaired abstraction, impaired theory of mind and impaired linguistic processing of information (with a relative strength in visual processing).

Abstraction is the gift that allows us to recognise like and similar and gradients of things. An impairment in abstraction manifests as the black-and-white thinking characteristic of people with ASD. Impaired abstraction makes understanding homonyms extremely difficult, such as understanding the difference between a tear in your eye and a tear in your pants. As an interesting exercise, think about a fluffy white cat and a small fluffy white dog. Then, without relying on the abstract notion of 'catness' and 'dogness', describe each on a piece of paper and see if you can identify the difference. While subtle, abstraction is the core unifying element in neurotypical thinking. It provides the glue, or central coherence. The gift of abstraction is the basis of generalisation.

Theory of mind is the gift that allows neurotypical thinkers to know that every person has a mind, that each mind is unique and hence different from each other. The ability to make a guess of what other people are thinking, using context and a self-referential process, is central to neurotypical thought. This is the process of imagining oneself in the other person's shoes and projecting an understanding that, if in that context I would feel *x*, there is a good chance the other person may be experiencing this, and this is the gift of theory of mind.

Theory of mind is impaired in people with ASD. The impairment is on a spectrum from the assumption that if I think it that all people think it, to knowing that other people have a mind separate from one's own, but being mystified by what others are thinking and feeling and what motivates their behaviour. Theory of mind is a central capability in social competence, and impaired theory of mind is manifested in the impaired social communication characteristic of ASD. This manifests in the symptoms of a deficit in the ability to engage in reciprocal conversation. In mental health reciprocal conversation, in which you put your thoughts out there and then modify your thinking based on the feedback of others, is the essence of reality testing (Cashin 2016).

Neurotypical thinkers are linguistic processors of information. Heidegger famously wrote 'to know the world is to name it' (Heidegger 1962). In typical thought information is stored based on the stories one tells themselves about the world. The coding would perhaps be most accurately written of as a type of mentalese, as opposed to what we understand to be language, but fundamentally it is a linguistically mediated process (Pinker 1997). This form of processing allows typical thinkers to build conceptual knowledge about abstract or non-concrete entities such as emotions. This is opposed to visual coding where the thing coded needs to be something concrete that can be seen to allow it to be coded.

Neurotypical thinkers can label emotions in themselves and others. The ability to recognise symptoms of the presence of emotions, and the emotions themselves, are purely a linguistic construct. You can easily describe symptoms of being happy, but you cannot produce and show someone 'a happy' as an example. This is because it is an abstract entity. The knowledge of emotions allows typical thinkers to self-monitor for the presence of these abstract entities and to regulate their behaviour based on this monitoring. People with ASD have a relative strength in visual coding of information and a relative deficit in linguistic processing. Even before we consider the compounding effect of the combination of the three impairments, the impact of the deficit in linguistic processing becomes clear. Impaired linguistic processing is linked to impaired self-regulation of behaviour, based on the self-monitoring enabled through identifying emotions.

These impairments in thinking and information processing each by themselves have clearly associated disability. However, the greatest impact comes from the combination of all three impairments globally in the process of thinking and information processing.

The world is unpredictable in many ways and presents each person with a succession of novel circumstances. The novelty may be a truly new situation or a variant of something experienced before. Adaptation, by definition, is the process of adapting in the context of novelty or changed circumstances (Cashin & Yorke 2017). As discussed earlier, society is socially mediated, and adaptation relies on a high degree of social competence.

When an individual is placed in a novel situation, they experience a surge in anxiety. This anxiety is the motivating factor to adapt. A neurotypical thinker is able, often without even being aware of the process, to gather clues to establish context and then reach into their unified in-head filing cabinet and pull forward directions from the closest situation they have been in before. This means they have a clue of how to begin to adapt and their anxiety subsides a little. The person can apply the directions and look for clues as to whether it has been effective. If it is not effective anxiety will again surge and prompt modification of their coping response. The person will then attempt to change their response in what appears to be the most efficient manner. Anxiety will again drop, and they will look for evidence of success. If not successful, the process will continue until adaptation has occurred. The person has then succeeded in adapting and, what is more, they then add the new context and directions to their in-head filing cabinet of life information for future use (Cashin 2005).

In these situations, you will notice that, while perhaps initially a long way off the mark, the person had some clue. First the person needed to recognise context. This includes a mixture of concrete and abstract elements. The person then had to reach in their unified base of knowledge of the world to find a like or similar context to have a clue of where to begin and what behavioural direction or strategies to apply. Both the recognition of like and similar, and the presence of a unified base of knowledge about the world, is dependent on abstraction. To judge success of the behaviour and whether adaptation has occurred relies at least in part on the feedback of others through the social mechanism of communication. To recognise anxiety and respond in a targeted manner of focused adaption, as opposed to being pushed into non-adaptive behaviour and thought, such as ritual and obsession, requires a recognition and labeling of the feeling (Cashin 2018). The final step of saving the information for future use and expanding the unified knowledge of the world requires again recognition of like and similar to store the information in a coherent and accessible manner.

When in novel situations people with ASD can in effect not have a clue where to begin. The anxiety, while not monitored for and hence recognised and labelled, still exists. Anxiety is designed to push, as in the flight and fight mechanism, and will push the person even if not acknowledged. While anxiety is not recognised, the flight or fight system biologically remains unimpaired. There is a link between increased anxiety and increased restrictive and repetitive behaviours, with the behaviours increasing in intensity and frequency as anxiety goes up (Cashin & Yorke 2018). The restrictive and repetitive behaviours have a filtering function where the focus shifts to managing the communicated demand to adapt as opposed to adapting (Cashin & Yorke 2016).

In terms of symptoms of mental illness, people with ASD experience a disproportionately high prevalence of comorbid mental illness. This includes high rates of anxiety disorders, which makes sense given the above description. It also appears that there is a high rate of depression, although much less studied (Vannucchi et al. 2013). People with ASD also experience high rates of psychosis, with up to 30% of people with ASD experiencing psychotic phenomenon (Cashin 2016). The comorbidity in some cases may be reactive and related to adaption. There is also a strong chance of shared, as yet undefined, biological mechanisms.

CONSUMER'S STORY 17.1

Martin

Martin was a 16-year-old male with a diagnosis of ASD in Year 10 at a public school in Victoria. Martin received his diagnosis when he was 7 years old. Martin had an IQ of 74 when last tested in Year 7 and was attending mainstream classes with homeroom support from a special education teacher and teacher aids. He was taking no medication and had no history of illicit drug use.

Martin had few friends at school and spent most breaks in his homeroom.

Martin became increasingly focused on the idea that males at the school were taking steroids. The intensity of Martin's beliefs increased in the context of acute stress when his parents separated. All of Martin's routines changed as he and his siblings lived between the family home and his father's new apartment. Martin had become panicked when out with his family when he saw males from the schools and explained it as a fear of being near steroid-takers. While able to describe his idea as a fear, Martin was not able to clarify it further and was not ameliorable to any other points of view when his parents tried to discuss it with him. Without warning, first thing on a Wednesday morning Martin walked into the playground and physically attacked a boy. When asked why he attacked the boy Martin claimed the boy was a steroid-taker.

The attack resulted in a suspension from school and full health assessment. Martin felt no empathy with the boy who he attacked and could not identify if the boy would have been scared or worried. Martin stated that he had been told one year earlier by an older boy that the boy he attacked was 'on steroids'. Martin ruminated over this idea even though the boy described was small and of slight build. Martin had become preoccupied with this thought over the year, but it had increased in intensity since his social situation changed. He was having difficulty falling to sleep because he could not get the thought out of his head.

Martin's thoughts were not sequential, and he had difficulty focusing on the discussion, often going onto tangents. Martin said that he infrequently heard voices calling his name when no one was in the room. Martin had no suicidal or homicidal ideation plan or intent and no recent history of physical ill health or injury.

Martin was prescribed risperidone 0.5 mg nocte and was able to return to school in one week after making a written agreement to not attack fellow students. The medication was titrated to 1 mg nocte 2 months later in the context of increased stress-related behaviour at school.

Healthcare staff worked with the family to develop firm routines that were made explicit, and if the routine was to change to show Martin with as much warning as possible what the change was and where it fitted. Through discussion, behavioural warning signs of increased stress (Martin does not label his feelings so cannot rate his own anxiety) were identified and management strategies formed and rehearsed.

Martin, although agreeing to not attack anyone, and able to give a historical account of the evolution of the idea, remained suspicious that it may be true that the boys was on steroids and resented the fact the boy was given a citizenship award at school for not fighting back.

Adapted from Cashin 2016

Intellectual disability

A concrete exercise to elucidate the vast number of choices we are continually confronted with, and the information we need to extract to optimise outcomes, is to write down each choice that was made and the action followed from the time you woke this morning up until the time you left the house for work or study. Of course, it is best to choose a morning when you left early because the information you will record will be voluminous.

The exercise may begin with choices such as to hit snooze or not on the alarm, what side of the bed to get out of, what leg to put weight on first as you stand, and so on. Our lives are full of choices, and we are constantly bombarded by stimuli (Gergen 2000). Many of the choices go underground as they become subconscious, and this is a way of managing the volume. Prejudice or pre-judgement is a typical way of also managing the volume of choice (Gadamer 1960/1985). It may come as a surprise that prejudice is a natural part of typical thought processes and that it has a function in making the volume of choice we are confronted with manageable. A good example is favourite foods, which make choices presented on a menu manageable. An even better example may be coffee choices, in what is often a time-limited rush into the coffee shop to grab a takeaway while often simultaneously engaged in other activities such as a phone call or checking social media updates. Of course when pre-judgements extend to races or groups of people, including those with intellectual disability, it is incumbent on us to make our prejudices as known to ourselves as is possible, to allow us to become aware of what we can modify, as needed, to be consistent with our overall worldview.

Even with prejudices, and many choices moving below the conscious level, it is clear that people are confronted with huge volumes of information that needs to be managed and often simultaneously and quickly. Any impairment of the volume of information that can be handled at any one time and the speed in which information can be processed and acted on, will result in serious functional impairments. Even self-care tasks consist of chains of behaviours each preceded by choices. Think of the simple activity of brushing your teeth. An exercise of writing out the chain of steps in brushing your teeth will show how a simple task, taken for granted by typical thinkers, is in fact quite complex.

People with intellectual disability also have a disproportionate prevalence of mental illness (Department of Developmental Disability Neuropsychiatry 2018). This burden may arise from the challenge and stress of adaptation but also plausibly be related to shared causative biological mechanisms.

Historical anecdote 17.2: A dark chapter in the history of nursing

Autism, intellectual disability and mental ill health have been used by nurses and other health professionals as justification for taking part in mass sterilisation and extermination. At the start of the 20th century the philosophy of 'eugenics' was developed by social policy experts and scientists in the United States. This philosophy suggested that people with disabilities or mental illness should be eradicated from society. From the 1920s to the 1960s, the influence of this ideology led to government policies that facilitated the involuntary sterilisation of more than 60,000 people with mental and physical disabilities in North America. The philosophy of eugenics was then used by Hitler and the Nazi regime in Germany to justify the extermination of more than 200,000 disabled people during World War II. Much of the extermination was carried out by nurses and doctors in hospitals like Hadamar in Germany.

Read more about it: *Iredale R 2000 Eugenics and its relevance to contemporary health care. Nursing Ethics 7(3): 205–14*

Physical health and ASD and intellectual disability

People with ASD and intellectual disability experience a higher burden of chronic ill health than the general population of people without either disability (Cashin et al. 2018; Trollor et al. 2018). It would appear that obesogenic factors are prevalent, particularly in the domains of diet and physical activity. The risk for ill health is particularly challenging related to inequitable access to health care and accessible information on self-care.

Autism spectrum disorder

There is a marked lack of research focused on the physical health of adults with ASD (van Dooren et al. 2016). The research with children has highlighted the need to focus intervention on the commonly experienced obesogenic factors and to be aware of ASD-related factors that exacerbate these, including restricted diet and reduced physical activity, such as when engaged in some obsessional behaviours (e.g. gaming) or avoidance of physical activity based on the social demands of participation (Curtin et al. 2014). People with ASD were identified internationally in a systematic review of related studies to carry a higher risk of mortality than the population without ASD (Woolfenden et al. 2012). This finding was repeated in a sample of people with ASD in New South Wales, with mortality 2.06 times more than the population without ASD (Hwang et al. 2019). This information is important to guide intervention and particularly from a mental health nursing perspective when prescribing or administering medications associated with an increased risk of chronic illness such as type 2 diabetes, that may further compound the risk of ill health. There is evidence of disparities in access to services for people with ASD (Nicolaidis et al. 2012).

Intellectual disability

People with intellectual disability experience a higher burden of ill health both physically and mentally to that of the population without intellectual disability (McCarthy & Duff 2019; Trollor et al. 2018). The impact is made even more significant by inequitable access to services. In New Zealand, within the context of limited statistical information, the life expectancy is 22.9 years less for people with intellectual disability than those without (McCarthy & Duff 2019).

Challenges exist both in the New Zealand and Australian contexts related to the identification of intellectual disability in mental health policy ranging from exclusion to inadequate acknowledgement of the unique needs of the group (Dew et al. 2018; McCarthy & Duff 2019). The policy context as it exists perpetuates both issues with access to services and an inadequate focus on teaching the required adjustments to provide adequate services to this group, and practitioners need this policy change for services to improve.

CONSUMER'S STORY 17.2

Margaret

Margaret is a 35-year-old woman who normally lives with her mother and has limited support needs. She has a small vocabulary but can understand much of what is said to her. She can perform self-help tasks and has developed competencies in occupational, leisure and social skills. Diagnostic overshadowing played a large part in the delay between the onset of severe symptoms and diagnosis for this client.

The police brought Margaret into the emergency department late one Sunday after local residents reported that she had been lying on the road outside a shopping centre. Margaret was very distressed and crying, and when asked why she was on the road replied: 'You will get run over lying on the road and go to heaven, sorry Mr Policeman'. She was able to give her name, phone number and address to the attending mental health nurse and a subsequent phone call found that Margaret lived at home with her mother and had gone to the local shops for bread. The mental health nurse and the duty psychiatrist decided that Margaret could go home to the care of her mother because there was no history of mental illness and she was able to say where she lived.

Lying on the road was dismissed as 'behaviour' due to her intellectual disability. This proved to be diagnostic overshadowing.

Two days later, Margaret's mother Jean telephoned the mental health service staff to say that a local shopkeeper had brought Margaret home after he had found her lying on the road. Jean was told that someone from the mental health team would visit in the next couple of days, but this was not regarded as high priority because the behaviour was seen as part of Margaret's intellectual disability. The following afternoon, community mental health nurses visited and questioned Margaret, who became tearful and repeated: 'I'll get run over and go to heaven'. Jean told the staff that she had heard Margaret crying at night and that she had been awake early in the morning and needed to be told to shower. This was unlike Margaret, but Jean said that she had been sad since her grandmother died 3 months ago and seemed to lack motivation.

On their way back to the community mental health centre the nurses called in to the local shops and discovered that Margaret had been lying on the road intermittently for the past 4 weeks. At first, she would get up as soon as someone called out to her, but over the past 2 weeks she would cry: 'No, I'll get run over and go to heaven'. The staff, recognising her behaviour as suicidal, arranged for Margaret to be admitted to the mental health unit as an involuntary patient (i.e. she was deprived of her right to discharge herself from hospital on the grounds that there was a reasonable risk that she would harm herself).

In Margaret's case, nursing and medical staff found that she was uncommunicative upon admission to the mental health unit and that she sat gently rocking and averting her gaze from staff. Fortunately, the staff were able to engage Jean in the process of taking a history and for some of the assessment process. After medical staff had performed a physical examination of Margaret, it was decided to take her to her bedroom and continue the assessment process once she had familiarised herself with her new environment. In the interim, a nurse was able to start brief conversations with Margaret using gentle open-ended questions. Margaret was subsequently asked to unpack her suitcase and engage in self-care activities independently.

Margaret lived at home and, in such cases, it is important to work with the family to gain their trust, to ensure the optimal outcome for the client and to obtain a reliable history of the client's mental and physical status. Over the course of the next hour, the nurse was able to ascertain from Jean that Margaret was uncharacteristically withdrawn and that her movements were much slower than usual. Jean also revealed that Margaret's concentration had deteriorated in recent weeks, and Margaret was able to add that she felt terrible and that she didn't 'want to live anymore'. Apart from these typical signs of clinical depression staff noted that Margaret's rocking had continued and that she made low, barely audible noises. Jean confirmed that rocking and moaning were atypical signs of Margaret's depression because they were not normally part of her behavioural repertoire.

Having gained the confidence of the new patient, the nurse was able to interview Margaret alone and, after some encouragement, found that she had retained her plan to kill herself by lying down in the middle of a road and being run over by a car. She did not have any other plans for her own death but repeated that what she really wanted was to die and go to heaven to see her grandmother. Eventually the nurse was able to complete the initial assessments for Margaret, including a physical assessment, mental status assessment, risk assessment, assessment of strengths and assessment of Margaret's risk of vulnerability to exploitation and abuse, and was able to write admission notes that described her signs and symptoms including the atypical signs of depression.

Margaret was subsequently placed on half-hourly general observations with 4-hourly observations. Although primary nursing was not a part of the unit's policy on patient care, Margaret was allocated a single nurse for each subsequent morning and afternoon 'shift' on the first 2 days of her admission to facilitate communications and to assist in the process of ongoing assessment. Despite these arrangements Margaret remained largely uncommunicative and chose to speak only with a few of the staff.

Apart from the interventions outlined above, the management of Margaret's depression was much like that afforded to other patients. While she was being stabilised on an antidepressant (in this case, fluoxetine), Margaret was offered grief counselling to help her to cope with the loss of her grandmother. Although Margaret was quick to understand that she needed to take her medication with her morning and evening meals until her doctor said to stop, she was unable to grasp education given to her by staff about the physiology of her depressive illness and the need to be vigilant regarding the symptoms of relapse. She also had a very limited understanding of the way in which her medication was helping her.

At the suggestion of Margaret's mother, and with Margaret's permission, it was decided to devise a mental health support plan to disseminate information about Margaret's management strategies to the people in her circle of support when she was discharged. The plan featured possible relapse signs (such as social withdrawal and 'rocking') and management strategies should Margaret again decide to harm herself (such as removing Margaret from harmful circumstances, clarifying Margaret's intentions and contacting the community mental health team if Jean required assistance).

Key points related to assessment

The good news related to the required adjustments to be discussed in this section of key points related to assessment, and in the following section on interventions, is that incorporating these adjustments into general practice will strengthen the delivery of truly person-centred care.

Before discussing specific adjustments is important to acknowledge that an assessment is not an interrogation designed to extract information to allow the formulaic construction of a diagnostic picture. An assessment is an opportunity for the assessor and assessee to build an understanding of the context, in the form of recent and more extensive history, and the personal experience of living within that context. How that understanding is co-constructed needs careful attention. The interview, as discussed earlier, includes coming to consensus on not only what the experience is but also how it is labelled (refer to choices on language).

In regard to working with a person with ASD it is imperative to take into consideration their thinking and information-processing style. Without being mindful of this it can be like speaking different languages, and while the words may appear common, it can impair the ability to develop shared understanding.

Regarding impaired abstraction it is important to check if the person makes sense of emotions and self-monitors for these. It may make more sense to explore symptoms of anxiety such as increased engagement in restrictive and repetitive behaviours than ask the person if they feel anxious. Don't assume rating scales such as 1–10 when discussing the experience of emotions make any sense to the person. Check this out thoroughly with them. If someone presents as sad, again, rather than discussing being depressed, it may make more sense to explore changes in usual behaviours such as sleeping, eating and activity. When discussing the experience of assessment, discuss what will happen in a linear fashion in the order that it will occur. If the person appears distracted, reground the interview by discussing where you are at in the order things, and what will occur next, with reference to what happened immediately before, what will happen now and what will follow. Don't expect the person to generalise from past experiences, particularly if these occurred in a different visual context such as a different emergency department. Even with a history of past assessments for the person this may be a novel situation. Be concrete in what is being asked. Be careful that your questions will result in discussion of the target information. A good example is the question: Do you hear voices? Unless experiencing a hearing deficit the answer would be yes; that is, if they heard the question. If exploring auditory hallucinations, a rephrased question such as, 'Do you hear voices when no one is around and there are no devices capable of delivering sound on?' can help.

In terms of theory of mind, at the outset it needs to be surfaced that the interview is a social process. On top of whatever challenge to health brought the person to the interview, the interview itself can generate significant anxiety. Affect is an important element of a mental health assessment. People with ASD may have a limited range of affect and reduced prosody (variance in pitch and tone) in the voice. Both affect and prosody are learned behaviours, and the learning is mediated in the social process, beginning with the child–parent relationship and expanding from there, by theory of mind. What the person with ASD is feeling on the inside (e.g. scared) may not be expressed externally through changes in affect or prosody. Ask the person clearly what they are feeling in the concrete context of enquiry. Don't rely on eye contact as a sign of attention. Lack of eye contact may be related to the social aspect of this, or equally that looking and listening is overwhelming and not looking allows full concentration on what is said. When exploring empathy, don't rely on the ability of the person with ASD to guess what others are thinking and feeling and to consider this perspective.

As the person with ASD is not primarily a linguistic processor of information, it is easy to become overwhelmed by words. If the person is appearing confused, reduce the volume of words. If giving instructions, make sure the person with ASD understands what is required and what order it is to be done in. Don't be afraid of doodling and drawing to augment understanding. The art does not have to be high quality; it just needs to promote understanding. Write down any key instructions and what is to happen next because, unlike spoke words, writing and drawing is not transitory.

In regard to intellectual disability all of the ASD adjustments will be important. In addition, become familiar with characteristic patterns of speech (particularly in people with a higher degree of intellectual impairment) such as echolalia. Be clear that the person is not just repeating the question rather than taking it as a form of confirmation. Be very mindful of changes to usual activity and behaviours, and explore plausible causes thoroughly. For non-verbal individuals, find out how they usually communicate and how this can be incorporated in the assessment. Work closely with family and carers to establish meaning making.

For people with ASD and people with intellectual disability, ensure a thorough physical examination is conducted. Be mindful that they may not describe discomfort or pain in the typical manner or, unless asked, may not disclose it all.

One common issue that warrants discussion is diagnostic overshadowing. This is the situation where everything is attributed to the primary diagnosis (such as ASD or intellectual disability) and this diagnosis overshadows other important understandings of what is happening. This leads to missing treatable comorbidities and is largely contributing to the increased morbidity and mortality in these groups. This overshadowing can lead to lack of exploration of provisional diagnosis. An example would be the failure to diagnose delusions in people with ASD due to an assumption that because people with ASD think differently, delusional beliefs must be normal for this group. Or that a rise in self-harming behaviour in someone with intellectual disability may just be an increase in self-stimulatory behaviour and have no relationship with self-harming, even though this is a new behaviour for this person.

Interventions

Interventions designed to work on thinking of course need to be modified to be accessible by the participants.

Psychotherapies used in typical populations all need adjustments to work with people with ASD and intellectual disability. As an example, modified narrative therapy has been effective in a trial with a small sample of young people with ASD (Cashin et al. 2013). The therapy was adjusted based on the principles discussed above to work on the problems of daily living (Cashin 2008). Similar modifications have occurred with cognitive behaviour therapy.

If we accept that talking therapies are needed by the neurotypical population, there is no logical reason why such therapy is not needed by people with ASD and intellectual disability. Mental health nurses are ideally situated to deliver the therapy but need to be mindful of the adjustments required to make them accessible and functional for people with ASD and intellectual disability. The health disparity between people with ASD and intellectual disability and the neurotypical population in general is large. Nurses have a role in reducing this and understanding the thinking and information-processing styles is all that is needed to make creative adjustments that can be trialled and evaluated.

Deinstitutionalisation

In the mid- to late 20th century nurses performed a central role in the care of people with ASD and intellectual disabilities in both Australia and New Zealand. Deinstitutionalisation with the move to community care progressively saw a decline in the involvement of nurses in the care of these groups (Trollor et al. 2018). Institutional living was, in many ways, undesirable (Burghardt 2018; Robinson 2013), and with the evolution of the diagnostic construct of ASD in particular, even if the return was seen as an answer it would not service a large proportion of those diagnosed. However, the return of nursing as a central component of care would undoubtedly lead to better health outcomes.

Chapter summary

Every nurse can make a difference in the lives of people with autism and intellectual disability. This can be in each clinical encounter and through advocacy to make adjustments to practice so that services can be more accessible. Participation in policy and practice related to inclusion criteria for services, at a local and national level is also an area where nurses can make an impact. Such adjustments are predicated on understanding the thinking and information processing style inherent in ASD, and the thinking and processing challenges experienced in intellectual disability. The link between thinking and behaviour once understood leads to both accessible and hence more effective assessment and intervention.

Useful websites

Autism Science Foundation: https://autismsciencefoundation.org/
Autism Spectrum Australia: http://www.autismlaunchpad.org.au/
Carer Gateway (Australian Government): https://www.carergateway.gov.au/
National Autistic Society (UK): https://www.autism.org.uk/
Raising Children.net: https://raisingchildren.net.au/
Research Autism: http://www.researchautism.net/
University of New South Wales – Department of Developmental Disability Neuropsychiatry (3DN): https://3dn.unsw.edu.au/content/disability-professionals-elearning

References

American Psychiatric Association, 2013. Diagnostic and Statistical Manual of Mental Disorders, fifth ed. APA, Washington DC.

Bettleheim, B., 1990. Recollections and Reflections. Thames and Hudson, London.

Burghardt, M., 2018. Broken: Institutions, Families and the Construction of Intellectual Disability. McGill-Queen's University Press, Montreal.

Cambridge English Dictionary, 2020. Society, Cambridge University Press. Online. https://dictionary.cambridge.org/help/. (Accessed 14 March 2020).

Cashin, A., 2018. Why do some people with autism have restricted interests and repetitive movements? [Online]. The Conversation. Available: https://theconversation.com/why-do-some-people-with-autism-have-restricted-interests-and-repetitive-movements-94401. (Accessed 26 June 2018).

Cashin, A., 2016. Autism spectrum disorder and psychosis: a case study. J. Child Adolesc. Psychiatr. Nurs. 29, 72–78.

Cashin, A., 2008. Narrative therapy: a psychotherapeutic appraoch in the treatment of adolescents with Asperger's Disorder. J. Child Adolesc. Psychiatr. Nurs. 21, 48–56.

Cashin, A., 2005. Autism: understanding conceptual processing deficits. J. Psychosoc. Nurs. Ment. Health Serv. 43, 22–30.

Cashin, A., Barker, P., 2009. The triad of impairment in autism revisited. J. Child Adolesc. Psychiatr. Nurs. 22, 189–193.

Cashin, A., Browne, G., Bradbury, J., et al., 2013. The effectiveness of Narrative Therapy with young people with autism. J. Child Adolesc. Psychiatr. Nurs. 26, 32–41.

Cashin, A., Buckley, T., Trollor, J.N., et al., 2018. A scoping review of what is known of the physical health of adults with autism spectrum disorder. J. Intellect. Disabil. 22, 96–108.

Cashin, A., Gallagher, H., Newman, C., et al., 2012. Autism and the cognitive processing triad: a case for revising the criteria in the Diagnostic and Statistical Manual. J. Child Adolesc. Psychiatr. Nurs. 25, 141–148.

Cashin, A., Heartfield, M., Bryce, J., et al., 2017. Standards for practice for registered nurses in Australia. Collegian 24, 255–266.

Cashin, A., Yorke, J., 2018. The relationship between anxiety, external structure, behavioral history and becoming locked into restricted and repetitive behaviors

in autism spectrum disorder. Issues Ment. Health Nurs. 39, 533–537.
Cashin, A., Yorke, J., 2017. Conceptualization of a heuristic to predict increase in restricted and repetitive behaviour in ASD across the short to medium term. Autism Open Access 7 (1), doi:10.4172/2165-7890.1000200.
Cashin, A., Yorke, J., 2016. Overly regulated thinking and autism revisited. J. Child Adolesc. Psychiatr. Nurs. 29, 148–153.
Committee on Children with Disabilities, 2001. Technical report: the pediatrician's role in the diagnosis and management of autistic spectrum disorder in children. Pediatrics 107, e85.
Croen, L., Zerbo, O., Qian, Y., et al., 2015. The health status of adults on the autism spectrum. Autism 19, 814–823.
Curtin, C., Jojic, M., Bandini, L., 2014. Obesity in children with autism spectrum disorder. Harv. Rev. Psychiatry 22, 93–103.
Department of Developmental Disability Neuropsychiatry, 2018. Recommendations from the National Roundtable on the Mental Health of People with intellectual disability 2018. Sydney: University of NSW.
Dew, A., Dowse, L., Athanassiou, U., et al., 2018. Current representation of people with intellectual disability in Australian mental health policy: the need for inclusive policy development. J. Policy Pract. Intellect. Disabil. 15, 136–144.
Feinstein, A., 2011. A History of Autism: Conversations With the Pioneers. John Wiley & Sons, West Sussex.
Gadamer, H., 1960/1985. The discrediting of prejudice by the enlightenment. In: Mueller-Vollmer, K. (Ed.), The Hermeneutics Reader. Basil Blackwell, Oxford.
Gergen, K., 2000. The Saturated Seld. Basic Books, New York.
Girimaji, S., Pradeep, A., 2018. Intellectual disability in international classification of Diseases-11: a developmental perspective. Indian J. Soc. Psychiatry (Suppl. S1), 68–74.
Heidegger, M., 1962. Being and Time. Blackwell Publishing, Malden.
Hwang, Y.I., Srasuebkul, P., Foley, K.R., et al., 2019. Mortality and cause of death of Australians on the autism spectrum. Autism Res. 12 (5), 806–815.
Iredale, R., 2000. Eugenics and its relevance to contemporary health care. Nurs. Ethics 7 (3), 205–214.
Kanner, L., 1943. Autistic disturbances of affective contact. Nerv. Child 2, 217–250.
McCarthy, J., Duff, M., 2019. Services for adults with intellectual disability in Aotearoa New Zealand. BJPsych. Int. 16 (3), 71–73.
Nicolaidis, C., Raymaker, D., McDonald, K., et al., 2012. Comparison of healthcare experiences in Autistic and Non-Autistic adults: a cross-sectional online survey faciltated by n academic- community partnership. J. Gen. Intern. Med. 28, 761–769.
Nursing Council of New Zealand, 2016. Competencies for registered nurses. Wellington: Nursing Council of New Zealand.
Nylander, L., Lugnegard, T., Hallerback, M., 2008. Autism Spectrum Disorders and Schizophrenia Spectrum Disorders in adults - is there a connection? A literature review and some suggestions for future clinical research. Clin. Neuropsychiatry 5, 43–54.
Pinker, S., 1997. How the Mind Works. W.W. Norton and Company, New York.
Robinson, S., 2013. Preventing the Emotional Abuse and Neglext of People With Intellectual Disability. Stopping Insult and Injury. Jessica Kingsley Publishers, London.
Shakes, P., Cashin, A., 2018. Identifying language for people on the autism spectrum: a scoping review. Issues Ment. Health Nurs. 40 (4), 317–325.
Trollor, J., Eagleson, C., Turner, B., et al., 2018. Intellectual disability content within pre-registration nursing curriculum: how is it taught? Nurse Educ. Today 69, 48–52.
van Dooren, K., McPherson, L., Lennox, N., 2016. Mapping the needs of adults with autism and co-morbid intellectual disaility. Curr. Dev. Disord. Rep. 3 (1), 82–89.
Van Naarden Braun, K., Christensen, D., Doernbeerg, N., et al., 2015. Trends in the prevalence of autism spectrum disorder, cerebral palsy, hearing loss, intellectual disability, and vision impairment, metropolitan Atlanta, 1991– 2010. PLoS ONE 10, e0124120.
Vannucchi, G., Masi, G., Toni, C., et al., 2013. Clinical features, developmental course, and psychiatric comorbidity of adult autism spectrum disorders. CNS Spectr. 19, 157–164.
Woolfenden, S., Sarkozy, V., Ridley, G., et al., 2012. A systemic review of two outcomes in autism spectrum disorder - epilepsy and mortality. Dev. Med. Child Neurol. 54, 306–312.

CHAPTER 18

Physical health

Andrew Watkins

KEY POINTS

- Maintaining physical health is multifaceted and is essential to wellbeing.
- Nurses play an important role in assessing, treating and preventing physical health issues.
- It is essential to assess and treat mental and physical health issues simultaneously.
- Physical health issues are often overlooked when the person has a mental illness.
- Partnerships and collaboration are key to improving physical and mental health.
- Most premature deaths among people with mental illness are from preventable physical health issues.

KEY TERMS

- Cardiometabolic health
- Cardiovascular disease
- Metabolic screening
- Metabolic syndrome
- Nutrition
- Obesity
- Obstructive sleep apnoea
- Oral health
- Physical activity
- Premature mortality
- Sexual health
- Type 2 diabetes

LEARNING OUTCOMES

The material in this chapter will assist you to:

- recognise the relationship between mental health and physical health
- identify the physical health issues that are commonly experienced by people with mental illness
- develop an understanding of the experience of people with both physical and mental health issues
- describe the nurse's role in assessing physical health
- describe interventions for improving the physical health of people with mental illness
- explain the importance of assessing physical health
- implement nursing interventions relevant to physical health issues identified.

Introduction

People living with mental illness experience much poorer physical health outcomes compared with the general population. A life expectancy gap of more than 20 years was first shown in consumers with severe mental illness (SMI) such as schizophrenia and bipolar disorder. Now there is clear evidence that individuals across the range of mental disorders have a significantly reduced life expectancy compared with the general population (Firth et al. 2019). In contrast with the commonly held misconception, nearly four in every five of these premature deaths are associated with preventable physical health conditions and not suicide (Correll et al. 2017). There is a multitude of reasons for high levels of physical morbidity among people with mental illness. Many of the psychotropic medications prescribed to people with SMI are associated with adverse effects on physical health, including weight gain and endocrine changes. In addition, the symptoms of many mental illnesses, like the negative symptoms of schizophrenia, can contribute to withdrawal, isolation and increased likelihood of living a sedentary lifestyle. The Australian National Psychosis survey identified that one in three people with SMI were sedentary and the large majority of the remaining two-thirds engaged in low levels of physical activity (Morgan et al. 2012). People with SMI also have greater susceptibility to other risk factors for chronic illness, including poverty, smoking, alcohol and drug use, homelessness, unemployment, dental disease, sexually transmitted infections, sleep disorders, and a poor-quality diet (Hayes et al. 2017; Jones et al. 2014; Tanskanen et al. 2018).

The World Health Organization (WHO) describes mental health as 'a state of well-being in which every individual realises his or her own potential, can cope with the normal stresses of life, can work productively and fruitfully, and is able to make a contribution to her or his community' (WHO 2013, p. 38). WHO also acknowledges a universal right to health that includes the right to control one's health and body, to be free from interference, also including the right to a system of health protection that gives everyone an equal opportunity to enjoy the highest attainable level of health (WHO 2008). Historically, the physical health care of people with mental illness has been neglected (Thornicroft 2011). In both Australia and New Zealand mental health commissions have made clear calls for the physical health of mental health consumers to be better addressed (Mental Health Commission New Zealand 2012; National Mental Health Commission 2013). In both countries Equally Well has been established with the primary purpose of taking initiatives and creating change to achieve physical health equity for people experiencing mental health issues. Nurses are well placed to take the lead in ensuring that people with mental illness have their physical health needs considered and adequately addressed from the initial assessment and right through a person's mental health journey. It is therefore vital that nurses practise in a holistic way that incorporates physical health care by 'keeping the body in mind'.

Historical anecdote 18.1: Health care or money making?

History teaches us that nurses need to remain wary of how swindlers and big business may seek to take advantage of mental health care. One example during the 18th century was a treatment known as 'mesmerism'. Developed in Vienna by Franz Anton Mesmer (1734–1815), the treatment promoted that idea that there was an invisible fluid called 'animal magnetism' flowing through all living things. When a person's level of animal magnetism was balanced, they experienced health; when it became unbalanced, they experienced illness. Patients attended group sessions in ornately furnished treatment rooms where they would be instructed to grab hold of metal rods protruding from a tank of magnetised water. During treatment some people experienced what appeared to be convulsions, while others were reportedly 'mesmerised' into hypnotic states. Mesmerism made its practitioners huge money until it was eventually disproved by Benjamin Franklin using one of the earliest placebo experiments in history.

Read more about it: *Darnton R 1968 Mesmerism and the end of the enlightenment in France. Harvard University Press, Cambridge*

It is beyond the scope of this chapter to address all the physical illnesses that are experienced by people with mental illness. The authors have therefore chosen to focus on physical health issues that negatively impact on life expectancy, which are most prevalent, and those that most markedly affect wellbeing and quality of life. Factors contributing to physical health risks are shown in Fig. 18.1. This chapter will discuss metabolic syndrome, diabetes, cardiovascular disease, respiratory diseases, oral health, sleep and sexual health. These physical health issues require action, and we believe nurses are well positioned to make a difference to the current trends.

Physical health neglect in the mental health system

People with comorbid serious mental and physical illness frequently fall through the gaps between physical and mental healthcare systems (Lawrence et al. 2013). The

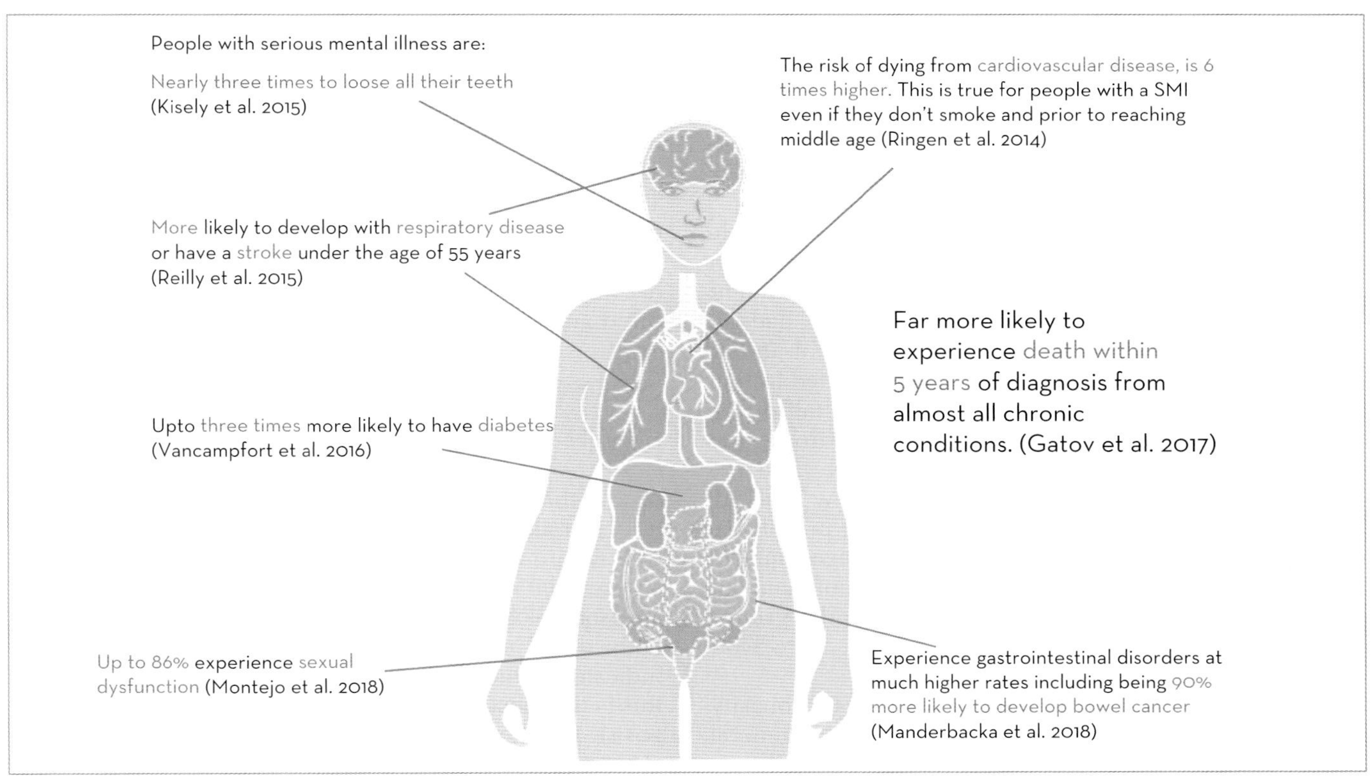

Figure 18.1
Factors that may contribute to physical health risks in people with severe mental illness People with serious mental illness are:
Courtesy of National Women's Health Information Center

healthcare systems in Australia and New Zealand are often divided between services for physical and mental health care, with a lack of integration. In mental healthcare systems, clinicians may focus on symptoms of mental illness often to the detriment of other health issues, a phenomenon referred to as 'diagnostic overshadowing' (Thornicroft 2011). Physical health symptoms regularly go unnoticed or are not addressed, even when people with mental illness report them to health professionals (Galletly et al. 2012). Often nurses and others working in mental health do not consider addressing physical health issues as fundamental to their duty of care or lack the confidence to undertake a physical assessment. In the wider health system, there is often a lack of confidence in working with people who have mental illness. Many services such as medical specialists and allied health services are commonly financially unavailable to this population. Any of these issues can form an extremely challenging obstacle to care for people with complex chronic comorbid conditions such as schizophrenia and diabetes. Therefore, this very vulnerable population can be marginalised from health services that are a human right and essential to attaining wellbeing.

Access and availability are not the only barriers to good health faced by people with SMI. The higher rate of physical illness among people with SMI not only leads to a much shorter life expectancy but also causes a secondary effect of ongoing physical illness on top of a mental illness such as schizophrenia and diabetes. These comorbidities increase the challenge of people being able to actively participate in the workforce and create an increased risk of poverty and welfare dependency. Despite having much higher rates of morbidity than most others in the community, people with SMI are less likely to have their physical health needs met (Morgan et al. 2012). A comorbid physical health issue can put extra demands on family, friends and carers of people with mental illness by expanding this role to include physical health care.

Metabolic syndrome

Obesity is associated with metabolic syndrome, which is a clustering of abnormalities that results in an increased risk of developing type 2 diabetes mellitus and cardiovascular disease (CVD) (Alberti et al. 2005). Metabolic syndrome includes a cluster of abnormal clinical and metabolic findings that are predictive for CVD (Kaur 2014).These abnormal findings include visceral adiposity, insulin resistance, increased blood pressure, elevated triglyceride levels and low-level high-density lipoprotein (HDL) cholesterol levels (Alberti et al. 2005). The complications of metabolic syndrome involve multiple body systems including the cardiovascular, hepatic, endocrine and central nervous systems. Meeting the criteria for metabolic syndrome causes a fivefold increase in the risk of developing type 2 diabetes and twofold increase in the risk of developing CVD over the next 5–10 years (Kaur 2014). Assertive intervention is therefore required when metabolic syndrome risk factors are present.

According to the 2010 National Survey of People Living with Psychotic Illness in Australia, of more than 1,800 people aged 18–65, three-quarters were overweight or obese, around half had hypertension, 50% had an abnormal lipid profile with low HDL-cholesterol and/or elevated triglycerides, and one in three had elevated fasting glucose level (Galletly et al. 2012). More than half of the people surveyed met criteria for metabolic syndrome (see Table 18.1), a rate two to three times higher than the general population (Morgan et al. 2012). In New Zealand, mental health service users also have higher prevalence of severe chronic physical conditions and an age-adjusted mortality rate twice the rate of the general population, but evidence gaps around Māori and Pacific Islander groups remain (Cunningham et al. 2014; Lockett et al. 2017; Scott et al. 2006).

People with SMI have much higher rates of obesity and abdominal obesity in comparison with the general population. This occurs even in the early phase of illness with or without medication (Correll et al. 2009). Similarly, to the general population obesity in people with SMI is associated with lifestyle factors such as a poor diet and lack of physical activity (Hjorth et al. 2014). There are a number of mental illness–related features such as sedation, amotivation and disorganisation that exacerbate the likelihood of negative lifestyle factors that promote weight gain (Cimo & Dewa 2018). There is also evidence of medication-induced effects on appetite and food intake (Cuerda et al. 2014).

Weight gain is a well-established side effect of antipsychotic medications. It is most pronounced at the beginning of treatment and generally continues with long periods of treatment (Alvarez-Jiménez et al. 2008). Mental health consumers identify weight gain as the most common distressing antipsychotic side effect (Cooper & Reynolds 2016). Weight gain is usually greatest with clozapine and olanzapine, while quetiapine, risperidone and paliperidone cause a more moderate gain (Bak et al. 2014). Aripiprazole, asenapine and ziprasidone are likely to cause less weight gain (Bak et al. 2014). Without interventions all antipsychotic medications have been found to result in significant weight gain when they are first initiated (De Hert et al. 2011). The Healthy Active Lives declaration (see Box 18.1) sets out standards of physical health expectations for people newly diagnosed with a psychotic illness. This important declaration and the algorithm will help nurses to integrate mind and body nursing care.

Screening for metabolic health

In order to identify metabolic syndrome and allow for early treatment it is vital to screen for the presence of factors that increase the risk of CVD and type 2 diabetes (Gates et al. 2015). Screening for metabolic syndrome is well within the scope of nurses and should be viewed as an essential activity. Metabolic screening involves taking a person's blood pressure, height and weight, and calculating body mass index (Cooper & Reynolds 2016). The best indicator of metabolic health is waist circumference, and this is the most important measure to screen (Curtis et al. 2012). In addition to these measures, fasting lipids and glucose completes the metabolic screening process (Cooper & Reynolds 2016). Screening should occur every 3 months, with the exception of when someone is starting a new medication or if there are concerns about a person's health (Curtis et al. 2012). More details about how to undertake a metabolic screen are provided in Box 18.2.

Diabetes

Type 2 diabetes is a progressive condition in which the body becomes resistant to the normal effects of insulin and/or gradually loses the capacity to produce enough insulin in the pancreas (Rathmann et al. 2015). Type 2 diabetes greatly increases the risk of CVD, renal failure, amputation and blindness, lowering life expectancy by 10 or more years (Gordon-Dseagu et al. 2015). The prevalence of type 2 diabetes in people with schizophrenia as well as in people with bipolar disorder is two to three times higher

TABLE 18.1 International Diabetes Federation Metabolic Syndrome Criteria

CENTRAL OBESITY (WAIST CIRCUMFERENCE IN CENTIMETRES)			PLUS ANY TWO OF:	
Ethnicity	Male	Female	Triglycerides	≥ 1.7 mmol/L
Europid	≥ 94	≥ 80	HDL	< 1.03 (males) mmol/L < 1.29 (females)
S/SE Asian Japanese	≥ 90	≥ 80	Blood pressure	≥ 130/85 mmHg
Central and South America	≥ 90	≥ 80	Fasting blood sugar	≥ 5.6 mmol/L

Adapted from Alberti et al. 2005

Box 18.1 Healthy Active Lives declaration

A group of clinicians, service users, family members and researchers from more than 10 countries joined forces to develop an international consensus statement on improving the physical health of young people with psychosis. The statement, called Healthy Active Lives (HeAL), aims to reverse the trend of people with SMI dying early by tackling risks for future physical illnesses proactively. Compared with their peers who have not experienced psychosis, young people with psychosis face a number of preventable health inequalities including:

- a lifespan shortened by about 15–20 years
- two to three times the likelihood of developing CVD, making it the single most common cause of premature death (more so than suicide)
- two to three times the likelihood of developing type 2 diabetes
- three to four times the likelihood of being a smoker.

The HeAL statement reflects international consensus on a set of key principles, processes and standards. It aims to combat the stigma, discrimination and prejudice that prevent young people experiencing psychosis from leading healthy active lives and to confront the perception that poor physical health is inevitable. It does this by:

- being tailored to each person
- having a longer duration, with more frequent face-to-face contact
- using multidisciplinary teams (including allied health practitioners).

The HeAL declaration sets out 5-year targets aimed to reduce future cardiovascular risk in youth with psychosis.

HeAL can be downloaded free of charge at http://www.iphys.org.au/

Box 18.2 Screening for metabolic health

WEIGHT

- First ask the person to remove their shoes, any items from their pockets and bulky clothing.

HEIGHT

- With their shoes removed, make sure feet are flat on floor and the person is looking straight ahead.

BODY MASS INDEX

- Calculate by dividing the person's weight by their height squared (normal range 18.5–25):

$$\frac{\text{weight}}{\text{height}(\text{m})^2}$$

- A useful online calculator is available at http://www.heartfoundation.org.au/healthy-eating/Pages/bmi-calculator.aspx

WAIST CIRCUMFERENCE

Waist measurements should be taken after exhaling. Consumers should be encouraged to relax and to not contract any abdominal muscles. Align the tape measure at the level of the belly button and circle the whole way around the body and back to the starting point.

- Make sure the tape is parallel to the ground and not twisted.
- The tape should be snug, without compressing the skin.
- Ask the person to breathe in and out twice and measure on the second out-breath.

BLOOD PRESSURE

- Ensure the correct cuff size.
- Measure the person when they are relaxed.
- Measure with their arm resting at the height of their heart.

PATHOLOGY

- Ensure the person has fasted. Test for:
  - lipid profile (including HDL/LDL)
  - glucose
  - liver function.

than in the general population (Stubbs et al. 2015). The risk of type 2 diabetes in people with anxiety depression or depressive symptoms is also elevated compared with those without depression (Hasan et al. 2014; Smith et al. 2018).

There are a multitude of reasons for the elevated risk of type 2 diabetes among people with SMI, including lifestyle factors, genetic predisposition and disease- and treatment-specific effects (Stubbs et al. 2015). Antipsychotic medications carry an increased risk of developing type 2 diabetes, with olanzapine and clozapine particularly noted as carrying an increased risk (Holt & Mitchell 2014).

Despite a high prevalence of type 2 diabetes among people with SMI, screening rates remain low. This leads to prolonged periods of raised blood glucose levels, hastening the negative consequences associated with type 2 diabetes (Holt & Mitchell 2014). Once diagnosed, people with SMI are more likely to be suboptimally treated and have poor glycaemic control (Galletly et al. 2012). Even when young, after being diagnosed with type 2 diabetes people with SMI experience a rapid decline in health and premature death (Ribe et al. 2014).

CONSUMER'S STORY 18.1

Judy

I started taking olanzapine in mid-2008 when I was 20 years old, and within 4 months I had gained over 20 kg! I was shocked. I was starting to recover from a serious episode of psychosis, but I became fat so quickly. I didn't feel at all comfortable with my new body shape and started to avoid people because I was ashamed. I found myself being very hungry nearly all of the time and craving food that was fatty and sugary. No one mentioned to me anything about the fact that I'd feel this hungry or put on this much weight.

Over the next few years I tried to lose the weight I had put on, but I couldn't seem to shift it. In fact, I continued to gain weight, although at a slower rate. In 3 years I put on another 15 kg. This was something that was very strange for me, I'd always been a fit and healthy person, and at that point I'd hit 105 kg, a far cry from the 68 kg I was prior to starting medication. I become resigned to the fact that I was going to be fat and there was nothing I could do about it.

I then met a mental health nurse who spoke to me about what my goals in life were. I had already got back into the workforce full time, so I told her that it was my physical health I wanted to work on. She told me that she'd be very happy to help and measured my weight, took my waist measurement and blood pressure and organised for a blood test. Together we looked at areas that could be improved and she assisted me to find out information on what were the best exercises to do and how I could improve my diet.

My blood test came back and showed a higher than normal cholesterol level. This really had me concerned and I expressed this to my nurse – I was worried that this was going to kill me. She told me that sometimes medications could cause these problems in addition to weight gain. She reassured me that it was possible to make changes to my health, even though things I'd tried in the past had not worked. She came with me to my next doctor's appointment and helped advocate for a change in medication. The doctor agreed and switched me to aripiprazole.

My nurse then suggested we work on some goals that were short term. We started with trying to stop my weight gain and then developed more goals that increased my fitness levels and improved my nutritional intake. I started to find that I could lose weight. I found this support and encouragement gave me a lot of motivation where I had previously given up.

Two and a half years later I have managed to take off all of that weight and am now about the same as I was before I started seeing mental health services. I feel so much happier and have lots more energy now. My cholesterol has returned to normal and I am not feeling burdened by physical health issues like I was.

Critical thinking challenge 18.1

Imagine you have just gained 20 kg in the past 2 months. Most of the weight gain is around your abdomen. How would you feel?

Consider your current lifestyle. What changes to your life would occur?

Imagine now that you have also been diagnosed with a psychotic disorder. What changes to your life would occur? How might your psychosis and weight gain affect your self-esteem? What might that do to your ability to recover? Would you continue to take medication if you thought that it caused you significant weight gain? Why or why not?

Cardiovascular disease

The term 'cardiovascular disease' refers to any disease that affects the heart and blood vessels (Langan & Smith 2014). Coronary heart disease and cerebrovascular disease are the primary components of CVD (Schoepf et al. 2014). The major risk factors for CVD are smoking, obesity, hypertension, raised blood cholesterol and type 2 diabetes (Todd et al. 2014). Other factors that increase the risk include genetic factors, an unhealthy diet, physical inactivity and low socioeconomic status (Ignaszewski et al. 2015).

CVD is the most common cause of death in people with SMI, with prevalence rates approximately twice that of the general population (Correll et al. 2017). In younger people with SMI, CVD rates are three times higher when compared with matched controls (Ringen et al. 2014). People with SMI have significantly higher rates of several of the modifiable risk factors when compared with controls; they are more likely to be overweight or obese, to have type 2 diabetes, hypertension or dyslipidaemia and to smoke (Stubbs et al. 2015).

Despite the high CVD mortality among people with SMI, they receive less of many specialised interventions or circulatory medications (De Hert et al. 2011). Evidence suggests that people with schizophrenia are not being adequately screened and treated for dyslipidaemia and hypertension (Galletly et al. 2012). Depression is also noted as being an independent risk factor for worsening morbidity and mortality in coronary heart disease (Lichtman et al. 2014).

People with SMI have considerably lower rates of surgical interventions such as stenting and coronary artery bypass grafting (Mather et al. 2014). This poorer quality of medical care contributes to excess mortality for people with SMI after heart failure (Schoepf et al. 2014). An additional significant barrier is the low level of care sought by people with SMI, even during acute cardiovascular events (Reininghaus et al. 2015).

In addition to weight gain and obesity-related mechanisms, there appears to be a direct effect of antipsychotics that contributes to the worsening of CVD risk (Bak et al. 2014). Type 2 diabetes antagonism can be caused by antipsychotics having a direct effect on developing insulin resistance (Stubbs et al. 2015). Higher antipsychotic doses predict greater risk of mortality from coronary heart disease and cerebrovascular incidents (Lin et al. 2014). Most antipsychotics and some antidepressants are associated with a change in the heart's electrical cycle known as QTc prolongation (Erlangsen et al. 2017). A prolonged QTc puts a patient at significant risk of torsade de pointes, ventricular fibrillation and sudden cardiac death (Glassman & Bigger Jr 2014).

Critical thinking challenge 18.2

Who should be responsible for screening and intervention of physical health problems in people with SMI? Consider the registered nurses' scope of practice, competencies and code of professional conduct. How do these standards influence your thoughts and actions on responsibility?

Management of cardiometabolic health

While screening for metabolic health is important, it serves little benefit if no action is taken after problems are identified. It is vital that nurses 'don't just screen but intervene' for metabolic health (Watkins 2014). At the centre of managing cardiometabolic health is lifestyle interventions. Nurses are well positioned to advise, encourage and implement lifestyle interventions around tobacco cessation (see Nurse's story 18.1), physical activity and healthy nutrition. People with SMI can benefit enormously from even small lifestyle changes. A positive cardiometabolic health algorithm has been developed to help guide clinicians in managing the leading causes of mortality of people with SMI (Curtis et al. 2012). See Fig. 18.2

Critical thinking challenge 18.3

Consider the HeAL declaration (Box 18.1) then use the cardiometabolic algorithm in Fig. 18.2 and the screening for metabolic health information in Box 18.2 to develop a nursing care plan for a young person who has just started taking antipsychotic medications. What information do you need to tailor the plan to the individual? How will you get this information? What do you consider most important? Why?

Core nursing interventions

TOBACCO-RELATED ILLNESS AND SMOKING CESSATION

Very high smoking rates are observed among people with SMI. Two in three people with mental illness are tobacco smokers compared with less than 13% of the general Australian population (Galletly et al. 2012; Morgan et al. 2012; 2013). People with mental illness also smoke more cigarettes per day and inhale more deeply than other smokers, achieving higher blood levels of nicotine than smokers without SMIs (Rüther et al. 2014).

Tobacco-related diseases made up approximately half of total deaths seen in people with SMI, and tobacco use represents the highest single factor that contributes to premature death (Brown et al. 2010; Callaghan et al. 2014). The high smoking rates among people with SMI increases their risk of developing cancer and respiratory diseases. Tobacco smoking may be particularly problematic because it amplifies the increased risk of CVD alongside the centralised weight gain associated with using atypical antipsychotic medications (Gartner & Hall 2015).

The high rate of smoking among people with SMI can be attributed to a high smoking take-up rate that occurs early in life, often before a mental health diagnosis, combined with fewer and less successful quit attempts (Myles et al. 2012, Smith et al. 2014). Addressing tobacco use in people with SMI is a major clinical and public health issue. There is also evidence of positive neurocognitive effects from cigarette smoking in people with schizophrenia, which is linked to stimulation of nicotine receptors (Wing et al. 2012). However, studies have shown improvements in depressed mood when transdermal nicotine patches are used (Mineur & Picciotto 2010). Despite evidence showing positive neurocognitive effects, addressing tobacco use in people with SMI is a major clinical and public health issue, and there is limited clinical attention devoted to tobacco use in these groups (Callaghan et al. 2014).

There is a common misconception that people with SMI do not wish to quit smoking (Lum et al. 2018). Despite this misconception, there is a strong interest in smoking cessation in people with SMI who are motivated for the same reasons as other smokers – to improve their health (Aschbrenner et al. 2015; Morgan et al. 2012). An additional motivation to quit is the substantial financial cost of cigarette smoking for people who often have very low incomes, largely derived from social welfare (Ashton et al. 2013).

Smoking cessation can be successfully delivered within mental health programs for both adult and youth populations successfully (Curtis et al. 2018; Gilbody et al. 2015). Substantial mental health benefits can be gained from quitting smoking, including reduced symptoms of depression and anxiety (Taylor et al. 2014). Symptoms of mental illness do not appear to deteriorate after quitting smoking (Rüther et al. 2014).

Nurses can play a vital role in smoking cessation, influencing tobacco-related mortality. People with SMI are likely to experience more severe withdrawal symptoms compared with the general population and require extra support during cessation attempts (Rüther et al. 2014). It is important to realise that people with SMI respond to smoking cessation treatment as well as the general population in the short term, although they generally have worse long-term outcomes (Peckham et al. 2017).

A person's current smoking status, nicotine dependency and previous quit attempts should be assessed. Assessing nicotine dependency will help predict the level of withdrawal symptoms the patient is likely to experience upon quitting. Smoking cessation is best initiated when

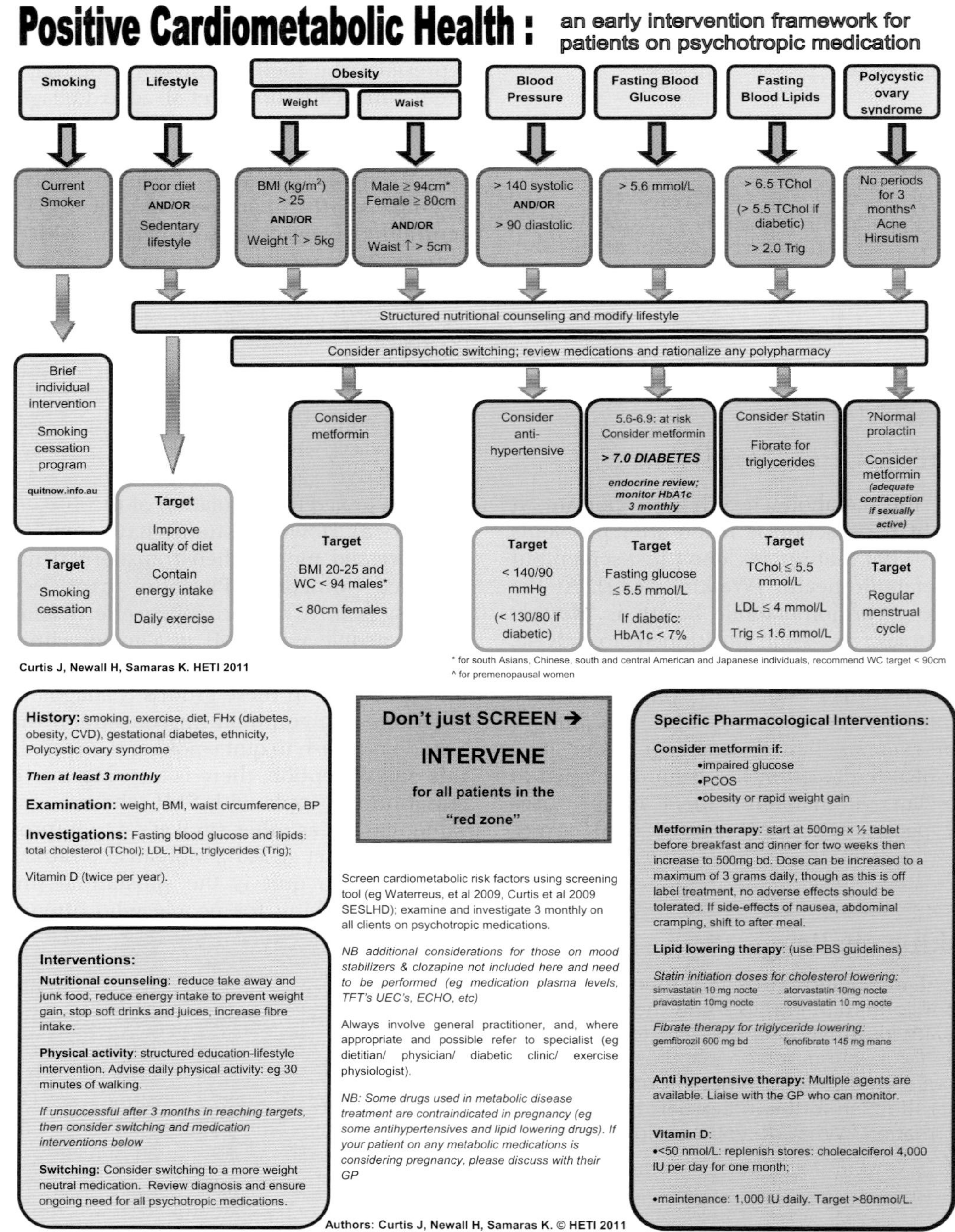

References: Alberti K, Zimmet P, Shaw J. "The metabolic syndrome - a new worldwide definition". *Lancet.* 2005; 366: 1059-62. Correll, C. U., P. Manu, et al. "Cardiometabolic risk of second-generation antipsychotic medications during first-time use in children and adolescents". *JAMA.* 2009; 302: 1765-1773. De Hert M, Dekker JM, Wood D, et al. "Cardiovascular disease and diabetes in people with severe mental illness position statement from the European Psychiatric Association (EPA), supported by the European Association for the Study of Diabetes (EASD) and the European Society of Cardiology (ESC)". *European Psychiatry.* 2009; 24: 412-24. Newall H, Myles N, Ward PB, Samaras K, Shiers D, Curtis J. "Efficacy of metformin for prevention of weight gain in psychiatric populations: a review". *Int Clin Psychopharmacol.* 2012; 27: 69-75. Newcomer JW, Hennekens CH. "Severe Mental Illness and Risk of Cardiovascular Disease". *JAMA.* 2007; 298: 1794-6. Waterreus AJ, Laugharne JD. "Screening for the metabolic syndrome in patients receiving antipsychotic treatment: a proposed algorithm". *MJA.* 2009; 190:185-9. Wu, R. R., J. P. Zhao, et al. "Lifestyle intervention and metformin for treatment of antipsychotic-induced weight gain: a randomized controlled trial". *JAMA.* 2008; 299: 185-193.

For online access to this fact sheet, please visit http://www.heti.nsw.gov.au/cmalgorithm

Figure 18.2
Positive cardiometabolic health algorithm
Source: Curtis et al. 2010

a person is in a stable mental state (Rüther et al. 2014). Consumers should be thoroughly informed on the processes that assist quitting smoking, enabling the person to formulate their individual quit plan and take ownership of their own quit attempt. Involvement in their quit attempt gives people the best chance of quitting successfully (Peckham et al. 2017).

A person should be supported in their quit plan with cessation counselling that includes advice about what to expect with withdrawal symptoms (e.g. depression and restlessness) and how to cope when these symptoms arise (Gartner & Hall 2015). Pharmacological support should be offered and could include nicotine replacement therapy or bupropion when there is even mild tobacco dependence (Rüther et al. 2014). Ceasing tobacco use can affect the way some medications (e.g. olanzapine, clozapine) are metabolised (Peckham et al. 2017). This should not be an impediment to encouraging quitting but requires careful monitoring for potential increases in side effects from psychiatric medication (Rüther et al. 2014).

Along with approaches to illicit drug use, advice on smoking to people with SMIs should also include advice on harm reduction (Gartner & Hall 2015) – for example, reducing the frequency or strength of cigarettes or switching to alternative methods of nicotine delivery (Rüther et al. 2014). This advice is especially relevant for people with SMI who are not yet ready to quit smoking or have faced significant challenges in past quit attempts (Peckham et al. 2017).

Factors such as socioeconomic disadvantage and cognitive impairment are common for people with SMI (Lum et al. 2018). When combined with an absence of social support for abstinence from family and peers, some people will find quitting smoking much more difficult (Gartner & Hall 2015). In some people with schizophrenia, nicotine may be used as self-medication to reduce the negative symptoms of their illness, improve their cognition or ease the side effects caused by antipsychotic medication (Lucatch et al. 2018).

Alongside smoking cessation, exercise should be promoted among people with schizophrenia to combat weight gain and increased metabolic risk. Nurses should carefully monitor patients' medication and fluctuations in weight for a minimum of 6 months after quitting smoking (Gartner & Hall 2015). Helpful advice and support is available via government websites in Australia (www.quitnow.gov.au) and in New Zealand (www.quit.org.nz).

NURSE'S STORY 18.1

Malcolm

Malcolm has been a nurse for 27 years and now works on an acute inpatient mental health unit. He has been leading a project to help people admitted to the mental health unit in dealing with smoking withdrawal and encouraging them to quit.

'When I first started working as a nurse in mental health, I was a smoker. The senior nurses I was working with at the time told me that a great way to build a relationship with the patients on the unit was to chat to them while we were all having a smoke.'

Malcolm ceased smoking 15 years ago after witnessing his aunt dying from lung cancer.

'I saw what my aunty was going through and it was horrible. She was in so much pain and distress. I decided at that time I needed to quit for my health. So, I quit. It wasn't easy at all, especially being around people smoking while I was at work. I persisted though and my health has improved out of sight.'

Malcolm decided he wanted to support the patients he was working with to experience the same benefits that he gained after quitting smoking. When he heard about the smoking ban in mental health units, he thought it was an ideal opportunity.

'I thought to myself: if they are not allowed to smoke while they are on the unit, they may as well use it as a launching pad to quit smoking. The worst part of nicotine withdrawal is the first couple of days, so it would make sense if they could make it through that, why couldn't they quit altogether? So, I got myself skilled up on withdrawal symptoms from nicotine and learnt how to adequately prescribe nicotine replacement therapy.'

As Malcolm built up the intervention, other nurses took an interest and became involved with the program. This led to a much more comprehensive approach to addressing smoking and not just when Malcolm was on shift.

'The key to the intervention was giving patients who were in nicotine withdrawal support. Nicotine replacement therapy doesn't completely stop the cravings, and talking to patients about how they are going with the withdrawal was really helpful.'

The program has become quite a success, with many people successfully quitting and not taking the habit up again. Malcolm and the program have also been recognised with awards.

'Just banning smoking is cruel but giving people "smoking leave" from the unit would just restart the withdrawal process again. What's the point in making people withdraw if there is no benefit for the person in the end? What we found was that many people actually wanted to quit and had found it really hard in the past. No one likes withdrawal symptoms, but in hindsight they were often very thankful that we supported them to actually start the quitting process properly.'

Critical thinking challenge 18.4

Discuss the following question: 'People with mental illness don't have much enjoyment in life, so why would you want to take another enjoyment away and encourage them to quit cigarettes?'

NUTRITION

Nutritional therapy in mental health treatment is a rapidly growing area in both the academic and clinical fields, with experts calling for nutritional medicine to be mainstream in mental health services (Sarris et al. 2015). People experiencing SMI have poorer diets when compared with the general population (Firth et al. 2018). This is a significant and, importantly, a modifiable factor that contributes to severe weight gain, subsequent poor cardiometabolic health and mortality gap in this population.

People with SMI commonly have diets lower in fruit and fibre and higher in saturated fat compared with the general population (Teasdale et al. 2019). Studies that assessed caloric intake found higher intakes in those with SMI (Firth et al. 2018), while evidence also demonstrated that the diets of those with SMI are lower in vegetable, legumes and dairy (Teasdale et al. 2019).

People receiving antipsychotic therapy commonly complain of significantly increased hunger and an inability to sense satiety (feeling full), particularly on clozapine and olanzapine (Kraus et al. 2014). These medications can affect ghrelin and leptin hormones, which regulate hunger and satiety (Potvin et al. 2015). The highest increases in leptin levels are seen in patients using antipsychotics that produce the most weight gain (Kraus et al. 2014).

Combining these factors with constant cravings for sugary or processed oily foods, low food preparation skills, low levels of motivation and often-restricted budgets provides a potent mix for weight gain and poor metabolic health. Additionally low mood and depression can also lead to overeating and 'comfort' eating (de Wit et al. 2015). Furthermore, people with SMI have lower basal metabolic rate than the general population, contributing to rapid weight gain (Cuerda et al. 2013). Additional dietary considerations for this population include fast-eating syndrome, disordered eating habits such as only eating one main meal per day, constipation and higher levels of dental and coeliac disease (Teasdale et al. 2017).

Given these dietary patterns and nutritional side effects, interventions that aim to reduce caloric intake and improve diet quality by increasing core foods and reducing discretionary foods can be seen as key factors in improving the physical health of those with SMI. Core foods in Australia reflect the five food groups: (1) vegetables, (2) fruit, (3) milk, cheese, yoghurt and alternatives, (4) lean meat, fish, poultry, eggs, seeds and nuts, and (5) grains, with some healthy oils such as olive oil. Discretionary foods reflect those that are high in energy (kilojoules/calories) and low in nutrients and are generally highly processed and refined foods (National Health and Medical Research Council 2013). Evidence has emerged demonstrating that people following a higher quality diet have better mental health, while those whose diet quality is lower have poorer psychological functioning (Begdache et al. 2019).

An alternative dietary pattern shown to be beneficial for mental health by preventing and/or reducing depressive symptoms is the Mediterranean diet (Parletta et al. 2019). The Mediterranean diet focuses on fruits and vegetables, fish, nuts/seeds, wholegrains, legumes, olive oil, feta cheese and moderate intakes of red wine, particularly with meals. In addition to improvements in mental health, this pattern of eating is protective for both type 2 diabetes and CVD (Estruch et al. 2013).

Key nutrients of concern in SMI include caffeine, omega-3 fatty-acids, folate and magnesium. Caffeine overconsumption is common in patients experiencing schizophrenia – they are twice as likely to consume more than 200 mg (2 cups of coffee) per day (Teasdale et al. 2019). There is currently no acceptable daily intake value for caffeine in Australia; however, a review performed by Food Standards Australia New Zealand suggests increased risk of anxiety at 95 mg (one cup of coffee or two cans of cola) per day for children and 210 mg for adults (Smith et al. 2000). Low levels of omega-3 fatty-acids, folate and magnesium have been linked with depression, with increased intake (oral or supplemented) proving to be an effective part of treatment (Casper 2011; Forsyth et al. 2012).

Nutrition interventions in people with SMI to date have generally been scarce; however, studies have demonstrated that nutrition interventions in both early intervention and longer term illness have reduced health risks (Teasdale et al. 2016; 2017). Although future studies need to assess the long-term impacts on anthropometric, biochemical and lifestyle (nutrition and exercise) measures, as well as quality of life, mental health symptomatology and readmission rates, there is enough evidence to support the use of nutrition interventions in combination with exercise as core components of mental health services.

Nutritional advice and support should be integrated into routine nursing care. When providing nutrition interventions it is crucial to provide both educational and practical components to ensure adequate knowledge but to also improve shopping, label reading, food safety and culinary (food preparation) skills. With patients particularly vulnerable to increased hunger, reduced satiety and cravings for high caloric convenience foods and drinks with little nutritional value, mindfulness-based activities may also prove to be an adjunctive intervention.

PHYSICAL ACTIVITY

Physical activity can be defined as any bodily movement produced by skeletal muscle resulting in an increased energy expenditure. The term 'physical activity' encompasses both structured forms of activity such as exercise and unstructured forms such as incidental activity. People experiencing mental illness are known to be less physically active than the general population and engage in prolonged periods of sedentary behaviour (Schuch et al. 2017; Stubbs et al. 2016). Low levels of physical activity are an established risk factor for cardiometabolic dysfunction including diabetes and obesity. In addition to low levels of physical activity, people with mental illness have poorer cardiorespiratory fitness in comparison with the general population, which is an established risk factor for all-cause mortality and morbidity (Bort-Roig et al. 2019). Given the high rates of premature mortality linked to preventable CVD within this population, evidence-based physical activity interventions aimed at reducing sedentary time, increasing overall activity and increasing moderate–vigorous physical activity participation should be considered part of routine care for people living with mental illness (Vancampfort et al. 2015b).

Physical activity and exercise have been shown to have beneficial effects on psychiatric symptomatology regardless of diagnosis, while a growing body of research has reported on the benefits of exercise for improving cognition (Sommer & Kahn 2015). Longitudinal studies have also highlighted the bidirectional relationship between activity and depressive symptoms (Pinto Pereira et al. 2014), with evidence of a protective effect of being physically active (Mammen & Faulkner 2013; Pinto Pereira et al. 2014).

Evidence-based strategies to increase physical activity among people with mental illness include behavioural techniques such as motivational interviewing, face-to-face and group-based exercise sessions (Rosenbaum et al. 2014). In addition structured exercise prescriptions and individualised interventions reflect individual variations in mood, motivation and access to facilities and resources (Lederman et al. 2017). Exercise is not a one-size-fits-all intervention, and a range of individual factors should be considered when developing individualised exercise interventions. Aside from physical limitations, factors to be considered are severity of psychiatric symptomatology, previous exercise history, motivation and access to services or facilities that may affect the modality and intensity of exercise that individuals are able to undertake (Stubbs et al. 2017).

Exercise is a structured subset of physical activity, and exercise prescriptions are typically described according to the 'FITT' principle (frequency, intensity, time and type) while incorporating appropriate goal-setting strategies. The International Organization of Physical Therapists in Mental Health (IOPTMH) recommends that adults aim for 150 minutes per week of moderate intensity physical activity or 75 minutes of moderate–vigorous activity in addition to muscle strengthening activities on at least 2 days per week (Vancampfort et al. 2012). Further, the IOPTMH advocates that patients should avoid physical inactivity, noting that some level of physical activity regardless of intensity is better than none (Vancampfort et al. 2012). People with SMI should be supported and encouraged to adhere to physical activity recommendations; however, there is growing consensus that such recommendations may be aspirational and unrealistic for many people living with SMI. Positive messaging around pragmatic goals such as breaking up sitting time throughout the day and aiming to increase short-duration walking should be routinely promoted (Vancampfort et al. 2015a; 2015b). Mental health nurses are well positioned to provide exercise advice and physical activity counselling to mental health consumers (Happell et al. 2014; Stanton et al. 2015). Examples of pragmatic interventions include using objective monitoring devices such as pedometers (or commercially available accelerometers), individualised advice on ways to accumulate greater light physical activity such as rising from a chair and moving during television commercial breaks or adding 5-minute walks at structured and specified points throughout the day. This may include, for example, taking less direct routes while walking to dining rooms within inpatient facilities (Vancampfort et al. 2015b). Although such limited interventions may appear trivial, encouraging small and incremental changes may better position sedentary people with SMI to transition to brief bouts of moderate intensity activity that will help them to achieve guideline-specified targets.

Respiratory diseases

Respiratory diseases were the leading cause of death in psychiatric institutions up until the 1970s (Brown 1997). Today, respiratory diseases are still more prevalent in people with SMI, with approximately one in three people having either restrictive or obstructive lung disease, a rate double the general population prevalence rate (Partti et al. 2015). The likelihood of developing pneumonia is also considerably raised (Partti et al. 2015). Not only are these conditions far more common in people experiencing SMI but they are more likely to lead to mortality (Schoepf et al. 2014). Tobacco smoking is closely associated with an increased risk of respiratory diseases and, in particular, influences chronic obstructive pulmonary disorder in its development and progression as well as mixed forms of asthma (Schoepf et al. 2014).

Respiratory assessment is an essential component of a physical health assessment and nurses should be vigilant and maintain regular and timely screening for respiratory conditions. Additional support and referral may be required, with consideration given to modifiable risk factors such as tobacco smoking, which is closely linked to increased cardiometabolic health risk factors. Physical activity should be promoted, since it might delay decline in lung function (Gartner & Hall 2015). Influenza is a potentially manageable public health issue that can lead to serious respiratory disease and death. Routine influenza vaccination should be encouraged among people with SMI (Partti et al. 2015). Information about influenza vaccination is readily available on government websites in Australia (www.flusmart.org.au) and in New Zealand (www.influenza.org.nz), and nurses need to ensure patients who they work with are vaccinated.

Critical thinking challenge 18.5

You are a nurse working on a busy acute mental health unit who is aware of the importance of influenza vaccination. What strategies could you develop to improve the vaccination rates of the staff and patients on the unit?

CASE STUDY 18.1
'Keeping the Body in Mind'

The Early Psychosis Program is located at the Bondi Centre in Sydney. It works with young people between the ages of 15 and 25 in the early stages of psychotic illness. The team works with an interdisciplinary model within a community mental health service.

Nurses working with young people experiencing their first episode of psychosis at the Bondi Centre were extremely concerned that, while atypical antipsychotic medications were successful in alleviating people of many of the troubling symptoms of mental illness, they also appeared to be correlated with rapid weight gain and subsequent longer term risks of diabetes and heart disease.

'We responded to these alarms by developing an assessment tool to measure changes in weight and other metabolic abnormalities. What we found was that young people were all too commonly putting on 10–20 kg and sometimes more within their first year with the service and that alterations in a person's metabolic health deteriorated rapidly with this weight gain. These issues included elevated cholesterol and hypertension. Blood glucose levels in the body may become raised, putting these young people at much higher risk of developing diabetes.'

Nursing staff also noticed that the young people were experiencing increased rates of stigma and poor self-esteem. This was like a 'double whammy' because a young person who was dealing with a new mental health diagnosis, and the fact that they have to take psychiatric medication was also trying to deal with transformations to their body image. This affected their personal lives, impacting on work, study and socialisation.

'We realised that just assessing people's health was inadequate. We actually needed to make a difference and so we adopted a mantra of 'don't just screen, intervene'.'

Working in conjunction with a multidisciplinary team, nursing staff established a number of lifestyle interventions and a program called 'Keeping the Body in Mind' (KBIM). This program aimed to prevent weight gain and the accompanying deterioration in metabolic health that might in future lead to heart disease and diabetes. The program is coordinated by a clinical nurse consultant and utilises an exercise physiologist, a dietitian and a peer support worker. The lifestyle intervention program encompasses three elements including health coaching, dietetic support and a supervised exercise program, which are delivered with an interconnected approach. Each participant's intervention program is tailored to suit the individual.

The program was recently evaluated in a controlled study comparing it against another early psychosis service. The KBIM program was compared against a similar early psychosis program in Sydney, with the exception of the metabolic intervention. Participants in the KBIM group were provided 12-week individualised lifestyle program, while the comparison group (n = 12) received standard care. The evaluation study established that the KBIM group had considerably less weight gain at 12 weeks (an average of 1.8 kg over 12 weeks) compared with standard care (an average of 7.8 kg). Only 13% per cent of the intervention group experienced clinically significant weight gain (greater than 7% of baseline weight) compared with 75% in the non-intervention group.

Source: Curtis et al. 2015

Oral health

Oral health is integral to general health and essential for wellbeing. It influences eating, physical appearance, speech and other social and psychological factors (Moore et al. 2015). Oral health issues include hygiene, dental caries (cavities), periodontal disease, dental trauma and oral cancers (Kisely et al. 2011). Oral health also plays a vital role in cardiometabolic health, with periodontal disease increasing the risk of type 2 diabetes, coronary heart disease and stroke (Moore et al. 2015). People with SMI experience markedly higher rates of oral health problems compared with the general population (McKibbin et al. 2015). The reasons that this population have poorer oral health outcomes in comparison with the general population are multifaceted (Tang et al. 2015). Many psychotropic medications can reduce the amount of saliva the mouth produces, leading to a dry mouth or xerostomia (McKibbin et al. 2015). Xerostomia is associated with an increase in periodontal disease (Moore et al. 2015). Symptoms of mental illness such as depression, amotivation and cognitive impairment can lead to an apathy around dental hygiene, and considerably lower rates of regular teeth brushing and flossing is observed in people with SMI (McKibbin et al. 2015). People with SMI are also more likely to be smokers and consume sugary carbonated drinks, both of which increase the likelihood of dental disease (Kisely et al. 2015).

Nursing management of oral health

People with SMI are less likely to seek dental treatment than the general population, especially for preventative dental work (Tang et al. 2015). Given the higher risk of dental disease in this population, it is essential that people with SMI attend to dental care more frequently than general public recommendations (Moore et al. 2015). Mental health nurses have a clear role in encouraging and facilitating access to dental services. This is particularly important in Australia and New Zealand where most dental services are private and financially out of reach for many people with SMI; people will often require assistance in accessing public dental schemes. It is also important that nurses use clinical interactions as an opportunity to promote oral health as a vital part of general health. Health promotion that focuses on smoking, diet, alcohol use and dental hygiene should be routinely incorporated into mental health nursing care (Moore et al. 2015).

Critical thinking challenge 18.6

Consider and discuss the social and economic factors that influence an individual's oral health. Consider what nursing actions/strategies you could develop to change these factors.

Sleep

Good sleep is essential to good physical and mental health. Sleep disturbance is a symptom of almost every mental disorder from anxiety disorders through to mood disorders and psychosis (Spiegelhalder et al. 2013). Though its significance is often under-recognised (Tobin & Tobin 2017), sleep disturbance can be one of the more distressing and persistent symptoms of mental disorder. Sleep disturbance can also present as one of the first signs of mental illness exacerbation (Ruhrmann et al. 2010). Poor sleep can also independently contribute to causing a mental illness and impede recovery from mental illness (Plante & Winkelman 2008). Recognising and treating sleep disturbances can therefore be critical to the primary or secondary prevention of mental disorders and their treatment.

Sleep disturbance

What is normal sleep? Each person has a different sleep requirement and this changes over the life span. On average, most adults need 7–8 hours; children and adolescents 9–10 hours per night and children 11–13 hours or more, depending on their age (Colten & Altebogt 2006). **Insomnia** is the most common sleep disturbance and is a core feature of mood disorders; it frequently complicates anxiety disorders and psychosis. Anxiety and severe depression are commonly associated with sleep disturbance (Shanahan et al. 2014). In schizophrenia, the sleep cycle is often disturbed, with fragmented sleep throughout the cycle or even reversal of the sleep–wake cycle so that most sleep occurs during the day (Afonso et al. 2014). **Hypersomnia** (excessive sleep) is less common but can occur in depression and in some cases of bipolar disorder (Kanady et al. 2015). Hypersomnia can also occur secondary to some treatments of mental illness, which have sedative side effects.

Given the high rates of obesity in people with mental disorders, the risk of obstructive sleep apnoea in this population is high, so it is important to screen for and treat this disorder (Kalucy et al. 2013). Obstructive sleep apnoea is the most common form of sleep disorder breathing. Untreated, it is associated with high morbidity and mortality due to increased risks of cardio- and cerebrovascular disease, and worsening of diabetes and hypertension (Carroll et al. 2015)

Critical thinking challenge 18.7

In what ways might poor sleep impede a person's mental health recovery? What nursing strategies can you implement to improve sleep for some who is experiencing insomnia?

Nursing assessment and intervention of sleep disorders

The most important primary action for nurses is to ask about a person's sleep. Depending on the clinical setting, there may be an option for nurses to take an active role in diagnosing and managing sleep problems. There are a number of useful screening and diagnostic tools, the most simple of which is a sleep diary (freely downloadable from the internet e.g. http://yoursleep.aasmnet.org/pdf/sleepdiary.pdf) in which the person documents times spent sleeping and other influential activities such as caffeine and alcohol intake, exercise and sedentary activities such as electronic screen time.

In established sleep disorders, nurses may play an important role in encouraging patients to manage any lifestyle issues that could be contributing to their sleep problems (see Box 18.3) Sedative/hypnotic medications have a place but should not necessarily be the first form of treatment offered. Benzodiazepines have a propensity for addiction and are associated with an increased risk of falls among other serious potential side effects (see Chapter 19 for more about medications and their sedative effects).

Sexual health

Sexuality and sexual health are important aspects of every person's health and wellbeing. Sexuality is a complex issue

Box 18.3 Principles of sleep hygiene

- Go to sleep and wake up at roughly the same time each day.
- Maintain regular meal times.
- Avoid daytime naps.
- Don't eat a big meal or exercise within 2 hours of going to bed.
- Avoid caffeinated drinks after midday.
- Minimise alcohol and cease smoking.
- Ensure the bedroom is comfortable, dark, quiet and safe and used for only sleep and sex.
- Engage in exercise (avoid this at night) and exposure to bright outside light each day, preferably in the morning.
- Do not share the bed with children or pets.
- If sleep is not achieved within 20–30 minutes of going to bed, get up and do something relaxing for a few minutes and then try again when feeling sleepy.
- Ensure medications are taken as directed because some can cause sedation or arousal.
- Avoid stimulating activities before bedtime such as watching a violent TV program or exposure to the blue light emitted by computer or tablet screens.

Adapted from Malcolm 2005

that encompasses not only the physical activity of sex but also gender identity, values and beliefs (Urry et al. 2019). Contrary to common belief, most people with SMI show an interest in sex that differs little from the general population (de Boer et al. 2015). High-risk sexual behaviours are more likely to be observed in people with SMI, including unprotected intercourse, multiple partners, involvement in sex work and illicit drug use (Pandor et al. 2015). The rates of blood-borne viruses such as HIV and hepatitis C have been found to be higher among people with SMI (Essock et al. 2014).

Social and interpersonal impairments commonly occur in people with SMI and limit the development of stable sexual relationships. Men with SMI in particular have poorer social outcomes, less frequent (sexual) relationships and fewer offspring than the general population (de Boer et al. 2015). Women with SMI are more likely to have relatively chaotic patterns of sexual behaviours and a higher rate of non-consensual sex than their counterparts without SMI (Pandor et al. 2015). An Australian study indicates that women with SMI were far less likely to use effective contraception methods and had on average three unplanned pregnancies (Hauck et al. 2014).

Another study based in New Zealand identified that mental health nurses don't ask about sex-related topics, with the authors concluding that mental health staff need to commit to being responsive to this important aspect of a person's wellbeing and health (Davison & Huntington 2010). This was echoed in an Australian report that found mental health nurses are reluctant to bring up the topic of sexual health (Quinn et al. 2011). To enable you to feel comfortable and confident to discuss sexual health you will need to identify any personal issues that affect your ability to openly discuss sexual health and increase your knowledge of sexual issues. Common issues that affect a person's sexuality and sexual health include sexually transmitted infections, body image, gender identity, physiological changes, medications and stigma (de Boer et al. 2015).

Critical thinking challenge 18.8

Consider and discuss social, cultural and religious beliefs that influence a person's sexuality.

Consider your own personal beliefs about sexuality. Do you have any preconceived ideas about mental illness and sexuality? Do you have any concerns about conducting a sexual health assessment?

Medication and sex

Medication-induced sexual dysfunction is a common but largely ignored side effect of most psychotropic medications (Urry et al. 2019). Psychotropic medications are linked with sexual dysfunction including low libido, delayed ejaculation, orgasm problems like anorgasmia, and impaired erection (Bella & Shamloul 2013; de Boer et al. 2015). Medication-induced sexual dysfunctions can lead to issues with relationships, medication adherence and quality of life (Hendry et al. 2018). Despite people with SMI considering sexual health issues to be highly relevant, it is important to remember that it is likely that issues like sexual dysfunction are unlikely to be discussed, often due to the reluctance of health professionals and mental health nurses to talk about sex (Hendry et al. 2018). This often leads to an underestimation of their prevalence and contributing to decreased adherence to treatment (de Boer et al. 2015). Chapter 19 discusses psychotropic medication and its side effects.

Sexual health screening

Health screening includes preventative testing or investigation to prevent or ameliorate future problems. Sexual health screening includes breast, prostate, cervical and sexually transmitted infection screening. Mental health nurses can play an important role in health screening, particularly when access to services is challenging for the person with mental illness. Mental health nurses can refer people directly to a health screening service or they can provide the health assessment. Nurses can offer advice about preventing the contraction and spread of sexually transmitted infections by providing education on safe sex such as the correct use of condoms (Pandor et al. 2015).

Breast, prostate and cervical screening services are generally offered by public health services. Given the vulnerability of clients with SMI around their sexual health, it is essential that nurses include sexual health screening as part of holistic care. Nurses should reflect on any personal attitudes or beliefs that might be creating barriers that impede a thorough sexual health assessment.

When psychiatric symptoms are not a mental illness

Confusion, vision problems, and behaviour changes can be common symptoms for many mental illnesses, but they are also common symptoms of brain tumours, infectious diseases and dehydration. Correct assessment that includes history taking and checking with relatives will lead to correct diagnoses and not missing a physical health issue (see Chapter 7 for more details of accurate assessment). Other medical conditions that may present with psychiatric conditions include Wilson's disease (a hereditary metabolic disorder), Graves' disease and HIV (McKee & Brahm 2016). Chapter 16 discusses the symptom similarities that can occur with depression, delirium and dementia.

Chapter summary

People who experience SMI have far higher rates of morbidity and mortality across nearly all chronic health conditions. This chapter has highlighted the importance of promoting, assessing and maintaining optimum physical health for people with SMI. Specific health assessments have been highlighted – sexual health, oral health, sleep, metabolic syndrome, CVD, diabetes and respiratory disease; however, it is important to remember that a full physical assessment, including routine health screening, is an essential element of holistic mental health care.

The vital role that nurses can play in improving preventable illness and disease is clear. People with SMI have physical health outcomes that are far worse than the general population. If we are to improve the unacceptable life expectancy gap that is currently experienced by those with an SMI, mental health nurses need to address this important issue with primary health messages and interventions. Smoking cessation, diet and exercise advice are core interventions crucially required for preventing premature CVD. Awareness and advocating for the screening and intervention of other areas of physical health, especially respiratory, sexual, oral and sleep, is extremely important to improve overall quality of life. Early intervention and prevention of physical health conditions is key to improving the outcomes of people with mental illness. Mental health nurses need to prioritise physical health care as one of their primary responsibilities, and this involves taking the time to listen and support people's needs in a holistic way.

EXERCISES FOR CLASS ENGAGEMENT

1. Maintaining optimum physical health is multifaceted and essential to wellbeing, and nurses play an important role in assessing, treating and preventing physical health issues. Working in groups discuss the following statements:
   - Sexual health is a human right.
   - Metabolic syndrome is preventable.
   - Oral health is an important part of overall health.
   - People with schizophrenia are likely to die 20–25 years earlier than the general population.
   - SMI is as much a risk factor of cardiovascular risk as a diagnosis of diabetes.
2. Working with your group, develop nursing interventions and strategies to ensure the issues listed in the statements are assessed, treated and not overlooked. Consider what resources you will need to implement the strategies you have identified. Are there any barriers? How can these barriers be overcome?

Useful websites

Australian Dental Association: http://www.ada.org.au/.
Equally Well Australia: https://www.equallywell.org.au.
Equally Well New Zealand: https://www.tepou.co.nz/initiatives/equally-well-physical-health/37.
International Diabetes Federation: http://www.idf.org/.
Keeping the Body in Mind in Youth with Psychosis: http://www.iphys.org.au/.
Mental Health Foundation of Australia: http://www.mhfa.org.au/main.htm.
Mental Health Foundation of New Zealand: http://www.mentalhealth.org.nz/.
New Zealand Dental Association: http://www.healthysmiles.org.nz/.
Sexual Health & Family Planning Australia: http://www.shfpa.org.au/.
Sleep diary: http://yoursleep.aasmnet.org/pdf/sleepdiary.pdf.
The New Zealand Sexual Health Society Incorporated: http://www.nzshs.org/.
World Health Organization: http://www.who.int/en/.

References

Afonso, P., Figueira, M.L., Paiva, T., 2014. Sleep–wake patterns in schizophrenia patients compared to healthy controls. World J. Biol. Psychiatry 15 (7), 517–524.
Alberti, K., Zimmet, P., Shaw, J., 2005. The metabolic syndrome – a new worldwide definition. Lancet 366 (9491), 1059–1062.
Alvarez-Jiménez, M., González-Blanch, C., Crespo-Facorro, B., et al., 2008. Antipsychotic-induced weight gain in chronic and first-episode psychotic disorders:

a systematic critical reappraisal. CNS Drugs 22 (7), 547–562.
Aschbrenner, K.A., Brunette, M.F., McElvery, R., et al., 2015. Cigarette smoking and interest in quitting among overweight and obese adults with serious mental illness enrolled in a fitness intervention. J. Nerv. Ment. Dis. 203 (6), 473–476.
Ashton, M., Rigby, A., Galletly, C., 2013. What do 1000 smokers with mental illness say about their tobacco use? Aust. N. Z. J. Psychiatry 47 (7), 631–636.
Bak, M., Fransen, A., Janssen, J., et al., 2014. Almost all antipsychotics result in weight gain: a meta-analysis. PLoS ONE 9 (4), e94112.
Begdache, L., Chaar, M., Sabounchi, N., et al., 2019. Assessment of dietary factors, dietary practices and exercise on mental distress in young adults versus matured adults: a cross-sectional study. Nutr. Neurosci. 22 (7), 488–498.
Bella, A.J., Shamloul, R., 2013. Psychotropics and sexual dysfunction. Cent. European J. Urol. 66 (4), 466.
Bort-Roig, J., Briones-Buixassa, L., Felez-Nobrega, M., et al., 2019. Sedentary behaviour associations with health outcomes in people with severe mental illness: a systematic review. Eur. J. Public Health 30 (1), 150–157.
Brown, S., 1997. Excess mortality of schizophrenia: a meta-analysis. Br. J. Psychiatry 171, 502–508.
Brown, S., Kim, M., Mitchell, C., et al., 2010. Twenty-five year mortality of a community cohort with schizophrenia. Br. J. Psychiatry 196 (2), 116–121.
Callaghan, R.C., Veldhuizen, S., Jeysingh, T., et al., 2014. Patterns of tobacco-related mortality among individuals diagnosed with schizophrenia, bipolar disorder, or depression. J. Psychiatr. Res. 48 (1), 102–110.
Carroll, J.E., Irwin, M.R., Merkin, S.S., et al., 2015. Sleep and multisystem biological risk: a population-based study. PLoS ONE 10 (2), e0118467.
Casper, R.C., 2011. Diet and mental health: an up-to-date analysis. World Rev. Nutr. Diet. 102, 98–113.
Cimo, A., Dewa, C.S., 2018. Symptoms of mental illness and their impact on managing type 2 diabetes in adults. Can. J. Diabetes 42 (4), 372–381.
Colten, H.R., Altebogt, B.M. (Eds.), 2006. Sleep Disorders and Sleep Deprivation, an Unmet Public Health Problem. The National Academies Press, Washington, DC.
Cooper, S.J., Reynolds, G.P., 2016. BAP guidelines on the management of weight gain, metabolic disturbances and cardiovascular risk associated with psychosis and antipsychotic drug treatment. J. Psychopharmacol. (Oxford) 30 (8), 717–748.
Correll, C.U., Manu, P., Olshanskiy, V., et al., 2009. Cardiometabolic risk of second-generation antipsychotic medications during first-time use in children and adolescents. JAMA 302 (16), 1765–1773.
Correll, C.U., Solmi, M., Veronese, N., et al., 2017. Prevalence, incidence and mortality from cardiovascular disease in patients with pooled and specific severe mental illness: a large-scale meta-analysis of 3,211,768 patients and 113,383,368 controls. World Psychiatry 16 (2), 163–180.
Cuerda, C., Velasco, C., Merchan-Naranjo, J., et al., 2014. The effects of second-generation antipsychotics on food intake, resting energy expenditure and physical activity. Eur. J. Clin. Nutr. 68 (2), 146–152.
Cuerda, C., Velasco, C., Merchán-Naranjo, J., et al., 2013. The effects of second-generation antipsychotics on food intake, resting energy expenditure and physical activity. Eur. J. Clin. Nutr. 68, 146–152.
Cunningham, R., Sarfati, D., Peterson, D., et al., 2014. Premature mortality in adults using New Zealand psychiatric services. N. Z. Med. J. 127 (1394), 31–41.
Curtis, J., Newall, H.D., Samaras, K., 2012. The heart of the matter: cardiometabolic care in youth with psychosis. Early Interv. Psychiatry.
Curtis, J.E., Newall, H., Samaras, K., 2010. Positive cardiometabolic health: an early intervention framework for patients on psychotropic medications. Early Interv. Psychiatry 4 (Suppl. 1), 60.
Curtis, J., Watkins, A., Rosenbaum, S., et al., 2015. Evaluating an individualized lifestyle and life skills intervention to prevent antipsychotic-induced weight gain in first-episode psychosis. Early Interv. Psychiatry 10 (3), 267–276.
Curtis, J., Zhang, C., McGuigan, B., et al., 2018. y-QUIT: smoking prevalence, engagement and effectiveness of an individualized smoking cessation intervention in youth with severe mental illness. Front. Psychiatry 9, 683.
Darnton, R., 1968. Mesmerism and the End of the Enlightenment in France. Harvard University Press, Cambridge.
Davison, J., Huntington, A., 2010. 'Out of sight': sexuality and women with enduring mental illness. Int. J. Ment. Health Nurs. 19 (4), 240–249.
de Boer, M.K., Castelein, S., Wiersma, D., et al., 2015. The facts about sexual (dys) function in schizophrenia: an overview of clinically relevant findings. Schizophr. Bull. 41 (3), 674–686.
De Hert, M., Vancampfort, D., Correll, C.U., et al., 2011. Guidelines for screening and monitoring of cardiometabolic risk in schizophrenia: systematic evaluation. Br. J. Psychiatry 199 (2), 99–105.
de Wit, L.M., van Straten, A., Lamers, F., et al., 2015. Depressive and anxiety disorders: associated with losing or gaining weight over 2 years? Psychiatry Res. 227 (2), 230–237.
Erlangsen, A., Andersen, P.K., Toender, A., et al., 2017. Cause-specific life-years lost in people with mental disorders: a nationwide, register-based cohort study. Lancet Psychiatry 4 (12), 937–945.
Essock, S.M., Dowden, S., Constantine, N.T., et al., 2014. Blood-borne infections and persons with mental illness: risk factors for HIV, hepatitis B, and hepatitis C among persons with severe mental illness. Psychiatr. Serv. 54 (6), 827–835.
Estruch, R., Ros, E., Salas-Salvadó, J., et al., 2013. Primary prevention of cardiovascular disease with a Mediterranean diet. N. Engl. J. Med. 368 (14), 1279–1290.

Firth, J., Siddiqi, N., Koyanagi, A., et al., 2019. The Lancet Psychiatry Commission: a blueprint for protecting physical health in people with mental illness. Lancet Psychiatry 6 (8), 675–712.

Firth, J., Stubbs, B., Teasdale, S.B., et al., 2018. Diet as a hot topic in psychiatry: a population-scale study of nutritional intake and inflammatory potential in severe mental illness. World Psychiatry 17 (3), 365.

Forsyth, A.K., Williams, P.G., Deane, F.P., 2012. Nutrition status of primary care patients with depression and anxiety. Aust. J. Prim. Health 18 (2), 172–176.

Galletly, C.A., Foley, D.L., Waterreus, A., et al., 2012. Cardiometabolic risk factors in people with psychotic disorders: the second Australian national survey of psychosis. Aust. N. Z. J. Psychiatry 46 (8), 753–761.

Gartner, C., Hall, W., 2015. Tobacco harm reduction in people with serious mental illnesses. Lancet Psychiatry 2 (6), 485–487.

Gates, J., Killackey, E., Phillips, L., et al., 2015. Mental health starts with physical health: current status and future directions of non-pharmacological interventions to improve physical health in first-episode psychosis. Lancet Psychiatry 2 (8), 726–742.

Gatov, E., Rosella, L., Chiu, M., et al., 2017. Trends in standardized mortality among individuals with schizophrenia, 1993–2012: a population-based, repeated cross-sectional study. CMAJ 189 (37), E1177–E1187.

Gilbody, S., Peckham, E., Man, M.S., et al., 2015. Bespoke smoking cessation for people with severe mental ill health (SCIMITAR): a pilot randomised controlled trial. Lancet Psychiatry 2 (5), 395–402.

Glassman, A.H., Bigger, J.T., Jr., 2014. Antipsychotic drugs: prolonged QTc interval, torsade de pointes, and sudden death. Am. J. Psychiatry 158 (11), 1774–1782.

Gordon-Dseagu, V.L., Mindell, J.S., Steptoe, A., et al., 2015. Impaired glucose metabolism among those with and without diagnosed diabetes and mortality: a cohort study using health survey for England data. PLoS ONE 10 (3).

Happell, B., Stanton, R., Hoey, W., et al., 2014. Cardiometabolic health nursing to improve health and primary care access in community mental health consumers: baseline physical health outcomes from a randomised controlled trial. Issues Ment. Health Nurs. 35 (2), 114–121.

Hasan, S.S., Clavarino, A.M., Mamun, A.A., et al., 2014. Incidence and risk of diabetes mellitus associated with depressive symptoms in adults: evidence from longitudinal studies. Diabetes Metab. Syndr. 8 (2), 82–87.

Hauck, Y., Nguyen, T., Frayne, J., et al., 2014. Sexual and reproductive health trends among women with enduring mental illness: a survey of Western Australian community mental health services. Health Care Women Int. 36 (4), 499–510.

Hayes, J.F., Marston, L., Walters, K., et al., 2017. Mortality gap for people with bipolar disorder and schizophrenia: UK-based cohort study 2000–2014. Br. J. Psychiatry 211 (3), 175–181.

Hendry, A., Snowden, A., Brown, M., 2018. When holistic care is not holistic enough: the role of sexual health in mental health settings. J. Clin. Nurs. 27 (5–6), 1015–1027.

Hjorth, P., Davidsen, A., Kilian, R., et al., 2014. A systematic review of controlled interventions to reduce overweight and obesity in people with schizophrenia. Acta Psychiatr. Scand. 130 (4), 279–289.

Holt, R.I., Mitchell, A.J., 2014. Diabetes mellitus and severe mental illness: mechanisms and clinical implications. Nat. Rev. Endocrinol. 11 (2), 79–89.

Ignaszewski, M., Yip, A., Fitzpatrick, S., 2015. Schizophrenia and coronary artery disease. B. C. Med. J. 57 (4), 154–157.

Jones, D.R., Macias, C., Barreira, P.J., et al., 2014. Prevalence, severity, and co-occurrence of chronic physical health problems of persons with serious mental illness. Psychiatr. Serv. 55 (11), 1250–1257.

Kalucy, M.J., Grunstein, R., Lambert, T., et al., 2013. Obstructive sleep apnoea and schizophrenia: a research agenda. Sleep Med. Rev. 17 (5), 357–365.

Kanady, J., Soehnera, A.M., Harvey, A.G., 2015. A retrospective examination of sleep disturbance across the course of bipolar disorder. J. Sleep Disord. Ther. 4 (2), 193.

Kaur, J., 2014. A comprehensive review on metabolic syndrome. Cardiol. Res. Pract. 943162. doi:10.1155/2014/943162. [Epub 2014 Mar 11].

Kisely, S., Baghaie, H., Lalloo, R., et al., 2015. A systematic review and meta-analysis of the association between poor oral health and severe mental illness. Psychosom. Med. 77 (1), 83–92.

Kisely, S., Quek, L.H., Pais, J., et al., 2011. Advanced dental disease in people with severe mental illness: systematic review and meta-analysis. Br. J. Psychiatry 199 (3), 187–193.

Kraus, T., Haack, M., Schuld, A., et al., 2014. Body weight and leptin plasma levels during treatment with antipsychotic drugs. Am. J. Psychiatry 156 (2), 312–314.

Langan, J., Smith, D.J., 2014. Cardiovascular morbidity and mortality in schizophrenia: implications for primary care. Prim. Care Cardiovasc. J. 7 (1), 23.

Lawrence, D., Hancock, K.J., Kisely, S., 2013. The gap in life expectancy from preventable physical illness in psychiatric patients in Western Australia: retrospective analysis of population based registers. BMJ 346, f2539.

Lederman, O., Suetani, S., Stanton, R., et al., 2017. Embedding exercise interventions as routine mental health care: implementation strategies in residential, inpatient and community settings. Australas. Psychiatry 25 (5), 451–455.

Lichtman, J.H., Froelicher, E.S., Blumenthal, J.A., et al., 2014. Depression as a risk factor for poor prognosis among patients with acute coronary syndrome: systematic review and recommendations a scientific statement from the American Heart Association. Circulation 129 (12), 1350–1369.

Lin, S.T., Chen, C.C., Tsang, H.Y., et al., 2014. Association between antipsychotic use and risk of acute myocardial

infarction: a nationwide case-crossover study. Circulation 130 (3), 235–243.
Lockett, H., Bagnall, C., Cunningham, R., et al., 2017. Cardiovascular disease risk and management in people who experience serious mental illness. Int. J. Integr. Care 17 (3), A158.
Lucatch, A.M., Lowe, D.J.E., Clark, R., et al., 2018. Neurobiological determinants of tobacco smoking in schizophrenia. Front. Psychiatry 9, 672.
Lum, A., Skelton, E., Wynne, O., et al., 2018. A systematic review of psychosocial barriers to smoking cessation in people living with schizophrenia. Front. Psychiatry 9, 565.
Malcolm, A., 2005. The nurse role in managing and treating sleep disorders. Nurs. Times 101 (23), 34–37.
Mammen, G., Faulkner, G., 2013. Physical activity and the prevention of depression: a systematic review of prospective studies. Am. J. Prev. Med. 45 (5), 649–657.
Manderbacka, K., Arffman, M., Lumme, S., et al., 2018. The effect of history of severe mental illness on mortality in colorectal cancer cases: a register-based cohort study. Acta Oncol. (Madr) 57 (6), 759–764.
Mather, B., Roche, M., Duffield, C., 2014. Disparities in treatment of people with mental disorder in non-psychiatric hospitals: a review of the literature. Arch. Psychiatr. Nurs. 28 (2), 80–86.
McKee, J., Brahm, N., 2016. Medical mimics: differential diagnostic considerations for psychiatric symptoms. Ment. Health Clin. 6 (6), 289–296.
McKibbin, C.L., Kitchen-Andren, K.A., Lee, A.A., et al., 2015. Oral health in adults with serious mental illness: needs for and perspectives on care. Community Ment. Health J. 51 (2), 222–228.
Mental Health Commission New Zealand, 2012. Blueprint II. improving mental health and wellbeing for all New Zealanders. How things need to be. Wellington, MHCNZ.
Mineur, Y.S., Picciotto, M.R., 2010. Nicotine receptors and depression: revisiting and revising the cholinergic hypothesis. Trends Pharmacol. Sci. 31 (12), 580–586.
Montejo, A.L., Montejo, L., Baldwin, D.S., 2018. The impact of severe mental disorders and psychotropic medications on sexual health and its implications for clinical management. World Psychiatry 17 (1), 3–11.
Morgan, V., McGrath, J., Jablensky, A., et al., 2013. Psychosis prevalence and physical, metabolic and cognitive co-morbidity: data from the second Australian national survey of psychosis. Psychol. Med. 44 (10), 2163–2176.
Morgan, V.A., Waterreus, A., Jablensky, A., et al., 2012. People living with psychotic illness in 2010: the second Australian national survey of psychosis. Aust. N. Z. J. Psychiatry 46 (8), 735–752.
Moore, S., Shiers, D., Daly, B., et al., 2015. Promoting physical health for people with schizophrenia by reducing disparities in medical and dental care. Acta Psychiatr. Scand. 132 (2), 109–121.
Myles, N., Newall, H.D., Curtis, J., et al., 2012. Tobacco use before, at, and after first-episode psychosis: a systematic meta-analysis. J. Clin. Psychiatry 73 (4), 468–475.
National Health and Medical Research Council, 2013. Australian dietary guidelines. Canberra: NHMRC. Available from: https://www.nhmrc.gov.au/_files_nhmrc/file/publications/n55_australian_dietary_guideli.
National Mental Health Commission, 2013. A contributing life: the 2013 national report card on mental health and suicide prevention. Sydney, NMHC.
Pandor, A., Kaltenthaler, E., Higgins, A., et al., 2015. Sexual health risk reduction interventions for people with severe mental illness: a systematic review. BMC Public Health 15 (1), 138.
Parletta, N., Zarnowiecki, D., Cho, J., et al., 2019. A Mediterranean-style dietary intervention supplemented with fish oil improves diet quality and mental health in people with depression: a randomized controlled trial (HELFIMED). Nutr. Neurosci. 22 (7), 474–487.
Partti, K., Vasankari, T., Kanervisto, M., et al., 2015. Lung function and respiratory diseases in people with psychosis: population-based study. Br. J. Psychiatry 1, 9.
Peckham, E., Brabyn, S., Cook, L., et al., 2017. Smoking cessation in severe mental ill health: what works? an updated systematic review and meta-analysis. BMC Psychiatry 17 (1), 252.
Pinto Pereira, S.M., Geoffroy, M., Power, C., 2014. Depressive symptoms and physical activity during 3 decades in adult life: bidirectional associations in a prospective cohort study. JAMA Psychiatry 71 (12), 1373–1380.
Plante, D.T., Winkelman, J.W., 2008. Sleep disturbance in bipolar disorder: therapeutic implications. Am. J. Psychiatry 165 (7), 830–843.
Potvin, S., Zhornitsky, S., Stip, E., 2015. Antipsychotic-induced changes in blood levels of leptin in schizophrenia: a meta-analysis. Can. J. Psychiatry 60 (3 Suppl. 2), S26.
Quinn, C., Happell, B., Browne, G., 2011. Talking or avoiding? Mental health nurses views about discussing sexual health with consumers. Int. J. Ment. Health Nurs. 20 (1), 21–28.
Rathmann, W., Pscherer, S., Konrad, M., et al., 2015. Diabetes treatment in people with type 2 diabetes and schizophrenia: retrospective primary care database analyses. Prim. Care Diabetes 10 (1), 36–40.
Reilly, S., Olier, I., Planner, C., et al., 2015. Inequalities in physical comorbidity: a longitudinal comparative cohort study of people with severe mental illness in the UK. BMJ Open 5 (12), e009010.
Reininghaus, U., Dutta, R., Dazzan, P., et al., 2015. Mortality in schizophrenia and other psychoses: a 10-year follow-up of the æsop first-episode cohort. Schizophr. Bull. 41 (3), 664–673.
Ribe, A.R., Laursen, T.M., Sandbæk, A., et al., 2014. Long-term mortality of persons with severe mental illness and diabetes: a population-based cohort study in Denmark. Psychol. Med. 44 (14), 3097–3107.
Ringen, P.A., Engh, J.A., Birkenaes, A.B., et al., 2014. Increased mortality in schizophrenia due to cardiovascular disease – a non-systematic review of epidemiology, possible causes, and interventions. Front. Psychiatry 5, 137.

Rosenbaum, S., Tiedemann, A., Sherrington, C., et al., 2014. Physical activity interventions for people with mental illness: a systematic review and meta-analysis. J. Clin. Psychiatry 75 (9), 964–974.

Ruhrmann, S., Schultze-Lutter, F., Salokangas, R.K., et al., 2010. Prediction of psychosis in adolescents and young adults at high risk: results from the prospective European prediction of psychosis study. Arch. Gen. Psychiatry 67 (3), 241–251.

Rüther, T., Bobes, J., De Hert, M., et al., 2014. EPA Guidance on tobacco dependence and strategies for smoking cessation in people with mental illness. Eur. Psychiatry 29 (2), 65–82.

Sarris, J., Logan, A.C., Akbaraly, T.N., et al., 2015. Nutritional medicine as mainstream in psychiatry. Lancet Psychiatry 2 (3), 271–274.

Schoepf, D., Uppal, H., Potluri, R., et al., 2014. Physical comorbidity and its relevance on mortality in schizophrenia: a naturalistic 12-year follow-up in general hospital admissions. Eur. Arch. Psychiatry Clin. Neurosci. 264 (1), 3–28.

Schuch, F., Vancampfort, D., Firth, J., et al., 2017. Physical activity and sedentary behavior in people with major depressive disorder: a systematic review and meta-analysis. J. Affect. Disord. 210, 139–150.

Scott, K.M., Oakley Browne, M.A., McGee, M.A., et al., 2006. Mental-physical comorbidity in Te Rau Hinengaro: the New Zealand Mental Health Survey. Aust. N. Z. J. Psychiatry 40 (10), 882–888.

Shanahan, L., Copeland, W.E., Angold, A., et al., 2014. Sleep problems predict and are predicted by generalized anxiety/depression and oppositional defiant disorder. J. Am. Acad. Child Adolesc. Psychiatry 53 (5), 550–558.

Smith, K., Deschênes, S.S., Schmitz, N., 2018. Investigating the longitudinal association between diabetes and anxiety: a systematic review and meta-analysis. Diabet. Med. 35 (6), 677–693.

Smith, P.H., Mazure, C.M., McKee, S.A., 2014. Smoking and mental illness in the US population. Tob. Control 23 (e2), e147–e153.

Smith, P.F., Smith, Andrew, Miners, John, et al., 2000. Safety Aspects of Dietary Caffeine – Report from the Expert Working Group. Australia and New Zealand Food Authority. 20-3.

Sommer, I.E., Kahn, R.S., 2015. The magic of movement: the potential of exercise to improve cognition. Schizophr. Bull. 41 (4), 776–778.

Spiegelhalder, K., Regen, W., Nanovska, S., et al., 2013. Comorbid sleep disorders in neuropsychiatric disorders across the life cycle. Curr. Psychiatry Rep. 15 (6), 364.

Stanton, R., Reaburn, P., Happell, B., 2015. Barriers to exercise prescription and participation in people with mental illness: the perspectives of nurses working in mental health. J. Psychiatr. Ment. Health Nurs. 22 (6), 440–448.

Stubbs, B., Firth, J., Berry, A., et al., 2016. How much physical activity do people with schizophrenia engage in? A systematic review, comparative meta-analysis and meta-regression. Schizophr. Res. 176 (2–3), 431–440.

Stubbs, B., Koyanagi, A., Schuch, F., et al., 2017. Physical activity levels and psychosis: a mediation analysis of factors influencing physical activity target achievement among 204 186 people across 46 low-and middle-income countries. Schizophr. Bull. 43 (3), 536–545.

Stubbs, B., Vancampfort, D., De Hert, M., et al., 2015. The prevalence and predictors of type two diabetes mellitus in people with schizophrenia: a systematic review and comparative meta-analysis. Acta Psychiatr. Scand. 132 (2), 144–157.

Tang, L.R., Zheng, W., Zhu, H., et al., 2015. Self-reported and interviewer-rated oral health in patients with schizophrenia, bipolar disorder, and major depressive disorder. Perspect. Psychiatr. Care 52 (1), 4–11.

Tanskanen, A., Tiihonen, J., Taipale, H., 2018. Mortality in schizophrenia: 30-year nationwide follow-up study. Acta Psychiatr. Scand. 138 (6), 492–499.

Taylor, G., McNeill, A., Girling, A., et al., 2014. Change in mental health after smoking cessation: systematic review and meta-analysis. BMJ 348, g1151.

Teasdale, S.B., Ward, P.B., Samaras, K., et al., 2019. Dietary intake of people with severe mental illness: systematic review and meta-analysis. Br. J. Psychiatry 214 (5), 251–259.

Teasdale, S.B., Ward, P.B., Rosenbaum, S., et al., 2017. Solving a weighty problem: systematic review and meta-analysis of nutrition interventions in severe mental illness. Br. J. Psychiatry 210 (2), 110–118.

Teasdale, S.B., Ward, P.B., Rosenbaum, S., et al., 2016. A nutrition intervention is effective in improving dietary components linked to cardiometabolic risk in youth with first-episode psychosis. Br. J. Nutr. 115 (11), 1987–1993.

Thornicroft, G., 2011. Physical health disparities and mental illness: the scandal of premature mortality. Br. J. Psychiatry 199 (6), 441–442.

Tobin, T., Tobin, M.L., 2017. Staying awake and aware: the importance of sleep in psychiatric nursing practice. Issues Ment. Health Nurs. 38 (11), 924–929.

Todd, R.A., Lewin, A.M., Bresee, L.C., et al., 2014. Coronary artery disease in adults with schizophrenia: anatomy, treatment and outcomes. Int. J. Cardiol. Heart Vessel. 4, 84–89.

Urry, K., Chur-Hansen, A., Khaw, C., 2019. 'It's just a peripheral issue': a qualitative analysis of mental health clinicians' accounts of (not) addressing sexuality in their work. Int. J. Ment. Health Nurs. 28 (6), 1278–1287.

Vancampfort, D., Correll, C.U., Galling, B., et al., 2016. Diabetes mellitus in people with schizophrenia, bipolar disorder and major depressive disorder: a systematic review and large scale meta-analysis. World Psychiatry 15 (2), 166–174.

Vancampfort, D., Stubbs, B., Ward, P.B., et al., 2015a. Why moving more should be promoted for severe mental illness. Lancet Psychiatry 2 (4), 295.

Vancampfort, D., Stubbs, B., Ward, P., et al., 2015b. Integrating physical activity as medicine in the care of people with severe mental illness. Aust. N. Z. J. Psychiatry 49 (8), 681–682.

Vancampfort, D., De Hert, M., Skjerven, L., et al., 2012. International Organization of Physical Therapy in Mental Health consensus on physical activity within multidisciplinary rehabilitation programmes for minimising cardio-metabolic risk in patients with schizophrenia. Disabil. Rehabil. 34 (1), 1–12.

Watkins, A., 2014. Keeping the body in mind. Aust. Nurs. Midwifery J. 21 (11), 44–45.

Wing, V.C., Wass, C.E., Soh, D.W., et al., 2012. A review of neurobiological vulnerability factors and treatment implications for comorbid tobacco dependence in schizophrenia. Ann. N. Y. Acad. Sci. 1248 (1), 89–106.

World Health Organization (WHO), 2013. Mental health Action Plan 2013–2020, WHO, Geneva.

World Health Organization (WHO), 2008. The right to health: fact sheet no. 31. Geneva: WHO. https://www.who.int/hhr/activities/Right_to_Health_factsheet31.pdf?ua=1.

CHAPTER 19

Psychopharmacology

Kim Usher and Simeon Evans

KEY POINTS

- Psychotropic medications play an important role in treating mental illness. Nurses play a pivotal role in medication administration, promoting adherence and educating consumers about medications. It is important for nurses to be aware of the uses, potential side effects and interactions of these medications.
- Many psychotropic medications are linked to physical health issues such as metabolic syndrome. It is important for nurses to be aware of these problems and to assess consumers prior to and during use of the medications.
- Nurses must be aware of the issues surrounding the administration of these medications to vulnerable groups such as children, pregnant women and the elderly.
- Polypharmacy is to be avoided where possible, especially the tendency to use medications from different classes at the same time.
- Issues related to as-needed (prn) medication administration are of contemporary relevance.
- It is important for mental health nurses to understand assessment and interventions related to psychopharmacological side effects.

KEY TERMS

- Akathisia
- Anticholinergic
- Atypical antipsychotic medication
- Collaborative prescribing
- Extrapyramidal side effects
- Informed consent
- Medication adherence
- Metabolic syndrome
- Mood-stabilising medication
- Neuroleptic malignant syndrome
- Neuroleptic medication
- Polypharmacy
- *pro re nata* (prn) medications
- Psychopharmacology
- QT prolongation
- Tardive syndromes
- Typical antipsychotic medication

LEARNING OUTCOMES

The material in this chapter will assist you to:

- describe the nurse's role in administering psychotropic medications and related interventions, including medication indications, interactions, side effects and precautions
- identify the important classes of psychotropic medication and the disorders for which they are used
- understand the issues for consumers requiring psychotropic medications
- understand the actions, use and side effects related to antianxiety/sedative hypnotic, antidepressant, mood-stabilising and antipsychotic medications
- understand the issues related to as-needed (prn) psychotropic medications and related interventions
- outline the relevant legal and ethical issues related to administering psychotropic medications
- understand the importance of monitoring physical health prior to and during treatment with psychotropic medications.

Introduction

This chapter provides an overview of the principles of psychopharmacology, which is the study of medications used to treat psychiatric disorders. Important information is discussed about medication indications, interactions, side effects, precautions, consumer experience and education, and the issues of adherence and as-needed or *pro re nata* (prn) medication administration.

Using medications that have a demonstrated ability to relieve the symptoms of psychiatric disorders has become widespread since the mid-1950s. The pharmacological agents used in current psychiatric practice are the antianxiety sedatives, antidepressants, mood-stabilising medications, antipsychotic medications and cognitive enhancers. Collectively, these medications are referred to as 'psychotropic medications' and are the focus of this chapter.

Psychotropic medications can be administered using a variety of methods such as oral, intramuscular and intravenous routes. It is important to remember that psychotropic medications are just one part of the consumer's treatment and on their own should not be considered a 'quick fix' or cure-all. In fact, psychotropic medications are not helpful to all people who experience the symptoms of mental illness and have many untoward effects that can cause discomfort and distress.

Psychotropic medications have the potential to improve quality of life for many people. However, it is also important to be aware that these medications have the potential to cause a number of serious side effects. Mental health nurses need to be aware of these effects and develop the appropriate skills to assess and monitor for them, including physical health and related issues (see Chapter 18), and to educate consumers and family/carers about potential issues related to psychotropic medication.

Skilful mental health nursing encompasses an understanding of the particular pharmacological actions of the psychotropic agents as well as an empathic understanding of the potential issues for the person taking these medications (see Nurse's story 19.1). Regardless of the treatment setting, which can range from inpatient to community, mental health nurses play a pivotal role in working with consumers and their families as they grapple with the issues surrounding these medications. It is important that nurses develop a comprehensive understanding of both the medications and their impact on an individual, as well as an understanding of the supportive and therapeutic nursing interventions that support medication adherence. Table 19.1 provides a list of commonly used terms related to psychopharmacology.

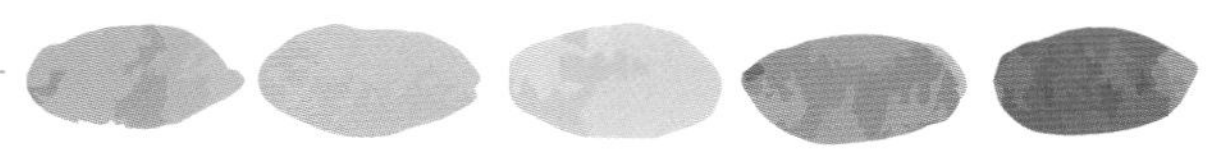

NURSE'S STORY 19.1

Diane

One day a consumer thanked me for looking after him and helping him to understand more about his medications and how they worked. This came as a surprise to me as I had never been thanked in this way before and thought it was my role to help consumers to better understand treatment options. While the older traditional antipsychotics were linked to many major side effects, the newer, second-generation treatments are better tolerated by consumers and have fewer reported side effects. However, it is easy to assume that, because of this, people no longer need to be informed and involved in their treatment decisions. It is important to recognise that the new antipsychotics do not provide a global effect for negative symptoms and in fact still have several unwanted side effects such as weight gain and metabolic disturbance. These side effects can be very distressing to the consumer and some have told me they think they are even worse off than before the treatment, even though it may have helped with their psychotic symptoms.

Reflecting on the incident described above I thought about how as nurses we often act in certain ways because of our own understanding or beliefs about an illness and its origins. For example, many nurses unwittingly propagate a pessimistic attitude to consumers with schizophrenia because of their belief that the disorder is caused by genetic factors. In such cases nurses may engage with consumers minimally and seek instead to do activities such as medication rounds. For me, it is important to try to work with consumers in ways that are free of assumptions and to focus on the needs of the consumer at all times.

Important pharmacological principles

Supportive and therapeutic nursing interventions enable the consumer to develop and maintain medication adherence and foster the consumer's understanding of their medications. Because mental health nurses play an important role in administering psychotropic medications, especially within psychiatric inpatient units, it is essential to have a sound working knowledge of psychotropic medications, including their pharmacology and relevant neurochemistry. This knowledge is important for nurses when offering medication education to consumers and their families.

TABLE 19.1 Commonly used terms

TERM	DEFINITION
Akathisia	Restlessness where the person cannot stay still
Anosognosia	Lack of insight
Antipsychotic medication	Medication prescribed to reduce psychotic symptoms
Ataxia	Lack of voluntary coordination of muscle movement
Atypical antipsychotic medication	Newer, second-generation antipsychotic medications
Cogwheeling rigidity	Type of rigidity seen in parkinsonism whereby the muscles respond with cogwheel-like jerks to the application of constant force in attempting to bend the limb
Dystonia	State of abnormal muscle tone
Extrapyramidal side effects	Drug-induced movement disorders
Half-life	The time until the serum level of a drug is reduced by half
Iatrogenic	An effect caused by a medication or by health personnel
Parkinson's syndrome	Imbalance between dopamine and acetylcholine, resulting in involuntary movements, reduced movements, rigidity and abnormal walking and posture
Polypharmacy	Use of multiple medications simultaneously
Pro re nata (prn)	As needed
Serotonin syndrome	A potentially life-threatening syndrome caused by excessive brain cell activity as a result of high levels of serotonin
Tardive dyskinesia	Involuntary movements of the tongue, lips, face, trunk and extremities related to taking antipsychotic medications
Tardive syndrome	Delayed-onset abnormal involuntary movement disorders caused by a dopamine-receptor blocking agent
Typical antipsychotic medication	Traditional type of antipsychotic medication

All medications are prescribed for particular effects or target symptoms that the prescriber and consumer hope to change. Therefore, it is important for nurses to be aware of the symptoms that particular medications target as well as the symptoms experienced by individual consumers. Correctly identifying symptoms is a key component of a thorough nursing assessment. Side effects, on the other hand, are the expression of effects for which the medication was not intended. Not all side effects are harmful, but some can be, so nurses need a sound working knowledge of this area of practice.

Nurses also need to be aware of polypharmacy. Polypharmacy involves the concurrent use of multiple psychotropic medications. Although polypharmacy might be useful at some stage for managing people with serious psychiatric disorders, it has negative connotations and is generally not advisable because it can increase the chance of adverse medication side effects and interactions. It can also be extremely problematic with certain groups of vulnerable people including the elderly, who are commonly prescribed several different medications concurrently (Hubbard et al. 2015).

An understanding of how psychotropic medications work is important for mental health nurses so they can better understand the issues surrounding the prescription and administration of these medications. The neuron is the basic functional unit of the brain and the central nervous system (CNS), and all communication in the brain involves neurons communicating across synapses at receptors. Receptors are the targets for the neurotransmitters or chemical messengers necessary for communication between neurons. The neurotransmitters acetylcholine, noradrenaline (norepinephrine), dopamine, serotonin (5HT) and GABA (gamma-aminobutyric acid) are implicated in developing mental illness.

Psychotropic medications produce their therapeutic action by altering communication among the neurons in the CNS. They alter the way neurotransmitters work at the synapse by modifying the reuptake of neurotransmitters into the presynaptic neuron, activating or inhibiting postsynaptic receptors, or inhibiting enzyme activity (Usher et al. 2009b). Generally, the major psychotropic medications are believed to act by altering the activities of the receptors, enzymes, ion channels and chemical transporter systems.

Important psychotropic medications

This section explores the most important groups of psychotropic medications in current use: the anxiolytics (antianxiety), antidepressants, mood-stabilisers and antipsychotics (neuroleptics). These groups of medications are listed in Table 19.2 with common examples from a local perspective.

TABLE 19.2 Classification of psychotropic medications

TYPE	MEDICATION GROUP	EXAMPLES
Antianxiety	Benzodiazepines	Chlordiazepoxide Diazepam Clonazepam Alprazolam Lorazepam
	Azapirones Beta-adrenergic blockers	Buspirone Propanolol
Antidepressant	Tricyclic and related medications	Amitriptyline Lofepramine Trazodone
	Selective serotonin reuptake inhibitors (SSRIs) and related medications	Fluoxetine Paroxetine
	Noradrenaline serotonin reuptake inhibitors (NSRIs)	Venlafaxine Mirtazapine
	Monoamine oxidase inhibitors (MAOIs)	Isocarboxazid Phenelzine Tranylcypromine
Mood-stabilising	Lithium	Lithium carbonate
	Anticonvulsants	Carbamazepine Valproate Topiramate Lamotrigine
Antipsychotic Typical (traditional)	Phenothiazines Thioxanthenes Butyrophenones Diphenylbutylpiperidines	Thioridazine Flupenthixol Haloperidol Pimozide
Atypical (second-generation)		Clozapine Risperidone Olanzapine Quetiapine Ziprasidone
Sedative-hypnotic	Benzodiazepines	Flurazepam Temazepam
	Cyclopyrrolones Imidazopyrimidines	Zopiclone Zolpidem

Antianxiety or anxiolytic medications

Anxiety is a common human experience that is a normal reaction to a threat of some kind. It leads to a fight-or-flight response in the individual. Anxiety is also the feature of many mental health problems. When anxiety becomes disabling, antianxiety medications may be useful (Bandelow et al. 2012). Antianxiety medications can be divided into benzodiazepines and non-benzodiazepines. Benzodiazepines are probably the most commonly prescribed medications in the world today. Although initially very effective in relieving anxiety symptoms, benzodiazepines are not recommended as first-line treatment for insomnia, panic disorders and anxiety (including anxiety with depression) (Psychotropic Expert Group 2013). This is due to the significant potential for dependence to develop, especially in those with a history of substance use disorders but also for many people when used regularly for longer than 12 weeks. Treatment for longer than 2–4 weeks is not recommended in most cases. Antidepressants are the primary treatment for anxiety disorders in Australia and New Zealand. These are discussed later in this chapter.

BENZODIAZEPINES

Indications for use

Benzodiazepines are thought to reduce anxiety because of their potentiation of the inhibitory neurotransmitter

GABA, which results in a clinical decrease in the person's anxiety by inhibiting neurotransmission (Usher et al. 2009b). Clinically they are used to treat anxiety, insomnia, alcohol withdrawal, skeletal muscle rigidity, seizure disorders, anxiety associated with medical disease and psychotic agitation. Therefore, although the discussion here primarily relates to these medications as antianxiety agents, they also have a sedative effect and are often used for that purpose.

Side effects

Side effects from benzodiazepines (see Table 19.3) are common, dose-related, usually short term and almost always harmless. They include drowsiness, reduced mental acuity and impaired motor performance. However, other effects such as headache, dizziness, feelings of detachment, nausea, hypotension and restlessness may also be experienced. Therefore, consumers should be warned of the risk of accidents and cautioned about driving a car or operating dangerous machinery. These medications generally do not live up to their reputation of being strongly addictive, especially if they have been used for appropriate purposes, if their use has not been complicated by other factors such as the addition of other medications and if their withdrawal is planned and gradual. However, a withdrawal syndrome can result (see Box 19.1) if ceased abruptly.

It is also important to remember that older consumers are more vulnerable to side effects because the ageing brain is more sensitive to the action of sedatives (Usher et al. 2009b).

Contraindications/precautions

Benzodiazepines should not be taken in conjunction with any other CNS depressants including alcohol. Their safety in pregnancy is not established.

TABLE 19.3 Managing benzodiazepine side effects

SIDE EFFECT	INTERVENTION
Drowsiness	Encourage appropriate activity but warn against engaging in activities such as driving or operating machinery
Dizziness	Observe and take steps to prevent falls
Feelings of detachment	Encourage socialisation
Dependency, rebound insomnia/ anxiety	Encourage short-term use Educate to avoid other medications such as alcohol Plan for withdrawal

Box 19.1 Symptoms of benzodiazepine withdrawal syndrome

- Agitation
- Anorexia
- Anxiety
- Autonomic arousal
- Dizziness
- Hallucinations
- Insomnia
- Irritability
- Nausea and vomiting
- Seizures
- Sensitivity to light and sounds
- Tinnitus
- Tremulousness

Interactions

Interactions may occur with alcohol, monoamine oxidase inhibitors (MAOIs), phenytoin, antacids and agents with anticholinergic activity.

Consumer education

Consumers should be educated about the following

- Driving or operating machinery should be avoided until the consumer knows how they react to the medication.
- Alcohol and other CNS depressants potentiate the effects of benzodiazepines and therefore should be avoided.
- Benzodiazepine use should not be stopped suddenly.
- The use of benzodiazepines during pregnancy is not recommended.

NON-BENZODIAZEPINE ANTIANXIETY MEDICATIONS

Buspirone is a potent non-benzodiazepine anxiolytic medication with no addictive or sedative properties. It is effective in treating anxiety and has no muscle relaxant or anticonvulsant properties. It is of no use in managing alcohol or other medication abuse or panic disorder. It generally takes 3–6 weeks before maximum anxiolytic effects are achieved.

Propranolol is a beta-blocker that is useful in treating anxiety. It blocks beta-noradrenergic receptors centrally as well as in the peripheral cardiac and pulmonary systems. Beta-blockers reduce certain physiological symptoms of anxiety, especially tachycardia, rather than working directly on the anxiety.

Antidepressant medications

Depression is a disorder characterised by symptoms such as depressed mood, lack of pleasure or interest, appetite disturbance, sleep disturbance and fatigue. Depression is associated with dysregulation of neurochemicals, particularly serotonin and noradrenaline. The physiological understanding of antidepressant medication action supports this theory. Antidepressant medications enhance the transmission of these neurochemicals in several ways – they block the reuptake of the neurotransmitters at the synapse, inhibit their metabolism and destruction and/or enhance the activity of the receptors. The action of these medications at the synapse is immediate but it takes several weeks for antidepressants to effect mood.

Historical anecdote 19.1: The evolution of methamphetamine

One of the earliest antidepressant medications of the 20th century was the amphetamine Benzedrine launched by the pharmaceutical company Smith, Kline & French in 1936. The company began advertising Benzedrine for treating mild depression in 1942 and by 1948 they were promoting the amphetamine as the 'antidepressant of choice'. In 1950 Smith, Kline & French released a hybrid amphetamine and barbiturate medication called Dexamyl, which was a combination of dextroamphetamine and the barbiturate amobarbital. The medication was promoted for its 'smooth and profound antidepressant effect'. By 1950 several pharmaceutical companies were marketing methamphetamine for its antidepressant qualities. The firm Burroughs Wellcome named its product 'Methedrine', while the company Endo Products called theirs 'Norodin'. Few people in the 1950s could have predicted that methamphetamine would go on to become one of the most tightly regulated and stigmatised drugs of the early 21st century - colloquially referred to as 'ice'.

Read more about it: *Hirschfeld RMA 2000 History and evolution of the monoamine hypothesis of depression. The Journal of Clinical Psychiatry, 61(Suppl6): 4–6*

Indications for use

Antidepressant medications are indicated in treating persistent depressive disorders, major depression, depression (maintenance treatment and prevention of relapse) and anxiety disorders such as panic disorder and obsessive-compulsive disorder. The medications elevate mood and alleviate the other symptoms experienced as part of depression. Choice of an antidepressant medication will depend on its symptom profile, side effects, comorbid medical conditions, concurrent medications and risk of medication interactions, and the individual's medication history. If the consumer responds to the course of treatment with a particular medication, they should continue taking the medication at the same dosage for up to 9 months. If they remain symptom-free during this time, the medication will be gradually withdrawn. Consumers whose depressive symptoms return after withdrawal of medication may need long-term maintenance (Usher et al. 2009b).

Contraindications/precautions

Caution is warranted in the use of all antidepressant medications. Suicidal ideation and related risk can be increased with antidepressant treatment both as an initial side effect but also once the medication starts to take effect and the consumer's mood lifts, potentially increasing their motivation to act on existing suicidal thoughts. SSRIs should not be combined with MAOI therapy. MAOIs should not be started within a week of tricyclic therapy and, conversely, tricyclic medications should not be commenced within 2 weeks of stopping a MAOI. The tricyclics are a special risk with depressed people because of their severe cardiac toxicity if taken in large doses. Caution is warranted in consumers with cardiac disease and with older consumers. Tricyclics may also impair reaction times, especially at the beginning of treatment. Alcohol may increase the sedative effects of tricyclics. Monotherapy with antidepressants risks precipitating hypomania in people with a bipolar mood disorder and can cause mood elevation for some people even without a recognised history of mood instability.

Consumer education

Inform the consumer of the time it will take for a marked effect to be experienced from the medication and that it is important for them to keep taking the medication even though they have not noticed an initial improvement in their condition.

Other information:

- Warn the consumer of problems when driving or operating machinery if sedation is experienced.
- Tell the consumer to discuss with their doctor if they become pregnant or intend to breastfeed.
- Warn the consumer about the effect that alcohol may have if combined with antidepressant medication.
- Inform the consumer about possible interactions with foods and other medications if taking MAOIs.

TRICYCLIC ANTIDEPRESSANTS

Side effects

The tricyclic medications, available on the market for many years now, are clinically similar, so their effects and side effects tend to vary little between individual medications. They work primarily by serotonin and noradrenaline reuptake inhibition. The blockade of reuptake leads to extra transmitters being available for receptor binding. Side effects include sedation, dry mouth, constipation, blurred vision, seizures and urinary retention. They may also cause postural hypotension and serious cardiac problems such as heart block and arrhythmias. Because of their serious side effects these medications can lead to life-threatening consequences if taken in large quantities, such as in suicide attempts, and if this is suspected, immediate action to support life must be instigated (Box 19.2 lists signs of overdose). In the case of severely depressed consumers where a potential for suicide is predicted, close supervision is required, and when the person is not an inpatient, the dispensing of small, sub-lethal quantities is recommended.

Box 19.2 Signs of tricyclic overdose

- Agitation
- Confusion, drowsiness, delirium
- Convulsion
- Bowel and bladder paralysis
- Disturbances with the regulation of blood pressure and temperature
- Dilated pupils

Source: Treatment Protocol Project 2004

CONSUMER'S STORY 19.1

Julie

When I began taking Amitriptyline for severe depression, I felt overwhelmed by side effects. My energy level was comparable to having severe flu. I experienced blurred vision, difficulty waking in the morning and an incredibly dry mouth that woke me many times throughout the night. The health professional listened to my concerns and was very understanding, patient and collaborative. He asked me to be patient because the side effects should lessen with time but explained that we could also experiment with adjusting the dosage, adding in other medications or, if necessary, changing the medication. Knowing of my anorexia diagnosis, he had also made me aware of the potential side effect of weight gain and allowed me to decide whether I could tolerate the risk of weight gain. It was good to feel heard and supported, and reassuring to know there were other options if the side effects continued to be unbearable. I don't think I should have to choose between living with terrible physical side effects or suffering from debilitating depression, but some health professionals don't appear to agree. It's important to me that they take the time and effort to find a good solution that minimises mental illness symptoms without creating unbearable physical side effects. Over time the side effects from Amitriptyline decreased; however, they remained intolerable, so my health professional and I agreed that I would cease taking it. As I had made many lifestyle changes to support my physical and mental health, and since my depression had lessened, we decided I would try managing without medication. There is always an option to try a different medication if I need to; however, it has not been necessary.

MONOAMINE OXIDASE INHIBITORS

MAOIs were the first group of antidepressant medications discovered. They remain very effective antidepressants; however, due to their potentially serious side effects, the newer antidepressant medications have mostly replaced their use. MAOIs work by inhibiting both types of the enzyme (MAO A and B) that metabolise serotonin and noradrenaline. Consumers taking these medications must avoid noradrenaline agonists, which include its dietary precursor, tyramine. Adverse effects include drowsiness or insomnia, agitation, fatigue, gastrointestinal disturbances, weight gain, hypotension, dizziness, dry mouth/skin, sexual dysfunction, constipation and blurred vision. The major concern with using these medications is their potential to interact with specific foods that contain tyramine and other amine medications such as those found in any cough preparation (see Box 19.3). Such an interaction can result in excessive and dangerous elevation in blood pressure, known as a hypertensive crisis.

Interactions

Hyperpyretic crisis, seizures or serious cardiac events may occur with MAOIs. They may prevent the therapeutic effect of some antihypertensives.

SELECTIVE SEROTONIN REUPTAKE INHIBITORS

The SSRI group of antidepressant medications inhibits the reuptake of serotonin at the presynaptic membrane. This leads to an increased availability of serotonin in the synapse and therefore at the receptors, thereby promoting serotonin transmission. These medications are as effective as the tricyclic antidepressants but safer because they cause less serious side effects and have decreased risk of death by overdose. While the actions and effectiveness of these

Box 19.3 Food and medications to be avoided by consumers taking MAOIs

Avoid:

- cheeses, especially matured cheeses
- pickled herrings, cured meats and beef extracts such as marmite
- liver and chicken livers
- whole broad beans, avocados (especially if overripe), soybean paste
- figs, especially if overripe
- large numbers of bananas
- alcoholic drinks, especially chianti and red wine
- other antidepressant medications, nasal and sinus decongestants, narcotics, adrenaline (epinephrine)
- stimulants, hay-fever and asthma medications.

medications are similar, they are all structurally different from each other, resulting in differences in their side effects. Side effects are similar to those of the tricyclic group except that they do not have the cardiovascular, sedative and anticholinergic side effects. Nausea, diarrhoea, anxiety and restlessness, insomnia, sexual dysfunction, loss of appetite, weight loss and headache are the most common side effects. They should not be stopped abruptly; the withdrawal syndrome includes symptoms such as dizziness, paraesthesia, anxiety, sleep disturbance, agitation and tremor. They should not be combined with MAOIs.

Interactions

Hypertensive crisis may occur if administered with many other medications including adrenaline, noradrenaline, reserpine, narcotic analgesics and vasoconstrictors. Consumers may also experience hypertensive crisis if tyramine-rich foods are ingested (see Box 19.3).

Alcohol may potentiate the effect of SSRIs. Use with cimetidine may result in increased concentrations of SSRIs in the bloodstream. Hypertensive crisis may occur if taken within 14 days of MAOIs.

NORADRENALINE SEROTONIN REUPTAKE INHIBITORS

NSRIs are a new class of antidepressant medications. They are considered more effective than SSRIs in some people. NSRIs block the reuptake of serotonin and noradrenaline, thus increasing the amount of these neurotransmitters available at the synapse. Common side effects associated with NSRIs include nausea, dry mouth, dizziness, excessive sweating, agitation and constipation.

Mood-stabilising medications

Mood stabilising medications are primarily used for treating bipolar disorder. Bipolar disorder is characterised by periods of major depressive disorder or dysthymia as well as periods of mania or hypomania. Treatment aims to stabilise a person's mood between these two 'poles'. Lithium, a naturally occurring salt, has been and largely remains the medication of choice for treating acute mania and for the ongoing maintenance of consumers with a history of mania. An Australian, John Cade, discovered its effectiveness as a treatment for mania in 1949 (see also Chapter 10). Just how lithium works is not clear, but it is known to mimic the effects of sodium, thereby compromising the ability of neurones to release, activate or respond to neurotransmitters. It does appear to reduce the sodium content of the brain and increase central serotonin synthesis and noradrenaline reuptake (Usher et al. 2009b). Lithium use has been decreasing in recent years due to concerns about side effects and long-term health impacts as well as an increasing number of other medications being used successfully, either alone or in combination with lithium, to control the symptoms of mania. A number of anticonvulsant medications are used very successfully to reduce mania and manage bipolar depression. Antipsychotics and particularly atypical antipsychotics are increasingly used to manage both acute mania and prophylactically to prevent relapse. Some atypical antipsychotics are also effective in treating bipolar depression. Antipsychotic medications are discussed later in this chapter.

LITHIUM

Indications for use

Lithium is the medication of choice for treating acute mania and the ongoing maintenance of people with bipolar disorder (Malhi et al. 2016; Royal Australian and New Zealand College of Psychiatrists 2015). It is also useful in treating unipolar depression, aggressive behaviour, conduct disorder and schizoaffective disorder.

Side effects

Side effects include drowsiness, a metallic taste in the mouth, difficulty concentrating, increased thirst, dizziness, headache, dry mouth, gastrointestinal upset, nausea/vomiting, fine hand tremor, hypotension, arrhythmias, polyuria, dehydration and weight gain.

Contraindications/precautions

Lithium is contraindicated with cardiac or renal disease, dehydration, sodium depletion, brain damage, pregnancy and lactation. Care should be taken with thyroid disorders, diabetes, urinary retention and history of seizures. The therapeutic range for lithium in Australia is 0.6–1.2 mmol/L for acute mania and 0.4–0.8 mmol/L for maintenance, while the recommended levels in New Zealand are 0.6–0.8 mmol/L but lower in maintenance and up to 1 mmol/L for severe symptoms (Royal Australian and New Zealand College of Psychiatrists 2015; Royal College of Pathologists of Australasia 2019). A lower therapeutic range is recommended for maintenance therapy because long-term administration of lithium can be associated with serious side effects such as renal and thyroid dysfunction. Symptoms of lithium toxicity rarely appear at levels below 1.2 mmol/L but are common above 2.0 mmol/L (Usher et al. 2009b). Therefore, as the therapeutic and toxic levels are so close, extreme care must be taken in monitoring the consumer's blood level regularly, especially during early phases of the treatment. If the level exceeds 1.5 mmol/L, the next dose should be withheld and the doctor notified. Levels are usually monitored weekly until stable and then monthly. The blood samples for testing should be taken 12 hours after the last dose when lithium has been taken for at least 5–7 days (Psychotropic Expert Group 2013; Usher et al. 2009b).

Interactions

Diuretics, ACE (angiotensin-converting enzyme) inhibitors, neuroleptics, non-steroidal anti-inflammatory medications, alcohol and caffeine may interfere with lithium absorption.

Consumer education

- Educate the consumer about the side effects and signs of toxicity (see Box 19.4 and Nurse's story 19.2) and the need for regular blood level checks.
- Encourage the consumer to include a regular intake of approximately 10 glasses of water every day.
- Remind the consumer to take their medication regularly, even when they are feeling well.
- Advise the consumer not to operate machinery until the initial drowsiness subsides.
- Discuss the risks of taking lithium during pregnancy or when considering pregnancy.

Box 19.4 Signs of lithium toxicity

- **Early stages** – anorexia, nausea, vomiting, diarrhoea, coarse hand tremor, twitching, lethargy, dysarthria, hyperactive deep tendon reflexes, ataxia, tinnitus, vertigo, weakness, drowsiness
- **Later stages** – fever, decreased urinary output, decreased blood pressure, irregular pulse, ECG changes, impaired consciousness, seizures, coma, death

Note: Lithium toxicity is a medical emergency.

NURSE'S STORY 19.2

Marnie

An older consumer was admitted to an inpatient unit for an episode of manic behaviour. She had experienced mania before and was on continuous treatment with lithium. The lithium dose was increased during the admission. The nurse returned to the ward after 2 days' leave and noticed that the consumer appeared unwell, had a coarse tremor, was confused, ataxic and had myoclonic jerks. She called the doctor on call, expressed her concern and told him she would withhold the evening dose of lithium. She asked him to see the consumer as soon as possible and to organise to have blood taken for a lithium level. The doctor refused to come to the ward and disagreed with the nurse's concern about the consumer. He insisted she give the evening dose of the medication and said he would see the consumer the next morning. The nurse refused to accept his decision and called her immediate supervisor and explained her concern for the consumer's wellbeing. The medication was withheld, and an urgent blood request determined that the consumer's lithium level was 2.2 mmol/L. The nurse had correctly diagnosed lithium toxicity and taken the correct action to advocate best care for the consumer.

ANTICONVULSANTS

Indications for use

Several anticonvulsant medications have been used to treat mania, especially when lithium is ineffective. These medications are now rapidly becoming the medication of choice for many consumers. Carbamazepine, valproate, lamotrigine and topiramate are examples of commonly used anticonvulsants. These medications have been found to have acute antimanic and mood-stabilising effects. Carbamazepine, valproate, topiramate (Vieta et al. 2008) and lamotrigine (Van der Loos et al. 2011) are recommended treatments for mixed or bipolar states, secondary mania, rapid cyclers and lithium refractoriness. Lamotrigine is identified as an effective alternative to antidepressants in treating bipolar depression, particularly in relation to concerns about antidepressant-induced mania.

Side effects

- **Carbamazepine** – blood dyscrasias, drowsiness, nausea, vomiting, constipation or diarrhoea, hives or skin rashes, hepatitis
- **Valproate** – prolonged bleeding time, gastrointestinal upset, tremor, ataxia, weight gain, somnolence, dizziness, hepatic failure, polycystic ovary syndrome in women
- **Topiramate** – cognitive impairment, sedation, nausea, weight loss, dizziness, vomiting, rash, agitation, paraesthesia
- **Lamotrigine** – blurred vision, rash, nausea, ataxia, drowsiness

Contraindications/precautions

Anticonvulsants are contraindicated with MAOIs and during lactation. Caution is required in older consumers, people with cardiac/renal disease and during pregnancy. Before commencing carbamazepine, a range of tests should be performed, including blood film examination, electrolytes, liver and kidney function and an ECG. Carbamazepine may also interfere with the metabolism and blood concentrations of other medications, so care is needed with oral contraceptives and other medications. There is a risk of fetal malformation, so it should not be taken during pregnancy.

Valproate should not be taken with aspirin and some antipsychotics. It may enhance the effects of alcohol and other CNS depressants. Polycystic ovary syndrome is more common among women treated with valproate; symptoms tend to emerge early, often within the first few months of treatment. Women should be informed of this risk before starting treatment.

Interactions

- **Carbamazepine** – erythromycin, isoniazid, oral contraceptives, theophylline, fluoxetine
- **Valproate** – may potentiate alcohol, carbamazepine, barbiturates; should not be taken with aspirin or antipsychotics

- **Topiramate** – concomitant use with lithium and valproate can cause cognitive impairment

Consumer education

- Inform the consumer about avoiding sudden cessation of the tablets.
- Encourage the consumer to report unusual symptoms to their doctor: spontaneous bruising, unusual bleeding, sore throat, fever, malaise, or yellow skin or eyes.
- Remind the consumer to take medications with meals if gastrointestinal upset occurs.
- Advise the consumer to avoid taking alcohol or non-prescription medications without consulting a doctor.
- Explain that pregnancy must be avoided while taking the medication. Alternative methods of contraception may be required if taking valproate, as oral contraception may not be effective.

Antipsychotic or neuroleptic medications

The traditional neuroleptic or antipsychotic medications (also known as the typical antipsychotics) have been an important treatment for psychotic disorders since their discovery in the 1950s. These medications revolutionised the treatment of mental illness and soon became the mainstay of treatment for most psychotic disorders (Usher et al. 2009a). Each group of the typical antipsychotics appears to be equally effective for reducing or eliminating the positive symptoms of psychosis (e.g. delusions, hallucinations, motor disturbances). However, the side effects profile of the typical antipsychotics are concerning because of their effect on quality of life and their link with non-adherence.

Historical anecdote 19.2: The evolution of phenothiazines

In the 1950s a French surgeon Henri Laborit used the antihistamine drug chlorpromazine to reduce the amount of general anaesthesia required by patients during surgery. Later, the calming effect of chlorpromazine was applied to psychiatric patients and, thanks to its tranquilising effect, it grew a reputation as the first 'typical antipsychotic' or 'major tranquillisers' belonging to the phenothiazine group, which includes thioridazine, trifluoperazine and fluphenazine. These drugs revolutionised management of the disruptive positive symptoms of schizophrenia. Although in recent years their use has been associated with problematic adverse reactions, back in the mid-20th century the phenothiazines provided new hope of successful illness management and even the prospect of independent living outside of the hospital setting.

Read more about it: *López-Muñoz F, Alamo C, Cuenca E, Shen WW, Clervoy P, Rubio G 2005 History of the discovery and clinical introduction of chlorpromazine. Annals of Clinical Psychiatry, 17(3): 113–35*

The newer, second-generation antipsychotics, commonly referred to as the 'atypical' or 'novel' antipsychotics, were introduced in the 1990s and have quickly become the medication of choice for psychotic symptoms. These medications are better tolerated and less likely to lead to problems with medication adherence (Usher et al. 2009a). Apart from clozapine, which has superior efficacy to the typical antipsychotics, their efficacy appears to be equal to that of the typical antipsychotics (Psychotropic Expert Group 2013) but they are more effective in reducing the negative symptoms of psychosis. Clozapine, risperidone, olanzapine and quetiapine remain the most widely used examples of the second-generation antipsychotics.

The typical antipsychotics are dopamine antagonists. They primarily block the postsynaptic D_2 receptors but also exert other synaptic effects. They reduce the positive symptoms of schizophrenia. Atypicals, on the other hand, have dopamine receptor subtype 2 (D_2) and serotonin receptor subtype 2 ($5HT_2$) blocking action.

Indications for use

Antipsychotics are indicated for treating acute and chronic psychoses, delusional disorder and severe depression where psychotic symptoms are present. Schizophrenia and schizoaffective disorders are the most common indications for antipsychotic medications. Some of the phenothiazine group has other uses, such as antiemetic in the case of prochlorperazine and treating intractable hiccups in the case of chlorpromazine. Many of the antipsychotic medications, especially the lower-potency ones such as chlorpromazine and haloperidol, have a prominent sedative effect. This effect is particularly conspicuous early in treatment, although tolerance usually develops quickly.

Side effects

The side effects of the typical antipsychotics are varied. They can affect every system of the body and range from effects on the CNS – including movement disorders, sedation and seizures – through to potentially life-threatening side effects such as neuroleptic malignant syndrome (NMS) (see Table 19.4 for an overview of the side effects of the typical antipsychotics). The most troubling of the side effects are the extrapyramidal reactions. These result from the effects of the antipsychotic medications on the extrapyramidal motor system. This is the same system responsible for the movement disorders of Parkinson's disease. Acute dystonia,

TABLE 19.4 Side effects of the typical antipsychotics

SIDE EFFECTS	KEY FEATURES	TIME OF MAXIMAL RISK	INTERVENTIONS
CNS extrapyramidal side effects			
Acute dystonic reaction	Painful muscle spasms in the head, back and torso; can last minutes to hours, occur suddenly; can cause fear	1–5 days	Administer antiparkinsonian medication quickly; respiratory support if needed; reassure and remain with the consumer
Akathisia	Restlessness, leg aches, person cannot stay still	5–60 days	Administer antiparkinsonian medication; change medication
Neuroleptic malignant syndrome	Potentially fatal with hyperthermia, severe extrapyramidal side effects, sweating, muscle rigidity, clouding of consciousness, elevated creatine phosphokinase	Weeks, usually	Supportive therapy; cease all medications; treat with bromocriptine or dantrolene
Parkinsonism	Rigid, mask-like facial expression; shuffling gait; drooling	5–30 days; can recur even after a single dose	Administer dopamine agonist; support the consumer
Seizures	Typical antipsychotics reduce seizure threshold, risk about 1% but greater with rapid titration or history of seizures	Early in treatment	May need to stop the medication, observe the consumer or manipulate the medication dose
Tardive dyskinesia	Usually results from prolonged use of typical antipsychotics; stereotyped involuntary movements (tongue, lips, feet)	After months or years of treatment (worse on withdrawal)	Assess the consumer often; change to atypical medications; no other treatment available
Other			
Anticholinergic	Dry mouth, blurred vision, orthostatic hypotension, tachycardia, urinary retention, nasal congestion		Observe, educate the consumer; provide support where needed; may need to change medication
Endocrine	Weight gain, diminished libido, impotence, amenorrhoea, galactorrhoea		Educate the consumer; reduce kilojoule intake; may need to change medication
Photosensitivity	Skin hyperpigmentation		Educate the consumer to avoid sun and wear protective clothing, sunscreen and sunglasses
Sedation	May be beneficial in agitated consumers; can be mistaken for cognitive slowing		Educate the consumer to avoid driving or operating machinery; rest periods; adjust dose

parkinsonism and akathisia occur early and can be managed by a variety of medications including antiparkinsonian and benzodiazepine medications. Tardive dyskinesia generally occurs later and has no effective treatment. The Abnormal Involuntary Movements Scale (AIMS) (see Box 19.5) is a useful tool for nurses to detect movement disorders in consumers. NMS, an idiosyncratic hypersensitivity to antipsychotic medications, is a rare but serious reaction that is potentially life-threatening (see Box 19.6).

Contraindications/precautions

Caution should be taken in administering antipsychotics to older people and to those who are medically ill or diagnosed with diabetes. Safety in pregnancy and lactation is not clear. They are contraindicated in people with a known sensitivity to one of the phenothiazines as a cross-sensitivity is possible. People taking typical antipsychotics should avoid extremes of temperature.

Box 19.5 Useful tools for assessing medication side effects

LUNSERS

The LUNSERS (Liverpool University Neuroleptic Side Effect Rating Scale) is a useful tool for assessing side effects. It is designed for self-administration but can also be a useful tool for nurses to help detect consumer reactions to changes in treatment (Morrison et al. 2000).

To access the scale, see: Day JC, Wood G, Dewey M et al. 1995 A self-rating scale for measuring neuroleptic side effects: validation in a group of schizophrenic patients. British Journal of Psychiatry 166(5): 650–3.

AIMS

The AIMS (Abnormal Involuntary Movements Scale) is a widely used tool for use with people on long-term antipsychotic medications. It is designed to assess for signs of tardive dyskinesia.

To access the scale, see: Munetz MR, Benjamin S 1988 How to examine patients using the Abnormal Involuntary Movements Scale. Hospital and Community Psychiatry 39(11): 1172–7.

Box 19.6 Neuroleptic malignant syndrome

NMS is a rare disorder that resembles a severe form of parkinsonism with coarse tremor and catatonia, fluctuating in intensity, accompanied by signs of autonomic instability (labile pulse and blood pressure, hyperthermia), stupor, elevation of creatinine kinase in serum, and sometimes myoglobinaemia. In severe forms it may persist for more than a week after ceasing the medication. The risk of death from this syndrome is high (more than 10%); therefore, immediate medical intervention is required if suspected. NMS is associated with higher number of antipsychotics used, use of first-generation agents (typical antipsychotics), and higher maximum doses. In particular, NMS is associated more highly with haloperidol, aripiprazole, depot flupenthixol decanoate and benzodiazepines.

Source: Su et al. 2014

Interactions

Concurrent use with antidepressants, antihistamines and antiparkinsonian agents may result in additional anticholinergic effects. Antacids and antidiarrhoeals may disrupt absorption of the antipsychotic. Alcohol may cause additional CNS depression.

Consumer education

The consumer needs education about the medication side effects and help with maintaining adherence. People taking typical antipsychotics should be careful in the sun and in extremes of temperature.

NURSE'S STORY 19.3

Lesley Douglas

Oculogyric crisis (OGC) is an acute dystonic reaction that is a side effect of some of the neuroleptic medications prescribed for psychosis. It is a distressing side effect characterised by prolonged involuntary upward deviation of the eyes.

Phil was a young man who had been admitted to an acute inpatient mental health unit as an involuntary patient to treat a first presentation psychosis. He was prescribed a neuroleptic medication (risperidone) by the psychiatrist. On the third day of pharmacological treatment, Phil was sitting in the unit corridor when I arrived for my shift. I noted him sitting stiffly in the chair with his eyes turned towards the ceiling, his neck flexed and his mouth open wide. These are classic symptoms of OGC and require immediate intervention.

Speaking with Phil, I realised he was distressed by the symptoms. Working quickly and quietly so as not to cause further anguish, benztropine was administered by intramuscular route as prescribed with the symptoms abating within 15 minutes. I sat with Phil for the next 30 minutes to ensure the efficacy of the prescribed medication, to describe in detail what had occurred and to allay his fears. During his 3-week admission to the mental health unit, Phil experienced further OGC episodes, all treated in the same manner.

Offering immediate assistance, support and ongoing education is imperative to ensure that appropriate treatment is provided. While OGC is not a common side effect from neuroleptic medications, it is experienced by young men in particular. As mental health nurses, we need to be able to recognise medication side effects and manage them effectively.

Atypical antipsychotics

Atypical antipsychotics are not all pharmacologically alike so they tend to have a diverse side effect profile. They do, however, have some similar side effects such as weight gain, constipation and dizziness, and are also linked to developing diabetes and metabolic syndrome (McDaid & Smyth 2015). Some may cause extrapyramidal side effects at higher doses, but they are not uniformly associated with parkinsonian symptoms, akathisia, dystonia or dyskinesia (Remington et al. 2013). Seizures may also occur with too rapid a titration associated with increase in dosage. In addition, cardiac problems such as atrial fibrillation, atrial flutter or myocarditis early in treatment, although uncommon, may occur.

Some of the side effects of individual medications include:

- **Clozapine** – more safety concerns than any other antipsychotic medication (Remington et al. 2013). A serious adverse effect is the potential for agranulocytosis, which occurs in 1–2% of consumers. Precautions must be taken to ensure swift detection of this side effect should it occur. Other side effects include constipation and paralytic ileus, hypersalivation (especially annoying during sleep) and tachycardia. Clozapine is one of the two most obesogenic antipsychotic medications (along with olanzapine).
- **Ziprasidone** – dizziness, tremor, dry mouth, hypotension
- **Risperidone** – insomnia, agitation, anxiety, headache, postural hypotension particularly at the start of treatment, drowsiness, weight gain, gastrointestinal upset, sexual dysfunction and extrapyramidal symptoms
- **Olanzapine** – drowsiness, weight gain, postural hypotension, peripheral oedema, extrapyramidal symptoms and anticholinergic side effects (dry mouth, hypotension, tachycardia)
- **Quetiapine** – mild somnolence, mild asthenia, dry mouth, limited weight gain, postural hypotension, tachycardia and occasional syncope.

Weight gain and the development of metabolic syndrome associated with the atypical antipsychotics is a serious issue (McDaid & Smyth 2015). Weight gain has been previously reported as predictable: a meta-analysis of weight change by Allison et al. (1999) found weight gain over 10 weeks of treatment with a standard medication dose, as follows: clozapine, 4.45 kg; olanzapine, 4.15 kg; risperidone, 2.10 kg; and ziprasidone, 0.04 kg – with insufficient data available to evaluate quetiapine. The weight gain usually occurs during the first 4–12 weeks of treatment. After the initial period the weight gain continues at a lower level over a prolonged period (Tschoner et al. 2007). Weight gain linked to atypical antipsychotics is typically associated with abdominal obesity and enhanced adiposity, which is linked with increased morbidity and mortality, as well as reduced quality of life (Tschoner et al. 2007). Together these changes make up what is referred to as 'metabolic syndrome', a cluster of metabolic abnormalities including hypertension, hyperlipidaemia, hyperglycaemia and abdominal obesity, which, when experienced together, lead to an increased risk of diabetes and cardiovascular disease. Thus, weight gain and metabolic disturbance linked to the atypical antipsychotics have become a major concern for clinicians and consumers (McDaid & Smyth 2015; Usher et al. 2013).

Previous Australian studies have found the prevalence rates of metabolic syndrome in people with schizophrenia to range between 51% and 68% (John et al. 2009; Tirupati & Chua 2007). Another Australian cohort study of people prescribed clozapine (Hyde et al. 2015) found higher prevalence rates for cardiovascular and metabolic events than previous Australian studies. The most common cardiovascular condition revealed was ECG-defined abnormalities (60%), while low high-density lipoprotein (HDL) cholesterol levels (69%) and high triglyceride levels (77%) were the most common metabolic abnormalities.

The weight gain and high rate of metabolic disturbance with the atypical antipsychotics is linked to several factors including impairment of the glucose metabolism system, which regulates appetite and weight management. Impairment of this system appears to be linked to developing type 2 diabetes and dyslipidaemia (Hepburn & Brzozowska 2016). However, while weight gain and cardiovascular risk has been attributed to modifiable risk factors including smoking, sedentary lifestyles, lack of exercise and substance misuse, there is evidence to suggest that autonomic dysfunction exists, even in medication-free individuals, and that some of the psychotropic medications can exacerbate cardiac risk in these individuals (Alveres et al. 2016).

Metabolic syndrome is diagnosed when a person has a girth measurement higher than recommended and any two of the following: raised triglycerides, reduced HDL cholesterol, raised blood pressure and raised fasting plasma glucose. Management of the syndrome includes lifestyle changes (improving nutrition and increasing exercise), ongoing monitoring and medication for dyslipidaemia, hypertension and glucose intolerance if required. Guidelines for assessing metabolic syndrome include baseline screening that includes girth measurement, weight, height, body mass index (BMI), blood chemistries and family and personal history, followed by regular monitoring. Thus, attention to the physical health of consumers is an important nursing role. This issue is covered in more detail in Chapter 18.

Early intervention for weight gain with the atypical antipsychotics should occur when the person begins taking the medication or when medication changes are made and should target reduced kilojoule intake and increased exercise, as these have been shown to have a positive ameliorating effect on weight gain. Several interventions have been introduced to manage the weight gain linked to these medications. For example, lifestyle interventions, education, weight loss medications and exercise have all been implemented and evaluated. However, research to date indicates significantly greater weight reduction in lifestyle intervention groups than in pharmacological intervention groups or standard care groups (Park et al. 2011).

Nurses should ensure consumers are regularly screened for weight gain, diet and exercise. Indeed, nurses are well placed to educate consumers about making healthy choices to prevent weight gain and metabolic symptoms such as diabetes and cardiovascular conditions (Edwards et al. 2010). It is important for nurses to be aware of the potential for weight gain with the atypical antipsychotics and to work with consumers when the medication is first introduced, rather than waiting until the weight gain becomes problematic (Park et al. 2011), as the weight gain associated with these medications is known to cause significant distress to consumers (Usher et al. 2013). However, while mental health nurses recognise working with consumers to manage weight gain and other medication side effects is an important nursing responsibility, they report lack of education and confidence (McDaid & Smyth 2015) to do so.

Contraindications/precautions

Clozapine

People taking clozapine must be made aware of the potential risk of agranulocytosis and be monitored regularly. Because of the medication's link to agranulocytosis it is restricted to those who have not responded to at least two other antipsychotics. Clozapine can be prescribed through the Clozaril Patient Monitoring System program only. The consumer's blood should be monitored weekly for 18 weeks and monthly thereafter. An immediate differential blood count must be ordered if the consumer reports flu-like symptoms. If during treatment an infection occurs and/or the white blood cell (WBC) count drops below 3,500/mm^3, or drops by a substantial amount from baseline, a repeat WBC and differential count should be completed. If the results confirm a WBC count below 3,500/mm^3 and/or reveal an absolute neutrophil count (ANC) of between 2,000 and 1,500/mm^3, the WBC and ANC must be checked at least twice weekly. If the WBC count falls below 3,000/mm^3 and/or the ANC count drops below 1,500/mm^3, clozapine must be withdrawn at once and the consumer closely monitored. Care should be taken when using these medications with older people.

Interactions

Medications known to have substantial potential to depress bone marrow function should be avoided concurrently with clozapine. Atypical antipsychotics may enhance the effect of alcohol and other CNS depressants.

Consumer education

Advice about having regular blood tests when taking clozapine should be provided. Consumers should also be told the importance of seeing a doctor immediately for any flu-like symptoms while taking clozapine. Information on possible side effects and medication interactions related to atypical antipsychotic medications should be provided.

While constipation is often considered as a minor medication side effect, it is a potentially serious side effect of clozapine. In fact, there have been several deaths associated with constipation resulting from clozapine. Other serious outcomes include paralytic ileus, bowel obstruction and toxic megacolon (Jessurun et al. 2013). It is essential for consumers to be warned of the potential for constipation, be educated about the need to monitor bowel habits and use interventions to manage constipation (e.g. drinking 6–8 glasses of water per day). See Box 19.7 for more interventions.

Box 19.7 Managing constipation side effects caused by psychotropic medications

Assess for:

- regular bowel movements
- current diet, exercise
- other medications.

Advise to:

- drink 6–8 glasses of water per day
- increase fibre in diet
- increase exercise
- use available pharmacological products as needed.

ANTIPARKINSONIAN MEDICATIONS USED TO TREAT TARDIVE SYMPTOMS

Antiparkinsonian medications, also referred to as anticholinergics, are used to reduce the extrapyramidal side effects or tardive side effects of antipsychotic medications. Antiparkinsonian medications with a central anticholinergic action act to reduce the symptoms associated with parkinsonism, acute dystonia and akathisia (which together make up the tardive symptoms experienced by some who take antipsychotic medications). They inhibit the action of acetylcholine and are presumed to decrease cholinergic influence in the basal ganglia and thereby help balance the effects of antipsychotic medication reduction of dopaminergic influence (Psychotropic Expert Group 2013). See Table 19.5 for examples of antiparkinsonian medications, action and side effects.

However, antiparkinsonians are not routinely administered, as many consumers taking antipsychotic medication do not experience extrapyramidal effects. The antiparkinsonian medications also have their own set of unwanted effects and there is considerable intentional misuse of these medications for euphoric and sometimes hallucinogenic effects.

Special issues with psychotropic medications

Serotonin syndrome

Serotonin is a chemical involved in communication between nerve cells in the brain. Too little serotonin is believed to be implicated in developing depression, while too much

TABLE 19.5 Antiparkinsonians: action and side effects

NAME	ACTION	GENERAL SIDE EFFECTS (DOSE-RELATED)
Benztropine mesylate	Antihistamine and sedating qualities, long acting	(Anticholinergic) Dry mouth, dilated pupils, urinary hesitancy, constipation, blurred vision, nausea
Benzhexol	Specific anticholinergic action; stimulant properties	Dizziness, hallucinations
Biperiden	Anticholinergic action	Euphoria, hyperpyrexia
Orphenadrine	Anticholinergic action	Delirium in older people

can cause excess cell activity leading to a potentially deadly expression of symptoms known as 'serotonin syndrome'. Serotonin syndrome may occur within hours of taking a new medication. Medications that affect any step in the serotonin metabolism or regulation pathways can provoke the syndrome. Antidepressants, especially SSRIs, are the most implicated. Symptoms of serotonin syndrome include confusion, agitation, dilated pupils, headache, nausea/vomiting, rapid heart rate, tremor, shivering, loss of muscle coordination and heavy sweating. Prompt treatment and discontinuation of the offending medications is vital. Most situations are self-limiting if the medication is ceased quickly; however, supportive care is required until the crisis is over.

Cognitive enhancers

Cognitive enhancers improve memory, boost energy and alertness levels, and increase concentration. These medications have been studied extensively over the last decade to improve cognitive function across a number of clinical conditions. Developmental conditions such as attention deficit/hyperactivity disorder are treated with methylphenidate and atomoxetine (Hussain & Mehta 2011). Side effects include high body temperature; increased activity; dry mouth; euphoria; decreased fatigue, drowsiness and appetite; nausea and headaches; and increased blood pressure and respirations (Australian Drug Foundation 2014). Neurodegenerative disorders such as Alzheimer's disease and Parkinson's disease are commonly treated with acetylcholinesterase inhibitors and memantine as standard practice. However, it is hard to determine whether these improve memory or alertness (Hussain & Mehta 2011). Side effects include nausea and other gastrointestinal upsets, and impairment of verbal and visual memory (Hussain & Mehta 2011).

Pro re nata antipsychotic medication administration

The need to rapidly reduce agitation, distress or aggression often results in the prescription and administration of a prn antipsychotic medication in inpatient mental health facilities. Antipsychotics and benzodiazepines are the main classes of medications used in this way. Generally, most prn medications are given in the first few days after admission and are most frequently administered during the evening shift, from 6pm onwards, and at weekends (Usher et al. 2009a). It appears that peaks in prn administration coincide with regular medication and mealtimes.

Reasons given for administering prn medications include agitation, threatening behaviour, irritability, abusiveness, insomnia, disruptiveness, assault and request by the consumer. Environmental influences have also been suggested. The study by Usher et al. (2007) proposed that the physical and psychological environment in which consumers were cared for had an effect on the individual's sense of security and adversely affected their mental health, causing anxiety, agitation and frustration, and ultimately aggression, which in turn affected the need to resort to prn medications.

When nurses give prn medications, they are often required to decide what to give from a range of medications, as well as the amount to give and when to administer (Usher et al. 2009b; 2010). This allows nurses to administer psychotropic medications rapidly in acute situations or at the request of the consumer. Unfortunately, while this is an area of relative autonomy for nurses, it is also an area of practice that has been criticised, with concerns raised about over-reliance on psychotropic medications, particularly prn medications. Mullen and Drinkwater (2011) claim that mental health facilities should offer a range of therapeutic options and ensure that prn medications are used sparingly, and their use is monitored regularly.

The medications most often prescribed for prn administration are the typical antipsychotics, particularly medications like haloperidol. There is evidence to suggest that the benzodiazepines are just as effective as the typical antipsychotics in managing acute agitation and disturbed behaviour and should therefore be the medication of choice (Taylor et al. 2018). However, examination of current practice indicates that this is not happening and that the typical antipsychotics are being used predominantly for prn management of psychotic disturbance (Usher et al. 2009a). An Australian study found that higher levels of prn psychotropic medications are associated with unstable staffing profiles, particularly the use of less-experienced staff, high staff turnover, the deployment of non-regular staff to the ward and staff unfamiliar with the ward. There was also evidence that cultural background influenced the administration of prescribed prn medications (Usher et al. 2009a; 2010).

Adherence and concordance with medications

Effective treatment for people with schizophrenia requires a commitment to taking medications on a regular basis. Adherence to a prescribed antipsychotic medication regimen is often an ongoing problem for consumers with schizophrenia. In the past, this issue has been referred to in the literature as noncompliance. However, the term 'compliance' implies a power differential between the consumer and the healthcare provider, as well as passive rather than active participation by the consumer in the management of their mental health, so the accepted term is now 'adherence'.

Non-adherence, when the consumer does not take their medications as prescribed, is often the cause of relapse and readmission to hospital. The issue of medication adherence is complex and multifaceted and rarely includes the voice of the consumer (Happell et al. 2004). When a consumer does not take their medication as prescribed, their symptoms may not improve at the rate expected. This can lead to assumptions by health professionals that the medication is not effective. In the long run, this can cause unnecessary treatment changes. However, taking these medications as prescribed can facilitate functional recovery and help prevent illness-related complications.

Causes of non-adherence are related to issues such as:

- medication side effects (the different side effects of the typical and atypical antipsychotic medications impact adherence differently), whereby the antipsychotic medication may have an adverse impact on the person's quality of life and may even cause more distress than the symptoms of the illness (Usher et al. 2013)
- anosognosia, or lack of insight into the illness and the relationship between the illness and the need to take medications
- personal preference.

Against advice, people sometimes stop taking their medications and, because they do not relapse immediately, fail to see the connection between the medications and their health.

To help overcome lack of adherence with antipsychotic medications, several strategies have been explored (see Box 19.8). Evidence suggests that an active relationship between the nurse and the consumer is essential for improving adherence (Brown & Gray 2015). Other helpful strategies to aid adherence include education about the medications and their side effects, providing medication dispensers (Clyne et al. 2011), frequent follow-up and support (Brown & Gray 2015) and motivational interviewing (Brown & Gray 2015). It appears that no strategy is sufficient on its own, and a mixed approach to adherence may in fact be best. A recent study sought to explore the views of mental health staff regarding adherence. The authors report a lack of clarity about who is responsible for adherence and a focus on personal belief rather than evidence when considering adherence strategies (Brown & Gray 2015).

Box 19.8 Interventions to help with adherence to medication

- Get to know the consumer well.
- Help the consumer to develop an understanding of why the medications have been prescribed.
- Spend time talking about medications and the decisions related to adherence.
- Ask about the side effects being experienced and offer strategies to manage side effects where possible.
- Help the consumer to discuss issues related to their medications with their doctor or nurse.
- Offer dispensers to assist with organising medications.
- Provide education sessions for family or significant others.

'Concordance' is a term now used to indicate an agreement between the consumer and a clinician regarding medication plans and choice. The key aspects of concordance are working together collaboratively and flexibly, understanding the consumer's beliefs about their condition and medications plans, and working towards agreed goals that end in shared decision making (Edward & Alderman 2013).

Discontinuation syndrome

Discontinuation syndrome can result from switching between or rapid withdrawal of one of the antidepressant or antipsychotic medications. Common symptoms of withdrawal include dizziness, paraesthesia, numbness, electric-shock-like sensations, lethargy, headache, tremor, nausea, sweating, anorexia, insomnia, nightmares, nausea, vomiting, diarrhoea, rhinorrhoea, irritability, anxiety, restlessness, agitation and low mood (Read 2009), as well as hyperthermia related to clozapine withdrawal (Cerovecki et al. 2013). Rapid-onset psychosis (also called 'hypersensitivity psychosis') occurs in some cases of discontinuation. As well as relapse of illness, sudden withdrawal of antipsychotic medications has been linked to rare but potentially life-threatening events including NMS (Kurien & Vattakatuchery 2013) and withdrawal catatonia (Thanasan 2010; Wadekar & Syed 2010). Case study 19.1 overviews a case of discontinuation leading to NMS and demonstrates the importance for mental health nurses to be educated and aware of the physical conditions that can occur as a result of withdrawal of psychotropic medications.

Box 19.9 How to avoid and manage discontinuation syndrome

- Switch between or withdraw from medications slowly – taper doses.
- Plan withdrawal and monitor closely.
- Prescribe hypnotics for insomnia.
- Prescribe antianxiety agents for other symptoms.

Source: Cerovecki et al. 2013

CASE STUDY 19.1

Discontinuation leading to neuroleptic malignant syndrome

A man in his 40s diagnosed with paranoid schizophrenia attended the emergency department. He reported recently discontinuing antipsychotic and antidepressant medication he had been taking for eight years (clozapine 225 mg daily and venlafaxine XL 225 mg daily). On presentation he was perplexed, sweaty and shaking, and told the nurse he was hearing 'voices'. Assessment revealed WBC count 20,600/mL (20,600 mm^3) and CPK 17361U, temperature 37.7°C, pulse 80–122 beats per minute and respirations 18–40 breaths per minute. He was diagnosed with NMS as a result of cholinergic rebound from clozapine and venlafaxine. He was transferred to the mental health unit and treatment included regular oral diazepam 20 mg and lorazepam 4 mg daily as needed. His mental and physical state improved gradually over the following 2 weeks. He was then recommenced gradually on clozapine and venlafaxine and his mental state improved.

Adapted from Kurien & Vattakatuchery 2013

Exactly why discontinuation syndrome occurs is unclear (Salomon & Hamilton 2014), but it is thought to be linked to cholinergic and/or dopaminergic blockade and subsequent rebound (Cerovecki et al. 2013). To avoid discontinuation syndrome, mental health nurses have an important role to play in educating and monitoring consumers (Salomon & Hamilton 2014). The important principle of education is gradual withdrawal or switching of medications. See Box 19.9 for more ways to minimise the occurrence of discontinuation syndrome.

Cardiac risks related to psychotropic medications

Mental health disorders are associated with an increased risk of all-cause mortality, most commonly related to cardiovascular disease where an estimated two- to three-fold increased risk of cardiovascular disease has been noted across disorders resulting in a reduction in life expectancy greater than that associated with heavy smoking (Alveres et al. 2016). Several psychotropic medications have been associated with prolongation of the electrocardiograph QT interval, which is linked to lethal arrhythmias such as Torsades de Pointes, especially in individuals with underlying medical issues. Torsades de Pointes, an uncommon ventricular tachycardia, is associated with QT prolongation, which can lead to sudden death.

It is important for clinicians to be vigilant about cardiovascular assessment of at-risk patients before treating with psychotropic medication or before an increase in medication level. In particular, ECG monitoring, and a careful analysis of other QT risk factors such as the consumer's other medications (other drugs may prolong the QT interval such as some antibiotics and methadone) is required. Collaboration with other members of the healthcare team can often identify simple solutions to allow for optimal medical and mental health treatment (Beach et al. 2018).

Those drugs implicated in this problem include antidepressants such as citalopram and escitalopram, as well as antipsychotics including thioridazine (causes the greatest QT prolongation), ziprasidone, haloperidol (particularly intravenous infusion medications) and iloperidone (Beach et al. 2018).

Consumer education

While antipsychotic medications may be associated with favourable clinical outcomes for people experiencing a mental illness, consumers do not always take medications as directed. Medication adherence is associated with lower use of acute care services and greater engagement with community services (Ascher-Svanum et al. 2009). However, medication adherence has been identified as a major issue for consumers. A qualitative study undertaken by Happell et al. (2004) found that consumers reported a general lack of understanding about the reasons for the prescription of antipsychotic medications and their side effects. Education about the need to take medications as prescribed has been identified as a key role for nurses. However, nurses report feeling inadequately prepared to educate others about psychotropic medications and many express concerns about their own knowledge deficit about these medications (Brown et al. 2007). While education about medication has been proposed as an important strategy for improving adherence, education alone is not always effective. Education programs designed for improving adherence with psychotropic medications are more effective when combined with behavioural aspects of taking medication or motivational approaches, family therapy, psychological therapy or counselling.

See case studies 19.2 and 19.3 for an example of non-adherence and nursing responses.

CASE STUDY 19.2

Non-adherence to psychotropic medications (Part A)

Tony was first diagnosed with paranoid schizophrenia 5 years ago. His symptoms were exacerbated by poor adherence to prescribed medications and 'self-medication' with cannabis. Despite it being objectively clear that cannabis use made him more paranoid, Tony felt it helped him relax and was dismissive of education about harm-minimisation or abstaining.

The main hurdle to adherence with prescribed medication for Tony was denial. Tony did not accept his diagnosis; consequently, he did not accept his treatment. If we accept that a diagnosis of schizophrenia would provoke a sense of loss (e.g. normalcy, altered levels of independence, re-evaluated life goals, decreased acceptance), we may be able to understand the denial as a component of grief. Tony certainly displayed other classic stages of grief, most notably anger (at his treating psychiatrist) and bargaining (with his community case manager about postponing or cancelling administration of depot medications).

Other contributing factors to Tony's non-adherence were: the illness itself – paranoia is a barrier to building trust and rapport with clinicians; lack of education/understanding about the illness and its treatment; and the side effects of the prescribed medications.

Critical thinking challenge 19.1

1. Denial is a commonly used defence mechanism when a person is faced with issues they are not yet able to cope with on a conscious level. Discuss the concept of denial as a component of grief and loss in relation to the diagnosis of a chronic mental illness. How does the concept of denial differ from that of insight? In part A of the case study (Case study 19.2), how could the nurse manage Tony's non-adherence while recognising the importance of denial as a coping mechanism?
2. Explore relevant strategies to address the other factors contributing to Tony's non-adherence, such as his paranoia, lack of education and understanding, and unwanted medication side effects.

CASE STUDY 19.3

Non-adherence to psychotropic medications (Part B)

A management plan was developed to address the factors contributing to Tony's non-adherence. Tony's outpatient care was assigned to a clinical nurse in the role of case manager. This nurse administered and monitored prescribed medications and worked to build a therapeutic alliance with Tony. When Tony was an inpatient, as occurred frequently during the first 3 years of diagnosis, he was assigned a primary nurse on the mental health unit, who collaborated with the case manager to provide continuity of care and another avenue for Tony to develop rapport.

Over time, Tony began to engage with his two primary carers, which provided an opportunity for education about his diagnosis and treatment options. In time, Tony became more accepting of the treating team as a whole and would discuss medication issues freely with his treating psychiatrist.

As Tony's acceptance improved, medication options were no longer restricted to depot injections, and oral medications were trialled. Tony was very sensitive to typical antipsychotics and developed extrapyramidal side effects at sub-therapeutic doses. Trials of other atypical antipsychotic medications also had problems – poor symptom control and marked weight gain. Twelve months ago, a trial of clozapine began. It took 4 months to stabilise the dose at 450 mg nocte (at night). In doing so, Tony's mental state also stabilised. He developed considerable insight into his condition and treatment and has developed a good degree of acceptance.

Nine months later, with encouragement from the treating team, Tony undertook a trial of abstinence from cannabis. Tony says he has used cannabis only twice since. This hasn't been objectively checked through urine samples, but his case manager has noted further improvement in symptom control and motivation to undertake activities of daily living and social interaction.

Tony has not required admission to the mental health unit for over 8 months now. If he remains stable until the new year, his case manager intends to assist Tony in seeking work.

The authors acknowledge this contribution from Paul McNamara, CNC, Consultation Liaison Team, Cairns Base Hospital, to this case study.

Critical thinking challenge 19.2

1. In part B of the case study (Case study 19.3), Tony was trialled on atypical antipsychotics. How does this group of medications differ from typical antipsychotics? Identify the benefits and disadvantages of each of these medication groups.
2. The incidence of extrapyramidal side effects varies according to the particular antipsychotic medication used. Identify the various extrapyramidal side effects and explore the most effective management for these.

3. Tony was trialled on clozapine. What are the benefits and disadvantages of using this medication? Why is it not necessarily the first medication of choice for consumers with psychosis?
4. Cannabis is commonly used by consumers with a mental illness. What are the reasons for this? What does the term 'self-medicating' mean? Explore the effect(s) of cannabis when a person has a psychosis.
5. Critically analyse the strategies in the management plan used for Tony's non-adherence. In your opinion, was the plan successful? If so (or not) explain the reason(s) for this.

Collaborative prescribing

The traditional role of prescribing is changing; and, the area of mental health practice is no different. In some countries, including Australia and New Zealand, medications that could once only be prescribed by medical practitioners are now being legally prescribed by other members of the multidisciplinary team (Hoti et al. 2011; Wheeler et al. 2012) including nurses, pharmacists and psychologists. Currently in Australia and New Zealand, mental health nurse practitioners can legally prescribe medications to mental health consumers in both inpatient and community settings in collaboration with other members of the multidisciplinary team. Collaborative practice is said to occur when multiple health professionals from different discipline areas work together with consumers, their families and others to deliver the highest quality care across diverse settings (World Health Organization 2010). Collaborative practice has a positive impact on consumer outcomes. It rests on the principle of involving consumers in all aspects of mental health service delivery to support them in making informed decisions (Chong et al. 2013), in this case, about medication prescription.

Informed consent and the ethics of psychotropic medications

The right of a consumer to determine his or her own treatment underpins the underlying values of beneficence and respect for an individual's autonomy and wellbeing. The elements of a valid informed consent include that the person has the capacity to consent, has received adequate information to consent and has given consent voluntarily and freely. It is not enough to assume a person lacks the ability to give consent based on their age, disability, appearance, behavior, medical condition (including presence of a mental condition), beliefs or apparent inability to communicate, or because the consumer does not agree with the clinician's decision. Competent people have the right to consent to treatment. At times, substitute decision-makers, including family and carers, can consent on behalf of an individual when that individual is deemed to lack the capacity to make an authoritative decision (Schachter et al. 2005). Informed consent regarding psychotropic medications can be very challenging. A consumer's mental illness may make it difficult for a consumer to make a competent decision regarding treatment and the clinician may be concerned about their ability to make appropriate decisions about the need to continue medication. This brings us to the issues of forcible or covert medication administration. Making consumers feel they have no option but to take a medication, or covertly (hiding the fact the consumer is being given a medication) administering a medication, is entirely unethical becausee it violates an individual's right to autonomy. However, if a consumer is deemed to lack the capacity to make a decision, the principle of autonomy is not violated as long as the treatment is deemed to be in the best interests of the consumer. It is therefore important that the clinician assesses whether the consumer has the capacity to agree to, or refuse, treatment as a matter of urgency, especially in emergency situations (Hung et al. 2012).

CASE STUDY 19.4
Ethical issues related to consent to psychotropic medication

Jill, a registered nurse, commences her medication round and enters the bay of four consumers with the drug trolley.

She approaches consumer A, who is lying down in long-sleeve pyjamas. Having drawn up the injection, she approaches A, who sits up in bed and rolls up his sleeve to expose the injection site. Jill administers the injection without saying anything.

Jill moves to consumer B, aged 10, who is 'groggy' from an anesthetic and swallows his medication after Jill asks him to take his tablets.

Jill moves to consumer C and as she hands over the tablets. The consumer asks what the various tablets are for. Jill says she does not know but says, 'You'd better take them because that's what the doctor ordered'.

Jill then moves to consumer D, and when handing the tablets to D the consumer says, 'I'm not taking them'. Jill replies: 'If you don't, then don't expect dinner.' D reluctantly takes the tablets.

Consent for these four consumers:

A. Consent can be expressed or implied. Rolling up the sleeve, for example, is an act consistent with giving *implied consent*.
B. No consent for two reasons. First the consumer does not have *legal capacity* due to being minor (under 18); and second, no mental capacity to make a decision due to the anesthetic.

C. Consent needs to be informed consent. C does not have the necessary information to make an *informed decision*.
D. Consent must be *freely* given without threat, inducement or coercion. Threatening to withhold a meal overrides the 'free will' of D.

Remember the four elements of a valid consent. To take medication the consumer must have:

1. competence/capacity (age and cognitive ability)
2. the consent is given voluntarily
3. the consent covers the medication in question
4. that the consumer was fully informed in making that decision.

The authors acknowledge this contribution from Dr Scott Trueman, RN.

Depot or long-acting intramuscular injectable antipsychotics

Depot or long-acting injectable antipsychotic preparations, introduced in the 1960s, are useful when there might be problems with adherence with oral medications, when the consumer is unable to take oral medications, if intestinal absorption is questioned or where accidental overdose is a possibility. Importantly, this strategy offers a more consistent treatment option (Smith & Herber 2014). There are also occasions where consumers express a preference for this form of treatment (Kane & Garcia-Ribera 2009). These long-acting, injectable forms of antipsychotic medications, produced mostly in decanoate esters dissolved in an oily base, are prescribed for up to 33% of people with schizophrenia and other mental health issues (Barnes et al. 2009). Mental health nurses are most commonly responsible for administering injectable antipsychotic medications; these may be delivered in both inpatient and community settings (Smith & Herber 2014). When administered by deep intramuscular injection, the medication is de-esterified to release the active medication, which slowly diffuses into the circulation. The injections are usually given every 2–4 weeks (Psychotropic Expert Group 2013) (see Table 19.6) and generally the release of medication must last at least 1 week to be considered a depot preparation. As depot injections involve large amounts of fluid, they should be injected into a large muscle using the z-track technique (McCuistion et al. 2014).

While this strategy is one way to manage adherence issues, it is important to remember that a strong nurse–consumer relationship can help promote medication adherence and that the consumer has a right to be involved in choosing the route of administration of prescribed medications wherever possible. A study explored the ethical issues experienced by mental health nurses in relation to administering depot or long-acting antipsychotic medications. The findings revealed that mental health nurses were conflicted by their desire to do what they believed to be in the best interests of the consumer, even if they thought this sometimes bordered on coercion, yet remaining aware of the need to protect the therapeutic relationship (Smith & Herber 2014). Unfortunately, several studies have indicated that community nurses report spending very little time with consumers at the time of administration of depot injections (Patel et al. 2005).

Medication for acute agitation

Acute agitation that may escalate to violence and aggression depends on a combination of internal factors (e.g. personality characteristics and intense mental distress) and external factors (e.g. the attitudes and behaviours of surrounding staff and service users, the physical setting and any restrictions that limit a person's freedom) (National Institute for Health and Care Excellence 2015). Acute agitation can occur in many different contexts, from a medical ward to psychiatric intensive care unit, and is not necessarily related to a mental illness or disorder. Initial approaches to managing agitation should be psychosocial, particularly because medication interventions are often coercive involving restraint and can be traumatising (Ministry of Health 2015). However, at times when psychosocial intervention is unsuccessful, medication may be needed to prevent harm occurring to the person themselves or to others including staff, family/carers and other patients.

Medications for acute agitation generally work as a result of their sedating, anxiolytic and tranquillising effects as opposed to treating an underlying cause. First-line intervention should be to offer oral medications with benzodiazepines due to the low level of side effects and their efficacy on modulating emotional responses cause by excessive amygdala output (Stahl 2013). Antipsychotics are very effective for managing agitated behaviour due to the neuroleptic effect of D_2 blockade as well as strong histamine binding (that causes sedation) with first-generation medications (e.g. haloperidol and droperidol) and second-generation medications such as olanzapine (Stahl 2013). Antipsychotic medications may also have the benefit of helping to treat underlying psychotic symptoms when agitation is related to psychotic processes. Fig. 19.1 outlines the choices of medications in different circumstances.

Psychotropic medication use in special populations

Pregnant and breastfeeding women

The management of women who are pregnant or breastfeeding poses a significant challenge for mental health nurses. The prescription and administration of psychotropic medications, if required during pregnancy

TABLE 19.6 Long-acting injectables (depot medications)

DRUG	TRADE NAMES	TEST DOSE	DOSE RANGE	INJECTION INTERVAL	COMMENTS
First-generation antipsychotics					
Flupenthixol decanoate	Depixol	5–20 mg injection	Usual dose range 20–40 mg every 2 to 4 weeks Higher doses of > 100 mg are used for treatment resistance	2–4 weekly	
Haloperidol decanoate	Haldol	Suggested 25 mg injection	50–300 mg	2–4 weekly	High prevalence of extrapyramidal side effects
Zuclopenthixol decanoate	Clopixol	100 mg injection	200–400 mg Higher doses are used for treatment resistance	Usually 2–4 weekly, although frequency can be increased	High prevalence of extrapyramidal side effects
Second-generation antipsychotics					
Aripiprazole monohydrate	Abilify Maintena	Establish tolerability with oral aripiprazole	300–400 mg	Usually 4 weekly Minimum of 26 days between injections	Requires 2 weeks of overlap with oral aripiprazole
Olanzapine pamoate	Zyprexa Relprevv	Establish tolerability with oral olanzapine	150–300 mg fortnightly to 405 mg monthly	2–4 weekly	Risk of post-injection syndrome Monitoring needed for at least 2 hours after administration
Paliperidone palmitate	Invega Sustenna	Establish tolerability with oral paliperidone or oral risperidone	25–150 mg	Monthly (after loading dose)	Loading dose schedule at initiation of treatment, 2 injections in first 8 days
Paliperidone palmitate	Invega Trinza	Only initiate after 4 months of treatment with Paliperidone Invega	175–525 mg	Every 3 months	Longest interval between administration of all long-acting injectables
Risperidone	Risperdal Consta	Establish tolerability with immediate release oral risperidone	25–50 mg	Every 2 weeks	Initiation needs to overlap with oral treatment due to delayed action

and breastfeeding, presents many risks to the unborn fetus or the newborn child. Antipsychotic medications, especially the atypical antipsychotics, commonly prescribed for women who experience psychoses during pregnancy or in the immediate postpartum period, have not been proved safe in pregnancy, and their use in pregnancy is not based on evidence from randomised clinical trials (Usher et al. 2009b). However, the consequences of untreated psychiatric disorders during pregnancy must be weighed against the risk of prenatal exposure to medications, as antenatal psychological distress is known to be linked to premature labour, low birth weight, smaller head circumference and inferior functional assessments in newborns (Kieviet et al. 2013).

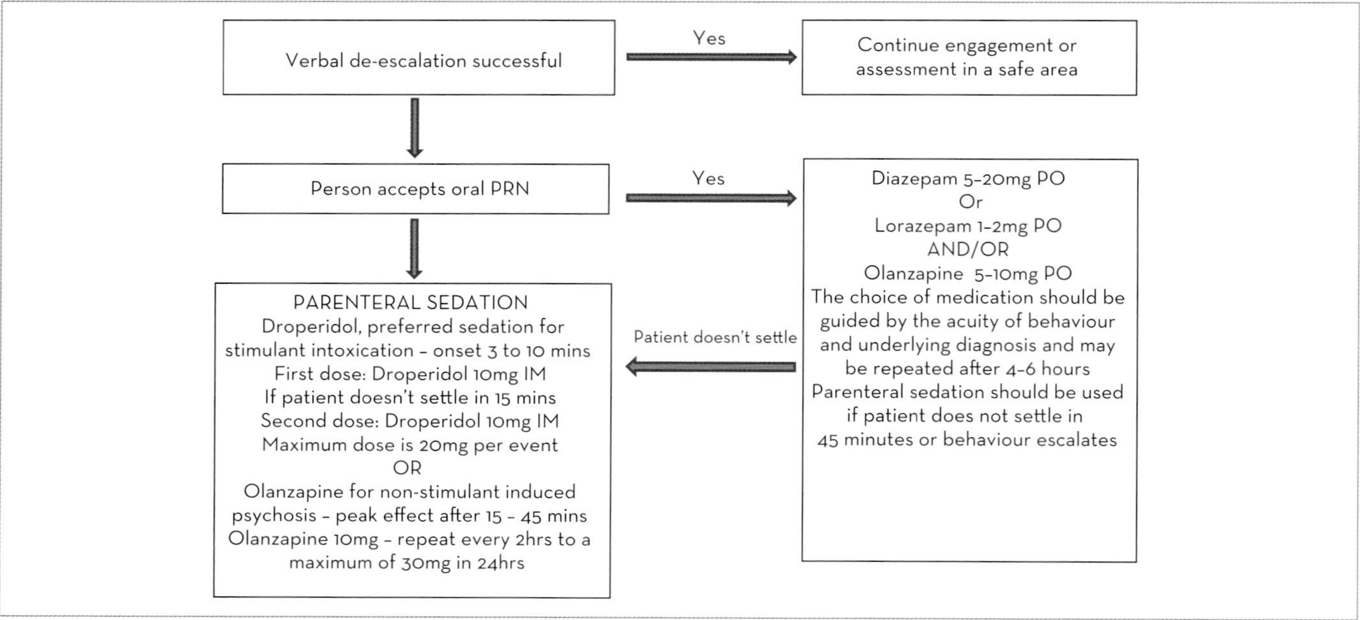

Figure 19.1
Pharmacological management of acute agitation and/or aggression: adults (under 65 years and/or no diagnosis of organic cognitive impairment)
Adapted from Galletly et al. 2016 and Ministry of Health 2015

The evidence of the teratogenic effects of psychotropic medications is mixed, and their use during pregnancy can expose the fetus to an increased risk of congenital malformation. Several psychotropic medications are known to have teratogenic effects in early pregnancy, as well as probable adverse effects on neonates late in pregnancy (Kieviet et al. 2013; Menon et al. 2008). Most antidepressants appear to be safe during pregnancy. However, as antidepressants and lithium are excreted in breast milk, at least in small quantities, the babies of mothers who choose to breastfeed should be monitored closely, especially in the first few weeks after birth (Bogan et al. 2012). Usher et al. (2005) proposed the following guidelines for psychotropic medication use in women who are pregnant or breastfeeding:

- Antipsychotics, including depot injections, should be avoided in the first trimester.
- Women using atypicals should change to typical antipsychotics as soon as pregnancy is diagnosed.
- Pregnant and breastfeeding women should be prescribed the lowest possible dose.
- Depot injections should be avoided in breastfeeding women.
- Only infants born at full term should be exposed to the potential to ingest medication via breast milk.

Children and adolescents

Although psychotropic medications have been used with children and adolescents for several decades, the use of these medications with this group should be monitored carefully. Second-generation medications are used to treat a variety of conditions in children and adolescents. While these and other psychotropic medications are used to manage numerous conditions such as autism, Asperger's syndrome, Tourette's syndrome and tic disorders, non-pharmacological options are the preferred treatment. However, if pharmacological agents are used, the atypical antipsychotics are usually chosen because they have less serious side effects in children and adolescents (Usher et al. 2009b). Antidepressants should be prescribed only with extreme caution in this group, as children are particularly vulnerable to the cardiotoxic and seizure-inducing effects of high doses of tricyclic compounds. Deaths have been reported in children after accidental or deliberate overdosage with as little as a few hundred milligrams of a tricyclic medication. Therefore, nurses must be particularly vigilant if working with children who are prescribed psychotropic medications.

Older people

Psychotropic medications are prescribed for older people for conditions such as mood and anxiety disorders, bipolar affective disorder, depression and dementia. Psychotropic medications have a role in managing these conditions (Usher et al. 2009b). However, particular care must be taken when psychotropic medications are considered for older consumers. It is generally considered that older people will experience more adverse effects from psychotropic medication use, especially people over the age of 70, due to slower medication metabolism and excretion. For example, benzodiazepines are more likely to cause dizziness, which can lead to falls and serious injury. Antidepressants in older people can be problematic and are more likely to cause dizziness, postural hypotension, constipation, delayed micturition, oedema and tremor (Usher et al. 2009b). There is also evidence that psychotropic medication prescription in the older person is linked to cognitive impairments such as delirium (Kaufman & Milstein 2013). It is important for mental health nurses to be aware of the special problems these medications may pose when used with older consumers and to be vigilant in supervising and monitoring side effects. Polypharmacy may have dire consequences for this group and should be avoided wherever possible. Older people are known to take more medications than younger people and often take more than one medication.

Psychotropic medication use is common in people with dementia; however, psychotropic medications have actually been reported as being of little use in managing the behavioural and psychological symptoms related to dementia even though their use is common in this population (Kaufman & Milstein 2013). However, a study of patterns of psychotropic medication use in several Australian nursing homes between 1993 and 2009 reported that rates of hypnotic, anxiolytic and antidepressant medication use are low compared with other countries (Snowdon et al. 2011).

Chapter summary

This chapter has presented an overview of the issues related to psychopharmacology, including the use of prn psychotropic medications, adherence with medications as prescribed and their use with special populations. To be effective practitioners, mental health nurses need to be equipped with knowledge and understanding of the distinct medication indications, interactions, side effects and precautions related to the four major psychotropic medication groups (antianxiety, antidepressant, mood-stabilising and antipsychotic). Mental health nurses need to have a working knowledge of psychopharmacology and related issues because administering these medications is a common but important nursing intervention. The information presented here will help to prepare mental health nurses to make well-informed treatment decisions and engage in successful consumer assessment and education. It will also help the nurse to detect and manage side effects from psychotropic medications, many of which can be harmful or even life-threatening.

EXERCISES FOR CLASS ENGAGEMENT

1. In a small group discuss the legal and ethical issues that a mental health nurse needs to consider when administering psychotropic medications. In particular, consider the issues related to consent regarding emergency situations.
2. In small groups, outline what you believe are the important issues related to medication adherence. How might your beliefs differ from those of consumers? Discuss your findings with the larger group.
3. In small groups, debate and respond to the following questions:
   - Discuss how you would manage a situation where you believed a consumer was being prescribed and administered a toxic level of a medication.
   - Describe how polypharmacy can be a problem for people taking antipsychotic medications and for members of vulnerable groups such as older people.
   - Describe the signs of a tricyclic overdose and list those who might be at high risk of such an outcome.
   - Anticonvulsant medications are used in the management of people with bipolar disorder. Describe the action of these medications and list their potential side effects.
   - Lithium is commonly used as a mood-stabilising medication. Outline why it is important to obtain regular blood tests for people taking this medication and outline the therapeutic range and signs of lithium toxicity.
   - Discuss the physical issues of importance when working with consumers taking psychotropic medications.

Useful websites

AIMS tool: http://www.cqaimh.org/pdf/tool_aims.pdf

Australian Prescriber – useful information on drugs: https://www.nps.org.au/australian-prescriber/

Glasgow Antipsychotic Side-effect Scale (GASS): https://mypsych.nhsggc.org.uk/my-psych-placement/tools/glasgow-antipsychotic-side-effect-scale-gass/

Healthline – drug interactions: https://www.healthline.com/health/what-is-a-psychotropic-drug#drug-interactions

Medsafe (New Zealand Medicines and Medical Devices Safety Authority): https://www.medsafe.govt.nz/

National Prescribing Authority (Australia): https://www.nps.org.au/

Pharmaceutical Management Agency of New Zealand (PHARMAC): https://www.pharmac.govt.nz/

References

Allison, D.B., Mentore, J.L., Heo, M., et al., 1999. Antipsychotic-induced weight gain: a comprehensive research synthesis. Am. J. Psychiatry 156 (11), 1686–1696.

Alveres, G., Quintana, D., Hickie, I., et al., 2016. Autonimic nervous system dysfunction in psychiatric disorders and the impact of psychotropic medications: a systematic review and meta-synthesis. J. Psychiatry Neurosci. 41 (2), 89–104.

Ascher-Svanum, H., Zhu, B., Faries, D.E., et al., 2009. Medication adherence levels and differential use of mental health services in the treatment of schizophrenia. BMC Res. Notes 2, 6.

Australian Drug Foundation, 2014. Cognitive enhancers (smart drugs). Available: adf.org.au/subscribe.

Bandelow, B., Sher, L., Bunevicius, R., et al., 2012. Guidelines for the pharmacological treatment of anxiety disorders, obsessive–compulsive disorder and posttraumatic stress disorder in primary care. Int. J. Psychiatry Clin. Pract. 16, 77–84.

Barnes, T.R.E., Shingleton-Smith, A., Paton, C., 2009. Antipsychotic long-acting injections: prescribing practice in the UK. Br. J. Psychiatry 195 (52), S37–S42. doi:10.1192/bjp.195.52.s37.

Beach, S., Celano, C., Sugrue, A., et al., 2018. QT prolongation, Torsades de Pointes, and psychotropic medications: a 5-year update. Psychosomatics 59 (2), 105–122.

Bogan, D.L., Sit, D., Genovese, A., et al., 2012. Three cases of lithium exposure and exclusive breastfeeding. Arch. Womens Ment. Health 15 (1), 69–72.

Brown, E., Gray, R., 2015. Tackling medication non-adherence in severe mental illness: where are we going wrong? J. Psychiatr. Ment. Health Nurs. 22, 192–198.

Brown, I., Stride, C., Psarou, A., et al., 2007. Management of obesity in primary care: nurses' practices, beliefs and attitudes. J. Adv. Nurs. 59, 329–341.

Cerovecki, A., Musil, R., Klimke, A., et al., 2013. Withdrawal symptoms and rebound syndromes associated with switching and discontinuing atypical antipsychotics: theoretical background and practical recommendations. CNS Drugs 27, 545–572.

Chong, W., Aslani, P., Chen, T., 2013. Multiple perspectives on shared decision-making and interprofessional collaboration in mental healthcare. J. Interprof. Care 27, 223–230.

Clyne, W., Mshelia, C., Hall, S., et al., 2011. Management of patient adherence to medications: protocol for an online survey of doctors, pharmacists and nurses in Europe. BMJ Open 1, 1.

Edward, K.L., Alderman, C., 2013. Psychopharmacology: Practice and Contexts. Oxford University Press, Melbourne.

Edwards, K.L., Rasmussen, B., Munro, I., 2010. Nursing care of clients treated with atypical antipsychotics who have a risk of developing metabolic instability and/or type 2 diabetes. Arch. Psychiatr. Nurs. 24 (1), 46–53.

Galletly, C., Castle, D., Dark, F., et al., 2016. Royal Australian and New Zealand College of Psychiatrists clinical practice guidelines for the management of schizophrenia and related disorders. Aust. N. Z. J. Psychiatry 50 (5), 1–117.

Happell, B., Manias, E., Roper, C., 2004. Wanting to be heard: mental health consumers' experiences of information about medication. Int. J. Ment. Health Nurs. 13, 242–248.

Hepburn, K., Brzozowska, M.M., 2016. Diabetic ketoacidosis and severe hyperlipidaemia as a consequence of an atypical antipsychotic agent. BMJ Case Rep. 2016, doi:10.1136/bcr-2016-215413.

Hoti, K., Hughes, T., Sunderland, B., 2011. An expanded role for pharmacisist: an Australian perspective. Aust. Med. J. 4 (4), 236–242.

Hubbard, R.E., Peel, N.M., Scott, I.A., et al., 2015. Polypharmacy among inpatients aged 70 years or older in Australia. Med. J. Aust. 202 (7), 373–378.

Hung, E.K., McNiel, D.E., Binder, R.L., 2012. Covert medication in psychiatric emergencies: is it ever ethically permissible? J. Am. Acad. Psychiatry Law 40 (2), 239–245.

Hirschfeld, R.M.A., 2000. History and evolution of the monoamine hypothesis of depression. J. Clin. Psychiatry 61 (Suppl. 6), 4–6.

Hussain, M., Mehta, M.A., 2011. Cognitive enhancement by drugs in health and disease. Trends Cogn. Sci. 15 (1), 28–36.

Hyde, N., Dodd, S., Venugopal, K., et al., 2015. Prevalence of cardiovascular and metabolic events in patients prescribed clozapine: a retrospective observational, clinical cohort study. Curr. Drug Saf. 10 (2), 125–131.

Jessurun, J.G., van Harten, P., Egberts, T.C.G., et al., 2013. The effect of psychotropic medications on the occurrence of constipation in hospitalized psychiatric patients. J. Clin. Psychopharmacol. 33 (4), 587–590.

John, A.P., Koloth, R., Dragovic, M., et al., 2009. Prevalence of metabolic syndrome among Australians with severe mental illness. Med. J. Aust. 190 (4), 176–179.

Kane, J.M., Garcia-Ribera, C., 2009. Clinical guideline recommendations for antipsychotic long-acting injections. Br. J. Psychiatry 195 (52), S63–S67.

Kaufman, D.M., Milstein, M.J., 2013. Kaufman's Clinical Neurology for Psychiatrists, seventh ed. Elsevier Saunders, London.

Kieviet, N., Dolman, K.N., Honig, A., 2013. The use of psychotropic medication during pregnancy: how about the newborn? Neuropsychiatr. Dis. Treat. 2013 (9), 1257–1266.

Kurien, R., Vattakatuchery, J.J., 2013. Psychotropic discontinuation leading to an NMS-like condition. Prog. Neurol. Psychiatry 17 (5), 11–12.

López-Muñoz, F., Alamo, C., Cuenca, E., et al., 2005. History of the discovery and clinical introduction of chlorpromazine. Ann. Clin. Psychiatry 17 (3), 113–135.

Malhi, G.S., Gershon, S., Outhred, T., 2016. Litiumeter: version 2.0. Bipolar Disord. 18, 631–641.

McCuistion, L.E., Kee, J.L., Hayes, E.R. (Eds.), 2014. Pharmacology: A Patient-Centered Nursing Process Approach, eighth ed. Elsevier Health Sciences, St Louis.

McDaid, T.M., Smyth, S., 2015. Metabolic abnormalities among people diagnosed with schizophrenia: a literature review and implications for mental health nurses. J. Psychiatr. Ment. Health Nurs. 22, 157–170.

Ministry of Health, 2015. Management of Patients With Acute Severe Behavioural Disturbance in Emergency Departments. NSW Government, Sydney.

Menon, S.J., et al., 2008. Psychotropic medication during pregnancy and lactation. Arch. Gynecol. Obstet. 277 (1), 1–13.

Morrison, P., Gaskill, D., Meehan, T., et al., 2000. The use of the Liverpool University Neuroleptic Side Effect Rating Scale (LUNSERS) in clinical practice. Aust. N. Z. J. Ment. Health Nurs. 9 (4), 166–176.

Mullen, A., Drinkwater, V., 2011. Pro re nata use in a psychiatric intensive care unit. Int. J. Ment. Health Nurs. 20, 409–417.

National Institute for Health and Care Excellence, 2015. Violence and aggression: short-term management in mental health, health and community settings (NICE Guideline 10). Available at: https://www.nice.org.uk/guidance/ng10.

Park, T., Usher, K., Foster, K., 2011. Description of a healthy lifestyle intervention for people with schizophrenia taking second generation antipsychotics. Int. J. Ment. Health Nurs. 20, 428–437.

Patel, M.X., De Zoysa, N., Baker, D., et al., 2005. Antipsychotic depot medication and attitudes of community psychiatric nurses. J. Psychiatr. Ment. Health Nurs. 12, 237–244.

Psychotropic Expert Group, 2013. Therapeutic Guidelines: Psychotropic, Version 7. Therapeutic Guidelines Limited, Melbourne.

Royal Australian and New Zealand College of Psychiatrists, 2015. Royal Australian and New Zealand College of Psychiatrists clinical practice guidelines for mood disorders. Aust. N. Z. J. Psychiatry 49 (12), 1–185.

Royal College of Pathologists of Australasia, 2019. Pathology manual: pathology results. Retrieved from: https://www.rcpa.edu.au/Manuals/RCPA-Manual/Pathology-Tests/L/Lithium. (Accessed 15 May 2019).

Read, J., 2009. Psychiatric Drugs: Key Issues and Service User Perspectives. Palgrave Macmillan, New York.

Remington, G., Agid, O., Foussias, G., et al., 2013. Clozapine's role in the treatment of first-episode schizophrenia. Am. J. Psychiatry 170 (2), 146–151.

Salomon, C., Hamilton, B., 2014. Antipsychotic discontinuation syndromes: a narrative review of the evidence and its integration into Australian mental health nursing textbooks. Int. J. Ment. Health Nurs. 23, 69–75.

Schachter, D., Kleinman, I., Harvey, W., 2005. Informed consent and adolescents. Can. J. Psychiatry 50 (9), 534–540.

Smith, J.P., Herber, O.R., 2014. Ethical issues experienced by mental health nurses in the administration of antipsychotic depot and long-acting intramuscular injections: a qualitative study. Int. J. Ment. Health Nurs. 24, 222–230.

Snowdon, J., Galanos, D., Vaswani, D., 2011. Patterns of psychotropic medication use in nursing homes: surveys in Sydney, allowing comparisons over time and between countries. Int. Psychogeriatr. 23 (9), 1520–1525.

Stahl, S.M., 2013. Stahl's Essential Psychopharmacology: Neuroscientific Basis and Practical Applications, fourth ed. Cambridge University Press, New York.

Su, Y-P., Chang, C-K., Hayes, R.D., et al., 2014. Retrospective chart review on exposure to psychotropic medications associated with neuroleptic malignant syndrome. Acta. Psychiatr. Scand. 130 (1), 52–60.

Taylor, D.M., Barnes, T.R.E., Young, A.H., 2018. The Maudsley Prescribing Guidelines in Psychiatry, thirteenth ed. Wiley Blackwell, London.

Thanasan, S., 2010. Clozapine withdrawal catatonia or lethal catatonia in a schizoaffective patient with a family history of Parkinson's disease. Afr. J. Psychiatry 13, 402–404.

Tirupati, S., Chua, L.E., 2007. Obesity and metabolic syndrome in a psychiatric rehabilitation service. Aust. N. Z. J. Psychiatry 42 (2), 606–610.

Treatment Protocol Project, 2004. Management of Mental Disorders, fourth ed. World Health Organization Collaborating Centre for Mental Health and Substance Abuse, Sydney.

Tschoner, A., Engl, J., Laimer, M., et al., 2007. Metabolic side effects of antipsychotic medication. Int. J. Clin. Pract. 61 (8), 1356–1370.

Usher, K., Baker, J., Homes, C., 2010. Understanding clinical decision making for prn medication in mental health inpatient facilities. J. Psychiatr. Ment. Health Nurs. 17, 558–564.

Usher, K., Baker, J., Holmes, C., et al., 2009a. Clinical decision-making for 'as needed' medications in mental health care. J. Adv. Nurs. 65 (5), 981–991.

Usher, K., Foster, K., Bullock, S., 2009b. Psychopharmacology for Health Professionals. Elsevier, Sydney.

Usher, K., Foster, K., McNamara, P., 2005. Antipsychotic drugs and pregnant or breastfeeding women: the issues for mental health nurses. J. Psychiatr. Ment. Health Nurs. 12 (6), 713–718.

Usher, K., Holmes, C., Baker, J., 2007. Enhancing the Understanding of Clinical Decision Making for PRN Medications Within Mental Health Facilities. Final report to the Queensland Nursing Council (QNC), Brisbane.

Usher, K., Park, T., Foster, K., 2013. The experience of weight gain as a result of taking second-generation antipsychotic medications: the mental health consumer perspective. J. Psychiatr. Ment. Health Nurs. 20, 801–806.

Van der Loos, M.L., Mulder, P., Hartong, E.G., et al., 2011. Long-term outcome of bipolar depressed patients receiving lamotrigine as add-on to lithium with the possibility of the addition of paroxetine in nonresponders: a randomized, placebo-controlled trial with a novel design. Bipolar Disord. 13, 111–117.

Vieta, E., Cruz, N., Garcia-Campayo, J., et al., 2008. A double-blind, randomized, placebo-controlled prophylaxis trial of oxcarbazepine as adjunctive treatment to lithium in long-term treatment of bipolar I and II disorder. Int. J. Neuropsychopharmacol. 11, 445–452.

Wadekar, M., Syed, S., 2010. Clozapine withdrawal catatonia. Psychosomatics 51 (4), 355.

Wheeler, A., Crump, K., Lee, M., et al., 2012. Collaborative prescribing: a qualitative exploration of a role for pharmacists in mental health care. Res. Soc. Adm. Psychiatry 8 (3), 179–192.

World Health Organization, 2010. Framework for action on interprofessional education and collaborative practice. Retrieved from: https://www.who.int/hrh/resources/framework_action/en/. (Accessed 15 May 2019).

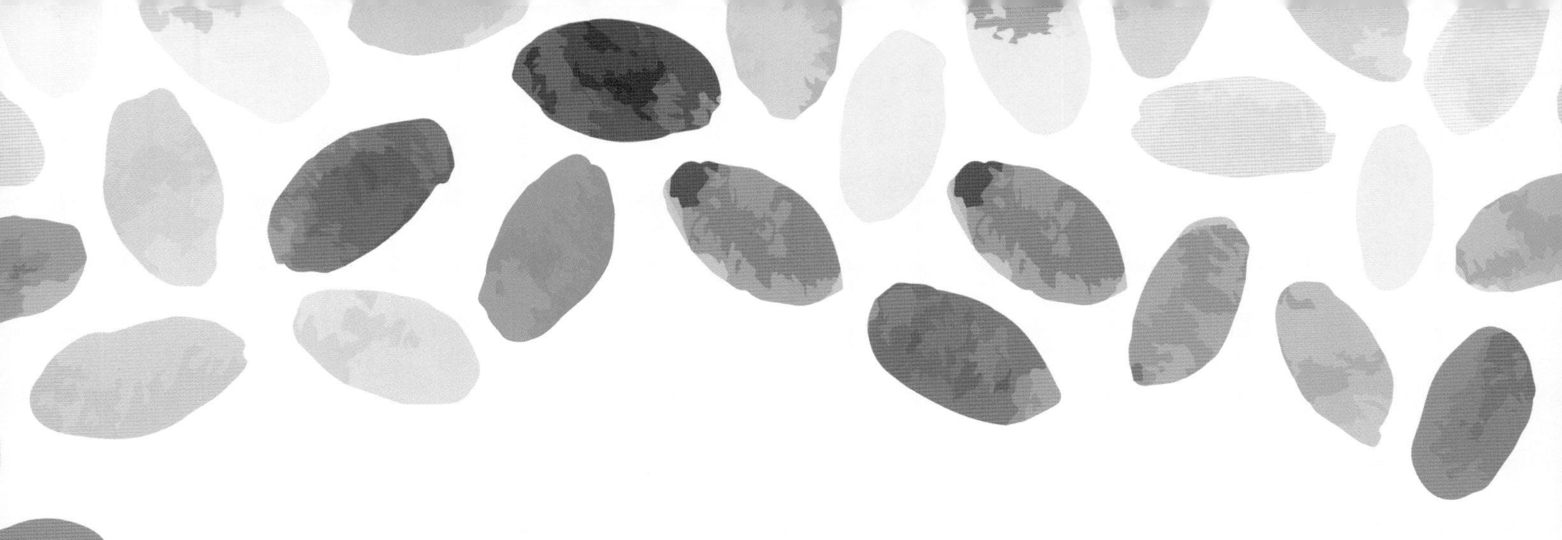

PART 3

Contexts of Practice

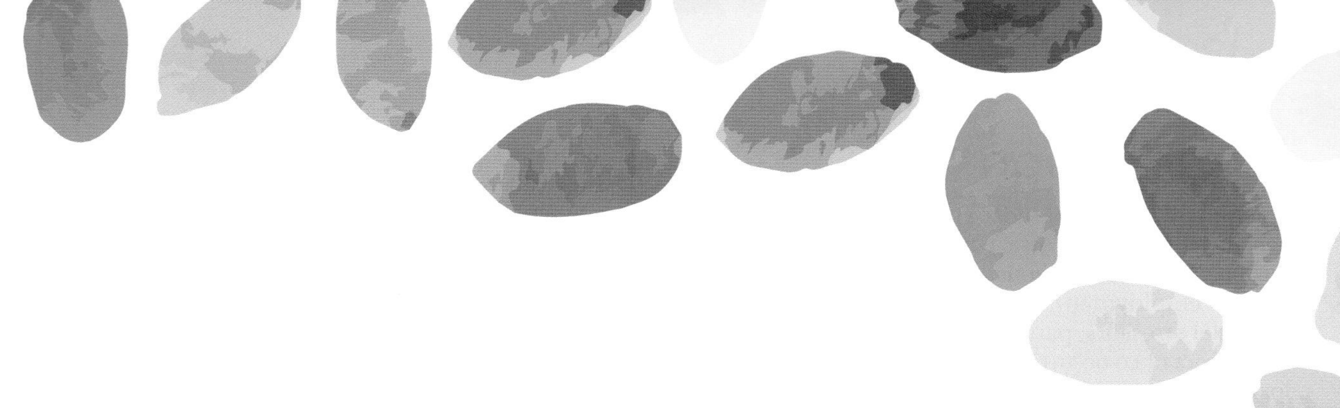

CHAPTER 20

Mental health in every setting

Peta Marks

KEY POINTS

- People experiencing mental health issues, mental illness and mental distress present to all health settings.
- Mental health service delivery occurs across the service spectrum in a stepped-care model that is person-centred and recovery-oriented.
- The stepped care model matches interventions to meet the person's needs.
- In a stepped care model, generalist nurses use fundamental mental health knowledge and skills, and mental health nurses use specialised mental health knowledge and skills.
- All nurses need to develop their mental health nursing knowledge and skills relevant to their clinical setting and scope of practice.

KEY TERMS

- Holistic care
- Mental distress
- Mental health issues
- Mental health service delivery
- Mental illness
- Stepped care

LEARNING OUTCOMES

The material in this chapter will assist you to:

- orientate yourself to Part 3 of this textbook that describes how mental health nursing skills can be applied across all care settings and services
- describe how mental health service delivery is integrated across the health service spectrum in Australia and New Zealand.

Lived experience comment by Jarrad Hickmott

The reflection points in this chapter provoke thought about what the consumer may be experiencing when they are engaging with the healthcare system. Such thoughts help to promote the therapeutic relationship, which is of utmost importance, and speak to the importance of strengths-based and trauma-informed care.

Introduction

As you will have read in Part 1 of this text, there are many social determinants of a person's mental and emotional wellbeing – including housing security, educational opportunities, employment, social connection opportunities, financial stressors, parenting and family issues, as well as the impact of co-occurring drug and alcohol use and misuse, loss and grief and other critical events. These are issues that affect all of us at various times in our lives. What this means for us as nurses is that no matter which clinical setting we choose to work in, we will encounter people experiencing a mental illness or who are in crisis and experiencing mental distress. We will work with people who may be struggling with any number of issues related to the social determinants outlined above, or who have a life-changing experience as the result of physical or mental illness, who are gravely ill, or who die from disease or injury. Box 20.1 includes some questions that will help you to reflect on what the role of the nurse might be regarding a person's emotional or mental wellbeing in a range of different circumstances.

This chapter introduces and sets the scene for Part 3, Chapters 21–27, and introduces the concepts that will be expanded and addressed in these chapters. This chapter will briefly overview how mental health care is integrated across the healthcare system and how nurses provide mental health care in a stepped care model. You will notice that chapters in this section are quite different in style to Parts 1 and 2 of the text. The following chapters have been written by clinicians who describe common scenarios relevant to their area of practice as they relate to mental health. They explore a range of presentations, a range of healthcare contexts, and demonstrate a range of effective nursing practice in mental health related to the person's story. These chapters are practical rather than theoretical and are designed to demonstrate how mental health skills can be applied in various clinical settings – at times describing the role of the mental health nurse working within a particular mental health setting using advanced mental health nursing skills, at other times, describing the fundamental mental health related knowledge and skills required of nurses working in other areas. Some new elements that you will encounter in this section include 'scenarios' and 'red flags'.

Box 20.1 Reflection points

Consider how you might feel in the following situations – what you might be worried about and what you would need and expect from a nurse.

- Imagine you are about to undergo an operation to remove your appendix and you are all alone outside theatre – how would you feel?
- What if you presented to your local emergency department because you'd been experiencing chest pain and you had to wait? What if you'd been sacked from your job that morning?
- What if you got your test results back and you were diagnosed with leukemia?
- How might you feel if you were having your first pap smear, or your baby contracted whooping cough and was struggling to breathe, or you discovered your teenager had self-harmed?
- What if your usually gentle grandfather became delirious after surgery to remove a hernia and was becoming aggressive and swearing? Or your mum was admitted to a residential aged care facility?
- What might you be worried about if you realised you'd been drinking too much for too long?
- How might you feel if you'd had unprotected sex with someone whose sexual history you weren't sure about? Or if you were presenting with injuries as a result of domestic violence?
- What if you were so worried about an upcoming exam that you experienced a panic attack? Or you had a previous experience of depression and had just discovered you were pregnant?

SCENARIO

Each chapter in Part 3 includes two scenarios developed by the authors that demonstrate typical presentations they might encounter in the respective healthcare settings. The scenario developed may demonstrate the physical health needs of a person with mental illness (which are often overlooked and contribute to the poor physical health outcomes of people with mental illness) or the mental health needs of a person with a physical illness (which are often ignored and impact on physical *and* mental health outcomes).

RED FLAGS

At the end of each scenario you will find a section outlining the 'red flags' that the scenario presents. These are elements of the person's background or clinical presentation that would highlight that a mental health issue may be present. They demonstrate the type of issues that should prompt you to consider the mental health needs of the individual concerned and the mental health nursing knowledge and skills you might need in order to provide comprehensive nursing care in these situations.

In demonstrating how you think about 'mental health' in every setting, Part 3 aims to support you to provide more holistic nursing care to all people you come in contact with during your nursing career – whether they have a diagnosed mental illness or not. As you read through these chapters, identify any knowledge or skill gaps that you may have that relate to the scenarios presented, then review the chapters from Parts 1 and 2 to help you to develop your practice.

INTEGRATING MENTAL HEALTH ACROSS THE SERVICE SPECTRUM

Mental health promotion and illness prevention occurs in the community, in schools and in primary care settings. For example, the reciprocal relationship between physical and mental health is well known, so if someone presents to general practice with a physical condition that places them at high risk for developing mental health issues, then raising that potential with the person, discussing how they might maintain good mental health in the face of the healthcare challenge and encouraging them to talk about any symptoms they may experience will increase the chances that the person will present early with any mental health issues. Once a person has identified that they are experiencing mental distress, or that they have a mental health issue, intervention at the person's level of need is required.

Mental health service delivery in Australia and New Zealand occurs in primary, community and hospital settings. While hospital and bed-based services have dominated mental health care in the past, deinstitutionalisation and a focus on recovery mean community-based services are the preferred site for contemporary mental health service delivery.

Services are provided by government (public), non-government and private organisations; they can be generalist or specialist mental health services and provide mental health assessment, management and treatment across the lifespan – from the perinatal and infant period, through to childhood and adolescence and on to adulthood and older age. It is also essential to consider the mental health and emotional needs of families and significant others when supporting a loved one in any healthcare setting – they may be frightened, distressed, angry or upset (or all of those).

At all times and in all settings, mental health services must be provided using a 'least restrictive' model of care – that is, one which enhances the person's autonomy, respects their rights, individual worth, dignity and privacy, and where any limitations placed on the person are the minimum necessary, enabling the person to participate as much as possible regarding all decisions that affect them. The philosophy of providing the least restrictive treatment option guides the choice of clinical setting and is one of the World Health Organization's Ten Basic Principles of Mental Health Care Law (1996). It requires that, in determining where a person will be treated, the health professional considers the disorder the person is experiencing, the treatments available, their level of autonomy, acceptance and cooperation with treatment, and the potential for harm to be caused to themselves or to any others.

As we have discussed in this textbook, in a person-centred healthcare system services should be organised around the needs of people rather than people having to organise themselves around the system. As a person's needs increase, the healthcare team should expand to include different support providers; and as people's needs decrease, the number of people involved will also decrease, with connection being maintained throughout by a general practitioner, the person's family and other key supports.

A stepped care approach

As described in Chapter 1, in Australia and New Zealand a 'stepped care' model of matching an individual's needs with evidence-based staged interventions (from least restrictive to most intensive) forms the framework of mental health service delivery. Stepped care services range from no-cost and low-cost options for people with common mental health issues such as anxiety and depression, through to support and wraparound services for people with severe and persistent mental illness such as psychotic illness, with the aim that all can live contributing lives in the community (National Mental Health Commission 2014). In a stepped care approach, a person is matched to the intervention level that most suits their current need – they don't have to start at the lowest, least intensive level of intervention in order to progress to the next 'step'; rather, they enter the system and have their service level aligned with their requirements.

You can see how the stepped care approach integrates well with a person-centred and least-restrictive model of care. The stepped mental health care model also aligns with providing a continuum of mental health care services – across primary, community, acute, subacute and extended care (rehabilitation) settings – that respond to the person's level of need. Table 20.1 demonstrates how these concepts integrate and the role nurses in particular might take regarding mental health care and managing mental and emotional distress at each point in the mental health service continuum. Of course, these are not the only care settings or nurses that need to respond to a person's mental health needs; these are merely some of the most common settings.

CARE SETTINGS AND NURSES' ROLES

Primary care services include general practice and mental health clinicians working in private practice (e.g. credentialled mental health nurses and mental health nurse practitioners, psychiatrists and psychologists). They also include services such as the Royal Flying Doctor Service (RFDS), Aboriginal and Torres Strait Islander and Māori health services, and rural and remote mental health services.

In Australia, primary health-based mental health services are funded by the Commonwealth Government, either through services commissioned by Primary Health Networks and rolled out within a particular geographical

Table 20.1 Nursing, mental health and a stepped care response

PERSON'S MENTAL AND EMOTIONAL DISTRESS	PERSON'S NEED FOR SUPPORT	ELEMENTS OF CARE	CARE SETTING	NURSES INVOLVED
Severe distress	*Very high level of need* Risk to life; severe self-neglect	Assessment Risk assessment Manage critical incidents Acute mental health care Medication Treatment	Acute mental health services Acute care teams	Mental health nurse practitioners Credentialled mental health nurses Mental health nurses
		Assessment Risk assessment Manage critical incidents Medication Arrange admission	Emergency departments	Consultation-liaison mental health nurses Mental health nurse practitioners
				Emergency department nurses
Moderate to severe distress	*High level of need for support* Recurrent, atypical and those at significant risk; complex care needs	Assessment and risk assessment Brief psychological interventions Psychological therapy Medication education and management Social support and care coordination	Inpatient mental health Acute care teams Community mental health	Mental health nurse practitioners Credentialled mental health nurses Mental health nurses
			Primary health	Mental health nurse practitioners Credentialled mental health nurses
		Assessment Risk assessment Brief interventions Medication education and management Referral	Emergency departments	Consultation-liaison mental health nurses Mental health nurse practitioners Emergency department nurses
			Acute alcohol and other drug services	Alcohol and other drug nurses
Moderate distress	*Moderate level of need for support* Moderate or severe mental health problems	Brief psychological interventions Psychological therapy Medication education and management Rehabilitation services	Community mental health Primary health Forensic mental health	Mental health nurse practitioners Credentialled mental health nurses Mental health nurses Forensic mental health nurses
		Identifying distress Appropriate referral Social support	Medical settings Primary health General practice	Emergency department nurses Alcohol and other drug nurses Nurses working in chronic disease Nurses working in primary health General practice nurses
Mild to moderate distress	*Low level of need for support* Mild mental health problems	Guided self-help Brief psychological interventions	Primary health headspace General practice	Mental health nurse practitioners Credentialled mental health nurses
		Identifying distress Raising awareness Flagging risk Watchful waiting	Medical settings Primary health General practice	Emergency department nurses Alcohol and other drug nurses Nurses working in chronic disease Nurses working in primary health General practice nurses
Minimal to mild distress	*Need for wellbeing and resilience promotion*	Recognition of risk and distress Mental health literacy Mental health promotion	All healthcare settings	All nurses in all settings

Legend

Blue: *generalist nurses, who use fundamental mental health knowledge and skills*

Green: *mental health nurses, who use specialised mental health knowledge and skills*

area or provided nationally through Medicare-funded psychological services. In New Zealand, local private primary health organisations provide overall management of primary health services including general practice and are largely funded or subsidised by the Ministry of Health. In both Australia and New Zealand, nurses are also employed in school-based settings with a focus on improving the mental health of students and responding to mental health crisis.

Community health, community mental health and acute care services (e.g. crisis teams, mobile assessment teams) are funded and managed by state-based mental health services. Non-government community-based services are often grant-based (state or Commonwealth) or funded through religious or philanthropic organisations.

One of the major ways nurses working in primary and community health settings promote optimal mental health and wellbeing is to engage with the person around the environment in which they live, work, play and interact, and to support them to connect with services or supports within the community that can provide culturally appropriate assistance or support where required. Nurses in these settings need to understand how to identify clients who are particularly at risk for developing mental health problems and to recognise and intervene appropriately when people present with mental health symptoms, chronic disease or other comorbid mental health needs and physical illnesses. They need to be able to collaborate with and refer to mental health clinicians to ensure people experiencing mental health conditions receive the level of specialist care they require. They can also work with a person's family or other support network to help identify and respond to unmet needs, which may be financial, emotional or practical/physical (Temple & Dow 2018). Chapter 21 will help you recognise how to adequately consider a person's mental health when delivering care in the primary care and community setting and help you to identify how to apply mental health nursing skills to improve the overall health and quality of life of all clients.

Bed-based services include emergency departments, general hospitals and inpatient mental health units, as well as rehabilitation units. Emergency departments are the key access point for health emergencies of all types, including psychiatric emergencies. In addition, people who require attention after self-harm frequently present for care to emergency departments and may require ongoing care in a general hospital.

In an emergency department or in a general medical setting, a nurse may use a mental health screening or a risk assessment tool or identify the possibility that mental health symptoms are present and make the appropriate referral within their service context. Nurses provide person-centred and consumer-focused therapeutic approaches and deliver specialised, recovery-oriented, evidence-based care to people across diverse life stages, cultures and settings. Targeted integrated clinical and social support helps people to maintain connections with family and community. The focus is on keeping people out of acute care (or getting them back to their community as rapidly as possible) by working with them to identify what it is they are experiencing and assisting engagement with the level of mental health services and treatments that they need.

The collocation of mental health units into mainstream general hospitals has resulted in staff who are working in general hospitals having increased contact with service users and clinicians from mental health services, and, of course, people with mental illness experience the same physical illnesses as the rest of the population and require treatment in general medical settings. Chapters 22 and 23 will give you some insight into the mental health needs of people you are likely to come across in these settings and in particular regarding assessing and responding to alteration in a person's mental state to promote optimal wellbeing.

Inpatient mental health units provide a range of services relevant to a person's care needs, presenting circumstances and age. For example, they might focus on children and adolescents, adults or older adults, or they may be considered suitable for acute or subacute presentations, and will provide varying levels of observation, supervision and restriction. They may only accept admissions of people who present voluntarily for treatment, or they may see people who are being detained and treated under mental health legislation; they might be locked or open units. Chapters 24, 25 and 27 provide scenarios that describe some of these variations, and Chapter 26 overviews forensic mental health services for people requiring a secure care setting. Mental health rehabilitation units, which can be provided in hospital or community settings, provide longer term admission (e.g. 3–12 months) for people with complex needs or enduring mental health symptoms who require intensive treatment and support to develop skills that will support recovery, independent living and improve quality of life.

Increasingly, health care is provided in community settings, so it is the person's family, partner and/or friends who often take on an informal carer role. Regardless of whether the person they are caring for has a physical or mental health concern (or both), the caring role has adverse health and mental health impacts on carers themselves (Loi et al. 2015). Research shows that carers of people experiencing a mental health crisis describe feeling rejected and overlooked by health professionals and that they can become socially isolated by trying to protect others in their social network from the burden they perceive in sharing their stress and distress (Albert & Simpson 2015). As such, it is essential that nurses in all service settings provide families and carers with support. This can take the form of acknowledging and validating their role, providing advice and education about mental health and illness and its management, making linkages with resources in the community to assist carers with day-to-day issues, and encouraging carers to monitor and respond to their own health and mental health needs (Albert & Simpson 2015). Families also require information about relevant services and payments they may be entitled to if they are providing care for their loved one, including voluntary and non-government services that might assist them. Often, it is a person's family or carers who will be providing the individual with the most informal care and support, and who will be the one liaising with health and other services on behalf of the person, especially when the person is acutely unwell. As such, to be able to provide families and carers with all the information they require, an awareness of what these services are in your local community should be part of every nurse's local knowledge. For more detailed information about working with families and carers, see Chapter 5.

Chapter summary

The social ecological or holistic approach to mental health nursing requires that nurses are as competent in recognising and responding to emotional distress and the mental health needs of a person as they are in identifying signs of physical deterioration or a treatment side effect, and that acknowledging the impact of a person's environment and experiences on their health and health outcomes is an important part of understanding their overall health.

The interdependence between all aspects of personhood – including biological, psychological, social and spiritual dimensions – requires that all nurses consider a person's mental health as part of their core business. The chapters in the following section have been designed to provide you with some insight into how fundamental mental health nursing skills are required and can be used across common clinical care settings, as well as to describe the specialist role that mental health nurses might take in a given clinical situation.

Useful websites

Australian College of Mental Health Nurses: http://www.acmhn.org/.
headspace: https://headspace.org.au/.
Mental Health Australia: https://mhaustralia.org/.
Primary Health Network mental health tools and resources: https://www1.health.gov.au/internet/main/publishing.nsf/Content/PHN-Mental_Tools.
SANE Australia: https://www.sane.org/.
Te Ao Maramatanga (New Zealand College of Mental Health Nurses): https://www.nzcmhn.org.nz/.

References

Albert, R., Simpson, A., 2015. Double deprivation: a phenomenological study into the experience of being a carer during a mental health crisis. J. Adv. Nurs. 71 (12), 2753–2762.

Loi, S.M., Dow, B., Moore, K., et al., 2015. The adverse mental health of carers: does the patient diagnosis play a role? Maturitas 82 (1), 134–138.

National Mental Health Commission, 2014. The National Review of Mental Health Programmes and Services. NMHC, Sydney.

Temple, J.B., Dow, B., 2018. The unmet support needs of carers of older Australians: prevalence and mental health. Int. Psychogeriatr. 30 (12), 1849–1860.

World Health Organization, 1996. Mental health care law: ten basic principles, WHO Geneva. https://www.who.int/mental_health/media/en/75.pdf.

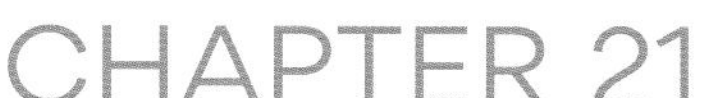

Primary care and community

Elizabeth Halcomb, Christopher Patterson and Ros Rolleston

KEY POINTS

- Mental health issues arise in all clinical settings. Primary and community care settings provide an important opportunity for the early identification of mental health symptoms and implementation of appropriate therapeutic interventions.
- While nurses need to perform within their individual scope of practice, primary and community nurses should be confident in talking to clients about their mental health, competently undertake an initial assessment of mental health issues and identify where referral to specialist services is required.
- Primary and community care nurses need to be vigilant to identify mental health issues opportunistically when providing care for physical health issues, as well as in those with established metal illness.
- People living with mental health issues also have a high risk of poor physical health. Nurses can improve health outcomes by ensuring these people have adequate access to physical health services including metabolic and preventative health screening.
- Stigma still plays a substantial role in people accessing mental health services. Non-judgemental care and value-free language is important to reduce stigma.
- Nurses should talk openly with people about their mental health symptoms in order to build a relationship of trust.

KEY TERMS

- Communication
- Community care
- Counselling
- General practice
- Primary care
- Stigma

LEARNING OUTCOMES

The material in this chapter will assist you to:

- understand the importance of a person-centred approach to both physical and mental health within primary and community care
- recognise the need to ensure mental health is adequately considered when delivering care in the community
- consider how primary and community nurses can influence the recovery of people with enduring mental health conditions and short-term mental health issues
- appreciate that support for mental health can improve clients' overall health and quality of life.

Lived experience comment by Jarrad Hickmott

The scenarios in this chapter acknowledge the difficulty people experiencing mental health concerns can have in putting forward their concerns and perspectives. Pharmacology is not the be-all and end-all, but rather a cog in the wheel that makes up the mental health sector. Providing consumers with the breadth of services and options out there is of the greatest benefit. Identifying the role the media plays in the portrayal and pedalling of mental health stigma is extremely important.

Introduction

This chapter provides an overview of the key considerations regarding mental health in the primary and community setting. In reading this chapter you will explore mental health as an important aspect of holistic health care for everyone. While for some people mental health problems are enduring, for others, mental health issues occur at various points in their life and are often related to situational crises. Regardless of the nature or severity of the mental health issue, early identification, assessment and intervention is likely to offer the best outcomes. This chapter will help you to understand that although every nurse may not choose to develop specialist mental health nursing skills, all nurses have an important role to play in supporting mental health in our community.

Specialist mental health nurses have expert skills and knowledge in the area of mental health that extends their scope of practice in this area. However, every nurse has a responsibility to practice safely within their scope of practice to deliver mental health screening, assessment, referral and support (Halcomb et al. 2018). A recent review of randomised trials of primary care nurse-delivered interventions for adults with a mental illness reported that while there was only a small number of trials, these interventions were acceptable to consumers and health professionals and many demonstrated significant improvement in symptoms (Halcomb et al. 2019). This highlights the important role of primary and community care nurses in supporting mental health.

Presentations to primary and community care settings

Although there are differences in access to primary and community care services across metropolitan and rural areas and barriers exist for some population groups, most people in Australia and New Zealand attend primary and community care settings. For example, in 2016–17 the Australian Institute of Health and Welfare (AIHW) (2018) identified that 83% of Australian adults had seen a general practitioner in the previous 12 months. For this reason, primary and community care settings are important, particularly in terms of mental health promotion for all, identifying those at risk of mental ill health and early identification of those with symptoms (see Chapters 1 and 3, which provide more information about a stepped care approach in mental health and what this means for mental health care across the spectrum of experiences). In addition, we know that primary and community care settings are essential to supporting the physical health of people with mental illness.

While many people who live with mental illness experience good physical health and long, productive lives, there is significant evidence linking mental illness diagnoses and poor physical health (Roberts et al. 2018). People living with severe mental illnesses have been demonstrated to, on average, have a life expectancy some 12–17 years shorter than the general community (Benson et al. 2018; Roberts et al. 2018; Ward et al. 2018). While only some 13% of the total Australian population access mental health–related treatment through the Medical Benefits or Pharmaceutical Benefits Schemes, they represent half of those who die prematurely from physical health conditions (Australian Bureau of Statistics (ABS) 2017). The ABS (2015) reports that 80% of people diagnosed with a mental illness also have a physical illness that affects their mortality. Indeed, 10 people living with a mental illness die prematurely as a consequence of a physical illness such as cancer or cardiovascular or respiratory diseases for every one person living with a mental illness who dies as a result of suicide (ABS 2017). There is a similar situation in New Zealand, where an estimated two-thirds of premature mortality in those with mental illness is attributable to preventable and manageable physical health issues (Ministry of Health 2019b). Optimising physical health in people experiencing mental illness is becoming a priority area for governments and policymakers (Ministry of Health 2019b).

There is an important role for nurses supporting people living with mental illness to manage their physical health as well as their mental health. Importantly, nurses should believe people with mental illness when they talk about their physical and emotional symptoms. People with a mental illness often have their opinions disregarded and their voices silenced (Geiss et al. 2018). Further, it is recognised that a historical or current diagnosis of mental illness may overshadow coexisting physical conditions, potentially leading to inadequate treatment of the presenting problems.

Nurses can make an important contribution by educating individuals, their families and carers living with mental illness to understand the medications that they are taking, their side effects and ways to manage these adverse reactions (Ward et al. 2018). Nurses have an important role in supporting people to engage in and maintain a healthy lifestyle (Ward et al. 2018). Lifestyle risk factors such as inadequate diet, limited physical activity and smoking add to a higher risk of cardiovascular disease, stroke and respiratory diseases in this group. Nurses can help to evaluate a person's readiness to change their lifestyle risk factors, support people to identify and implement change actions and reinforce the value of small and sustained changes. The value of positive reinforcement, encouragement and emotional support should never be underestimated.

It is also essential for nurses to consider the mental health of people presenting to primary and community care with physical health problems and to keep alert to the fact that the person may be experiencing a mental health issue. For example, when people visit their primary care practitioner for a mental health issue, they are more likely to describe physical manifestations. Indeed, pain is one of the most frequent initial complaints among mental health presentations in primary care. Or, a person may be experiencing a physical health condition that has a known impact on mental health. For example, depression is a relatively common mental health condition that affects around one in four adults during their lifetime (Moxham et al. 2018). Compared with the wider population, people with chronic diseases such as diabetes and cardiovascular disease are twice as likely to experience major depression (Pols et al. 2017).

Keep in mind too that men are less likely than women to seek help for mental health concerns (Thompson et al. 2016) but are no less likely to experience mental health issues. Many people who die by suicide have attended primary health care in the 12 months leading up to their death and up to 50% of them in the month prior to their death (Joyce & Piterman 2009). As such, it is incumbent upon nurses to notice and act on 'red flags' and to open conversations about mental health to help people communicate their mental health needs. Keep mental health in mind at all times and understand that, regardless of the reason a person presents to primary or community care, they may be at high risk of metal health issues or experiencing mental health symptoms. Nurses should not only seek to pick up on cues and ask appropriate and effective probing questions but also initiate conversations about mental health – in the same way that nurses should explore the physical health of people with mental illness. It is also imperative that nurses seriously consider the presence of suicidal ideation and intent and ask people directly. Nurses may worry that asking about suicide will cause people to act. That attitude and belief is a myth. Suicide can be a real concern across the lifespan regardless of a person's background, education or financial status. Ignoring the topic of suicide won't make it go away but having an honest and respectful conversation about how a person is feeling might just save their life. To read more about suicide and risk assessment see Chapter 7.

The Australian College of Mental Health Nurses' (2018) *Mental Health Practice Standards for Nurses in Australian General Practice* are aligned with (and follow the same domains as) the Australian Nursing and Midwifery Federation's (2014) *National Practice Standards for Nurses Working in Australian General Practice*. This document provides a broad framework that articulates how nurses working in primary and community care settings can contribute to the mental health and wellbeing of Australians.

The following scenarios (21.1 and 21.2) describe how the application of a 'mental health' lens can be applied to people presenting to primary and community care settings.

SCENARIO 21.1

Jack

Jack is a 70-year-old man with a long history of hypertension and cardiovascular disease. He has come into the general practice for his routine health assessment and care plan review. Last year, while playing golf, Jack had a significant heart attack that necessitated bypass surgery and left him in hospital for several weeks. Even though it has been more than 8 months since he came home, Jack hasn't played golf since his heart attack and says he does not see his golfing mates much anymore. The nurse observes that Jack looks tired and, when asked, he says that he isn't sleeping well and that he lacks energy. Jack describes how everything seems to take so much more effort than it used to. He says he just can't get going. The nurse notes that Jack has lost 8 kg since last year and looks dehydrated. Jack says that his weight loss is good because the nurses at the hospital told him that he needed to watch his weight to improve his heart health. He then jokes that it has been easy to lose weight as he doesn't really have much of an appetite or even desire to eat or drink much these days.

RED FLAGS

- Everyone has periods of low mood from time to time. However, when low mood affects a person's usual functioning or lasts longer than 2 weeks, the nurse needs to think about depression being present.
- Not engaging in usual activities, experiencing a lack of energy, having difficulty sleeping and poor food and fluid intake related to Jack's diminished desire to eat should prompt the nurse to ask some probing questions about Jack's mental health and emotional wellbeing.
- The fact that Jack is not engaging with his friends at golf and not seeing them much should also prompt consideration of whether Jack has become socially isolated.
- Because it is unclear whether Jack has much family support, the nurse should also explore this further.

PROTECTIVE FACTORS

- Social support can reduce symptoms of depression in individuals with cardiovascular disease, as well as improving the person's coping ability and promoting the uptake of positive health behaviours (Su et al. 2018). Conversely, a lack of social support has been demonstrated to diminish quality of life and increase morbidity (Hawkes et al. 2013; Hori et al. 2015).
- Social support can include practical or emotional support and can be provided by a range of people including family members, friends, neighbours and acquaintances. People with cardiovascular disease who live with a spouse or partner perceive higher levels of

social support and less depression than those living alone (Su et al. 2018). Unfortunately, as the population ages, many people no longer have a spouse or partner and are left to rely on other sources of social support. See Chapter 5 for more information about working with families in mental health.
- Primary and community care nurses have an important role in assessing social support and linking individuals who have social support needs with social groups and community services that can assist in building networks. Notably primary and community care nurses can also provide social support in the form of emotional support.
- While he hasn't been in contact for a while, Jack does have a social network within the golfing community that he might be able to reconnect with.

KNOWLEDGE

- As many as one in five people are affected by depression afte.r a cardiac bypass, acute coronary syndrome or chronic heart failure (Richards et al. 2018).
- The presence of depression can have significant consequences following a myocardial infarction because of its impact on the recovery process and behavioural modification (Martin 2010; Su et al. 2018) by decreasing motivation and interest, reducing energy, lessening enjoyment of life and causing poor sleep and appetite.
- Someone who is depressed may lack the desire to engage in physical rehabilitation and participate in programs such as cardiac rehabilitation, which will improve long-term physical and mental health outcomes. It becomes clear, therefore, that ongoing depression increases mortality and has a negative effect on quality of life in people with cardiovascular disease (Oranta et al. 2011; Richards et al. 2018).
- Depression in people with cardiovascular disease increases healthcare costs and precipitates more unscheduled episodes of care (Richards et al. 2018).
- Detecting and appropriately managing depression in people with cardiovascular disease is an important strategy to optimise cardiac rehabilitation.
- Many people still do not receive enough support and treatment to effectively manage depression following a cardiac event, despite recognising importance and the availability of interventions based on robust evidence (Richards et al. 2018).
- While some interventions can be delivered via cardiac rehabilitation and hospital outreach programs, these programs do not reach all potential people who would benefit from the interventions. Therefore, individuals presenting to primary and community care providers following cardiovascular events need to be carefully screened and assessed to enable referral to the most appropriate health professionals to provide effective depression management.

ATTITUDES

- Attitudes towards people with mental illness remain poor and consequently they are among the most marginalised and vulnerable people in society. Although this has changed over the years, stigma is still very prevalent (Perlman et al. 2018).
- Experiencing stigma, whether from members of the broader community, health professionals or self-stigma, is often a barrier to people seeking help (Clement et al. 2015). It is often because of these widely held negative attitudes that people like Jack don't seek help for mental health symptoms.
- The attitude of the nurse is vitally important. People with a mental health issue describe feeling judged by health professionals and are often highly attuned to health professionals holding negative attitudes.
- All people should be treated with unconditional positive regard, and the care and treatment provided by nurses should be value- and judgement-free.

MENTAL HEALTH SKILLS

A basic mental health assessment

While clients with cardiovascular disease may receive psychological assessment and/or intervention from cardiovascular services following an acute cardiac event, many do not. In many cases mental health symptoms appear after the person has left the acute hospital setting. Additionally, some clients may feel more comfortable seeking help from community-based care providers with whom they trust and have long established relationships (Halcomb et al. 2015).

It is vital that primary and community nurses feel confident in talking to clients about their mental health and that they can competently undertake a basic assessment of mental health issues using a validated assessment tool (Halcomb et al. 2018).

Standardised screening tools such as the Kessler Psychological Distress scale (K10) (Kessler et al. 2003) and the Primary Care PTSD Screen (PC-PTSD) (Prins et al. 2016) can help primary and community nurses to undertake initial mental health screening. The K10 is widely used to measure clients' mental state and to identify people potentially requiring further assessment for depression and anxiety. However, it is also important for nurses to recognise their individual scope of practice, its limitations, and when referral to specialist services is required (Halcomb et al. 2018; Martin 2010).

Establish trust and a therapeutic relationship

When working with someone like Jack it is important that nurses do the following:

- Listen! Listening helps to identify the person's concerns about symptoms and their possible impact on daily life.
- Open up the conversation in a matter of fact way, to show that the person's mental health is of equal importance to their physical health and that it can be discussed.
- Be open, factual and speak without negative judgement or using value-laden statements (e.g. telling people they have nothing to be anxious about or telling people they have no reason to be depressed).

This demonstrates that the nurse can help to address the issues they are currently facing and that doing so will optimise their mental and physical health and recovery.
- Demonstrate a manner that facilitates an ongoing trustful and therapeutic relationship to be maintained between the patient and the nurse. For example, the nurse might ask Jack about why he isn't playing golf or seeing his mates to understand what his concerns are.
- In Jack's case, if appropriate, offer a referral to cardiac rehabilitation, which may include opportunities to review his diet and nutrition and link him to social supports such as the local men's shed or a seniors' walking group.

RELEVANT TREATMENT MODALITIES AND CONSIDERATIONS

Talking therapy

- Not everyone who has depression will be prescribed medication.
- Counselling or talking/psychotherapy is also very effective and a referral to a mental health specialist may be required. See Chapter 10 for a detailed description of the type of therapies that can be useful for people with mood disorders.
- e-mental health internet treatment programs can be helpful for common mental health conditions – these might be offered in a self-help or guided self-help (with a mental health clinician) format (Orman & O'Dea 2018). While these may often be considered most appropriate for younger people, older people should be individually assessed to determine if an internet intervention is appropriate.

Medication

Medication is often prescribed for people with depression (see Chapter 19 for more information about psychopharmacology).

The role of the primary and community care nurse regarding medication management will be to speak with Jack and ask him:

- how he is managing with his medication
- whether he is taking medications as prescribed
- importantly, about any side effects he may be experiencing. Understanding side effects is important because if these are unpleasant, they may result in Jack not taking his medication.

If Jack is experiencing side effects, work with him to establish effective strategies to manage these. It is important that Jack is part of goal setting and identifying the solution.

Working *with* people in managing their mental health issues will elicit better outcomes than taking a paternalistic approach and telling them what to do.

Social and emotional support

- Primary care nurses can provide social support and offer emotional support. This is also an effective treatment modality.
- Providing emotional support to Jack includes validating his feelings and actively listening to what he has to say.
- Talk with Jack about ways he can improve his mood and work with him to set attainable goals.
- Demonstrate to Jack the difference between negative self-talk and constructive self-talk.
- Talk to Jack about relaxation or mindfulness activities, and let him know that physical activity can help lift his mood. Help Jack to develop a schedule for these kinds of activities and identify who might support him to undertake these activities.
- Most importantly do not dismiss his concerns nor diminish their impact. Saying things like 'You really have a lot to be happy about' or 'It will pass ... just get on with it' isn't helpful.

SCENARIO 21.2

Fiona

Fiona is a 45-year-old Aboriginal woman who was diagnosed with paranoid schizophrenia in her mid-20s. She is currently working with a care coordinator from the community mental health team but receives her monthly paliperidone palmitate depot injection through the general practice. She currently lives in a rented house with her mother, after her father died five years ago. Since her father died, Fiona doesn't leave the house much and has been admitted to hospital twice due to threats of self-harm, thought disorder and increasing level of paranoia. Her admissions lasted for several months each time because of her fixed belief that the police were tracking her through the TV.

While she was previously working in a supermarket, her recurring mental health symptoms have meant she is currently unemployed. Over previous visits to the Aboriginal Medical Service her symptoms of thought disorder, auditory hallucinations and paranoia have been fairly well under control and she has been adherent with her antipsychotic medications. Fiona has in the past been on a community treatment order but not anymore. She successfully stopped drinking alcohol a year ago but continues to smoke a packet of 30 cigarettes each day. She has tried to give up three times.

Physical observations reveal that Fiona's blood pressure is elevated (150/90), her random blood glucose is 9.8 mmol/L and that she has put on 6 kg in the past 4 months.

Fiona is quite guarded when she speaks and fears that she may end up back in hospital. She does not describe the admission in a positive way. She is reluctant to speak to anyone about her thoughts until she has built up rapport and feels as though she can trust the person. Fiona has been ridiculed about her mental health in the past.

Fiona's current mental state is stable, and she describes herself as being in a good stage of her personal recovery. She continues to hear voices but her beliefs about being tracked by the police have subsided. Fiona says the voice she hears says nice things, but she wished sometimes the voice – who is called 'Tim' – would be quiet. She has to shout at him sometimes to 'shut up' and that upsets her mother.

When asked, Fiona says she is not thinking about self-harm or suicide.

RED FLAGS

- The physical examination revealed several red flags. The combination of hypertension, raised random blood glucose and increased body weight all highlight a need for further investigation of Fiona's physical health status and cardiometabolic health.
- Further investigation of lifestyle risk factors such as smoking, alcohol, nutrition (dietary intake) and physical activity is required to identify additional risks to physical health.
- Antipsychotic medication will also contribute to a risk of developing metabolic syndrome.

PROTECTIVE FACTORS

- Despite the growing recognition of the importance of monitoring for metabolic syndrome among mental health professionals, this remains inconsistently applied in clinical practice. Rates of metabolic monitoring have been reported as low as 3% (McKenna et al. 2014) in some studies despite being undertaken in specialist inpatient settings; however, others have reported monitoring rates of 36% (Happell et al. 2016) to 43.4% (Tso et al. 2017). This highlights the need for primary care providers to be alert and ensure that this monitoring is occurring.
- Regular monitoring provides opportunities for early detection of abnormalities and treatment to reduce risk and is a demonstration to the person that the primary care nurse cares about their health.
- People like Fiona who take antipsychotic medications should undergo regular metabolic screening including:
  - an annual electrocardiograph
  - 3-monthly blood tests (full blood count, urea, electrolytes, fasting blood glucose and lipids, liver function tests and prolactin)
  - monitoring of physical parameters such as weight, waist circumference, blood pressure and body mass index (Benson et al. 2018; Ward et al. 2018).
- Monitoring a person's physical health also provides a good opportunity to discuss their mental health in a non-threatening way. A person-centred, holistic and culturally appropriate approach would indicate that the two should always be undertaken together.

KNOWLEDGE

- General practice manages mental health issues 1.3 times more frequently for Indigenous Australians than the rest of the community (AIHW 2015).
- Indigenous people are also twice as likely to be admitted to hospital for a mental health issue than non-Indigenous people (AIHW 2015).
- The rate of suicide among Indigenous Australians is between two (adults) and five (15–19-year-olds) times that of non-Indigenous people (AIHW 2015). A similar picture can be seen in New Zealand, with Māori people 1.6 time more likely to experience a mental health issue than non-Māori (Ministry of Health 2019a).
- For an Indigenous woman like Fiona, the lower life expectancy of Indigenous Australians (9.5 years lower than non-Indigenous women) places her at additional disadvantage (AIHW 2015).

Metabolic syndrome

- A key marker of physical health in people with mental illness is metabolic syndrome.
- Metabolic syndrome is a cluster of symptoms that include hypertension, central obesity, dyslipidaemia and impaired fasting blood glucose (Benson et al. 2018). When clustered together these symptoms significantly increase an individual's risk of developing diabetes, stroke and cardiovascular disease (Ward et al. 2018) and lead to high rates of morbidity and mortality (Benson et al. 2018).
- The risk of metabolic syndrome is increased by prescription of antipsychotic medications, predominantly as a result of weight gain and other metabolic disturbances.
- The positive and negative symptoms experienced by people living with schizophrenia (see Chapter 12 for description of signs and symptoms), as well as stigma and social isolation, can impair their ability to participate in activities that would enhance physical health and reduce the risk of metabolic syndrome (Ward et al. 2018).

Modifiable risk factors

- As the severity of negative symptoms of schizophrenia increases there is likely to be weight gain (which may be related to medication), as well as reductions in engagement with activities to promote good health such as diet and exercise.

- Prochaska et al. (2017) identifies that people living with mental illness have a disproportionally high prevalence of smoking, being two to three times more likely to smoke than the general population. While reductions in overall smoking rates have been seen in the general population, these have not been mirrored in people living with mental illness (Prochaska et al. 2017). It is important to remember that smoking also decreases the efficacy of some medications.

ATTITUDES

- People living with mental illness, and psychotic disorders in particular (especially paranoid schizophrenia), are often portrayed negatively in movies and the media. Additionally, people *without* mental illness but who commit violent crimes and take out their anger on others are often described as 'psycho' or even 'schizo'. This kind of stereotyping, as well as discriminatory and stigmatising language, serves to alienate people with mental illnesses even further.
- People with mental illness are more likely to be victims of crime than they are to be perpetrators (US Department of Health and Human Services 2017).
- As a result of pervasive stigmatising attitudes and inaccurate and sensationalist media portrayal in the community, nurses can also be fearful of people who experience psychotic disorders such as schizophrenia (Reavley et al. 2016).
- Nurses who subscribe to negative beliefs can provide care underpinned by stigmatising or discriminatory attitudes, leading to less-than-ideal nursing care.
- It is important that primary care nurses engage in self-reflection and self-awareness, reflecting on the attitudes that they hold towards people with mental illness.
- In a relatively professionally isolated environment such as primary and community health care settings, nurses might benefit from mentoring and clinical supervision to help them to develop professional skills in this area of practice.

MENTAL HEALTH SKILLS

The therapeutic relationship

- Develop and maintain a positive rapport with Fiona, building a therapeutic relationship based on trust and mutual respect. Fiona is far more likely to speak truthfully if she trusts and respects the nurse.
- Speaking freely to Fiona about her experience of auditory hallucinations in a curious and matter-of-fact way will help build trust.
- Ask Fiona about 'Tim'. What is he saying? When does he stop talking? Does he command her to do things? Can she resist his commands?
- Even though Fiona denies having thoughts of suicide or self-harm, ask her again about this. Creating a safety plan with her might be appropriate (see Chapter 7 and the 'Useful websites' link at the end of this chapter).
- Ask Fiona if she thinks anyone wants to harm her.
- Ask Fiona if she feels there is anything she needs help with regarding her mental health or other aspects of her life that relate to her health and emotional wellbeing more broadly.
- Open honest communication is always best.

NURSING ACTIONS AND INTERVENTIONS

Collaborative care planning

- Where it is decided that Fiona would benefit from referral to other health professionals such as exercise physiology, dietetics or a credentialled diabetes educator to help her to address the various health issues that she is facing, a care plan will be developed.
- Care should be taken to negotiate such a plan with Fiona to build trust rather than appear paternalistic or demanding to promote uptake of the plan.
- Fiona may need ongoing support from the nurse to encourage uptake of these referrals because barriers to engagement with health professionals may be present.
- With her permission, discuss Fiona's history with the other healthcare providers to ensure she receives appropriate interventions that meet her needs.

Physical health assessment and monitoring

- The nurse should conduct a full physical health assessment, including an electrocardiograph if one has not been done in the preceding year.
- In addition to assessing physical parameters such as blood pressure, waist circumference, serum lipids, blood glucose level, oxygen saturation, weight and body mass index, the nurse should carefully assess lifestyle risk factors and Fiona's readiness to change.
- An assessment of Fiona's nutrition and physical activity will also be crucial considering the elevated blood glucose and hypertension.
- With Fiona's permission, contact with the community health team will be valuable.
- The nurse should also refer Fiona to a general practitioner for appropriate blood tests and pharmacology review.

RELEVANT TREATMENT MODALITIES AND CONSIDERATIONS

Talking therapy

- Clinicians used to think that talking about symptoms with people who had a psychotic illness such as paranoid schizophrenia should be avoided. These days, evidence suggests that verbal and social interventions are showing some promise when used with an appropriate medication regimen.
- In schizophrenia, family intervention has been shown to reduce rates of relapse and enhance social functioning (McFarlane 2016).
- Adapted cognitive behaviour therapy can be a positive treatment for people experiencing positive psychosis symptoms (Hofmann et al. 2012).

- When aimed at improving memory and attention, interventions such as social skills training and cognitive remediation can assist in managing negative symptoms (Mahmood et al. 2019; Turner et al. 2017).
- These treatment modalities can help improve motivation or poor confidence, which can help to improve social and workplace skills.
- See Chapter 12 for detailed information about treatment relevant to people who experience psychosis.

Physical health and lifestyle

- Monitoring Fiona's physical health and metabolic risk factors as outlined above will be essential.
- Fiona should be supported to consider lifestyle changes, at her own pace, using a motivational approach.
- Supporting people to quit smoking is an ongoing process and often requires prescription pharmacotherapy. However, interventions by primary and community nurses using motivational interviewing can effectively assist in supporting smoking cessation and lifestyle risk factor reduction (Zwar et al. 2015).

Chapter summary

This chapter has provided some information about mental health within the primary and community care context through exploring two clinical scenarios. Several actions and interventions have been described that will assist you in developing confidence in working with people who experience mental illness. Some of these strategies apply to specific situations; however, there is always a way of effectively working with people experiencing challenging mental health issues. Some are more technical than others and require further education and practice to master, but many of the skills outlined here can be learned and applied to the interactions you will experience now as a novice nurse and later as your clinical experience develops. The main thing to remember is to be caring and authentic and to listen to the people in your care. See Chapter 2 for more detailed explanations of the interpersonal skills and mental health interventions that should be applied by nurses in all clinical settings.

Novice nurses frequently express their concern that they might 'say the wrong thing' and make the situation more challenging for the person in their care. If you take a caring and thoughtful approach that avoids the generous delivery of advice, it is unlikely that you will cause harm. Be genuine and authentic – people can tell when you aren't – and always come from a place of 'naïve enquirer'. However, if you practise specific skills such as active listening and validating feelings, and understand the models underpinning your practice, you are likely to feel more confident and to understand the goals of your interaction. It is also hoped that, through reading this chapter, you have developed a sense of the importance of responding to people with mental health concerns with unconditional positive regard and respect. Value them as people and plan care *with* them, not *on* or *for* them. Take note of their lived experience; after all, they are the experts of their own life, including their experience of health and illness. One in four people live with a mental health issue (Moxham et al. 2018), and everyone experiences challenges to their emotional wellbeing at times, so it is wise to develop your mental health knowledge and skills to be able to provide truly holistic nursing care.

Useful websites

Australian College of Mental Health Nurses Mental Health Practice Standards for Nurses in Australian General Practice: http://www.acmhn.org/images/Resources/1-32_GPN_Standards18_NEWsc2.pdf

Beyond Blue Safety Planning: https://www.beyondblue.org.au/get-support/beyondnow-suicide-safety-planning/create-beyondnow-safety-plan

Black Dog Institute: https://www.blackdoginstitute.org.au/

Blue Knot Foundation: National centre of excellence for complex trauma: https://www.blueknot.org.au/

eMHprac – e-mental health in practice: https://www.emhprac.org.au/

headspace youth mental health: https://headspace.org.au/

Primary Health Network mental health tools and resources: https://www1.health.gov.au/internet/main/publishing.nsf/content/phn-mental_tools

SANE Australia: https://www.sane.org/

Te Oranga Hinengaro Māori Mental Wellbeing (2018): https://www.hpa.org.nz/sites/default/files/Final-report-TeOrangaHinengaro-M%C4%81ori-Mental-Wellbeing-Oct2018.pdf

UK Mental Health Triage Scale: https://ukmentalhealthtriagescale.org/

University of Melbourne Recovery Library: https://recoverylibrary.unimelb.edu.au/

References

Australian Bureau of Statistics, 2017. Mortality of People Using Mental Health Services and Prescription Medications. Analysis of Data 2011. ABS, Canberra.

Australian Bureau of Statistics, 2015. National Health Survey: Mental Health and Co-existing Physical Health Conditions, Australia 2014–15. ABS, Canberra.

Australian College of Mental Health Nurses, 2018. Mental Health Practice Standards for Nurses in Australian General Practice. ACMHN, Canberra.

Australian Institute of Health and Welfare (AIHW), 2018. Patient experiences in Australia in 2016-2017. Cat. No. HPF 34. Canberra: AIHW.

Australian Institute of Health and Welfare (AIHW), 2015. The health and welfare of Australia's Aboriginal and Torres Strait Islander peoples: 2015. Cat. no. IHW 147. Canberra: AIHW.

Australian Nursing and Midwifery Federation, 2014. National Practice Standards for Nurses in General Practice. Australian Nursing and Midwifery Federation, Melbourne.

Benson, C., Kisely, S., Korman, N., et al., 2018. Compliance of metabolic monitoring at rehabilitation facilities. Australas. Psychiatry 26, 41–46.

Clement, S., Schauman, O., Graham, T., et al., 2015. What is the impact of mental health-related stigma on help-seeking? A systematic review of quantitative and qualitative studies. Psychol. Med. 45, 11–27.

Geiss, M., Chamberlain, J., Weaver, T., et al., 2018. Diagnostic overshadowing of the psychiatric population in the emergency department: physiological factors identified for an early warning system. J. Am. Psychiatr. Nurses Assoc. 24, 327–331.

Halcomb, E.J., McInnes, S., Moxham, L., et al., 2019. Nurse-delivered interventions for mental health in primary care: a systematic review of randomised controlled trials. Fam. Pract. 36, 64–71.

Halcomb, E., McInnes, S., Moxham, L., et al., 2018. Mental Health Practice Standards for Nurses in Australian General Practice. Australian College of Mental Health Nurses Inc, Canberra.

Halcomb, E., Salamonson, Y., Cook, A., 2015. Consumer satisfaction and comfort with nursing in Australian general practice. Collegian 22, 199–205.

Happell, B., Platania-Phung, C., Gaskin, C.J., et al., 2016. Use of an electronic metabolic monitoring form in a mental health service – a retrospective file audit. BMC Psychiatry 16, 109.

Hawkes, A.L., Patrao, T.A., Ware, R., et al., 2013. Predictors of physical and mental health-related quality of life outcomes among myocardial infarction patients. BMC Cardiovasc. Disord. 13, 69. doi:10.1186/1471-2261-13-69.

Hofmann, S.G., Asnaani, A., Vonk, I.J., et al., 2012. The efficacy of cognitive behavioral therapy: a review of meta-analyses. Cognit. Ther. Res. 36, 427–440.

Hori, R., Hayano, J.-i, Kimura, K., et al., 2015. Psychosocial factors are preventive against coronary events in Japanese men with coronary artery disease: the Eastern Collaborative Group Study 7.7-year follow-up experience. Biopsychosoc. Med. 9 (1), 3. doi:10.1186/s13030-015-0030-8.

Joyce, C.M., Piterman, L., 2009. Farewell to the handmaiden?: profile of nurses in Australian general practice in 2007. Aust. J. Adv. Nurs. 27 (1), 48–58.

Kessler, R.C., Barker, P.R., Colpe, L.J., et al., 2003. Screening for serious mental illness in the general population. Arch. Gen. Psychiatry 60, 184–189.

Mahmood, Z., Clark, J.M., Twamley, E.W., 2019. Compensatory cognitive training for psychosis: effects on negative symptom subdomains. Schizophr. Res. 204, 397–400.

Martin, F., 2010. The impact of depression on recovery and rehabilitation following STEMI. Br. J. Card. Nurs. 5, 58–63.

McFarlane, W.R., 2016. Family interventions for schizophrenia and the psychoses: a review. Fam. Process 55, 460–482.

McKenna, B., Furness, T., Wallace, E., et al., 2014. The effectiveness of specialist roles in mental health metabolic monitoring: a retrospective cross-sectional comparison study. BMC Psychiatry 14, 234. doi:10.1186/s12888-014-0234-7.

Ministry of Health, 2019a. NZ Health Survey 2017–18 Annual Data. Ministry of Health, Wellington.

Ministry of Health, 2019b. Office of the Director of Mental Health and Addiction Services. Annual Report 2017. Ministry of Health, Wellington.

Moxham, L., Hazelton, M., Muir-Cochrane, E., et al., 2018. Contemporary Psychiatric-Mental Health Nursing: Partnerships in Care. Pearson Australia, Sydney.

Oranta, O., Luutonen, S., Salokangas, R.K.R., et al., 2011. The effects of interpersonal counselling on health-related quality of life after myocardial infarction. J. Clin. Nurs. 20, 3373–3382.

Orman, J., O'Dea, B., 2018. e-Therapy in primary care mental health. Aust. J. Gen. Pract. 47 (4), 168–172.

Perlman, D., Brighton, R., Patterson, C., et al., 2018. Stigmatization and self-determination of preregistration nurses: a path analysis. Int. J. Ment. Health Nurs. 27, 422–428.

Pols, A.D., Schipper, K., Overkamp, D., et al., 2017. Process evaluation of a stepped-care program to prevent depression in primary care: patients' and practice nurses' experiences. BMC Fam. Pract. 18, 1–14.

Prins, A., Bovin, M.J., Smolenski, D.J., et al., 2016. The primary care PTSD screen for DSM-5 (PC-PTSD-5): development and evaluation within a veteran primary care sample. J. Gen. Intern. Med. 31, 1206–1211.

Prochaska, J.J., Das, S., Young-Wolff, K.C., 2017. Smoking, mental illness, and public health. Annu. Rev. Public Health 38, 165–185.

Reavley, N.J., Jorm, A.F., Morgan, A.J., 2016. Beliefs about dangerousness of people with mental health problems: the role of media reports and personal exposure to threat or harm. Soc. Psychiatry Psychiatr. Epidemiol. 51, 1257–1264.

Richards, S.H., Dickens, C., Anderson, R., et al., 2018. Assessing the effectiveness of Enhanced Psychological Care for patients with depressive symptoms attending cardiac rehabilitation compared with treatment as usual (CADENCE): a pilot cluster randomised controlled trial. Trials 19, 1–18.

Roberts, R., Lockett, H., Bagnall, C., et al., 2018. Improving the physical health of people living with mental illness in Australia and New Zealand. Aust. J. Rural Health 26, 354–362.

Su, S.F., Chang, M.Y., He, C.P., 2018. Social support, unstable angina, and stroke as predictors of depression in patients with coronary heart disease. J. Cardiovasc. Nurs. 33, 179–186.

Thompson, A.E., Anisimowicz, Y., Miedema, B., et al., 2016. The influence of gender and other patient characteristics on health care-seeking behaviour: a QUALICOPC study. BMC Fam. Pract. 17, 38.

Tso, G., Kumar, P., Jayasooriya, T., et al., 2017. Metabolic monitoring and management among clozapine users. Australas. Psychiatry 25, 48–52.

Turner, D.T., McGlanaghy, E., Cuijpers, P., et al., 2017. A meta-analysis of social skills training and related interventions for psychosis. Schizophr. Bull. 44, 475–491.

US Department of Health and Human Services, 2017. Mental Health Myths and Facts [Online]. Available: https://www.mentalhealth.gov/basics/mental-health-myths-facts. (Accessed 3 July 2019).

Ward, T., Wynaden, D., Heslop, K., 2018. Who is responsible for metabolic screening for mental health clients taking antipsychotic medications? Int. J. Ment. Health Nurs. 27, 196.

Zwar, N.A., Richmond, R.L., Halcomb, E.J., et al., 2015. Quit in general practice: a cluster randomized trial of enhanced in-practice support for smoking cessation. Fam. Pract. 32, 173–180.

CHAPTER 22

Emergency care

Justin Chia and Timothy Wand

KEY POINTS

- Many people presenting to emergency departments have mental health issues, either as the primary reason for their presentation or in conjunction with a physical health issue for which they have presented.
- Physical symptoms such as chest pain and breathlessness should be medically investigated before assuming they are due to anxiety or panic.
- The nursing skills required for responding to mental health presentations are the skills of therapeutic engagement.
- Therapeutic interventions such as solution-focused therapy are useful in helping consumers to identify previous stressful situations they have managed successfully.

KEY TERMS

- Assessment
- Anxiety
- Engagement
- Self-harm
- Trauma
- Therapeutic relationships

LEARNING OUTCOMES

The material in this chapter will assist you to:

- identify mental health assessment skills for use in emergency departments
- understand the need for therapeutic engagement with people presenting to an emergency department
- understand the relationship between acute physical symptoms and psychological distress
- identify useful nursing approaches and therapeutic interventions for responding to acute distress.

Lived experience comment by Jarrad Hickmott

The prevalence of trauma in those who experience mental health concerns is extremely high. Acknowledging and discussing trauma-informed care and supporting the person to develop coping strategies are important elements of strength and recovery models. It's important to consider an alternative to the term 'patient'. General consensus among lived experience circles is that 'consumer' is the preferred term. Noting this, everyone will have their own perspectives and options about how they prefer to be referred to.

Introduction

Presentation rates for people with mental health problems to emergency departments (EDs) are increasing, and this is an international phenomenon. General hospital EDs are frequently the first point of contact for people accessing mental health services. This necessitates a change in thinking and practice and a reorientation of resources to meet this change in demand. While it is important for EDs to have access to additional specialist resources on-hand to provide timely care and support ED staff, the knowledge and skills of ED nursing and medical staff also need to expand to address this clinical need.

Using two clinical examples, this chapter provides an overview of the key considerations in responding to people presenting to an ED in a state of agitation or mental distress. What classifies as a 'mental health' presentation in the ED context is not clearly defined, and the mental health of all people accessing health care should always be considered. For example, the incidence of depression is generally higher for people with medical illnesses such as heart disease, hypertension, cancer and diabetes. There are common types of mental health–related presentations in EDs including:

- anxiety and panic
- self-harm
- suicidal ideation and suicide attempts
- depression
- psychosis
- physical health issues causing mental distress
- pain (acute and/or chronic)
- situational crisis
- cumulative stress
- drug- and alcohol-related issues.

Approaches to mental health presentations in the emergency setting

In mental health, assessment is considered a central clinical activity. For nurses, assessment is a continuous process integrated within routine interactions with consumers. While the word 'assessment' carries a fairly procedural connotation, it is important to remember that effective assessment and data gathering hinges on effective therapeutic engagement (Shea 2017) and that holistic, person-centered engagement is central to the practice of nursing (Santangelo et al. 2018). See Chapter 7 for more detailed information about mental health assessment in nursing.

Conducting formalised risk assessments had until recently dominated mental health services. However, it is now recognised that there is no evidence that clinical risk assessment and management practices have any impact on reducing acts of harm. For instance, there is no evidence that a focus on risk factors (e.g. plans or means) has any impact on circumventing suicide (Large et al. 2011; 2016), and no form of risk stratification (high, medium, low) is warranted for determining the need for clinical services or follow-up (Carter et al. 2016). While suicidal thoughts and plans are common, the act of suicide is statistically rare. Moreover, in the emergency setting mental health consumers have expressed an aversion for being asked the same questions repeatedly and consider many questions about their developmental history irrelevant to their current health challenges. Instead consumers have identified a preference for a therapeutic response and emphasised the fundamental benefits of being listened to and understood (Wand et al. 2016). This does not have to constitute lengthy interaction. Listening to a person and conveying that you appreciate the challenges they are facing can be achieved in a short exchange. Shea (2017) points out that for some people experiencing suicidal ideation, feeling comfortable to share this painful experience with a fellow human being who cares may represent hope the person has not experienced before, or at least in recent memory.

Additionally, simple gestures such as providing information and reassurance as well as basic comforts such as seating, food and drink can ameliorate anxiety and distress and improve engagement between clinicians and consumers. The following scenario illustrates the importance of appreciating that most people with mental health challenges have experienced some form of trauma or adversity, particularly in early childhood, and this is common in people who frequently attend EDs. This perspective also recognises that people who have experienced trauma are more likely to experience distress and re-traumatisation as a result of encountering the healthcare system (Reeves 2015). See Chapter 2 for more information about a trauma-informed approach in mental health.

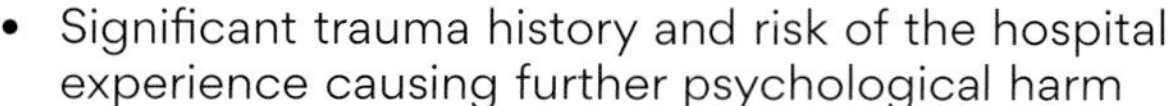

RED FLAGS

- Significant trauma history and risk of the hospital experience causing further psychological harm
- Bariatric/obese individual with respiratory and cardiac comorbidities
- Aggression risk
- Risk of harm to herself (potential future harm and possible harm already inflicted such as an as-yet undisclosed overdose)
- Absconding risk

PROTECTIVE FACTORS

- While this is not an uncommon scenario for Rachel, she has previously responded well to verbal de-escalation strategies using a trauma-informed approach from clinicians she is familiar with.
- While not always the case, she has also previously responded well to clinicians reminding her of the various distress tolerance and other psychological strategies she speaks to her psychologist about.

SCENARIO 22.1

Rachel

Rachel is a 27-year-old woman who has been brought in by ambulance to the ED having called a telephone counselling crisis line. She said she was having thoughts of killing herself by taking an overdose of her prescribed medication, so the crisis line worker called emergency services.

Rachel is well known to the ED, the toxicology service at the hospital and to the local mental health service. She carries a diagnosis of complex post-traumatic stress disorder secondary to childhood trauma and has a history of longstanding suicidal ideation, difficulty managing her emotions and frequent episodes of both deliberate self-harm and serious suicidal behaviour. She has previously taken large overdoses requiring intubation and intensive care admissions. While Rachel's care is coordinated by the local community mental health service, she presents regularly to the ED under similar circumstances and frequently accesses the local mental health acute care team after hours.

Rachel also has significant medical comorbidities. These include morbid obesity (weight of 147 kg and a body mass index of 57), type 2 diabetes mellitus, obstructive sleep apnoea, sinus tachycardia and chronic knee and back pain.

On arrival at the ED, Rachel is lying on the ambulance stretcher swearing at staff, screaming 'Let me the fuck out of here!' She is agitated and thrashing her arms and legs against the stretcher's seatbelt restraints. Rachel has been transported under the Mental Health Act due to her reluctance to attend hospital and the suicidal thoughts she has continued to voice in the ambulance.

- While Rachel has an extensive history of deliberate self-harm and suicidal behaviour, she also has a history of seeking help, either when feeling at risk of engaging in these behaviours or shortly after engaging in these behaviours. It is important to note that for some consumers, accessing help shortly after engaging in self-harm or suicidal behaviour may represent a significant improvement in coping compared with their past patterns of behaviour.

KNOWLEDGE

General knowledge

- General principles of a trauma-informed care approach
- Contribution of physical health problems to a consumer's mental health

Managing agitation and distress

- Verbal de-escalation knowledge and skills to manage Rachel's clear agitation and distress
- Possible need for sedation in response to Rachel's behaviour if verbal de-escalation is ineffective (in this instance, it is important to consider obesity-related risk of respiratory, airway or other complications from sedation)

Protocols

- Knowledge of protocol around medications used for acute sedation of behavioural disturbances – for example, the New South Wales *Guidelines for management of patients with acute severe behavioural disturbance for adults under 65 years old* (NSW Ministry of Health 2015):
  - First preference – offer oral sedation (diazepam 5–20 mg PO or lorazepam 1–2 mg PO and/or olanzapine 5–10 mg PO)
  - If not accepting of oral sedation, move to parenteral sedation (first dose droperidol 5–10 mg IM)
  - If not settled in 15 minutes, then a second dose of droperidol (10 mg IM/IV), with a maximum dose of 20 mg per event
- Knowledge of the record-keeping requirements for restraint and sedation mandated by the facility or health department policy, and by the relevant jurisdiction's legislation
- Knowledge of the service protocols related to:
  - the legal procedure for reviewing people detained under the Mental Health Act
  - whether the ED makes provisions for senior ED medical officers to review and discharge someone detained under the Mental Health Act where they consider psychiatry consultation is not required (this may be the preferred option if the person is adamant they want to leave and will require significant physical restraint and sedation to ensure they stay).

The risks of engaging in further coercive treatment and complications of sedation should be weighed against the benefits of keeping Rachel in hospital for further review, and the risks associated with discharge from ED without waiting for psychiatry review. While it may not apply directly to Rachel in this instance, it has been asserted that, contrary to some published guidelines, not every consumer who presents to an ED with suicidal thinking needs to be seen by a mental health professional. In some cases, a senior ED clinician can decide to discharge the person without a formal psychiatric assessment (Ryan et al. 2015).

Staffing

- Capacity of the ED to provide the high level of care Rachel requires given the resources available and

competing workload/acuity demands on the department as a whole. For example:
  - Rachel may respond to verbal de-escalation and low-dose oral sedation so could be cared for in a more open space with a 1:1 nurse.
  - If sedation is indicated, Rachel may require a resuscitation bay level of observation given the increased risk of complications.
- Access to psychiatry staff:
  - On-site psychiatry staff can provide a quick response for a psychiatrist review.
  - If psychiatry staff are on site but limited (few in number or because of a high demand for service) there could be delays in conducting a psychiatry review.
  - If psychiatry staff are off-site but contactable via phone or videoconference, this could result in delays.

ATTITUDES

- A calm, non-judgemental, empathetic, validating approach is required. Consider Rachel's trauma history including possible trauma she may have experienced in the hospital environment when accessing health care previously.
- Rachel's presentation may be the psychological equivalent of a serious medical emergency and her care should be prioritised as such.
- Be mindful that Rachel has several medical comorbidities that also require consideration in the emergency/acute setting. Neglecting the physical health of people with mental illness is common.

SKILLS

Engagement and a person-centred approach

Engage with Rachel from a person-centred approach: 'In person-centered interviewing the patient is not viewed as the problem but as a unique individual filled with solutions to the many problems that life invariably brings to all of us. There is a humbleness to a person-centered interviewer. It is the wisdom that, even at our best, we do not know all the answers, for we do not even know all the questions. Thus, it is intensely important to listen to what our patients have to teach us and the questions that they bring us' (Shea 2017, p. 9).

Verbal de-escalation

- Use a trauma-informed approach to minimise the chance of re-traumatisation.
- Engage verbal de-escalation skills with Rachel.
- Convey empathy and validation to start building a therapeutic rapport.
- Convey a genuine interest in hearing what Rachel has to say in an effort to understand what her experiences mean for her.
- Be mindful of your non-verbal communication (posture, gestures, eye contact, facial expression and rate, pitch and tone of your voice).

Safety

- Consider variables in the physical environment such as ready access to IV lines/poles, sharps or other implements that Rachel could use to cause harm to herself or others. Generally, EDs are noisy, busy places. Is there a suitable place in the department that is lower stimulus and clinically appropriate to care for Rachel?
- Using the above considerations to positively affect our bedside manner facilitates an environment that is both physically and psychologically safe. This enables a person's neurologically based fear response to be calmed, thereby maximising engagement and promoting recovery (Parnas & Isobel 2017).
- Use your knowledge and skills to engage in the process of safe physical restraint and administration of parenteral sedation where required and when verbal de-escalation and therapeutic engagement have been insufficient to reduce the risk of harm associated with Rachel's current behaviour.

TREATMENT MODALITIES AND CONSIDERATIONS

Solution-focused brief therapy

A person-centred, strengths-based approach to engage Rachel and attempt to verbally de-escalate her initial agitation and distress can be used. Once calmed, a solution-focused brief therapy (SFBT) approach may be useful in engaging Rachel and collaboratively working out a reasonable outcome to her presentation. SFBT is a strengths-based approach that has a strong evidence base. The approach empowers the consumer by inviting them to explore their own resources and past success as solutions to achieve their identified future hopes and goals (Franklin 2015; Franklin et al. 2016; Gingerich & Peterson 2013).

SFBT assumes the consumer is their own expert on what is helpful for them. The SFBT approach draws attention to those occasions in the past where individuals have successfully coped with a challenging or stressful situation and assists them in articulating, to clinicians and themselves, how they achieved that. It also assists the individual to build a positive picture of what their life will look like without their current problems and the ways their current life is even a bit like that preferred future.

A consistent, coordinated approach

A consistent, coordinated approach across all service delivery locations and teams involved in Rachel's care are crucial aspects of her treatment given the multitude of services she accesses concurrently. This could take the form of an inter-service agreement document briefly outlining her background history, a consistent approach to be taken by all teams/clinicians, and specific strategies to use in each setting.

Examples of possible agreed aims or general principles for the plan could be:

- supporting Rachel to develop safe ways of coping with stress as opposed to her current ones that put her at significant risk of harm

- supporting Rachel's recovery within the community
- facilitating psychotherapy within the community to support recovery
- reducing hospital and ED presentations and admissions
- providing a consistent and coordinated approach between services if admission is required
- allocating a lead clinician who is readily accessible for consultation by other clinicians to discuss Rachel's care.

Examples of a strategy specific to the ED context might be:

- prompt review by an ED medical officer (senior medical officer only) on arrival, with or without a mental health nurse
- early liaison with the lead clinician on every presentation to ED during the lead clinician's operating hours
- a reminder of the importance of using a calm, empathetic, validating approach when engaging with Rachel
- using examples of treatment strategies from other services aimed to assist in the ED setting
- having the lead clinician support the acute care team and the ED mental health clinicians in providing a consistent approach to Rachel.

SCENARIO 22.2

Yasmina

Yasmina is a 40-year-old woman of Turkish background. She has presented to the ED several times over a 2-week period reporting dizziness, palpitations, shortness of breath, dry mouth, tingling in the fingers and gastrointestinal discomfort. She has undergone numerous investigations during her ED visits including vital signs, ECGs, a chest x-ray, full blood count and thyroid function. Yasmina has also been referred to the neurology outpatient 'dizzy clinic'.

Yasmina is a non-smoker and does not consume alcohol or any illicit substances such as cannabis or amphetamines. She drinks minimal coffee and tea and doesn't consume 'energy drinks', which also have a high caffeine content. Yasmina is referred to the mental health nurse in the ED for a review.

With little prompting, Yasmina recognises that stress has played a role in her symptoms. She has a supportive husband, two small children and works full time as a community pharmacist. Yasmina acknowledges that she tends to worry, especially about her children. She often fears that something bad such as an illness or accident will happen to them. Yasmina explains that her mother died from cancer when she was 10 and that her father died from a heart attack when she was 16. Yasmina was essentially raised by her grandmother, who she describes as highly anxious and 'overprotective'. Recently Yasmina's grandmother was admitted to intensive care in a hospital in Turkey and was not expected to survive. Yasmina flew to Turkey to see her grandmother; however, she had panic symptoms during the flight over. She has not experienced any difficulty flying in the past. The hospital where she visited her grandmother was the same hospital in which her mother was treated and died. Returning to that hospital and seeing her grandmother in the ICU caused great distress for Yasmina. She also missed her husband and children and decided to fly home only 2 days after arriving in Turkey.

RED FLAGS

- Panic symptoms can mimic many medical conditions including cardiovascular and respiratory conditions, hyperthyroidism and others.
- Comorbid cardiac and respiratory conditions also increase with panic.
- Many of the symptoms associated with coronary artery disease are common with panic.
- Even if a history of anxiety is known, clinicians should not discount the potential for comorbid coronary disease.
- For people presenting with chest pain, a focused history, physical examination, ECG and judicious use of diagnostic tests should occur to rule out acute life-threatening conditions.

PROTECTIVE FACTORS

- Yasmina has a supportive husband and family.
- She is educated, has full-time employment, has stable housing and no financial stress.
- Her diet and lifestyle do not predispose her to any serious physical conditions.
- Yasmina is seeking help and recognises that stress plays a role in her symptoms.

KNOWLEDGE

Anxiety and panic symptoms are widespread in the general population. Data from the Australian Institute of Health and Welfare (2018) identifies that 14.4% of the population have an anxiety-related condition. Moreover, it is estimated that 35–50% of adults will experience a panic attack at some point in their lives (Treatment Protocol Project 2013). See Chapter 9 for a more detailed discussion of anxiety.

The nature of anxiety and panic symptoms

The acute symptoms of anxiety and panic are manifestations of the fight-or-flight response. These symptoms are the result of both an increase in release of catecholamines and a consequence of hyperventilation, which have overlapping symptom profiles. During the fight-or-flight response catecholamines are released from the adrenal medulla and the sympathetic nerve terminals, which precipitates behavioural and physiological changes that prepare the body to overcome a stressor.

The catecholamines adrenaline and noradrenaline play a vital role in the fight-or-flight response, acting as both neurotransmitters and hormones, producing cardiovascular, respiratory and metabolic effects. They increase two- to tenfold during times of stress and act as powerful cardiac stimulants, raising the heart rate and increasing the force of myocardial contraction and coronary blood flow. Another manifestation of the fight-or-flight response is increased respiration, which occurs via connections between the limbic system and hypothalamus to the brainstem respiratory centre. Hyperventilation is one of the physiological responses most frequently seen in panic attacks. During hyperventilation individuals exhale excessive carbon dioxide precipitating an acute respiratory alkalosis with a drop in arterial partial pressure of carbon dioxide ($PaCO_2$) and an elevation in pH. Patients who chronically over-breathe may develop a compensated respiratory alkalosis with near normal pH and a decrease in bicarbonate (HCO_3^-).

Alkalosis increases calcium binding to albumin and a decreased ionised calcium as well as shifting potassium into cells leading to serum hypokalaemia. This hypocapnia-induced respiratory alkalosis produces a variety of symptoms. Increased neuro-excitability as a result of hypocalcaemia causes paraesthesia (tingling in lips and extremities) and carpopedal spasm. Tachycardia can result from the physiological changes that occur in respiratory alkalosis including hypokalaemia and increased sympathetic activity. Chest pain may be caused by coronary vasospasm or decreased myocardial oxygen delivery and may also be the result of overuse of chest wall muscles in overbreathing, rather than using the diaphragm as in normal breathing. Feeling hot, flushed and sweaty is attributed to hyperventilation, leading to increased work in breathing· Gastrointestinal symptoms occur in acute respiratory alkalosis including nausea, vomiting and increased gastrointestinal motility. Peripheral and central nervous system symptoms include dizziness, vertigo, anxiety, forgetfulness and clumsiness.

ATTITUDES

- It is important that symptoms are not dismissed, even if due to psychological stress.

SKILLS

Psychoeducation

- Information on the nature of anxiety, the fight-or-flight response, the role of hyperventilation and fears and cognitive reactions commonly held by those who panic are the first steps in supporting people to address anxiety and panic symptoms.
- Hearing of common fears associated with anxiety and panic can provide reassurance and normalise the person's experience. For example, people who experience panic attacks often report that they are 'going mad' or 'losing control'. Reassurance that this is a fear held by many people who experience panic attacks can be immensely therapeutic.

Screening

- Screen for substances and medications that are associated with anxiety and panic symptoms such as alcohol, nicotine, caffeine (including energy drinks), cannabis, amphetamines, cocaine, antidepressants, steroids, thyroxine and phenytoin.

TREATMENT MODALITIES AND CONSIDERATIONS

- The recommended approaches for resolving anxiety and panic symptoms are non-pharmacological.
- People should be encouraged to engage in activities and interests that they find relaxing and shift attention from their physical and cognitive symptoms – for example, yoga, meditation or gardening.
- Metabolism-altering exercise (e.g. brisk walking, running, swimming or cycling) has proven effectiveness for discharging the nervous energy associated with anxiety and panic, thereby reducing symptoms.
- There is mounting evidence that walking in nature, or simply exposure to natural settings, has a positive impact on mental and emotional wellbeing (Frumkin et al. 2017; James et al. 2015; Keniger et al. 2013; Tucker et al. 2015). Nature is even being 'prescribed' by doctors in the United States and the United Kingdom.

Chapter summary

Working effectively in a busy emergency care setting requires consideration of the inextricable interrelationship between physical and mental health and sensitivity to the heightened states of physical and emotional arousal in people presenting. Therapeutic care in the ED need not entail lengthy and in-depth discussions with consumers. Indeed, an approach that is mindful of non-verbal responses, that conveys an attitude of humility and respect and is focused on providing reassurance and support can be immensely therapeutic. While risk issues do need to be considered, the underlying philosophy of person-centred therapeutic engagement is the key to maximising positive outcomes for consumers accessing care in an ED. A solution-focused perspective provides a practical framework in the emergency setting for engaging consumers in conversations that surface current strengths, coping skills and assist in orienting people towards a future focus.

Useful websites

Blue Knott Foundation – support for adults traumatised as children: https://www.blueknot.org.au/.

Breathe App by Reach Out – free app for iOS that provides coaching for deep-breathing exercises: https://au.reachout.com/tools-and-apps/reachout-breathe.

Head to Health – information on anxiety disorders, with useful information and links to other useful websites and apps: https://headtohealth.gov.au/mental-health-difficulties/mental-health-conditions/anxiety-disorders.

References

Australian Institute of Health and Welfare, 2018. Mental health services in Australia. Retrieved from: https://www.aihw.gov.au/reports/mental-health-services/mental-health-services-in-australia/report-contents/hospital-emergency-services.

Carter, G., Page, A., Large, M., et al., 2016. Royal Australian and New Zealand College of Psychiatrists clinical practice guidelines for the management of deliberate self-harm. Aust. N. Z. J. Psychiatry 50, 939–1000.

Franklin, C., 2015. An update on strengths-based, solution-focused brief therapy. Health Soc. Work 40 (2), 73–76.

Franklin, C., Zhang, A., Froerer, A., et al., 2016. Solution focused brief therapy: a systematic review and meta-summary of process research. J. Marital Fam. Ther. 43 (1), 16–30.

Frumkin, H., Bratman, G.N., Breslow, S.J., et al., 2017. Nature contact and human health: a research agenda. Environ. Health Perspect. 125 (7), 075001.

Gingerich, W.J., Peterson, L.T., 2013. Effectiveness of solution-focused brief therapy: a systematic qualitative review of controlled outcome studies. Res. Soc. Work Pract. 23 (3).

James, P., Banay, R., Hart, J., et al., 2015. A review of the health benefits of greenness. Curr. Epidemiol. Rep. 2 (2), 131–142.

Keniger, L.E., Gaston, K.J., Irvine, K.N., et al., 2013. What are the benefits of interacting with nature? Int. J. Environ. Res. Public Health 10 (3), 913–935.

Large, M., Kaneson, M., Myles, N., et al., 2016. Meta-analysis of longitudinal cohort studies of suicide risk assessment among psychiatric patients: heterogeneity in results and lack of improvement over time. PLoS ONE 11 (6), e0156322.

Large, M., Sharma, S., Cannon, E., et al., 2011. Risk factors for suicide within a year of discharge from psychiatric hospital: a systematic meta-analysis. Aust. N. Z. J. Psychiatry 45, 619–628.

NSW Ministry of Health, 2015. Management of Patients With Acute Severe Behavioural Disturbance in Emergency Departments. Ministry of Health, North Sydney. Retrieved from: https://www1.health.nsw.gov.au/pds/ActivePDSDocuments/GL2015_007.pdf.

Parnas, S., Isobel, S., 2017. Navigating the social synapse: the neurobiology of bedside manner. Australas. Psychiatry 26 (1), 70–72.

Reeves, E.A., 2015. Synthesis of the literature on trauma-informed care. Issues Ment. Health Nurs. 36, 698–709.

Ryan, C.J., Large, M., Gribble, R., et al., 2015. Assessing and managing suicidal patients in the emergency department. Australas. Psychiatry 23, 513–516.

Santangelo, P., Procter, N., Fassett, D., 2018. Mental health nursing: Daring to be different, special, and leading recovery-focused care? Int. J. Ment. Health Nurs. 27 (1), 258–266.

Shea, S.C., 2017. Psychiatric Interviewing: The Art of Understanding, third ed. Elsevier, Edinburgh.

Treatment Protocol Project, 2013. Management of Mental Disorders, fifth ed. Clinical Research Unit for Anxiety and Depression. University of New South Wales School of Psychiatry, Darlinghurst.

Tucker, A., Norton, C.L., DeMille, S.M., et al., 2015. The impact of wilderness therapy: utilizing an integrated care approach. J. Exper. Educ. 39 (1), 15–30.

Wand, T., D'Abrew, N., Acret, L., et al., 2016. Evaluating a new model of nurse-led emergency department mental health care in Australia; perspectives of key informants. Int. Emerg. Nurs. 24, 16–21.

CHAPTER 23

Generalist inpatient settings

Catherine Daniel and Cynthia Delgado

KEY POINTS

- Patients with physical or mental ill health will experience alterations in mental state of varying degrees and duration.
- Clinical manifestations of ill health and alterations in mental state present as changes in the person's usual behaviour, emotional expression, thinking and/or cognitive state in addition to physiological changes.
- Inpatient care in generalist settings should include mental health care and promotion of optimal wellbeing.
- All nurses working in generalist inpatient settings have a role in providing quality care for patients. This comprises a biopsychosocial focus in care, including assessment and nursing interventions for people experiencing mental ill health.

KEY TERMS

- Alteration in mental state
- Biopsychosocial
- Consultation-liaison psychiatry
- Holistic care
- Mental ill health
- Mental illness
- Mental state
- Optimal wellbeing
- Physical ill health

LEARNING OUTCOMES

The material in this chapter will assist you to:

- identify, describe and discuss contributing factors to a person's deterioration in mental state
- discuss the complexity of care in comorbid physical and mental ill health conditions
- identify the role of nurses in assessing deterioration in mental state
- describe interpersonal strategies to assist a person with emotional distress and related behaviour
- differentiate the clinical features of mental illness and/or organic disorders and identify principles of management
- identify the role of consultation-liaison psychiatry in assessing and supporting people who experience deterioration in their mental state.

Lived experience comment by Jarrad Hickmott

Recovery is much more than being asymptomatic – many people continue to live a meaningful life while maintaining varying degrees of symptoms. While we are all human beings, everyone is individual, unique and maintains a different pacing and timeline for their recovery. Promoting self-efficacy (when safe to do so) is well grounded in strength and recovery models and is beneficial for nurses and consumers alike.

Introduction

A physical health condition is usually the primary reason for people presenting or being admitted to a general hospital. The ill-health experience and physical condition can significantly affect a person's thoughts as well as their emotional, behavioural and cognitive state. For example, a usually calm person who experiences pain can also experience emotional distress. This may manifest as fear, frustration or anger (alteration in emotional state), hypermotor activity and verbal abuse (alteration in behavioural state) and an inability to focus or concentrate (alteration in cognitive state). That is, the person experiences an alteration in their mental state.

There is a complex bidirectional relationship between mental and physical ill health (Doherty & Gaughran 2014; Reyner et al. 2014). Mental ill health is associated with higher risk of physical ill health. Mental illnesses, including psychotic, mood, anxiety and personality disorders, have a high prevalence of comorbid serious physical health conditions including cardiovascular disease, diabetes, chronic obstructive pulmonary disease, cancer and dental problems (De Hert et al. 2011; Jayatilleke et al. 2018). Consequently, people who have a mental illness are likely to have physical ill health conditions that will require hospitalisation and treatment in general inpatient settings. A person with a mental illness who is hospitalised for a physical health condition may experience an exacerbation of symptoms related to their mental illness due to or in conjunction with their physical health condition. This does not automatically mean they will require input from psychiatric mental health services. It is important to consider that a person with a past or present diagnosis of mental illness may not experience active symptoms of their mental illness during hospitalisation. Additionally, people with a mental illness often achieve optimal overall wellbeing while continuing to experience some symptoms of mental ill health but do not experience adverse impacts from these.

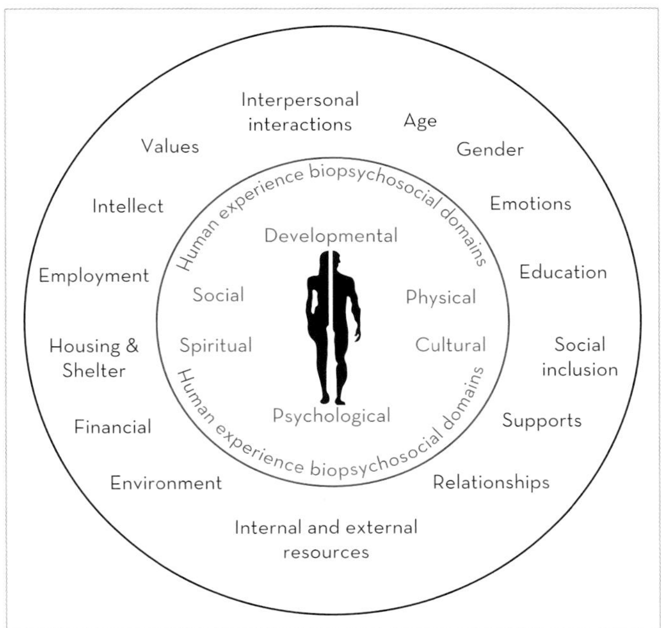

Figure 23.1
Biopsychosocial domains and factors that affect and influence health and wellbeing

Ill-health experiences

A person's ill-health experience often signifies an episode of diminished wellbeing that may have an impact on the whole person. As has been described in Chapters 1 and 2 of the text, this includes disruptions to any of the biopsychosocial domains – that is, the person's physical, developmental, psychological, social, cultural and/or spiritual experience (Fig. 23.1). An experience of ill health may affect a person's relationships, ability to study or work, or the way they cope. Conversely, factors closely aligned with the social determinants of health and the conditions in which people grow, live and age can also affect and influence a person's overall health and wellbeing (World Health Organization 2008). Depending on the person's individual experiences, supports and ability to develop, maintain or access resources, these factors may be protective against or increase their risk and vulnerability for developing, or recovering from ill health. In addition to assessing and identifying the signs and symptoms of illness, conditions or risk factors (Box 23.1) that may contribute to the person's experience of ill health, protective factors (Box 23.1) should also be identified. Protective factors can impact positively on the person, improve their mental state and contribute to their recovery, and therefore should also be assessed for, identified and incorporated into their care, treatment and discharge plan. For example, a supportive family can provide financial and emotional support and resources to aid recovery. In contrast, families may also contribute to risk if there is history of family violence, substance misuse or conflict.

Mental state

A person's mental state reflects their overall state of being. Mental state is closely linked to biopsychosocial aspects of the person's experience. Fluctuations in mental state are a normal aspect of a person's individual adaptation to changes in their internal or external experience, environment and circumstance. Every person's mental state is demonstrated differently through their verbal and non-verbal communication at various points in time based on their overall functioning and (positive or negative) experiences. A person's thoughts, cognitive and emotional experience is expressed through their behaviour. The way a person responds to others, conducts themselves or acts is therefore directly reflective of their mental state.

> **Box 23.1** Defining risk and protective factors in health and wellbeing
>
> In everyday life, we all experience situations, interactions and events that may impact positively or negatively on our whole being. Across the lifespan there are risk and protective factors that may be present, develop or occur that can affect and influence our health and wellbeing. Risk and protective factors are also discussed in the chapters in Part 1 of this book.
>
> Risk factors may increase the likelihood that:
>
> - mental health problems, physical/mental illness or diminished overall biopsychosocial health and wellbeing will occur in the short or long term
> - existing issues may become more severe and last longer (Everymind 2017).
>
> Examples of risk factors may include chronic physical illnesses and conditions, psychological trauma, lack of social support, poor interpersonal relationships, loss, stigma, stress and homelessness.
>
> Protective factors may:
>
> - enhance and protect a person's biopsychosocial health and wellbeing
> - be preventative against, or reduce the likelihood of, developing a mental illness
> - minimise the impact of ill health
> - enhance a person's capability to manage stressful life events and improve their resistance to risk factors (Everymind 2017).
>
> Examples of protective factors include supportive close personal relationships, employment, positive interpersonal interactions, sense of humour and engagement in hobbies and interests.
>
> Risk and protective factors are closely linked to the social determinants of health and can occur or exist in individual, biopsychosocial, cultural or environmental contexts (Commonwealth Department of Health and Aged Care 2000).

ALTERATION IN MENTAL STATE

An alteration in mental state occurs when a person's mental state has deviated or changed from their usual (cultural/social) norms. In the healthcare context, changes to a person's mental state signify a disruption to their biopsychosocial homeostasis and can often be the first sign of ill health. The type, severity and duration of alteration in mental state are highly dependent on the individual – their ill-health condition and symptoms (physical/mental or both), treatments and existing biopsychosocial contributing factors such as coping style, internal/external resources and supports, personal circumstances and acuity in their existing condition and situation.

Every person is different and therefore changes to mental state may develop slowly and subtly or very quickly and suddenly. Depending on the person's ill-health experience, changes to mental state may resolve very quickly or intermittently last for days, weeks or months, and fluctuate or remain the same for the duration of the episode of care. As a person's health condition and situation improves, however, their mental state also improves (at varying rates) and should return to their usual baseline (homeostasis). In general health care settings, a commonly observed condition that causes significant fluctuating alteration in mental state, particularly in older people, is delirium. Delirium is an acute confusional state characterised by disturbed consciousness, cognitive function and sleep–wake cycle, altered perception and changes to a person's emotional state (Australian Commission on Safety and Quality in Health Care 2016; Inouye et al. 2014). For example, an older person whose emotional expression and behaviour (emotional state) is usually very calm, pleasant, and able to have a coherent conversation may suddenly become confused, fearful and irritable when experiencing delirium. These cognitive and emotional changes may lead to changes in behaviour, such as becoming hyperalert, restless, aggressive, or, conversely, completely withdrawn. The changes are usually sudden and episodic; a person could return to their usual mental state during one shift and change in the next. This fluctuating alteration in mental state could last for days or weeks, depending on the cause and how long treatment begins to work. Delirium in older people can often be caused by a urinary tract infection. As the infection is treated, the person's mental state returns to their usual baseline.

ASSESSING FOR DETERIORATION IN MENTAL STATE

In any general hospital setting, you are likely to be working with people of all ages (and their families) experiencing an alteration in their mental state. As part of holistic care, it is good practice to assess and document your observations of a person's mental state (thoughts, cognition, emotional and behavioural state) when they first arrive and as part of your observations on a shift-to-shift basis. When able, it is also helpful to gain an understanding about what the person's premorbid mental state is usually like (this can be achieved by asking the person or obtaining corroborative information from family and/or other care providers). This enables you as a nurse to accurately detect any fluctuations and changes that could indicate a deterioration or improvement to the person's mental state and health condition. Regular assessment of mental state is also helpful in monitoring for triggers or patterns that may be contributing to changes in a person's mental state and health condition.

Like every person admitted to or receiving treatment in general health care, people with a pre-existing mental illness who have physical ill health may also experience some deterioration in their mental state. This does not necessarily mean the person will experience a relapse of their mental illness or experience deterioration in their

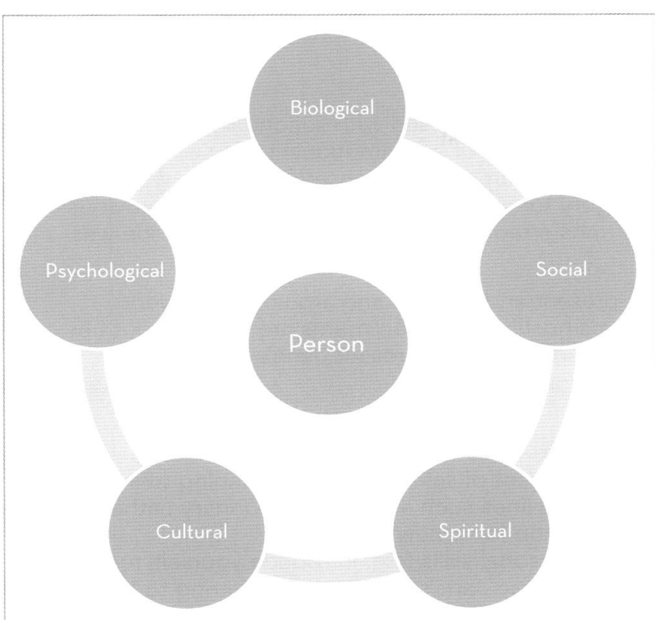

Figure 23.2
Biopsychosocial assessment

overall mental health and wellbeing. In every instance, initial and ongoing biopsychosocial assessment of the individual person's experience, severity and duration of symptoms, and impacts on the person's healing and recovery in the context of their physical health condition and treatment, is needed (see Fig. 23.2).

For any person experiencing a marked and/or prolonged alteration in mental state, or who is experiencing deteriorating symptoms of a mental illness, consultation-liaison psychiatry services (Box 23.2) or another mental health service that provides a service to the general hospital can be contacted for further assessment and consultation about care planning, intervention or treatment.

In the following scenarios, the principles of a holistic approach to care in conducting a biopsychosocial nursing assessment, mental state assessment and recommended nursing actions and interventions have been illustrated.

Box 23.2 Consultation-liaison psychiatry – a resource for general health settings

Consultation-liaison psychiatry is a subspecialty of psychiatry mental health. Consultation-liaison psychiatry multidisciplinary teams include psychiatrists, psychiatric registrars, mental health nurses and allied mental health staff who provide mental health services to and within a general health setting (Sharrock & Happell 2000; The Royal Australian & New Zealand College of Psychiatrists (RANZCP) 2016). The services provided by the consultation-liaison psychiatry team (see Box 23.3 later in this chapter for examples) include assessment, education, consultation, care and treatment planning support.

These services are offered to non-mental health staff and treating teams in relation to the care and treatment of people who may be experiencing mental ill health in a general hospital setting. This includes people who experience alteration of their mental state due to a physical ill health condition and who may or may not have a comorbid mental illness.

Consultation-liaison psychiatry teams work in partnership with the patient's treating team(s) and provide consultation through direct involvement with the patient (e.g. assessment or psychological support and counselling), or indirectly by liaising, educating and working with general health staff involved in the patient's care, with the aim of enhancing and providing the best patient-centred care (RANZCP 2016; Sharrock & Happell 2000).

Consultation-liaison psychiatry nurses often provide a significant component of liaison, assisting staff at the local and wider health service level in developing and providing education, quality improvement projects and policy development for safe holistic practice (Sharrock et al. 2008). Due to individual complexities and those of the working environment, consultation, assessment and intervention processes can be provided at any time of a person's admission. For example, obtaining collateral information, providing support to family/carers, and health staff advice and education on treatment and intervention related to the patient's care can be given, even in instances where the person receiving care may not be fully conscious.

The role of consultation-liaison psychiatry nurses has been articulated by the Australian College of Mental Health Nurses (2018) consultation-liaison nurse special interest group and includes:

- working with patients and their relatives, providing expert mental health assessment and intervention
- providing guidance, education and support to generalist staff caring for the patient and collaborating with them to develop a care plan
- being a positive role model to generalist staff in mental health care and practice
- working with the organisation or department as a mental health resource on mental health-related projects, education and policy development
- providing a link between generalist and mental health services (public and private, hospital and community).

SCENARIO 23.1

Jane

Jane is a 38-year-old woman with breast cancer who has recently been diagnosed with secondary brain cancer. She had been home when her family noted sudden changes in her behaviour and emotional state such as staying awake all night, increased amount of speech and irritability, and she became more focused on charity work, which is something she has not done previously. She also required surgery for a wound that was not healing (previous breast surgery) and high doses of prednisolone. Once she was transferred to the ward, staff noted that she was irritable and abusive towards her family and staff.

You have been allocated to take a handover from ICU; Jane is present and irritable and arguing with every comment the ICU nurse is making. Jane is orientated and appears hostile when comments are made about her mood. In front of her, the ICU nurse says, 'Psych need to be involved', and this increases Jane's agitation considerably. Now she wants to leave hospital.

RED FLAGS

- ICU admission is known to increase the risk of delirium.
- The use of prednisolone may precipitate changes in behaviour including clinical features of mania.
- There is a risk Jane may leave hospital and not get the required treatment.
- Irritability, agitation and using abusive language is not Jane's usual manner.

PROTECTIVE FACTORS

- There has been a clear precipitation to her change in behaviour (started prednisolone).
- Jane has a supportive family.
- Jane is alert and orientated.
- Jane is well known to the oncology team.
- Since transfer to the ward Jane will be cared for by staff who she is well engaged with.

KNOWLEDGE

- There are risks of behavioural changes with prednisolone.
- Emotional distress can be due to both the situation for the person and organic factors.
- Establish the patient's rights and responsibilities/ethical care.
- Consider the escalation pathway if agitation does not respond to supportive nursing care. This includes when to seek medical review, medications that may be used to manage clinical agitation and any further investigations.
- Potential organic causes such as hypoxia, urinary tract or respiratory infections that contribute to reversible changes to behaviour on transfer from ICU to ward bed should be investigated.

SKILLS

- Assessment of mental state
- Assessment of risk (leaving hospital, missing required treatment)
- Assessment of safety and care planning (minimise invasive lines such as indwelling urinary catheters, early escalation for review)
- Interpersonal skills (e.g. introduce yourself, respect privacy, use Jane's name when referring to her, respect personal space, explain care to Jane prior to commencing nursing care)
- Empathy about Jane's situation
- Emotional intelligence (recognising emotions in self and others, and emotional self-regulation)
- Assessment of Jane's capacity to understand what is happening to her, provide informed consent and make sound decisions in relation to her care, interventions and treatment

NURSING ACTIONS AND INTERVENTIONS

In the first instance:

- Respond to Jane's distress and listen to her content and concerns.
- Speak in a calm and soft manner.
- Avoid clinical conversations near Jane if this is distressing her but include her in handover communication.
- Do not debate, justify or argue.
- Allow time for communication and explain all care before it's provided.

Once handover is completed:

- Attend to orientation to the ward (Who will care for Jane? What will happen next?), ensuring she is comfortable.
- Conduct observations (pain, vital signs, review medications).
- Prioritise nursing care and group together tasks to avoid multiple interruptions.
- Consider current cognitive, behavioural and emotional state against Jane's usual behaviour, emotional expression and cognitive functioning (What is the alteration/deterioration in the patient's mental state?).
- Seek clinical review given her change in behaviour.

Involving the family:

- Prepare Jane's family for the change in her behaviour.
- Prepare the family to respond to Jane by providing education (e.g. don't argue, listen, don't collude with the content but acknowledge the distress, focus conversation on simple concepts, limit demands and decision making being placed on Jane).
- Review nursing resources required to care for Jane (Are there staff on shift who know her? Is there flexibility in the allocation of staff if Jane needs some additional time for reassurance?)

Assessment of potential contributing factors for alteration in mental state:

- Pain
- Sleep deprivation in ICU
- Dehydration
- Urinary tract infection (had an indwelling catheter in ICU)
- Emotional distress/fear (diagnosis and deterioration)
- Biochemical imbalance (review bloods)
- Potential for infection/collection at surgery site
- Delirium

Documentation:

- Observed behaviour and Jane's concerns
- Description of what happened and what helped
- Diet/food intake
- Nursing care plan
- Investigations pending such as results of blood tests for infections

Box 23.3 When to contact the consultation-liaison psychiatry team for Jane

Sometimes changes in a person's behaviour may lead the treating team to query if the person has a history of or is experiencing an episode of mental ill health. In this instance, it is highly likely that the consultation-liaison psychiatry team would be contacted with a request for a more comprehensive mental health assessment and/or recommendations for care planning, interventions and treatment. The consultation-liaison psychiatry team could support the medical team to confirm there is no history of mental illness by presenting assessment findings and providing a possible differential diagnosis or other reasons for the person's change in mental state. Given Jane's symptoms, the most plausible differential diagnosis would be delirium.

The consultation-liaison psychiatry would liaise with the relevant members of Jane's treating team (doctors, nursing staff and allied health) and recommend that delirium care pathways and management principles are applied. These include establishing if there are reversible causes such urinary tract infections or side effects of medication and providing ongoing review and liaison to the medical team. The consultation-liaison psychiatry team has expertise in managing agitation and can provide information on medications that can be used for agitation and also explore contributing factors to the change in a person's mental state.

SCENARIO 23.2

Rita

Rita is a 48-year old overweight woman with a history of bipolar 1 disorder who is admitted to a general ward after collapsing at home. Rita's partner Evan found her unconscious on their living room floor and called an ambulance. Evan reported that Rita had been 'fine' up until then. Rita is prescribed and is adherent with her medication regimen of quetiapine 300 mg and sodium valproate 600 mg PO twice daily. Rita also has type 2 diabetes treated with metformin 500 mg twice daily and consistently monitors her own blood sugar levels. Rita received intravenous fluids in the emergency department for rehydration and was commenced on intravenous antibiotics for a urinary tract infection. Rita is now on the ward in a four-bed bay for further observation and treatment.

You introduce yourself to Rita and explain you will be taking basic observations to monitor her pulse, blood pressure and blood sugar levels. Rita verbally responds by talking rapidly and incoherently. She is confused and disoriented to time and place. You note she has been incontinent of urine. She is fidgeting with her fingers, pulling at the bed sheet and looking around her. She starts repeatedly screaming 'Help me! Help me!' and suddenly jumps out of bed.

RED FLAGS

- Incontinent of urine
- Diabetes
- Dehydration
- Rapid, incoherent speech
- Fidgeting and pulling at sheets
- Screaming 'Help me'
- Confused and disoriented
- Recent loss of consciousness
- Prescribed sodium valproate
- Suddenly jumps out of bed

PROTECTIVE FACTORS

- Prior wellbeing
- Lives with a partner
- Responds to her name

- Is adherent with usual medication regimens
- Usually monitors her own blood sugar levels

KNOWLEDGE

- Rita's usual/baseline behaviour, emotional expression, cognitive functioning (mental state homeostasis)
- Differentiation between physical and mental ill health conditions and their expected/potential clinical manifestations (signs and symptoms of bipolar 1 disorder, diabetes, urinary tract infection, dehydration and how these may affect a person's mental state)
- Medications (interactions, indications, side effects)
- Recognising emotional distress
- Comorbid conditions
- Ward processes and alerts
- Contacts and escalation of care pathways
- Referral processes and pathways
- Patient's rights and responsibilities, ethical care

SKILLS

- Mental state and related risks and protective factors assessment
- Interpersonal communication (verbal and non-verbal)
- Empathy
- Emotional intelligence (recognising emotions in self and others, and emotional self-regulation)
- Safety and care planning (physical and mental)
- Performing procedures and administering treatment safely and sensitively
- Reporting and documentation
- Ability to prioritise needs
- Assessing Rita's capacity to understand what is happening to her, to provide informed consent and make sound decisions in relation to her care, interventions and treatment
- Recognising abnormal blood pathology (deviation from Rita's usual/baseline)

ATTITUDES

Behaviours and understandings that help to promote and maintain safety for the patient and others include:

- a non-judgemental approach
- professional curiosity
- objectivity
- empathy.

NURSING ACTIONS AND INTERVENTIONS

In the first instance:

- Assess for levels of safety in relation to Rita, other patients and yourself/staff members.
- Remain calm (role-modelling desired behaviour) and attempt to engage Rita by providing her with a little space, speaking in a soft, calm voice and addressing Rita by her preferred name. Acknowledge her distress, ask her what happened and let her know you're there to help. Use short sentences and provide brief information to reorient her, asking what she feels she needs and inviting her to sit down or, if able, to have a shower before returning to bed (because she has been incontinent and this could be a source of embarrassment).
- Ask for help from another nurse if needed.

When Rita is less distressed:

- Attend to basic observations. Observe her breathing, colour and level of consciousness and explain that her pulse, blood pressure and blood sugar levels need to be taken.
- Ensure that before each procedure (before touching the patient), you explain what the procedure will involve (e.g. 'I am going to put this cuff around your arm to take your blood pressure. It will feel a little tight on your arm for a bit but will pass quickly'). This is important to ensure Rita is given due respect and her dignity is maintained. It also minimises the possibility for her to become startled. Proceeding in this way will give Rita the opportunity to ask any questions if she's able and you the opportunity to observe for safety concerns and cues.
- If safe to do so, encourage Rita's self-efficacy by inviting her to attend to her own blood sugar level (she does this regularly at home) and assess her current capacity to understand what is happening to her and her ability to make sound/relevant decisions about her care.
- Consider Rita's current cognitive, behavioural and emotional state against her usual known and reported behaviour, emotional expression and cognitive functioning (What is the alteration/deterioration in Rita's mental state?).
- Consider Rita's current physical health status and any deviations from her usual experience of her physical condition.
- Plan with and offer Rita assistance with toileting if needed and take a urine sample for urinalysis.
- Change the bed or ask someone to assist with changing the bed linen if you are attending to Rita.

Assessment of potential contributing factors for alteration in mental state:

- Blood sugar level
- Dehydration
- Sodium valproate overdose
- Urinary tract infection
- Emotional distress/fear
- Active symptoms of bipolar disorder
- Unknown potential another infection or a related physical condition – look at blood pathology results (or ensure bloods are ordered)
- Delirium

Documentation:

- Observations of specific behaviour, emotional expression, thinking and physical assessments (including fluid input/output; food intake)
- Note what interventions and actions were taken and the outcomes from these

- Details of what and to whom referrals were made
- A clear and updated care plan

Referral:

- Refer Rita to the treating team for further medical review.
- Given Rita's history of mental illness and change in level of mental state alteration and deterioration, a referral to the consultation-liaison psychiatry team could be considered (Box 23.4).

Box 23.4 Referring Rita to the consultation-liaison psychiatry team

Rita has a known comorbid physical (type 2 diabetes) and mental illness (bipolar 1 disorder). Given that Rita's husband said she was 'fine' before her hospitalisation, it is likely that Rita's current alteration in her mental state, demonstrated predominantly as emotional and behavioural distress, is not due to her pre-existing mental illness. There is, however, a marked deterioration in Rita's mental state from her baseline. In this case, the consultation-liaison psychiatry team may be contacted to provide staff support and education about:

- Rita's mental illness – this would help the treating team and nursing staff become aware of how and what bipolar 1 disorder symptoms Rita experiences and may be differentiated from a physical cause
- psychotropic medication
- interpersonal interventions and strategies in effectively communicating and attending to Rita when she's experiencing high levels of distress
- care planning strategies aimed at engaging Rita and promoting her self-efficacy and recovery while she is hospitalised.

If Rita's mental state continues to deteriorate (see Box 23.5), the consultation-liaison psychiatry team may complete a further comprehensive mental health assessment of Rita, review her current psychotropic medication and may provide recommendations about any changes or additions to her current treatment. In this instance, the consultation-liaison psychiatry team may become regularly involved in more formalised care processes (such as case reviews) and may also take a role if needed in coordinating Rita's care and discharge planning (including advocacy and referral to the relevant care provider upon discharge).

If Rita's deterioration in mental state was caused by a physical health condition, it is important to note that, as her physical health improves, her mental state will also improve and return to baseline. If this happens quickly, the consultation-liaison psychiatry team may not need to be involved.

Box 23.5 Useful tips to engage with patients who have a deterioration in mental state

- As soon as possible in their admission, explore and discover what the person's usual way of being is (What is their usual baseline mental state?) and clearly document this.
- Develop an awareness of the person's usual functioning (Do they live alone? Are they independent? Are any regular healthcare services involved? What are their personal preferences for food, fluid and personal items?).
- Speak to the patient, even if they are experiencing alteration in their mental state. Ask direct questions and try to talk *to* them rather than *about* them.
- Monitor for patterns or triggers that may contribute to changes in a person's mental state. Don't assume the behaviour is due to mental illness. It can often be the first or main feature or sign of ill health (Could it be due to pain, delirium or other reversible causes?).
- Don't focus on the diagnosis but ask yourself: 'What care is required here?' Patients depend on healthcare staff to advocate for evidence-based care.

The patient's capacity to consent and refuse treatment may need to be determined. Be aware that a person with capacity will not necessarily make decisions you agree with.

Chapter summary

In this chapter we have identified contributing factors to a person's deterioration in mental state and explored the nursing care provided. The interpersonal interventions to assist a person with emotional distress and related behaviour have been described and applied to clinical examples. Nursing assessment to differentiate clinical features of mental illness and/or organic disorders and identify the key principles of nursing management has been described. The role of consultation-liaison psychiatry in assessing and supporting people who experience deterioration in their mental state has been outlined.

Web resources

Australian College of Mental Health Nursing – Consultation Liaison Nurses Special Interest Group: http://www.acmhn.org/index.php/home-clsig

Australian Commission on Safety and Quality in Health Care: https://www.safetyandquality.gov.au/standards/nsqhs-standards/recognising-and-responding-acute-deterioration-standard/detecting-and-recognising-acute-deterioration-and-escalating-care

Victorian Department of Health and Human Services physical health framework: https://www2.health.vic.gov.au/about/publications/policiesandguidelines/equally-well-in-victoria-physical-health-framework-for-specialist-mental-health-services

Victorian specialling guidelines: https://www2.health.vic.gov.au/mental-health/practice-and-service-quality/service-quality/nursing-observation-through-engagement-in-psychiatric-inpatient-care

References

Australian College of Mental Health Nurses, 2018. Consultation Liaison Special Interest Group. [online] Available at: http://www.acmhn.org/index.php/home-clsig. (Accessed 30 March 2020).

Australian Commission on Safety and Quality in Health Care (ACSQHC), 2016. Delirium Clinical Care Standard. Sydney: ACSQHC.

Commonwealth Department of Health and Aged Care, 2000. National Action Plan for Promotion, Prevention and Early Intervention for Mental Health. Mental Health and Special Programs Branch. Commonwealth Department of Health and Aged Care, Canberra.

De Hert, M., Correll, C., Bobes, J., et al., 2011. Physical illness in patients with severe mental disorders. I. Prevalence, impact of medications and disparities in health care. World Psychiatry 10 (1), 52–77.

Doherty, A.M., Gaughran, F., 2014. The interface of physical and mental Health. Soc. Psychiatry Psychiatr. Epidemiol. 49 (5), 673–682.

Everymind, 2017. Prevention First: A Prevention and Promotion Framework for Mental Health. Everymind, Newcastle.

Inouye, S.K., Westendop, R.G.J., Saczynski, J.S., 2014. Delirium in elderly people. Lancet 383, 911–922.

Jayatilleke, N., Hayes, R., Chang, C., et al., 2018. Acute general hospital admissions in people with serious mental illness. Psychol. Med. 48 (16), 2676–2683.

Reyner, L., Matcham, F., Hutton, J., et al., 2014. Embedding integrated mental health assessment and management in general hospital settings: feasibility, acceptability and the prevalence of common mental disorder. Gen. Hosp. Psychiatry 36, 318–324.

Sharrock, J., Bryant, J., McNamara, P., et al., 2008. Exploratory study of mental health consultation-liaison nursing in Australia: part 1 demographics and role characteristics. Int. J. Ment. Health Nurs. 17 (3), 180–188.

Sharrock, J., Happell, B., 2000. The psychiatric consultation-liaison nurse: towards articulating a model for practice. Aust. N. Z. J. Ment. Health Nurs. 9, 19–28.

The Royal Australian & New Zealand College of Psychiatrists (RANZCP), 2016. Service Model for Consultation-Liaison Psychiatry in Victoria. RANZCP Victorian Branch, Melbourne.

World Health Organization, 2008. Closing the Gap in a Generation: Health Equity Through Action on the Social Determinants of Health. World Health Organization, Geneva.

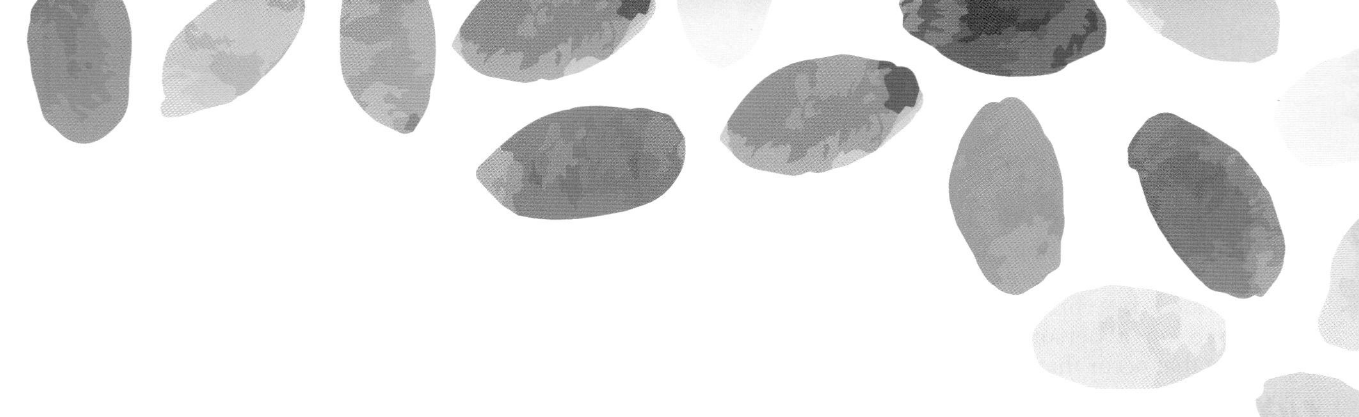

CHAPTER 24

Older age care

Melissa Robinson-Reilly and Sharon Rydon

KEY POINTS

- Mental health issues affect older age people. These may be pre-existing mental health disorders or the development of a new disorder that has occurred from a life event or experience.
- All people age differently, and physical changes have an impact on the mental health of older people. Chronic illnesses are also implicated with mental health disorders such as depression, dementia and delirium. Physical inactivity or a sedentary lifestyle contributes to poorer health outcomes.
- Caring for people of older age requires that nurses have an awareness of issues associated with longevity and health and be able to identify factors that contribute to mental health disorders. Health literacy of the older age person, as well as stereotyping and stigma associated with ageing, can lead to stress and anxiety.
- Nurses caring for older people are well situated to promote meaning, purpose and connectedness for that individual.

KEY TERMS

- Chronic illness
- Connectedness
- Health literacy
- Older age care
- Quality of life

LEARNING OUTCOMES

The material in this chapter will assist you to:

- understand the impact of mental health and the older age person
- consider the implications of living longer and the physical limitations that contribute to mental health disorders, including health literacy and the ability to seek help
- identify strategies to support an older age person to recovery
- reflect on nursing practice to promote rapport and quality of life.

Lived experience comment by Jarrad Hickmott

The sexuality of older adults is an important topic that isn't always discussed. The hefty discussion around stigma and attitudes that affect the care and treatment of older adults is so important. Stressing the importance of relationship, communication and person-centred care is also of great benefit. Remaining cognisant of these facts leads to a decrease in stigma and better treatment of older adults.

Introduction

This chapter builds on the key considerations discussed in Chapter 16 regarding mental health care of older age people. Older age care is multifaceted and can be complicated by chronic illness and events that have impacted on a person's life. There are often physical changes that occur that can risk stereotyping an individual, such as greying hair, stooped posture or requiring a mobility aid, without considering the experiential impact of ageing.

Although a person may have a strong awareness of their mortality, this is underpinned by their individual life circumstance, as you will read in the two case scenarios presented. Health literacy and decision making can be compromised by the person's present needs. Loss of physical independence and financial changes can contribute to how an older person perceives their value in the community. From exploring Chapter 16 you have come to understand there are many transition points in life that are relevant to older adults including the death of a spouse, cognitive changes and isolation. Although depression, dementia and delirium are often considered as manifesting in older age, these illnesses can in fact occur in younger people.

While working though the scenarios provided, consider the cognitive assessment tools that may assist in assessing an older age person in your care (there are a variety of tools available, so it is important to ensure the tool chosen is appropriate for the evaluation and your level of experience).

Having an awareness of the factors contributing to a person's behaviour and an understanding of the underlying circumstances surrounding the behaviour is the initial approach to care. Gathering all the cues contributes to your assessment and informs the management/interventions to be undertaken to provide the best outcome. This may include a referral to a specialist mental health team as within a stepped care strategy. It is important to be cognisant of the organisations and specialist teams that can support the individual in higher levels of care and/or to restore or maintain independence, and how this complements your role.

SCENARIO 24.1

Bill

Bill is an 80-year-old man who cares for his elderly wife and his 51-year-old son, who has bipolar disorder. Bill was previously a mechanic working 7 days a week and rarely took holidays. His working life ended after an industrial accident 16 years ago where he sustained a right shoulder injury (the proximal humerus was fractured causing irreversible nerve damage) and despite multiple surgeries he has never regained full function of his right arm. Bill often contemplates leaving his home or hopes for his life to end given the impact of his physical disabilities, health, loss of income as a pensioner and the stress of maintaining the household. He drives his wife, who has a chronic illness, to her appointments, three times a week.

Bill refuses home help. He tries to keep daily order and feels external interference would interrupt his routine. At times his own health deteriorates because he cannot afford his own medications that he feels 'do not help anyway'. His adult son has manic episodes and on occasion is violent towards Bill. Bill is struggling to manage his finances. He is reduced to tears and becomes emotionally distraught when asking for help. He tries to have enough money available for scheduled utility payments, but any unexpected expenses can affect his ability to make these payments. He often voices that his pension falls out of sequence with the payments he needs to make and has trouble trying to organise himself. Bill feels his general practitioner, who is aware of his home life situation, is often dismissive of the symptoms he describes, even when his weight fluctuates with unexplained loss or he has unusual feelings of no physical strength.

RED FLAGS

- **Ageism and longevity:** Life is ever changing, and living longer (longevity) can impact on one's role. Not all older age people experience the same issues though, they may experience similar circumstances that they say cause stress and affect their ability to perform as previously. Be aware of presuming Bill's issues are the same as other older people's.
- **Suicidal ideation:** Bill is voicing suicidal ideation, which should be considered as a red flag that he needs help. The contributing factors that are affecting him may not be obvious to him or those around him.
- **Overwhelm:** Several issues are influencing how Bill feels he is coping. It is important to understand and explore these issues because of Bill's suicide ideation, given the difficulties he describes in caring for his wife and son and having to do all the household chores, as well as manage on his pension, in addition to experiencing his own health issues.
- **Age:** Bill's age (80 years) places him close to the highest risk age group for suicide – mental ill-health and suicide incidence is higher in males over the age of 85 years (Australian Bureau of Statistics 2017) – so the fact that Bill is experiencing suicide ideation in the context of absence of caring for own health, social isolation, financial stress and his difficult home life should prompt further exploration of his mental health.

- **Symptoms:** Bill is clearly overwhelmed and struggling with his life circumstances and likely to be experiencing depression.

PROTECTIVE FACTORS

- It is important to identify Bill's current supports, including any other family members or friends who might help, as well as identifying the appropriate team to assist him to feel a greater sense of agency, and to support his recovery.
- Although he has described him as dismissive, Bill is still connected to his general practitioner (GP). There may be an opportunity to support Bill to see an alternative GP in the same practice.

KNOWLEDGE

Older people at risk of suicide

- Related factors that contribute to increased suicide risk in older adults include being male, poor socioeconomic standing, chronic pain and illness (Australian Bureau of Statistics 2017).
- Suicidal ideation and behaviour in individuals over the age of 65 years has been attributed to physical illness and functional disabilities (Fässberg et al. 2016).
- Research also suggests caregivers may be in the high-risk group (Anderson et al. 2019; Joling et al. 2018).
- Although risk factors for suicide include feeling lonely, lack of social supports, hopelessness and having a mental disorder, it is important to consider the current mental state of the person and what factors may be impacting at that point in time.
- Studies identify that older age people often consult their GP within weeks before death (Ahmedani et al. 2017; Fässberg et al. 2016).

Age-related considerations

- Cognition and health literacy should also be considered for older age people because this may affect a person's decision-making and problem-solving abilities (Conejero et al. 2018).
- Depression in older people is common and underdiagnosed. Untreated, it may impact negatively on the person's ability to enjoy the end years of life (Conejero et al. 2018). There is also evidence to support depression coexisting with suicide ideation (Joling et al. 2018). It is more common in older males and in those with diminished physical function.

Physical health

- Screening for thyroid dysfunction and vitamin B_{12} deficiency should also be conducted to rule these out as causal factors. Low-functioning thyroid has been implicated in depressive symptoms (Wildisen et al. 2019), and vitamin deficiency B_{12}, in particular, is implicated in cognitive decline in the elderly (da Rosa et al. 2019).

Carer responsibilities

- As a carer, quality of life is impacted by the increased responsibility needed to care for the family member and can become challenging and burdensome (Gilbertson et al. 2019; Joling et al. 2018).
- Independent risk factors such as family conflict and loss of employment can reduce social integration and the feeling of belonging (Conejero et al. 2018).

ATTITUDES

- Stereotyping older people as frail, incompetent or impaired is not uncommon, and even older people often expect this is how they are or should be perceived, which may contribute to their inability or reluctance to seek help. There is a notable difference between those living independently at a higher functioning capacity, contrasted with those who may be frail aged and living in the residential aged care environment. Clearly, this has contributed to stereotypical attitudes with all 'older aged being (considered) the same, and therefor treated the same' (Ross et al. 2018, p. 194).
- Caring for predominately frail aged or physically ill older people is associated with negative stereotyping of the elderly (Ross et al. 2018). To gain an understanding of what it is like to be an older aged person, consider how you would want to be treated as you age. Ask yourself this, or how you would want your parents or grandparents treated.
- Too often, for example, as clinicians are talking with older aged people, their voices are raised, they use slowed, simple speech that can feel patronising and contributes to the maintenance of stereotypical attitudes that infer that older aged people are deaf and have difficulties understanding; this contributes to lowering a person's self-esteem (Schroyen et al. 2018).
- Older aged people are often perceived to have mental illnesses such as depression or dementia, or are considered inept, and assumptions are made that they will be unable to complete activities of daily living due to frailty (Fullen et al. 2018).
- Our attitudes about older people, particularly if developed at an early age, potentially continue and remain with us throughout our career in nursing.
- It is also suggested that negativity towards becoming old is impacted by the assumption that one will experience illness, become isolated from lifelong friends and family, and lose independence (Gale & Cooper 2018).

As you read in Chapter 16, mental health of the older age is affected by the person's life trajectory and interrelated with physical changes and loss. Considering Bill, a stance of taking a negative attitude and seeing him in a stereotypical way because of his age and his presentation increases the risk of poor management of his needs. Early exploration of the red flags is a proactive approach, including knowing and addressing your own beliefs and bias. Thus, a nurse's positive attitude and a willingness to demonstrate care will influence behaviour and support actions that are intended to help.

SKILLS

Assessment

- Mental health assessment should be structured and comprehensive.
- Exploring previous attempts of suicide (risk factors) and substance misuse will help inform the most appropriate management.
- Understanding the health history includes a comprehensive physical and mental health history, understanding the medications the person has been prescribed and whether they adhere to the prescribed regimen.

Therapeutic relationship

- Establishing a rapport and gaining trust is vital to ensuring the person is comfortable disclosing personal information and will enable an open discussion.
- Using a person-centred approach will improve the person's confidence and have a positive impact on the relationship and on health outcomes (Ross et al. 2018).
- Listening is the simplest, yet most important action nurses can take. We can listen, non-judgementally, to the person in our care, when they share their stories and experiences. This is where we collect information that will guide us as to how to proceed with interventions and management. By listening, we are gaining an understanding of how the person feels and how they experience the environment they dwell in.
- The way you communicate is equally important. Do not use a patronising tone or condescending terms of endearment such as, 'lovey' or 'darl', and ask the person how they wish to be addressed.
- By listening, observing and communicating appropriately, you are further developing rapport and trust. These are essential elements before introducing any strategies to treat or manage and ensures the person's wants and needs are central to the process.

Mental health promotion

- Promoting wellness, resilience and a sense of belonging is an important part of care, and improving our own knowledge around these will improve our confidence in interacting with older aged people. It is appropriate for you to refer the person to a more experienced clinician or service if you feel out of your depth (Fullen et al. 2018).

Observation

- Observing the person's surroundings and the interactions they have with others can help build a picture of what may be occurring or contributing to how they are feeling.
- Enquiring about who the person's supports are and whether/how they are managing in the community will also inform management.

Useful tools

There are validated tools available that can be incorporated in your nursing actions and that can help you to identify what the focus of nursing interventions might be. For example:

- The UCLA Loneliness Scale is recommended when you suspect the person is experiencing loneliness, which may be contributing to the behaviours displayed (Akpan et al. 2018). This tool has three questions and can be easily incorporated into your discussion without needing a tick-box sheet for the person to complete. Enquiring about how often they feel (1 = lonely; 2 = left out; 3 = isolated from others) can enable the person to respond, with 'hardly ever' scoring 1, 'sometimes' scoring 2, or 'often' scoring 3. A total score of 6–9 indicates the person is 'lonely'.
- Once you have established this or ruled out loneliness, other tools such as the Geriatric Depression Scale short form (GDS-15 or GDS 5/15) can be used to assess mood in cognitively intact people (Sheikh & Yesavage 1986). Gain assistance and develop your skills if you are not familiar with this (or any other) tool.
- Screening or assessing for suicide intent can be based on the Patient Health Questionnaire (PHQ), though people can answer the questions with a 'no' and still have thoughts of suicide. Any indication by the older age person about suicide or suicide ideation should be considered as an indication of increased risk.

RELEVANT TREATMENT MODALITIES

Once all the assessments have been conducted and cues identified, a decision can be made on the most appropriate treatment modalities or strategies to assist. For example, identifying loneliness as an issue then prompts interventions and actions that increase social connection and reduce isolation and loneliness. The assessment will also determine if care requires escalation to support services. For Bill, getting a sense of how he understands his own health and health care is the first action.

- Talking to Bill and ascertaining what he wants and needs can help identify the goals of care.
- Bill's GP or primary care nurse should also be engaged early in determining how Bill's health is currently being managed and if there are any other underlying health causes.
- Understanding his current medications and whether he is adhering to the treatment regimen will help identify whether any changes are to be made or any additional treatments required.
- Non-pharmacological strategies – for example, cognitive behaviour therapy or acceptance and commitment therapy – should be used as a first-line approach, with antidepressant medication if psychological therapy alone is not effective.
- Antidepressant medication is a commonly used treatment for people who are depressed. Prescribing for the elderly must be planned and monitored carefully because of age-related physical changes that occur, such as renal function impairment (Australian Medicines Handbook 2019), and that can impact on therapeutic effect (and side effects). Bill will require support if commencing on antidepressant medication and should be started at a lower dose to minimise any

adverse effects such as falls risk (Australian Medicines Handbook 2019).

- In considering the initial red flags for Bill, referral to community-based team for support and services such as social work and counselling, aged care teams and supportive care should be considered.

Interprofessional practice provides varied specialisation and comprehensive mental health care (Neils-Strunjas et al. 2018).

- Involving his immediate family and friends can assist Bill in achieving his care goals.

SCENARIO 24.2

Mabel

Mabel is an 85-year-old woman who has been living in a residential aged care facility for 3 months. She has complex medical disorders including congestive heart failure and osteoarthritis in her left knee. She has been treated for hypertension, hyperlipidaemia and gastric reflux for some years. The diversional therapist at the aged care facility has worked with Mabel to provide a life story to help the healthcare team to get to know and understand Mabel as a person. Mabel never married after her fiancé was killed in a farming accident when he was 22 years old, a year before their planned wedding. As a young woman needing to support herself in the 1950s when options for women were limited, Mabel became a hairdresser and over time acquired her own salon that she owned and managed until she retired fully at 75 years of age. She has one brother who is married with three adult children, all of whom have been an important part of Mabel's life.

Mabel also had a companion, Betty, who lived with her for 25 years before her admission to the aged care facility. Betty is 10 years younger than Mabel and provided Mabel with daily care for about the past 7 years; she is now a daily visitor to the care centre. Betty continues to live independently in the home she previously shared with Mabel in a neighbouring area, though she now takes the bus to visit because she no longer feels confident driving. Mabel experiences daily pain from her osteoarthritis and requires the registered nurses to help manage this through pharmacological and non-pharmacological interventions. A multidisciplinary team review is coming up for Mabel because she has been in care for 3 months. Since admission to the aged care facility Mabel has struggled with multiple losses; her mobility is becoming increasingly limited, her independence regarding activities of daily living has been affected with her increasing pain on movement and her sleep is often of poor quality. She expresses a great sense of loss having been physically parted from Betty despite her almost daily visits. She misses the privacy of the home they shared, their dog Scamp and two cats, along with the meals they enjoyed cooking together and the friends who visited. Mabel remains cognitively unimpaired; however, since admission she has become increasingly anxious – partially related to financial and family pressures because her brother and nephew believe Betty should leave the home they shared so it can be sold to support Mabel's care. The staff have also noticed Mabel is increasingly reluctant to leave her room for meals or activities. Her disinterest in food has led to a 4 kg weight loss since admission, despite her diet being adjusted to provide her with more calories.

As per the aged care facility's policy, the registered nurse spent time with Mabel to undertake some advance care planning. During this conversation, Mabel expressed feelings of sadness and despair – particularly about her relationship with Betty, as she has confided that they were more than companions and were in an intimate relationship for many years. She desperately misses the intimacy of the relationship and dreads that it won't remain private now she is in care. She does not feel confident telling her brother and nephew that this is the reason she does not wish to sell the house Betty lives in. However, they have been increasingly pressuring her about this, wanting to ensure that Mabel has a valid will and advance care directive. They are making assumptions that they will be the primary recipients and executors of Mabel's will and will be the people she nominates as her enduring power of attorney. Betty cannot take Mabel to their home because of her limited mobility and Betty's inability to drive.

RED FLAGS

- Mabel is increasingly frail, and her complex issues are affecting her quality of life and her resilience as she copes with the transition to the aged care facility. For an older person, this may include a loss of identity, independence and autonomy.
- In the face of feelings of helplessness, social isolation and loneliness, it is difficult for Mabel to develop new fulfilling relationships with staff and others.
- The sensitive issues of love, intimacy and sex, which attract a great degree of stigma and discrimination in relation to older people (Bauer et al. 2016), are also weighing heavily on Mabel. Mabel fears she will be unable to keep her relationship with Betty private and her expectation is that having the relationship exposed to staff and other residents will mean she will not be accepted by others and that tensions will increase with her brother and his family.
- Mabel is at risk of being compromised nutritionally because of her low mood and isolation.

- Chronic pain affects her sleep quality and contributes to her feeling tired and less willing to socialise with other residents at mealtimes.
- A primarily pharmacological approach to supporting Mabel may contribute to a situation of polypharmacy and unintended consequences such as increasing her risk of falls.

KNOWLEDGE

Ageing

- Underpinning an effective toolbox of skills is knowledge of anatomy and physiology and an understanding of the process of ageing.
- Developing comprehensive assessment skills requires knowledge about specific physical systems (e.g. integumentary, oral, urinary, cardiovascular, respiratory, musculoskeletal) as well as knowledge about clinical reasoning, psychosocial assessment and ethico-legal and professional considerations (Bauer et al. 2018).
- Frailty is an important concept not linked specifically to age but to the increasing impact of ageing from disease processes on a person's functional and physical abilities, along with the potential decline in cognitive functioning and physical strength (Health Quality Safety Commission 2019).
- In residential aged care facilities, care to ensure quality of life must not be constrained by a person's physical or mental decline. Frailty should not be a barrier to providing interventions with the goal of improving the older person's health and quality of life (Burn et al. 2018).

Loss, grief and social isolation

- Loss is a significant issue for people admitted to residential aged care facilities, with the loss of relationships, independence, privacy and the ability to make decisions about daily routines, personal care and meals, belongings and pets.
- Experienced as sometimes the most difficult transition they have had to make, older people moving into a residential aged care facility experience significant mental health and wellbeing issues, with high rates of social isolation, loneliness and depression being well documented for residents in this setting (Franck et al. 2016).
- The decision to live in an aged care facility may be the result of increasing frailty and is sometimes preceded by a hospital admission for complex medical issues that may also mask emotional issues. It may also be related to the inability of a carer to continue providing adequate levels of care in the community setting. Older people may be experiencing distress related to the suddenness or unexpectedness of the need to move to residential aged care (Lee et al. 2013; McKenna & Staniforth 2017).

Sexuality and relationships

- Increasingly the population of residential aged care facilities will reflect the diversity of the communities they serve.
- The issues faced by heterosexual residents are amplified for residents from the LGBTIQ+ community. Studies identify that LGBTIQ+ people fear ageing and admission to residential aged care. They are subject to ageist attitudes around sexuality and intimacy and additionally are at risk of experiencing stereotypical and negative attitudes towards their sexuality.
- There is also a high degree of invisibility in residential aged care for anything other than heterosexual relationships, leaving those not in heterosexual relationships feeling vulnerable even when they have been comfortable and confident in their relationships outside this setting (Willis 2017).

Nutrition

- Nutritional needs are not always easily met for people living in residential aged care.
- While multivitamin supplementation can improve both nutritional status and bone quality in aged care residents and can be easily implemented (Grieger et al. 2009), residents experience food in very different ways.
- Food choice and food service satisfaction affect nutritional status and, conversely, dissatisfaction with food has been linked with poor food intake and a negative impact on quality of life.
- Residents will have a range of food practices prior to admission and have eaten and cooked for family and friends in diverse ways.
- Accommodating personal preferences is challenging when some residents will appreciate fresh food, some will enjoy unhealthy food, some will only consume a narrow range of foods and some will enjoy diversity (Bailey et al. 2017).
- Individuals eating the same food and portions will still experience the taste and fulfilment from the food differently, so while some may find food too salty, for others the food will seem to lack enough salt (Bailey et al. 2017).
- Person-centred care requires residents to have choice when it comes to the food and drinks they consume by identifying their preferences, so the challenge is to cater to the diverse individual preferences of residents who all prefer food they are familiar with and have consumed before living in an aged care facility.

ATTITUDES

- For some, the aged care environment is not considered an attractive option in nursing, making recruitment for aged care providers problematic. Historically nurses working in aged residential care have been paid less than those working in other settings and this, along with the lack of a focus on gerontology and the lack of an aged care specialisation in nursing degrees, has contributed to recruitment and retention issues in residential aged care (Lea et al. 2017).
- Nurses should be well prepared in physical care (such as wound dressings and more intimate tasks such as showering) and in mental health nursing skills, such as developing a good rapport with someone, mental health assessment in the context of older age,

communication skills and building relationships with residents including those with dementia.
- A small study of first-year nursing students' learning opportunities in residential aged care reported that students experienced the environment as supportive for developing confidence, competence, skills and knowledge because they were able to link theory to practice with available and encouraging mentors (Lea et al. 2014). The students expressed a greater interest in considering aged care as an option after graduation.

Ageism, sexuality and intimacy

- Ageist attitudes lead to assumptions from staff and families when addressing sexuality and intimacy for the older person in residential aged care.
- Older people continue to see sexuality and intimacy as important and contributing to their quality of life.
- Developing intimate relationships and other expressions of sexuality may be met with negative and discriminatory responses from staff, residents and family, resulting in the older person's sexuality and intimacy needs being constrained by the attitudes and expectations of how older people 'should' be.
- An ethical decision-making process that focuses on the privacy, wellbeing and quality of life of the resident in relation to their needs around sexuality and intimacy is required to navigate the barriers that exist to sexuality and intimacy needs being met.
- The attitudes and values of staff and families may differ, or staff and families may disagree about who best understands the resident's needs (Cook et al. 2017).
- The first action point for staff would be to engage in training focused on increasing staff awareness of their own attitudes and how they can provide culturally safe care for LGBTIQ+ residents.

SKILLS

Communication

- Highly developed communication skills are essential for nurses to effectively manage their healthcare team, work with residents, participate in the multidisciplinary team and interact with families.
- Ensuring privacy and the ability to have private space for interactions with family, friends and pets and to engage with children and animals in activities helps promote communication, prevent boredom and provides the opportunity to develop and engage in meaningful social relationships.

Individualised care

- Getting to know a resident by reading their notes or a life story helps staff to grow an understanding of the person. A life story may contribute more detail in terms of person-centred care such as preferences, their life journey and family and social history; however, both provide a richer understanding of the person and improve attitudes towards residents (Dennerstein et al. 2018).
- Assessing whether Mabel would benefit from additional support from an LGBTIQ+ community organisation needs to be determined in discussion with Mabel and Betty.
- For residents, feeling cared for, having the opportunity to reminisce about treasured memories and having professional support so they can safely express their grief and loss as well as being affirmed for their personal strengths, allows them to still set goals and engage in opportunities that continue to expand their life experiences (McKenna & Staniforth 2017).

Therapeutic relationship

- Mental health nursing knowledge, skills and attitudes will help develop the therapeutic relationship between nurses and residents in long-term care.
- Therapeutic use of self will enable the nurse to empathise with Mabel to establish an emotional connection and to demonstrate caring to support courageous conversations such as those required during the process of advance care planning.
- The ability to be self-aware, recognise verbal and non-verbal cues and to be compassionate and caring will support Mabel to express her immediate and long-term anxieties and concerns in developing approaches to sensitive issues such as her will, the enduring power of attorney, the tensions in her relationship with her brother and his family and her fear of being stigmatised and discriminated against because of her sexuality.

NURSING ACTIONS AND INTERVENTIONS

Assessment and care planning

- Because of the increasingly complex care needs of residents, nurses working in aged care need to exhibit a high level of nursing skills, especially in assessment, understanding the concept of frailty and recognising when residents are deteriorating.
- Assessment, including physical health assessment, mental health assessment and cognitive assessment, is key to delivering quality care to residents and nurses working in residential aged care. Nurses need to call on an extensive range of assessment skills that support a person-centred approach to care within a multidisciplinary team.
- Residents need an initial assessment to inform an initial care plan and then for a longer term care plan.
- Ongoing assessment is essential because the health status of older people changes and there will be times when a focused assessment and plan of care is required for a specific problem such as a delirium, a pressure injury or an infection.
- There will also be a need for urgent assessment when the resident experiences a specific event such as a fall or health deterioration from another disease process.

Observation and monitoring

- Monitoring intake is important because malnutrition in older aged people will impact on wound healing and increase their susceptibility to infection, anaemia,

fractures and pressure ulcers, hypotension and deterioration in mental acuity.
- Nutritional assessment tools (such as the MUST screening tool) need to be deployed to assess and prevent complications (Poulia et al. 2012).
- Dehydration will have a similar impact and additionally increase the risk of urinary tract infection or acute kidney injury (Health Quality Safety Commission 2019).

RELEVANT TREATMENT MODALITIES

Person-centred care

- A person-centred model of care allows those in residential aged care to exert as much choice over their lives as possible. Mabel's thoughts and perspective must be elucidated, and relevant external health practitioners should be involved as required to ensure a person-centred approach is maintained (Sankaran et al. 2010).
- Placing the resident at the centre of care facilitates their involvement in activities that contribute to them forming relationships with other residents and staff and attaining a sense of belonging.
- Promoting autonomy and independence for residents through choice (food, activities, clothing, personalising their own space with plants and personal effects) and facilitating the resident's ability to be involved in decision making in a wide range of aspects of daily life encourages a feeling of control.
- The basis for deciding on relevant treatment modalities for Mabel require the nurse to conduct a holistic assessment that reflects Mabel as a person as well as the complexity of her physical, social and mental health issues.
- Mabel's GP will be an integral part of the multidisciplinary team in the review process. However, other health professionals have much to offer residents, including nurses with specialties in gerontology and mental health of older people.
- The Eden Alternative TM is one model of care that has been identified as providing residents in residential aged care with the environment to enable them to continue to experience fulfilment in their life (Brownie & Horstmanshof 2012).

Psychotherapy

- Non-pharmacological interventions need to be considered for Mabel's emotional and social issues in the same way that non-pharmacological interventions for Mabel's pain and poor sleep are implemented.
- Because she is significantly concerned with the issues to do with her life partner and her family, it is likely that supporting Mabel to resolve some of her fears and concerns about this will help improve her mental health and emotional wellbeing.

Pharmacotherapy

- For the reasons explained in Scenario 1 and Chapter 16, minimising polypharmacy and careful prescribing is important in aged care.
- While Mabel may be exhibiting symptoms of anxiety and a mild depressive disorder, additional medication could increase the risk of falls as well as other physical complications (Lalic et al. 2016; Moore et al. 2014).

Chapter summary

Ageing is one of the non-negotiables of life and, regardless of the clinical setting, every nurse will work with older people. The two scenarios described in this chapter invite you to consider the importance of developing your knowledge, skills and confidence in providing nursing care to older age people and the importance of mental health nursing skills in working with people at this life stage. There are various approaches to care, though the context of care should be the focus. There are differences in providing care for those who are self-sufficient and living in their own home, in contrast to older people living within a residential aged care facility or nursing home, and who may depend on care providers. Both contexts present challenges that need to be approached with consideration and respect for the person as an individual. Working with the person to ascertain what it is they want and need will help to identify the goals of care. Considering mental health in older age is an opportunity to learn and develop your attitudes, beliefs and understanding of people's experiences as they age. It is also an opportunity to practise interpersonal communication and develop mental health nursing skills. Reflection is also a helpful strategy for developing self-confidence.

Be mindful that you alone cannot solve all the problems of one person and that a team or interdisciplinary approach is often the most effective, bringing a collaboration of skills together to attain the best outcome for the older person. The role you have will be to recognise that the person may be experiencing factors that affect their mental health or that there is a mental health–related concern or red flag impacting on the older person in your care, and to act accordingly.

References

Ahmedani, B.K., Peterson, E.L., Hu, Y., et al., 2017. Major physical health conditions and risk of suicide. Am. J. Prev. Med. 53 (3), 308–315.

Akpan, A., Roberts, C., Bandeen-Roche, K., et al., 2018. Standard set of health outcome measures for older persons. BMC Geriatr. 18 (1), 36.

Anderson, J.G., Eppes, A., O'Dwyer, S.T., 2019. 'Like death is Near': expressions of suicidal and homicidal ideation in the blog posts of family caregivers of people with dementia. Behav. Sci. (Basel) 9 (3), 22.

Australian Bureau of Statistics (ABS), 2017. Australian Demographic Statistics, June 2016. Cat. no. 3101.0. Canberra: ABS.

Australian Medicines Handbook, 2019. Australian Medicines Handbook. Online. https://amhonline.amh.net.au/.

Bailey, A., Bailey, S., Bernoth, M., 2017. 'I'd rather die happy': Residents' experiences with food regulations, risk and food choice in residential aged care. A qualitative study. Contemp. Nurse 53 (6), 597–606.

Bauer, M., Fetherstonhaugh, D., Winbolt, M., 2018. Perceived barriers and enablers to conducting nursing assessments in residential aged care facilities in Victoria, Australia. Aust. J. Adv. Nurs. 36 (2), 14–22.

Bauer, M., Haesler, E., Fetherstonhaugh, D., 2016. Let's talk about sex: older people's view on the recognition of sexuality and sexual health in the health-care setting. Health Expect. 19 (6), 1237–1250.

Brownie, S., Horstmanshof, L., 2012. Creating the conditions for self-fulfilment for aged care residents. Nurs. Ethics 19 (6), 777–786.

Burn, R., Hubbard, R.E., Scrase, R.J., et al., 2018. A frailty index derived from a standardized comprehensive geriatric assessment predicts mortality and aged residential care admission. BMC Geriatr. 18 (1), 319.

Conejero, I., Olie, E., Courtet, P., et al., 2018. Suicide in older adults: current perspectives. Clin. Interv. Aging 13, 691–699.

Cook, C., Schouten, V., Henrickson, M., et al., 2017. Ethics, intimacy and sexuality in aged care. J. Adv. Nurs. 73, 3017–3027.

da Rosa, M.I., Beck, W.O., Colonetti, T., et al., 2019. Association of vitamin D and vitamin B_{12} with cognitive impairment in elderly aged 80 years or older: a cross-sectional study. J. Hum. Nutr. Diet. 32 (4), 518–524.

Dennerstein, M., Bhar, S.S., Castles, J.J., 2018. A randomised controlled trial examining the impact of aged care residents' written life-stories on aged care staff knowledge and attitudes. Int. Psychogeriatr. 30 (9), 1291–1299.

Fässberg, M.M., Cheung, G., Canetto, S.S., et al., 2016. A systematic review of physical illness, functional disability, and suicidal behaviour among older adults. Aging Ment. Health 20 (2), 166–194.

Franck, L., Molyneux, N., Parkinson, L., 2016. Systematic review of interventions addressing social isolation and depression in aged care clients. Qual. Life Res. 25, 1395–1407.

Fullen, M.C., Granello, D.H., Richardson, V.E., et al., 2018. Using wellness and resilience to predict age perception in older adulthood. J. Couns. Dev. 96 (4), 424–435.

Gale, C.R., Cooper, C., 2018. Attitudes to ageing and change in frailty status: the English longitudinal study of ageing. Gerontology 64 (1), 58–66.

Gilbertson, E.L., Krishnasamy, R., Foote, C., et al., 2019. Burden of care and quality of life among caregivers for adults receiving maintenance dialysis: a systematic review. Am. J. Kidney Dis. 73 (3), 332–343.

Grieger, J.A., Nowson, C.A., Jarman, J.F., et al., 2009. Multivitamin supplementation improves nutritional status and bone quality in aged cared residents. Eur. J. Clin. Nutr. 63, 558–565.

Health Quality Safety Commission, 2019. Frailty Care Guides: Ngā Aratohu Maimoa Hauwarea. HQSC, Auckland.

Joling, K.J., O'Dwyer, S.T., Hertogh, C.M., et al., 2018. The occurrence and persistence of thoughts of suicide, self-harm and death in family caregivers of people with dementia: a longitudinal data analysis over 2 years. Int. J. Geriatr. Psychiatry 33 (2), 263–270.

Lalic, S., Jamsen, K.M., Wimmer, B.C., et al., 2016. Polypharmacy and medication regimen complexity as factors associated with staff informant rated quality of life in residents of aged care facilities: a cross-sectional study. Eur. J. Clin. Pharmacol. 72, 1117–1124.

Lea, E., Marlow, A., Altmann, E., et al., 2017. Nursing students' preferences for clinical placements in the residential aged care setting. J. Clin. Nurs. 27 (1–2), 143–152.

Lea, D., Marlow, A., Bramble, M., et al., 2014. Learning Opportunities in a resident aged care facility: the role of supported placements for first-year nursing students. J. Nurs. Educ. 53 (7), 410–414.

Lee, V.S.P., Simpson, J., Froggatt, K., 2013. A narrative exploration of older people's transitions into residential care. Aging Ment. Health 7 (1), 48–56.

McKenna, D., Staniforth, B., 2017. Older people moving to residential care in Aotearoa New Zealand: considerations for social work at practice and policy levels. Aotear. N. Z. Soc. Work 29 (1), 28–40.

Moore, K.J., Doyle, C.J., Dunning, T.L., et al., 2014. Public sector residential aged care: identifying novel associations between quality indicators and other demographic and health-related factors. Aust. Health Rev. 38, 325–331.

Neils-Strunjas, J., Crandall, K.J., Shackelford, J., et al., 2018. Students report more positive attitudes toward older adults following an interprofessional service-learning course. Gerontol. Geriatr. Educ. 12, 1–11.

Poulia, K.A., Yannakoulia, M., Karageorgou, D., et al., 2012. Evaluation of the efficacy of six nutritional screening tools to predict malnutrition in the elderly. Clin. Nutr. 31 (3), 378–385.

Ross, L., Jennings, P., Williams, B., 2018. Improving health care student attitudes toward older adults through educational interventions: a systematic review. Gerontol. Geriatr. Educ. 39 (2), 193–213.

Sankaran, S., Kenealy, T., Adair, A., et al., 2010. A complex intervention to support 'rest home' care: a plot study. N. Z. Med. J. 123 (1308), 41–53.

Schroyen, S., Adam, S., Marquet, M., et al., 2018. Communication of healthcare professionals: is there ageism? Eur. J. Cancer Care (Engl.) 27 (1), e12780.

Sheikh, J.I., Yesavage, J.A., 1986. Geriatric Depression Scale (GDS): recent evidence and development of a shorter version. Clin. Gerontol. 5 (1–2), 165–173.

Wildisen, L., Moutzouri, E., Beglinger, S., et al., 2019. Subclinical thyroid dysfunction and depressive symptoms: protocol for a systematic review and individual participant data meta-analysis of prospective cohort studies. BMJ Open 9 (7), e029716.

Willis, P., 2017. Queer, visible, present: the visibility of older LGB adults in long-term care environments. Hous. Care Supp. 20 (3), 110–120.

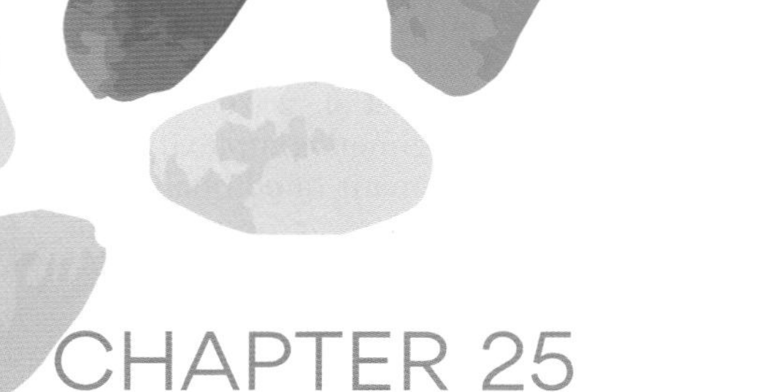

CHAPTER 25

Perinatal and infant mental health

Julie Ferguson

KEY POINTS

- The perinatal period is a time of rapid physical and mental change.
- During the perinatal period mental health disorders can surface for the first time.
- Changes during the perinatal period can trigger exacerbation of a pre-existing mental health problem.
- The perinatal period is an opportunity for mental health promotion, early identification, intervention and mental health treatment.
- A variety of therapies are regarded as very effective during this period including cognitive behaviour therapy, interpersonal psychotherapy, couples therapy, parent–infant psychotherapy and attachment-focused psychotherapy.
- Antidepressants and mood stabilisers are major classes of medication used during the perinatal period.

KEY TERMS

- Antenatal
- Care planning
- Ethics
- Lithium
- Medication
- Parent–infant dynamic
- Perinatal
- Postnatal
- Prenatal

LEARNING OUTCOMES

The material in this chapter will assist you to:

- describe the incidence of perinatal depression and anxiety
- identify who is vulnerable within the population at risk of developing perinatal difficulties
- identify risk factors to look for when screening women during the perinatal period
- describe the care-planning process when working with women with severe mental illness during the perinatal period
- describe risk assessment for the parent–infant dynamic
- understand the risk–benefit dynamic process used when deciding on medication options for women during the perinatal period
- understand the importance of working within an interprofessional collaboration framework in the perinatal period
- understand the importance of including the partner when assessing and treating a woman experiencing perinatal difficulties
- examine some of the therapeutic modalities used when working with women and their families during the perinatal period.

Lived experience comment by Jarrad Hickmott

Acknowledging trauma and the role it may play in someone's life, and the importance of interacting with this in a trauma-informed way that leads to a positive and safe outcome for those involved, is essential.

Introduction

The perinatal period is defined as the time from conception until the first year after birth (postnatal) (Austin et al. 2017). It is a time of great change both physically and mentally for women and their partners. For most women and their families, it is a time of great joy. As described by Scioli and Biller (2009), the arrival of a new baby is like a 'dance of hope' – the new child bringing promise and possibility that can re-energise parents, allowing them to reinvest in themselves and their family.

While many women feel joy about their pregnancy, not all women experience pregnancy and parenthood as a positive time. The experience of pregnancy is different for each woman and her relationships and psychosocial circumstances need to be considered. For some pregnant women, their previous experiences of miscarriage, traumatic delivery or the loss of a child can cause great distress. An unwanted or unplanned pregnancy, a teenage pregnancy, a difficult relationship with her partner (including domestic violence) or lack of support from her family can also cause increased stress. A history of trauma, sexual abuse or drug and alcohol dependence can also cause considerable concern during pregnancy and increase a person's vulnerability to developing a mental health concern during the perinatal period.

The perinatal period is also associated with increased risk of mental health conditions including antenatal depression/anxiety, the 'baby blues', postnatal depression and postpartum psychosis (see Chapter 10 for more detailed information) or the exacerbation of pre-existing mental health problems including anxiety disorders, bipolar disorder, psychosis and schizophrenia (Austin et al. 2017). Between 15 and 20% of women experience mood and anxiety disorders during their pregnancy (Shea et al. 2014); in the general perinatal population one in 10 women experience depression or anxiety and approximately one in six experience postnatal depression (Austin et al. 2017).

Some women are at higher risk of developing mental health problems during the perinatal period (Austin et al. 2017) – see Box 25.1.

The perinatal period offers a window of opportunity for intervention. Women see more health professionals during pregnancy and early parenting than at other times in their life. As suggested by Bowlby (1979), because relationships at this stage of the parent's development are in a state of change, it is a time when families will seek help and accept it. So, the perinatal period provides an important opportunity for intervention, not only for the parents but for the long-term outcomes of the child. There are many areas of nursing that come into contact with a woman and her family during the perinatal period – including midwives, child and family nurses, mental health nurses (inpatient, community, primary care), primary health and general practice nurses and, of course, specialist perinatal and infant mental health nurse specialists. All nurses and midwives, in all clinical settings, can make a significant difference to the mental health outcomes of women in the perinatal period, providing we are aware of the early warning signs and risk factors.

In this chapter we will explore two clinical scenarios to understand the complex presentations that can occur during the perinatal period and examine the nursing responses, medication treatments and psychological interventions that can help facilitate change.

Box 25.1 Women at increased risk of perinatal mental health problems

- **Indigenous women** are more likely to experience mental health problems. In a service in New South Wales up to 40% of the indigenous women accessing the service had a history of mental health problems. In an area of New Zealand one in three Maori women accessing the service experienced at least one mental health problem. In Canada, Aboriginal women are twice as likely to be depressed as non-Aboriginal women.
- **Migrant women** are at higher risk of developing perinatal depression, with refugee women at heightened risk of psychological morbidity.
- **Women experiencing intimate partner violence** are four times more likely to develop depressive symptoms and 10 times more likely to experience anxiety than the general perinatal population.
- **Women who experience life stressors** such as family problems, violence or loss are at higher risk of developing mental health problems postpartum.
- **Women from lesbian, gay, bisexual, trans and/ or intersex groups** are more likely to face discrimination and have their parenting abilities questioned.
- **Women who have experienced mental illness previously** and those with a family history of mental illness are more likely to be affected during the perinatal period.

Sources: Austin et al. 2017; Hartz & McGrath 2017

SCENARIO 25.1

Jane

Jane was a 30-year-old woman who was referred to a perinatal and infant mental health service following her 6-week postnatal appointment with a child and family nurse. During that appointment, the nurse asked Jane to complete an Edinburgh Perinatal Depression Scale (Cox et al. 1987). The EPDS is an important aspect of the routine 6-week postnatal check-up that child and family nurses conduct (and is also used during the antenatal period by midwives, which can alert them to the risk of the woman developing perinatal depression or anxiety). Jane scored 18, with a 2 on question 10 (which relates to self-harm), both of which indicate a risk of depression. The child and family nurse arranged a referral to the perinatal and infant mental health service.

This was Jane's first baby (a daughter) to her partner, Chris. It was not a planned pregnancy but was wanted once the couple had become accustomed to the idea of being parents. Jane had previously had two terminations of pregnancy to Chris due to her anxiety about not being ready to be a parent and worrying how she would cope with a child of her own.

Jane had a complex family history. She was the youngest child of five and her father died when she was only 3 years old. Jane's mother struggled to cope with the loss of her husband; she was diagnosed with bipolar disorder and hospitalised on many occasions throughout Jane's childhood. Over the past 20 years we have come to understand the important role fathers play in assisting children to modulate intense affect (Fischer 2012). Jane was often without enough adult emotional input to help her make sense of her world. Jane had a troubled adolescence; she dropped out of school early and often had difficulties with her peer group. Jane had, however, experienced a positive, supportive relationship with a counsellor during her adolescence.

RED FLAGS

- Jane had somehow slipped through the net of psychosocial screening in the antenatal stage of pregnancy despite that her history ticked many boxes for risk factors indicating struggles in the perinatal period.
- An EPDS score above 13 can indicate possible depression, and any score on question 10 (self-harm) will require further risk assessment. Jane scored 2 on question 10, which asks, 'The thought of harming myself has occurred to me...' Jane answered 'Sometimes'. When a person responds positively to this question, it is important to explore feelings of self-harm. In this circumstance Jane was able to describe her feelings of wanting to flee when her baby was distressed. She often felt overwhelmed, but not suicidal.
- Jane scoring 18 overall on the EPDS was a trigger for her being referred to a specialist mental health service, indicating that she was possibly experiencing depression and required further assessment.
- Complex family history with her mother having a diagnosed mental health problem (bipolar disorder) and regular hospital admissions, and the death of her father in early childhood, is another red flag.
- Jane had two previous terminations of pregnancy due to ambivalence about becoming a parent.
- If Jane is struggling, how is her partner coping?

KNOWLEDGE

Psychosocial screening during pregnancy

- All pregnant women should be routinely screened for depression and anxiety symptoms using the EPDS scale, as well as screening for psychosocial risk factors as early as possible in the pregnancy.
  - The EPDS has been used extensively throughout the perinatal period since its development in 1987 (Cox et al. 1987).
  - When a person scores above 13 on the EPDS, depression is indicated. When working with women from different cultural backgrounds, it is important to keep in mind that across studies of different cultural groups, this cut-off score varies considerably (Smith-Nielsen et al. 2018).
  - Any score on question 10 (self-harm) requires further assessment. Most people use self-harm as a way of coping with overwhelming feelings, not because they are experiencing suicidal thoughts (Hungerford et al. 2017).

BARRIERS TO SCREENING

Barriers to screening include:

- a woman's experience of stigma (e.g. feeling worried about being judged)
- normalising their emotional difficulties as being related to 'hormones' or the situation
- preferring to manage their feelings themselves
- not knowing what 'normal' feelings during the perinatal period are (Austin et al. 2017).

It is also important to consider the cultural background of a woman and her family and their beliefs about pregnancy, birth and parenthood, as well as about mental health and illness.

Reflection

Jane delivered her baby in a large public hospital, so did have psychosocial screening early in her pregnancy. (Many private hospitals have not offered routine psychosocial screening until recently (Austin et al. 2017).) So how did she slip through the net during the antenatal period? When Jane was contacted to make a follow-up appointment, she played down what was happening for her, saying she was okay, which is not uncommon for women who have had a difficult childhood and have learned to cope on their own.

SAFETY, RISK ASSESSMENT AND PROTECTIVE FACTORS

- Risk factors, which are described as vulnerabilities, are adverse factors that are present in a woman's life (Jomeen et al. 2017). The presence of risk factors may be used to highlight the possibility of a woman developing postnatal depression.
- Research has also explored the impact of protective factors that influence an individual's adaptation to life stressors. Recent evidence has suggested that there is an association between resilience and avoidance of postnatal depression (Jomeen et al. 2017). This raises questions about the possibility of treatment options for developing resilience in women during the perinatal period.

Assessing risk to the baby

When assessing the level of risk of suicide for a woman in the postnatal period, it is also important to assess any risk to her baby (Austin et al. 2017).

- The mother–infant interaction can be a valuable aspect of the risk assessment. If difficulties in the interaction are observed and if the woman has a significant mental health condition, further assessment will be required (Austin et al. 2017).
- Sometimes the risk of harm to the infant is related to the mother's suicide risk, but this is not always the case, and needs to be further assessed.
- This assessment would include psychosocial risk factors (see Box 25.2), infant factors, infant behaviours of concern (observed or reported), relationship factors (observed or reported), maternal factors and protective factors (Austin et al. 2017).
- If there is a risk to the baby, then the care planning will need to include other important supports from within the family or close friends, and referral to the relevant child protection agency may be necessary.
- A safety plan is essential to ensure that both the mother and baby are kept safe during this difficult time. Jane indicated no immediate risk to her baby during the assessment.

Box 25.2 Psychosocial risk factors

- Unresolved family-of-origin issues
- History of physical/sexual abuse, family violence or childhood neglect
- Past pregnancy loss or excess pregnancy concern
- Unplanned or unwanted pregnancy
- Was the mother able to touch the baby on the day of the birth?
- Did the mother have sole responsibility for the baby's care during the first week of life?
- Who else was involved in the baby's care?
- Availability of emotional/social/practical support
- How much time does the mother spend away from the baby?
- Is the mother excessively worried about the baby?

Perinatal mental health in partners

- The transition to parenthood occurs for both the mother and her partner. The change in relationship from a couple to a trio can be a difficult transition for some people.
- Whenever a woman is diagnosed with a perinatal mental health disorder, it is important to assess how her partner is coping. Research in Australia has shown that one in 10 men experience paternal depression between the first trimester of pregnancy and 1 year postpartum, and one in six fathers experience anxiety during the perinatal period (Austin et al. 2017).
- Untreated depression and anxiety in fathers during the perinatal period can have long-term effects on their relationships with their children as well as their partners.
- There is no data available for same-sex partners, suffice to say that all partners need to be included in the same way a father would be included in the assessment.

TREATMENT MODALITIES AND CONSIDERATIONS

Over the past 30 years we have gained a greater understanding of intergenerational trauma. Fallon and Brabender (2012) highlighted the importance of a woman working through her trauma history to develop a coherent narrative of her own childhood experiences, such that it allows her to go on to provide care for her baby and children. Austin et al. (2017) highlight that women with a history of trauma experience higher incidents of psychological distress during the perinatal period.

Treatment in the perinatal period is usually similar to that used to treat any depressive episode or significant anxiety problem, including cognitive behaviour therapy, interpersonal therapy and dialectical behaviour therapy, and are associated with good outcomes (Stephens et al. 2016). In addition, there are a few treatments specific to the perinatal period.

Parent–infant psychotherapy

There are many forms of parent–infant therapy available. When there has been relational trauma in the early relationship due to mental health problems such as depression, this repair work helps develop a secure relationship between the mother, partner and their child. The therapy addresses a range of conscious and unconscious factors that shape the individual parent's and infant's specific modes of being with each other, which focuses on the attachment relationship (Baradon & Joyce 2016).

Parenting training programs

A wide range of parenting programs are available. These are often run in the community by specialist parenting support services such as Tresillian and Karitane as well as other non-government services. Organisations and programs such as Circle of Security (Powel et al. 2016) and Triple-P (Sanders & Mazzucchelli 2018) focus on supporting positive parenting strategies.

Couples therapy

The transition from couple to trio can be a challenging time for parents. Couples therapy can provide a valuable space to process this change.

MEDICATION DURING PREGNANCY AND BREASTFEEDING

There is a great deal of misinformation circulating about antidepressant medication use during the perinatal period. It is vital for clinicians to be well informed about the research on antidepressant use during this period to accurately convey and translate the latest findings to women and their families (Galbally et al. 2014). Sudden discontinuation of pharmacological treatments leads to higher risk for relapse.

- When working with mothers who are pregnant or breastfeeding it is important to weigh up the risks and benefits of medication (Kendall-Tackett 2017). A mother who has moderate to severe depression or anxiety would most likely benefit from continuing antidepressant medication.
- It is important to consider the types of symptoms she is experiencing (or experiences when she is unwell) such as the symptoms of depression and her attitude towards taking medication.
- Women often worry about becoming addicted to medication or that the antidepressant medication could have a negative effect on their fetus or infant (Kendall-Tackett 2017). Studies have shown that many women cease antidepressant medication upon becoming pregnant due to concerns about fetal wellbeing (Galbally et al. 2014).
- Clinicians need to discuss with women the risk of ceasing antidepressant medication abruptly and that, if a medication is ceased, this needs to be done gradually with advice from a mental health professional (Austin et al. 2017). Einarson found that 70% of women who abruptly ceased their antidepressant medication experienced adverse effects and that 30% became suicidal (cited in Boyce et al. 2014).
- For many women with moderate to severe anxiety or depressive disorders, the first-line treatment is likely to be pharmacological, with psychological treatments introduced once medications have become effective (Austin et al. 2017). They suggest using a selective serotonin reuptake inhibitor (SSRI) as first-line treatment for moderate to severe depression and/or anxiety in pregnant women. The risk of transmitting SSRIs and tricyclic antidepressants through breastmilk is very low; the rate of transmission of larger molecule medication through the alveolar cells (milk ducts) reduces after the first three days postpartum when the milk matures (Hale 2019).
- In most instances, the most important determinant of drug penetration into milk is the mother's plasma level. This means that being aware of peak plasma levels (when the amount of medication in the plasma is at its highest) can help to reduce the infant ingesting the small amounts of medication found in breastmilk (Kendall-Tackett 2017).

ATTITUDES

- Sometimes nurses struggle to understand a woman's choice to have a baby when she has a mental illness.
- Nurses need to consider our attitudes towards the decisions clients make and any stereotypes or biases we may hold about this. Using clinical supervision to discuss these issues is important.
- Many women, including those with a history of mental illness, do not want to take medication while pregnant or breastfeeding. It is important to provide the woman with as much information as she needs to make an informed decision and, unless she or her infant is at great risk (in which case she may be treated under a mental health Act), decisions about medication are the woman's choice.

SKILLS

- **The therapeutic relationship** is the most important aspect of any treatment success.
- **Use the Mental State Examination (MSE)** to inform your practice (see Chapter 7). This can be a helpful way to formulate your care planning and facilitate communication between health professionals using shared language.
- **Safety for all.** In the postnatal period we need to consider the woman in context, understanding that the baby is both a protective factor and a risk factor, as well as understanding how mental health symptoms may affect a woman's impulsivity. Asking directly, with an empathic tone, is essential. For example: 'Are you worried that you are feeling so bad that you might hurt the baby?'
- **A family approach** is essential to all aspects of care for women in the perinatal period. Including fathers/ partners and extended family in the care planning process is vital to ensure the best outcomes for the woman and her family.
- **Psychoeducation** is a valuable tool, particularly concerning issues such as medication use during pregnancy and breastfeeding. This includes not suddenly ceasing medication during pregnancy due to the potential relapse of previous symptoms, or withdrawal symptoms.
- **Interprofessional collaboration** is crucial. During the perinatal period women see more health professionals than at any other time in their life. Taking a collaborative approach means that all professionals involved in the woman's care are working together to ensure the best possible outcomes (Psaila & Schmied 2017).
- **Accessing ongoing support.** Nurses can be pivotal in helping women and their families to access suitable treatment and ongoing support. One of the most helpful things you can do is to support mothers to get

help from longer term support systems. With modern technology this can mean accessing mothers' support groups online. Breastfeeding support, sleep and settling support as well as many other resources are often available 24 hours a day, as well as providing information for fathers.

SCENARIO 25.2

Helen

Helen was a 33-year-old woman referred to a perinatal infant mental health service by her general practitioner for preconception planning. Helen had been diagnosed with bipolar disorder following the birth of her first child (a son) three years previously. He had arrived at 30 weeks' gestation via emergency caesarean delivery and required admission to the neonatal intensive care unit (NICU) for some weeks. Helen felt traumatised by the event and became manic while she was expressing milk constantly to feed him. Her level of exhaustion as well as changing hormone levels contributed to the deterioration of Helen's mental state. When the baby was discharged from the NICU, Helen required a mental health hospital admission. After a trial of several different medications Helen's mood was stabilised on lithium carbonate (a mood stabiliser) and olanzapine (an antipsychotic). She kept taking the medications after discharge and has remained well. Helen is anxious about having another child, but she and her husband, Joe, always planned to have two children...

RED FLAGS

Given Helen's history, nurses during the perinatal period should aware of:

- medication management during pregnancy and breastfeeding
- Helen's previous traumatic delivery of a baby
- how to manage women diagnosed with bipolar disorder during pregnancy
- care planning including the partner and extended family to improve outcomes for the mother
- interprofessional collaboration.

KNOWLEDGE

Preconception planning for women diagnosed with mental illness

- Preconception planning should begin as soon as a woman of childbearing age is diagnosed with a mental illness (Austin et al. 2017).
- Pregnancy can be a complex process for any woman, with changes in hormonal levels, increased inflammation processes and fluctuations in biorhythms, all of which can cause relapse (Snellen & Malhi 2014).
- Preconception planning is particularly important for women diagnosed with schizophrenia, bipolar disorder and depression, as relapse is common (particularly when medication is ceased) and associated with a range of adverse outcomes (Betcher et al. 2019). For example, untreated bipolar disorder has been linked with pregnancy complications such as preterm birth, low birthweight and Apgar scores, induced labour and caesarean section delivery (Snellen & Malhi 2014).
- The management of pregnant women with mental illness can be complex for both obstetric and mental health services, suggesting that specific considerations be attended to and monitoring systems followed during the perinatal period (Snellen & Malhi 2014).
- There are important aspects to consider in preconception planning such as the woman's health literacy, family/partner support, the woman's living/social conditions and the complex issues related to medication use during pregnancy and breastfeeding (Austin et al. 2017).

Medication management during pregnancy and breastfeeding

- Each woman's treatment history should be considered individually (Snellen & Malhi 2014).
- When women are on medication during pregnancy it is essential that there is interprofessional collaboration (Psaila & Schmied 2017).
- Regarding antipsychotic medication during pregnancy, it is recommended that 'women who need to take an antipsychotic during pregnancy continue the antipsychotic that has been most effective for symptom remission' (Betcher et al. 2019, p. 17). Olanzapine, for example, is a second-generation antipsychotic medication that has not been associated with adverse pregnancy or infant outcomes (Betcher et al. 2019). However, given the increased risk of metabolic disorders associated with second-generation antipsychotics (Hirsch et al. 2017), this will need to be monitored closely during pregnancy. Monitoring the mother's blood sugar levels is a routine aspect of antenatal care.
- The risk of relapse following delivery, especially if medication has been ceased during pregnancy, is high (Snellen & Malhi 2014).
- In recent studies the relapse of bipolar disorder was twice as likely for women who have ceased mood stabilisation medication during the perinatal period (Austin et al. 2017). Women with schizophrenia who stop taking antipsychotic medication experience a 53% increased risk of relapse compared with a 16% relapse rate for women who continue medication (Betcher et al. 2019).

Anticonvulsant/mood stabilising medication

- There is a strong correlation of teratogenicity with the use of anticonvulsant medication such as sodium valproate during pregnancy; however, evidence shows the use of lithium during pregnancy is much lower risk (but not without risk) (Snellen & Malhi 2014).
- Austin et al. (2017) highlight the importance of monitoring lithium levels during pregnancy because lithium requirements change throughout the pregnancy. Lithium levels should be monitored monthly until 36 weeks' gestation, then weekly until birth (Snellen & Malhi 2014).
- Thyroid and renal function should be monitored during each trimester, and high-resolution ultrasound and Doppler flow studies for early cardiac assessment should be attended at 16 weeks' gestation due to possible malformation caused by lithium use in pregnancy (Snellen & Malhi 2014).
- A morphology scan at 20 weeks' gestation, with particular attention to a fetal echocardiogram, should be performed (Snellen & Malhi 2014).
- If lithium is prescribed during pregnancy it is recommended that the dose be reduced just prior to delivery, then reintroduced at the pre-pregnancy dose after delivery, providing the woman is not breastfeeding (Austin et al. 2017).
- It is recommended that lithium not be used while breastfeeding due to the transmission through breastmilk causing infant toxicity (Austin et al. 2017).

Ethical considerations and medication during pregnancy

There are many ethical considerations when weighing the risks and benefits of taking medication during pregnancy including:

- potential risk to the developing fetus exposed to medication in utero
- increased risk of the mother's mental state deterioration without medication, which can also cause risk to the fetus.

Referral to a specialist service such as 'Mother Safe' can provide the opportunity for a woman to weigh up the risks and benefits of continuing medication during pregnancy.

SCENARIO 25.2 continued

Helen

As part of her preconception planning, Helen chose to be under the care of a obstetrician who specialised in in-utero scan technology. This was important for Helen to ensure there was no fetal abnormalities due to taking lithium. Helen's psychiatrist referred her to 'Mother Safe' for consultation, providing a comprehensive history so the consultant was fully informed. It was unclear from Helen's previous history if she had developed bipolar disorder *during* the pregnancy, which may have contributed to the early and traumatic arrival of her son. Helen did experience psychotic phenomenon during the manic episode and had a re-emergence of psychotic symptoms each time olanzapine was ceased. As part of her preconception plan, Helen decided she would continue with lithium and olanzapine during her second pregnancy because she feared a relapse. And because breastfeeding her first baby had been a traumatic experience for Helen, she decided not to breastfeed with her second baby. Therefore, continuing lithium after delivery did not pose a concern.

KNOWLEDGE

Traumatic and preterm births

- Traumatic birthing experiences can have lasting effects on not just the woman but her partner as well (Thomson et al. 2017). This can lead to post-traumatic stress disorder.
- In recent research Thomson et al. (2017) highlighted the importance of having support systems in place and good care planning to reduce the risk of further birthing trauma for women.

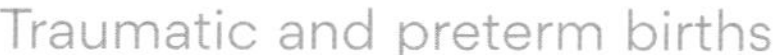

SCENARIO 25.2 continued

Helen

Helen's first delivery was certainly traumatic – she felt she had no control over the situation and did not feel she had enough explained to her about the delivery or risks. She also felt her husband was not included in the decision-making process. This increased her anxiety around the birth of her second baby. In consultation with her obstetrician a planned caesarean was arranged. Helen felt she was listened to by her health professionals and, because they were working as a team around her (all the clinicians involved in her care worked in different settings but communicated regularly through teleconferencing and written communication), Helen experienced the arrival of her second baby very differently.

A premature birth is one that occurs before 37 weeks' gestation. There are many aspects of infant care in a NICU that can be distressing for parents (Feeley 2017). Preterm infants can require hospitalisation for weeks or months, which can lead to mothers experiencing significant separation anxiety from their baby. Helen certainly experienced this with her son; her attempt to stay connected to him was by producing breastmilk for him. Expressing and breastfeeding can be difficult for some women, even under the best of circumstances.

Helen became obsessed with attempting to produce enough milk and so was awake most of the night trying to express, which contributed to the deterioration in her mental state. When Helen and her son were admitted to a mental health unit, she stopped trying to breastfeed so she could start taking lithium. Helen felt relieved but guilty for not breastfeeding her son.

Helen had private health insurance so was able to be admitted to a specialist mother–baby unit. In many states in Australia there are no specialist mother–baby units in the public sector, which causes further trauma for mothers requiring a mental health admission postnatally.

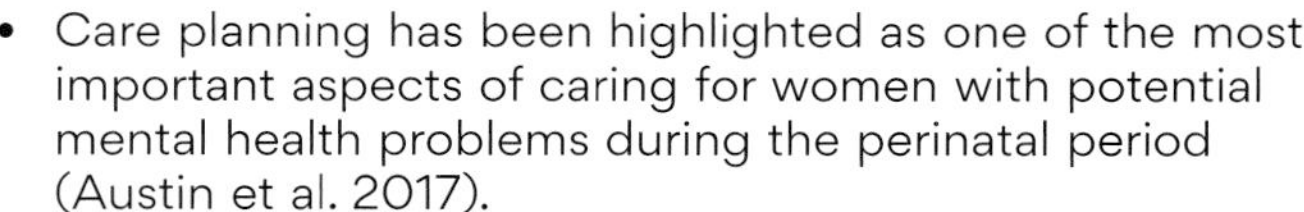

CARE PLANNING FOR DELIVERY AND POSTNATAL CARE

- Care planning has been highlighted as one of the most important aspects of caring for women with potential mental health problems during the perinatal period (Austin et al. 2017).
- All clinicians involved in a woman's care should be involved in the care planning process. This includes her general practitioner, a general practice nurse, an obstetrician, midwives (in the antenatal clinic, delivery suit and in the postnatal ward or visiting service), child and family nurses and other practitioners. In some cases, this may involve the hospital's consultation liaison psychiatry team, including a consultation liaison mental health nurse or an acute mental health team and a perinatal and infant mental health nurse if one is available.
- Care planning also provides the woman with an opportunity to discuss any worries about the upcoming delivery or parenting. Given Helen's experiences with a preterm delivery and trauma surrounding the delivery, having a space to process this can be very helpful.
- Including the woman's partner and extended family in the care planning process is essential for positive outcomes.
- It is important that all information about a woman's health care is communicated in writing to all the health professionals involved. Regular letters to her general practitioner, psychiatrist and obstetrician are necessary to keep everyone informed of her progress and any concerns.

ATTITUDES

- The role of nurses and midwives is to provide the best possible care to women by ensuring they are as informed as possible about their choices and treatment options in relation to their mental health during the perinatal period.
- All nurses and midwives need to reflect on whether they hold judgemental attitudes and biases about woman who experience mental illness (e.g. bipolar disorder or schizophrenia) choosing to have a baby. Clinical supervision is the appropriate place to consider this.

NURSING ACTIONS AND INTERVENTIONS

- Work with the woman, her partner and other members of the multidisciplinary team to avoid a hospital admission, but plan for that outcome should it be required.
- Monitor the woman's mental state by using the MSE and tools such as the EPDS and provide an update to all members of the treating team.
- Providing the team with a written care plan for delivery and immediate aftercare is a high priority. This would include a brief history of the mother's mental health experiences and medication regimen.
- Ensure the mother can recommence her medication at the pre-pregnancy dose as soon as possible after the delivery.
- Alert midwives and nursing staff in the maternity unit of the need to monitor the baby for any withdrawal from medication side effects. Including information about the mother's choice not to breastfeed is essential so she does not feel any pressure to do this, particularly when taking medication such as lithium.
- Helping women to develop anxiety management skills and ensuring adequate rest is also very important to reduce the risk of relapse. Asking someone other than the mother to take care of the baby overnight for the first few weeks can ensure she gets enough sleep, which reduces the risk of relapse.
- Including a woman's partner or the baby's father is also vital to ensure the woman has adequate post-delivery support. In Helen's case, helping Joe to understand how he could best support Helen after the delivery, as well as the early warning signs of deterioration in her mental state, would reduce the chance of relapse and

increase the likelihood of more rapid intervention if it did occur.

- Requesting a psychiatric review in the first few days after delivery can be beneficial. Many hospitals have consultation liaison psychiatry services that provide this.
- Monitor the mother closely for the first few months postnatally, with weekly reviews to ensure she receives timely treatment if her mental state does deteriorate.

TREATMENT MODALITIES

Treatment would include a range of therapeutic interventions such as cognitive behaviour therapy, interpersonal therapy, dialectical behaviour therapy, parent–infant psychotherapy, couples therapy and parenting training programs as described previously. The most important aspect of care is monitoring the mother's mental state and ensuring her safety with her baby and children.

In this situation Helen did not require another mental health hospital admission due to careful preconception planning, care planning and medication management.

Chapter summary

This chapter has considered the importance of early intervention and treatment in the perinatal period. Care planning that includes the woman and her partner/the father, the baby, other children and extended family is essential to positive outcomes.

Medication management and good care planning including interprofessional collaboration is necessary to improve the outcomes for women and their families.

Slade (2008) suggested that for parents to hold their children in mind, that we as health professionals need to hold the parents in mind. This can be for quite a long time.

Useful websites

Beyond Blue: https://healthyfamilies.beyondblue.org.au/
Centre of Perinatal Excellence (COPE): https://www.cope.org.au/
Dadvice (this is a website with valuable information for fathers): https://healthyfamilies.beyondblue.org.au/pregnancy-and-new-parents/dadvice-for-new-dads
Gidget Foundation: https://gidgetfoundation.org.au/
Good Beginnings: https://www.savethechildren.org.au/
Karitane: https://karitane.com.au/
Mothersafe: https://www.seslhd.health.nsw.gov.au/royal-hospital-for-women/services-clinics/directory/mothersafe
Moodgym: https://www.moodgym.com.au/
Mental Health in Multicultural Australia: http://www.mhima.org.au/
Post and Antenatal Depression Association (PANDA): https://www.panda.org.au/
Parent-Infant Research Institute (PIRI): http://www.piri.org.au/
Tresillian: https://www.tresillian.org.au/

References

Austin, M.P., Highet, N., the Expert Working Group, 2017. Mental Health Care in the Perinatal Period: Australian Clinical Practice Guideline. Centre of Perinatal Excellence, Melbourne.

Baradon, T., Joyce, A., 2016. The theory of psychoanalytic parent-infant psychotherapy. In: Baradon, T., Biseo, M., Broughton, C., et al. (Eds.), The Practice of Psychoanalytic Parent-Infant Psychotherapy: Claiming the Baby. Routledge, London.

Betcher, H.K., Montiel, C., Clark, C.T., 2019. Use of antipsychotic drugs during pregnancy. Curr. Treat. Opin. Psychiatry 6 (1), 17–31.

Bowlby, J., 1979. The Making and Breaking of Affectional Bonds. Routledge, London.

Boyce, P., Galbally, M., Snellen, M., et al., 2014. Pharmacological management of major depression in pregnancy. In: Galbally, M., Snellen, M., Lewis, A. (Eds.), Psychopharmacology and Pregnancy Treatment Efficacy, Risks, and Guidelines. Springer, Heidelberg.

Cox, J.L., Holden, J.M., Sagovsky, R., 1987. Detection of postnatal depression. Development of a 10 item Edinburgh Postnatal Depression Scale. Br. J. Psychiatry 150, 782–786.

Fallon, A.E., Brabender, V.M., 2012. A secure connection, the tethering of attachment and good-enough maternal care. In: Akhtar, S. (Ed.), The Mother and Her Child, Clinical Aspects of Attachment, Separation, and Loss. The Rowman & Littlefield Publishing Group, Inc, Maryland.

Feeley, N., 2017. Giving birth earlier than expected: mothers whose new-born requires neonatal intensive care. In: Thomas, G., Schmied, V. (Eds.), Psychosocial Resilience and Risk in the Perinatal Period: Implications and Guidance for Professionals. Routledge, London.

Fischer, N., 2012. Mother-infant attachment: the demystification of an enigma. In: Akhtar, S. (Ed.), The Mother and Her Child, Clinical Aspects of Attachment, Separation and Loss. The Rowman & Littlefield Publishing Group, Inc., Maryland.

Galbally, M., Lewis, A.J., Snellen, M., 2014. Introduction: pharmacological treatments of mental disorders in pregnancy. In: Galbally, M., Snellen, M., Lewis, A. (Eds.), Psychopharmacology and Pregnancy Treatment Efficacy, Risks, and Guidelines. Springer, Heidelberg.

Hale, T.W., 2019. Hale's Medications and Mothers' Milk 2019. Springer, New York.

Hartz, D., McGrath, L., 2017. Working with Indigenous families. In: Thomas, G., Schmied, V. (Eds.), Psychosocial Resilience and Risk in the Perinatal Period: Implications and Guidance for Professionals. Routledge, London.

Hirsch, L., Yang, J., Bresee, L., et al., 2017. Second-generation antipsychotics and metabolic side effects: a systematic review of population-based studies. Drug Saf. 40 (9), 771–781.

Hungerford, C., Hodgson, D., Bostwick, R., et al., 2017. Mental Health Care: An Introduction for Health Professionals in Australia, third ed. Wiley, Brisbane.

Jomeen, J., Fleming, S.E., Martin, C.R., 2017. Women with a diagnosed mental health problem. In: Thomas, G., Schmied, V. (Eds.), Psychosocial Resilience and Risk in the Perinatal Period: Implications and Guidance for Professionals. Routledge, London.

Kendall-Tackett, K.A., 2017. Depression in New Mothers; Causes, Consequences and Treatment Alternatives. Routledge, London.

Powel, B., Cooper, G., Hoffman, K., et al., 2016. The Circle of Security Intervention: Enhancing Attachment in Early Parent-Child Relationships. The Guilford Press, New York.

Psaila, K., Schmied, V., 2017. Interprofessional collaboration: a crucial component of support for women and families in the perinatal period. In: Thomas, G., Schmied, V. (Eds.), Psychosocial Resilience and Risk in the Perinatal Period: Implications and Guidance for Professionals. Routledge, London.

Sanders, M.R., Mazzucchelli, T.G., 2018. The Power of Positive Parenting: Transforming the Lives of Childern, Parents and Communities Using the Triple P System. Oxford University Press, New York.

Scioli, A., Biller, H.B., 2009. Hope in the Age of Anxiety. Oxford University Press, New York.

Shea, A.K., Nguyen, T.A.T., Brain, U., et al., 2014. Maternal and fetal factors that influence prenatal exposure to selective serotonin reuptake inhibitor antidepressants. In: Galbally, M., Snellen, M., Lewis, A. (Eds.), Psychopharmacology and Pregnancy Treatment Efficacy, Risks, and Guidelines. Springer, Heidelberg.

Slade, A., 2008. Working with parents in child psychotherapy: engaging the reflective function. In: Busch, F.N. (Ed.), Mentalization Theoretical Considerations, Research Findings, and Clinical Implications. The Analytic Press, Taylor & Francis Group, New York.

Smith-Nielsen, J., Matthey, S., Lange, T., et al., 2018. Validation of the Edinburgh Postnatal Depression Scale against both DSM-5 and ICD-10 diagnostic criteria for depression. BMC Psychiatry 18, 393.

Snellen, M., Malhi, G.S., 2014. Bipolar disorder, psychopharmacology, and pregnancy. In: Galbally, M., Snellen, M., Lewis, A. (Eds.), Psychopharmacology and Pregnancy, Treatment Efficacy, Risks, and Guidelines. Springer, Heidelberg.

Stephens, S., Ford, E., Paudyal, P., et al., 2016. Effectiveness of psychological interventions for postnatal depression in primary care: a meta analysis. Ann. Fam. Med. 14 (5), 463–472.

Thomson, G., Beck, C., Ayers, S., 2017. The ripple effects of a traumatic birth, risk, impact and implications for practice. In: Thomas, G., Schmied, V. (Eds.), Psychosocial Resilience and Risk in the Perinatal Period: Implications and Guidance for Professionals. Routledge, London.

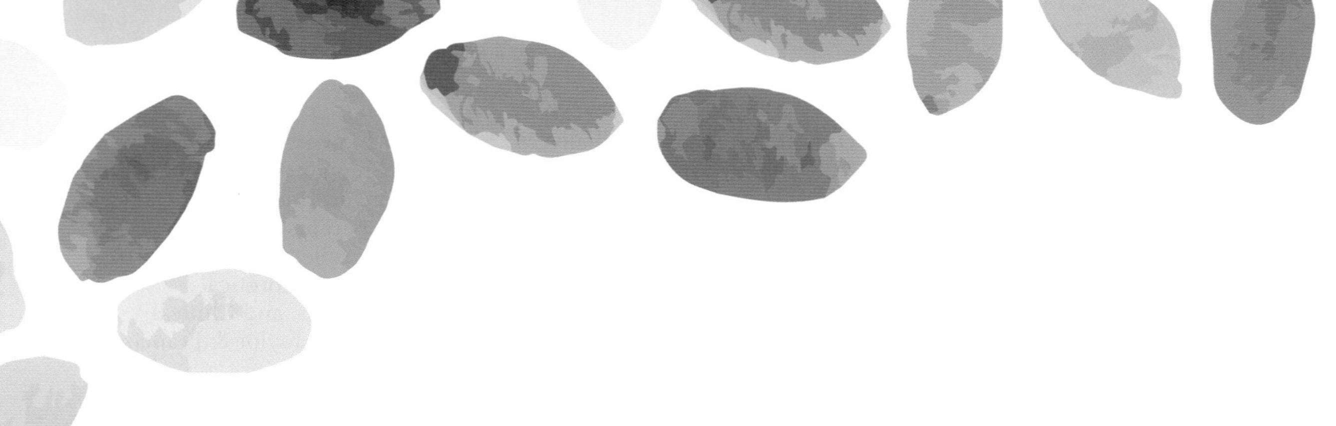

CHAPTER 26

Forensic mental health nursing

Tessa Maguire and Brian McKenna

KEY POINTS

- Mental health nurses have begun to identify the knowledge, skills and attitudes that are required to work with forensic mental health consumers.
- Forensic mental health consumers are a heterogeneous group of people who will often have a range of needs that will need to be addressed including offence-related issues.
- Risk assessment, treatment and management processes continue to develop and to be used by nurses to meet the needs of consumers and to ensure safety for the community.
- Forensic mental health nurses remain focused on recovery-oriented care in partnership with consumers and carers.

KEY TERMS

- Comorbidity
- Criminality and mental ill health
- Housing and homelessness
- Law and jail
- Recovery-oriented care
- Risk assessment
- Self-awareness
- Social justice

LEARNING OUTCOMES

The material in this chapter will assist you to:

- demonstrate awareness of the lived experience and needs of forensic mental health consumers
- identify specific nursing interventions for forensic mental health consumers
- discuss the skills, knowledge and attitudes that are central to forensic mental health nursing
- utilise the structured clinical judgement approach to risk assessment, treatment and management.

Lived experience comment by Jarrad Hickmott

It can be very easy to label someone as 'aggressive' without considering context. The authors of this chapter have carefully discussed aggression and violence, acknowledging that the consumer may be experiencing stressful factors that they find distressing, and which result in such behaviour. Stigma, especially the twin contributors of criminality and mental ill health, has flow-on effects and can impact on a person's identity and self-esteem.

Introduction

For many reasons, people experiencing mental illness are over-represented in the criminal justice system. Forensic mental health services have developed in Australia and New Zealand to provide containment, assessment, treatment and management of forensic mental health consumers. These services have grown from the recognition that neither the criminal justice system nor the mental health system can adequately provide services for forensic mental health consumers, and that the two systems must work in partnership to meet the needs of consumers and, at times, the need for community safety.

The criminal justice system includes the police who arrest people alleged to have committed a crime and the courts that are responsible for making determinations of guilt or innocence and for imposing penalties if the person is found guilty. Imprisonment and community-based sentencing options are possible penalties. When the person is thought to be experiencing mental illness, there are options for diversion from police custody, court or prison to mental health services for assessment and treatment. However, most mainstream mental health services do not have the structural security or available treatment and rehabilitation options to contain, assess, treat and manage certain forensic mental health consumers, and therefore forensic mental health services have been developed.

Forensic mental health services are generally independent of the criminal justice system and are managed within the health sector. Components of forensic mental health services include services within police custody centres, prisons and courts. Secure hospitals and community services are also essential components. Forensic mental health services, which have been traditionally custodial and involved in compulsory treatment and care, are being challenged to transform to recovery-oriented services.

As such, the call is to focus on the lived experience of the individual consumer, with the aim that the person leads a satisfying life irrespective of the difficulties imposed by mental health needs and secure services (Simpson & Penney 2011). Integrating a person-centred approach within a custodial environment remains a problematic but essential practice priority for contemporary forensic mental health nurses.

Australia and New Zealand do not particularly recognise specialties of nursing, but the term 'forensic mental health nurse' is used in this chapter to identify mental health nurses who specialise their practice in criminal justice or forensic mental health settings. Similar to other health fields, there are more nurses than other specialists in these settings. Nurses working in these settings must possess the knowledge, skills and attitudes that are required to provide comprehensive care for complex forensic mental health consumers.

Although this chapter focuses on nursing in criminal justice and forensic mental health settings, there is no doubt that nurses in mainstream services will, at some time, work in partnership with consumers to address their physical health, mental health or forensic mental health needs.

SCENARIO 26.1

John

John is 25 years old and has been admitted from prison onto an acute forensic mental health unit. He is on remand in prison, accused of stabbing his flatmate. On the day of the stabbing John had been up all-night drinking alcohol and ruminating about his flatmate stealing his belongings. John had become convinced his flatmate had been conspiring with another acquaintance in the thefts. When confronting his flatmate, John became enraged and attacked him with a kitchen knife. Prior to admission John had been in a management unit in prison (where prisoners are locked in a cell by themselves) due to repeated threats to kill prison officers. He had refused to speak with the mental health staff, saying he did not have a mental illness.

When John arrived at the hospital he was handcuffed and appeared anxious, hypervigilant, malnourished and would not make eye contact. During the initial assessment John said that he knew why he had been transferred but he didn't agree he had a mental illness. He said he came from a large Greek family that he has had no contact with since he was arrested. He attributed the lack of contact with his family to them not knowing how to get in touch with him. On initial assessment John reported a history of offending, often involving altercations with others. John reported drinking and alcohol use from a young age and 'getting around with the wrong crowd'. Several years ago, he was in a car accident and received a head injury and has been unable to work since. Although John has had contact with community mental health services in the past, he reported that they hadn't helped because he didn't have a mental illness. This is John's first admission to a mental health service, and he reports that he is worried about the other patients on the unit.

RED FLAGS

- Length of stay will determine what care mental health nurses are able to provide. If his stay is short term, the priority will be to stabilise John's mental state and provide him with skills to manage in the prison environment. If John's admission is longer, once his mental state has stabilised there may be the potential to address offence-related needs.
- The possibility of family contact will need to be explored.
- Building rapport with John will be necessary to assess his holistic health and to work in partnership with him. It is possible John will be facing a lengthy prison sentence and will therefore be involved with forensic mental health services in a secure hospital or in prison.

KNOWLEDGE

- Forensic mental health consumers have complex needs that forensic mental health nurses must thoroughly assess in order to provide holistic care, in partnership with consumers and their carers.
- Apart from the clinical need for treatment, many consumers have recovery needs related to social, cultural and adaptive malfunctioning and patterns of offending that can present as a risk to themselves or others.
- On admission, it is important to conduct a comprehensive assessment that includes biopsychosocial factors (e.g. mental state, family history, cultural/spiritual/religious needs, physical health, education employment) but also includes a detailed assessment of risk to self and others.
- It is also important to consider the impact of incarceration and how this may affect a person's mental, emotional and physical status (e.g. trauma associated with incarceration, inability to exercise, isolation from supports such as family and stress related to pending court issues).

The legal status of forensic consumers

- Forensic mental health consumers are subject to criminal justice legislation and policies that vary greatly between Australian states and territories and between countries, but the groups of forensic mental health consumers described in are commonly found.
- Defendants appearing in court must be fit to plead. If mental illness prevents a person from meeting certain criteria (including having an understanding of the nature of the charge and the trial, being able to enter a plea and being able to give instructions to the legal practitioner), then that person is likely to be ordered to receive treatment until they are fit to return to court. A small number of consumers are never fit, and other processes are put in place to ensure their treatment and supervision.
- Consumers are found not guilty by reason of mental impairment by the court when it has been proved that the person was so unwell at the time of the offence that they did not understand the nature and quality of the act (the offence), or did not know that the act was wrong. Consumers who are found not guilty due to mental impairment are required to undertake treatment; the duration and location of the treatment will depend on the severity of the offence and the risk status of the consumer.
- A prisoner experiencing mental illness may require a transfer to a secure hospital for treatment, if an adequate level of treatment and care cannot be provided at the prison or if the prisoner is unwilling to accept treatment. The policy in Australia and New Zealand is that prisoners cannot be treated involuntarily in prison because the potential for abuse of mental health treatment is possible in a coercive environment. Some offenders in prison who are experiencing mental illness can adhere to treatment and need an equivalent level of treatment and care to that available in the community, such as outpatient appointments with a nurse. This service may be provided by prison mental health in-reach teams. Some prisons have mental health units for assessing and treating prisoners. Some high-risk prisoners will be referred to either a forensic mental health hospital or a community team for as sessment and treatment following release from prison.
- Wherever forensic mental health nurses practice, it is their responsibility to understand the legislation that affects consumers. Forensic mental health consumers and their carers are sometimes confused by the legal processes and requirements. The nurse's knowledge of the law needs to be used proactively to assist forensic mental health consumers and their carers to understand

Box 26.1 Groups of forensic mental health consumers

- Offenders or alleged offenders referred by police, courts, legal practitioners or independent statutory bodies for psychiatric assessment and/or treatment
- Alleged offenders detained, or on conditional release, as being unfit to plead or not guilty by reason of mental impairment
- Offenders or alleged offenders with mental illness ordered by courts or independent statutory bodies to be detained as an inpatient in a secure forensic facility
- Prisoners with mental illness requiring secure inpatient hospital treatment
- Selected high-risk offenders with a mental illness referred by releasing authorities
- Prisoners with mental illness requiring specialist mental health assessment and/or treatment in prison
- People with mental illness in mainstream mental health services who are a significant danger to their carers or the community, and who require the involvement of a specialist forensic mental health service

Source: *Australian Health Ministers' Advisory Council 2006, pp. 3–4*

the function and impact of criminal justice legislation and policies, and to optimise care in the context of integrating security, safety and therapeutic intent. The nurse must also provide information to consumers and carers to ensure they are aware of their rights.

Demographic characteristics

- The forensic mental health population tends to be young, male, never married, of low socioeconomic status, unemployed, with poor educational achievement and in itinerant living situations prior to conviction. However, the number of imprisoned women is increasing and therefore the female forensic consumer population is growing in both Australia and New Zealand (Australian Bureau of Statistics 2018; Foulds & Monastario 2018).
- There is an over-representation of Indigenous peoples and post-colonisation immigrant populations in forensic mental health services.
    - Colonisation usurped the self-determination of Indigenous peoples and, similarly, immigrant populations are required to adapt to the social reality of the dominant culture. Such social adjustments place considerable pressure on disadvantaged groups.
    - These pressures are reflected in several adverse social indicators such as poor educational achievement, high unemployment rates, high crime rates and poor health statistics.
    - In New Zealand, Māori and Pacific Islander ethnicities are over-represented in New Zealand prisons. Although Māori comprise 16% of the general population and Pacific Islanders 6%, they make up 51% and 12% of the prison population respectively (Foulds & Monastario 2018).
    - In Australia Aboriginal and Torres Strait Islander peoples are over-represented in prison settings. In 2018 there were 11,849 prisoners who identified as Aboriginal or Torres Strat Islander, and there has been a 5% increase since 30 June 2017 (Australian Bureau of Statistics 2018).

Cognitive and social skills

- When a person's ability to think clearly and relate constructively to others is compromised by mental illness, the likelihood of antisocial behaviour including violence and offending is enhanced (Douglas et al. 2009).
- The reasons for compromised cognitive and social ability are complex and may not relate directly to mental illness. They may relate to diminished learning opportunities in the context of the family and environment; harsh or inconsistent parenting; delinquent peer associations; or acquired brain injury.
- A significant proportion of forensic mental health consumers have a history of traumatic childhood experiences (Egeressy et al. 2009) and acquired brain injury (Jackson & Hardy 2011). Therefore, the development of cognitive and social skills is a recovery requirement of forensic mental health services.
- Limitations in cognitive and social skills can militate against a socially positive response to life's challenges (Bennett et al. 2005).

Mental illness and risk to others

- Most people who experience mental illness are not violent and are not a risk to others. They are more likely to be the victim of a crime than the perpetrator of it.
- The relationship between mental illness and criminal behaviour is complex and varies between individuals.
- Nurses need to identify the unique relationship for each consumer so they can ascertain the risk and protective factors that need to be addressed in treatment and risk management strategies.
- Most offenders who progress from assessment to remain on the caseload of forensic mental health nurses experience serious mental illness (a psychotic illness or major depression).
- A seminal 20-year study undertaken by Wallace, Mullen and Burgess (2004) found that the overall frequency of violent offences was significantly higher among people experiencing schizophrenia than among the comparison community subjects (8.2% versus 1.8%). The rate of violent offending among people experiencing schizophrenia gradually increased over the years of the study, but there was no difference in the rate of increase when compared with the comparison subjects over the same period. Most people experiencing schizophrenia are not violent and do not commit criminal offences, and the risk might lie in specific symptoms such as paranoia.
- International studies have found modest increases in criminal and violent behaviour with serious mental illness but also note that there is no evidence that mental illness causes criminal behaviour; rather, several factors mediate mental illness and offending. These factors include antisocial tendencies of peers and alcohol or drug abuse (Hodgins 2008).

Substance use

- Substance abuse is common in forensic mental health and the community generally.
- Researchers consider that the major driver of crime and violence in people (with and without a mental illness) is substance misuse (Fazel & Baillargeon 2011). There is a high prevalence of prisoners who have a mental illness and who also abuse substances (Fazel & Baillargeon 2011).
- Forensic consumers have high rates of substance abuse (Miles et al. 2007; Young 2006) and these coexisting conditions have a link to offending and risk of violence

(Hodgins 2008). There is substantial evidence for substance misuse being a significant risk factor for violence and aggression for consumers who have a major mental disorder, particularly schizophrenia (Fazel et al. 2009).

- While the link between substance abuse and aggression/offending is widely recognised, the mechanisms are poorly understood, resulting from a complex process involving the interaction of the substances' active agents, the substance misuse, the context of the substance misuse and personal factors such as a predisposition to aggression.
- See Chapter 11 for more information about substance use and abuse, and their association with coexisting mental disorders.

Attitudes

At some point, most nurses will provide care and treatment for consumers with an offending history or who are at risk of offending. When a consumer has committed an offence and is experiencing mental illness, the nurse is expected to apply the core knowledge, skills and attitudes of nursing generally, mental health nursing specifically and the additional or enhanced skills that are required to work effectively with forensic mental health consumers.

For some nurses, the ability to provide care can potentially be compromised by the complex presentation of some forensic mental health consumers.

- Antisocial personality attributes that are not pleasant to relate to may present as a contributing factor that clouds the nurse's ability to place moral judgement to one side – for example, when the nurse becomes the target of hostile or threatening behaviour.
- Forensic mental health nursing research has articulated the difficulties that nurses face in confronting moral judgements concerning such behaviour. Poor judgements regarding this behaviour compromise the delivery of nursing care. For instance, framing a consumer as primarily 'bad' can result in a total absence of planned care in the form of care plans for this consumer (Mason et al. 2002).
- It is essential that nurses in general and forensic mental health nurses in particular recognise and manage their personal feelings and values related to the offences committed by forensic mental health consumers.
    - Nurses who focus on the offences and allow their feelings and values to dominate their clinical perspective of consumers will be ineffective in providing care. Often, professional dissonance is experienced.
    - Equally inappropriate is the belief that the offending behaviour is not a concern of the nurse. In such cases, nurses may choose to ignore offending behaviour because they find the personal and moral effects distressing. But by ignoring the offending behaviour, a significant forensic mental health consumer need is not addressed. It is offending and other antisocial behaviours that distinguish consumers within the forensic mental health setting.
- The professional response is to view offending behaviour as another need to be addressed during therapeutic engagement with the forensic mental health consumer. Consumers need to understand the factors associated with their offending behaviour in order to increase their personal choice and responsibility.

Mental health nursing actions and interventions

- Forensic mental health consumers generally have a mental illness, a history of offending and personality attributes and ways of acting and reacting that heighten their potential for risk of harm to self and others.
- Nurses working in forensic mental health hospitals are likely to be caring for consumers who consistently present with seriously challenging behaviours, including aggression and violence (Daffern et al. 2015).
- Aggression may be an inevitable outcome of providing treatment to involuntary forensic mental health consumers, some of whom will have limited skills to manage anger that is provoked by the ongoing demands, expectations and conflict of inpatient treatment (Martin & Daffern 2006).
- Nurses working within these facilities undertake assessment, assist with treatment and facilitate recovery.
- Forensic mental health nurses are obliged to consider the least restrictive alternatives in risk management and to reduce the use of restrictive interventions such as seclusion.

Although there are barriers that work against nurses in forensic hospitals being able to safely manage forensic mental health consumers, there are also opportunities such as:

- longer admissions, resulting in reduced access to illicit substances and increased access to treatment (Maguire et al. 2012)
- a higher staff–consumer ratio, providing the opportunity for nurses to work with consumers to undertake assessment, treatment and other environmental interventions (Timmons 2010)
- access to best-practice risk assessment and management approaches.

Risk assessment

Prevention and management of offending, especially violence, have become the focus of contemporary risk assessment in forensic mental health.

- Rigorous risk assessment processes are undertaken to identify factors that indicate risk to self or others and the protective factors that mitigate such risk.

- **Static risk factors** cannot be changed by clinical intervention (e.g. gender and age).
- **Dynamic risk factors** (e.g. substance use and social support from friends) are factors that are more open to clinical modification and can be altered through risk management.
- An emphasis on identifying **protective factors** diminishes the potential for adverse events (Allnutt et al. 2013).

- Planning of appropriate interventions is assisted through structured clinical judgement, which includes using validated risk assessment instruments. See Box 26.2 for more details.

In undertaking risk assessments, comprehensive information needs to be collected in a systematic manner. Some of the sources include:

- interviews and in collaboration with the forensic mental health consumer to facilitate their understanding
- interviews with the consumer's family/carers and any person with relevant information to contribute to the process
- a review of the clinical files
- other documentation such as legal reports and incident reports.

Following the assessment of risk, the plan to manage the assessed risk is clearly articulated, negotiated and documented with the person concerned.

Box 26.2 Risk assessment instruments

The two most used instruments for the short to medium term are the following:

- The Dynamic Appraisal of Situational Aggression (DASA) (Ogloff & Daffern 2006) – a short-term actuarial instrument for assessing the likelihood of imminent aggression. The instrument is used daily in inpatient settings and takes approximately 5 minutes to complete by a nurse. The DASA is intended not only to predict the risk of aggression but also to assist in managing the risk by prompting interventions (Maguire et al. 2018).
- The Short-Term Assessment of Risk and Treatability (START) (Webster et al. 2009) is a risk assessment instrument for the medium term. START considers more general risks beyond risk to others. It also assists in the identification and assessment of protective risk factors that, if present, could prevent or reduce the likelihood of an adverse event.

Cultural awareness

- There is a strong awareness in forensic mental health services of the cultural needs of the communities served and the necessity for an appropriate response to these needs.
- Forensic mental health nurses must pay attention to consumers' cultural and spiritual needs throughout the therapeutic process. Additional cultural and spiritual expertise may be needed to assist this – for example, including local Indigenous elders in forensic mental health consultation processes, community outreach and recovery plans.
- Central to any culture is the family. Family members have the potential to provide a vital link to the community for the consumer and to promote the consumer's wellbeing through supportive relationships. However, mental illness, and the nature of the offence and its consequences, may compromise this potential. For example, family members are more likely to be victims when perpetrators of serious violence have a mental illness (Canning et al. 2009).
- Containment of the consumer can have an impact on family function (emotional, financial or social). The nurse must be part of the multidisciplinary team endeavouring to assist in healing family relationships and maximising the potential of the family to be partners in addressing the needs of forensic mental health consumers.

RELEVANT TREATMENT MODALITIES AND CONSIDERATIONS

- Local legislation and policies will determine where the consumer is placed following arrest, sentencing and release and will identify the conditions, the duration of treatment and the rights of the consumer.
- Research in forensic mental health settings has demonstrated that a systemic approach to restrictive practice reduction can reduce both the frequency of the use of seclusion and its duration (Maguire et al. 2012).
- Validated risk assessment instruments are formally administered, ensuring coverage of the range of factors that need to be considered and for pattern recognition. They also enable clarification of those risk factors that are static and dynamic.
- Culturally competent and culturally safe practice is particularly critical in forensic mental health given the over-representation of Indigenous people and those from migrant cultures in forensic mental health services.

SCENARIO 26.2

Stacey

Stacey is an Indigenous woman who was exposed to a long history of abuse and victimisation during her childhood and dropped out of school when she was 12. She reported using drugs and alcohol from age 13 to cope with the abuse. Stacey gave birth to her daughter when she was 18 and reported struggling following the birth, feeling as if she had no one to talk to, being estranged from her family and having few friends. In the context of depression with psychotic features, 10 years ago Stacey was found not guilty by reason of mental impairment for the murder of her daughter.

It took 4 years for Stacey's mental illness to stabilise, but following intensive rehabilitation she is currently living in a low-secure forensic mental health unit and has applied for leave to transition to a supported community living arrangement. While Stacey's team feel she is ready to apply for leave, Stacey is anxious about the change. She has also applied for a part-time job but is anxious about having to disclose her illness and offence to a new employer.

Since her admission Stacey has gained 30 kg and has recently been diagnosed with type 2 diabetes. Weight gain has also had an impact on her self-esteem. Stacey hopes that she will be able to address her weight gain by attending a gym near her new housing arrangement.

RED FLAGS

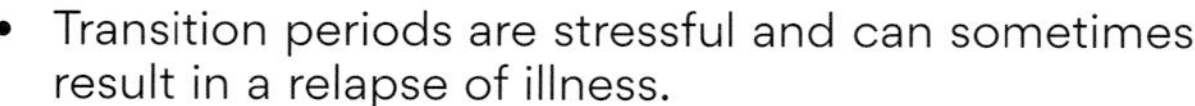

- Transition periods are stressful and can sometimes result in a relapse of illness.
- Stigma is an important issue for forensic mental health consumers, who can be disadvantaged by the negative appraisal of others; this can impact on their identity and self-concept.
- Forensic consumers may be vulnerable to poor physical health for a variety of reasons.

KNOWLEDGE

Imprisoned offenders constitute a small proportion of the sentenced population, with the criminal justice system favouring community sentencing options (Elias 2009). Little is known about the rates of mental illness in this population, although literature from the United Kingdom indicates that approximately 30% of the probation caseload have had formal contact with mental health services (Brooker et al. 2008). Consumers who offend and are placed on community-based orders are usually linked to general mental health services. Furthermore, general mental health services engage with consumers with complex needs who may have a forensic history or patterns of behaviour indicative of potential criminal involvement. Specialist community forensic liaison roles involving mental health nurses and psychiatrists have been piloted to assist mainstream mental health services to manage this group of consumers.

Specialist community forensic mental health teams have also been established to assist forensic mental health consumers with transitioning to the community from forensic mental health hospitals and prisons. The model of care of these teams often involves intensive case management, with the goal of eventual transfer to general mental health services. Forensic mental health community services provide assessment, consultation and ongoing treatment or shared care with general mental health services.

In Australia, there are numerous sources of referral to community forensic mental health services including forensic mental health hospitals, justice agencies (courts, prisons, community corrections or the parole boards) and legal aid centres. Forensic mental health consumers are not always well accepted by mainstream community mental health services and tend to be referred to community forensic mental health services, if they have a history of violence and other offending; high levels of anger, suspicion or hostility; poor response or non-adherence to treatment and service engagement; or substance misuse (Coffey 2012).

As case managers in community forensic mental health teams, nurses coordinate necessary services including health, legal, social, vocational, financial and accommodation services. They assist to manage mental illness, substance abuse, offending and other specific concerns to facilitate clinical recovery and support personal recovery. The community care of forensic consumers also requires working with families and carers. Collaboration is often required for joint management with other agencies to comprehensively address complex needs and avoid duplication in services (Coffey 2012).

Mental health nurses need to understand, plan for and respond in order to support consumers through difficult transition periods

MENTAL HEALTH NURSING ACTIONS AND INTERVENTIONS

Pre-release planning and relationship building

- The correct treatment, support and level of supervision are essential to assist forensic mental health consumers to maximise the opportunity for success

when transitioning from prison or a forensic mental health hospital to the community.
- Agencies that will work with the consumer after they leave custody should start building a relationship with them while they are still in prison or hospital. This ensures time for trust to be established, which makes engagement more likely once the consumer is in the community. It also makes recidivism less likely (McKenna et al. 2015).
- Crucial supports include:
  - early, meaningful engagement with mental health services and substance use agencies (McKenna et al. 2015)
  - the involvement of justice agencies if the consumer is on bail or parole or another order requiring ongoing justice involvement
  - assistance to address social care needs including the need for housing, food, financial assistance, employment and social supports (Freudenberg et al. 2005).

Addressing stigma and discrimination

- The possible outcome of consumers' engagement with forensic mental health services is double stigma: criminality and mental illness. Community attitudes towards both are misinformed, ignorant and fearful.
- The media, through which the public becomes 'informed', tends to present offenders with mental health problems in a manner that potentially feeds into this stigma (McKenna et al. 2007). This stigma in turn affects identity, self-concept and self-esteem (Livingston et al. 2011).
- Forensic mental health nurses need to be aware and provide support, education and advocate where necessary to address stigma and discrimination.
- It is crucial that forensic mental health nurses work in partnership with forensic mental health consumers in this regard.

Considering social disadvantage

- When assessing the needs of forensic mental health consumers, forensic mental health nurses must also consider the consumer's sociocultural context.
- The influences of cultural disadvantage and low socioeconomic status are especially important (Martin et al. 2013).
- Forensic mental health consumers are more at risk of victimisation compared with the general population. Victimisation includes being subjected to violence, intimidation, sexual exploitation and financial exploitation.
- Violence may be the reality of high-crime neighbourhoods where people experiencing mental illness often live. There is an indication that people experiencing mental illness move into, or fail to rise out of, low socioeconomic locations because of the impact of the social stigma attached to the illness (Constantine et al. 2010).

Promoting optimal physical health

- Forensic mental health nurses must consider risks and the consumer's needs when planning interventions to promote the physical health of consumers.
- A comprehensive nursing health assessment must include physical health and the nurse must work with the consumer, their family and the multidisciplinary team to develop, implement and evaluate treatment plans that promote and enhance optimal physical health (Martin et al. 2013).
- Forensic mental health consumers are at a high risk of developing metabolic syndrome and associated physical illnesses such as diabetes, cardiovascular disease and respiratory problems.
- Although a key contributing factor is the use of antipsychotic medications, restrictions on activities and lifestyle choices in custodial environments contribute to physical health deficits.
- Forensic mental health nurses must contribute to an environment that promotes a healthy lifestyle through health education and health-enhancing activities.

RELEVANT TREATMENT MODALITIES AND CONSIDERATIONS

- Pre-release planning and relationship building bring together a variety of possible supports in partnership with the consumer and should begin many months before a person is released from being detained. Through the pre-release planning process, it is more likely that all involved will clearly understand one another's roles and be able to demonstrate a clear commitment to the consumer following release.
- Integrated health, justice and social care agency responses are required for this population to attain acceptable levels of social functioning and quality of life (either in prison or in the community) and to avoid reoffending.
- In the literature, there are examples of mental health nurses initiating healthy living programs targeted to address physical health care concerns with forensic mental health consumers (for example, see Prebble et al. 2011).

Chapter summary

This chapter has sought to assist nurses to consider the practice reality of forensic mental health nursing. The challenges of this practice reality are characterised by 'complexity' relating to the needs of forensic mental health consumers, the configuration of services to meet these needs and the law that dictates service provision. All these present as challenges to forensic mental health nursing practice. However, satisfaction with nursing in this area is a direct corollary of this complexity. The challenges of the complexity can inspire nurses and create a passion for serving some of the most vulnerable and disadvantaged people in our society. The relationships nurses establish with forensic mental health consumers are pivotal to this work, although there is recognition that forensic mental health consumers often come to the relationship with a history of trauma, distrust and cynicism. Breaking through such barriers and meeting the challenge of recovery-oriented care are possible when nurses maintain therapeutic optimism and an ethical approach to care. Well-informed collaborative care planning, addressing stigma and discrimination, and supporting social and cultural connections are all essential during periods of transition from forensic services to community living.

Useful websites

Australia

Australasian Legal Information Institute (Austlii): http://www.austlii.edu.au/

Each state and territory has different legislation. The following sites may provide a good starting point.

Law and justice: http://australia.gov.au/topics/law-and-justice

Mental Health Review Tribunal: https://www.mhrt.qld.gov.au/

Queensland Forensic Mental Health Branch: https://www.health.qld.gov.au/public-health/topics/mental-health

Victorian Institute of Forensic Mental Health, Forensicare: https://www.forensicare.vic.gov.au/

New Zealand

Department of Corrections: https://www.corrections.govt.nz/

Mason Clinic (Auckland Regional Forensic Psychiatry Services, including an e-learning package): https://www.healthpoint.co.nz/public/mental-health-specialty/mason-clinic-regional-forensic-psychiatry/at/mason-clinic/

Ministry of Health New Zealand: http://www.moh.govt.nz/

Ministry of Justice: http://www.justice.govt.nz/

Other useful sites

International Association of Forensic Nurses: https://www.forensicnurses.org/

Statistics New Zealand: http://archive.stats.govt.nz/browse_for_stats/snapshots-of-nz/yearbook/society/crime/corrections.aspx

World Health Organization Mental Health Atlas Project: https://www.who.int/mental_health/evidence/atlas/profiles/en/

References

Allnutt, S., Ogloff, J., Adams, J., et al., 2013. Managing aggression and violence: the clinician's role in contemporary mental health care. Aust. N. Z. J. Psychiatry 47 (8), 728–736.

Australian Bureau of Statistics, 2018. Prisoners in Australia 2018. http://www.abs.gov.au/ausstats/abs@.nsf/mf/4517.0. (Accessed 16 February 2019).

Australian Health Ministers' Advisory Council, 2006. National statement of principles for forensic mental health, 2006. Available: https://www.aihw.gov.au/getmedia/e615a500-d412-4b0b-84f7-fe0b7fb00f5f/National-Forensic-Mental-Health-Principles.pdf.aspx. (Accessed 25 February 2019).

Bennett, S., Farrington, D.P., Huesmann, L.R., 2005. Explaining gender differences in crime and violence: the importance of social cognitive skills. Aggress. Violent Behav. 10, 263–288.

Brooker, C., Fox, C., Barrett, P., et al., 2008. A health needs assessment of offenders on probation caseloads in Nottinghamshire and Derbyshire. University of Lincoln, Lincoln.

Canning, A., O'Reilly, S., Wressell, L., et al., 2009. A survey exploring the provision of carers' support in medium and high secure services in England and Wales. J. Forens. Psychiatry Psychol. 20 (6), 868–885.

Coffey, M., 2012. Negotiating identify transition when leaving forensic hospitals. Health 16 (5), 489–506.

Constantine, R., Petrila, J., Andel, R., et al., 2010. Arrest trajectories of adult offenders with a serious mental illness. Psychol. Public Policy Law 16 (4), 319.

Daffern, M., Maguire, T., Carroll, A., et al., 2015. Workplace violence: a focus on the mental health sector. In: Day, A., Fernandez, E. (Eds.), Violence in Australia: Policy, Practice and Solutions. The Federation Press, New South Wales, pp. 104–116.

Douglas, K., Guy, L., Hart, S., 2009. Psychosis as a risk factor for violence to others: a meta-analysis. Psychol. Bull. 135 (5), 679–706.

Egeressy, A., Butler, T., Hunter, M., 2009. 'Traumatisers of the traumatised': trauma experiences and personality characteristics of Australian prisoners. Int. J. Prison. Health 5 (4), 212–222.

Elias, S., 2009. Blameless babes. Annual 2009 Shirley Smith Address. Wellington Branch of the NZ Law Society, Victoria University, Wellington.

Fazel, S., Baillargeon, J., 2011. The health of prisoners. Lancet 377 (9769), 965–966.

Fazel, S., Grann, M., Carlstron, E., et al., 2009. Risk factors for violent crime in schizophrenia: a national cohort study of 1806 patients. J. Clin. Psychiatry 70 (3), 362–369.

Foulds, J.A., Monastario, E., 2018. A public health catastrophe looms: the Australian and New Zealand prison crisis. Aust. N. Z. J. Psychiatry 52, 1019–1020.

Freudenberg, N., Daniels, J., Crum, M., et al., 2005. Coming home from jail: the social and health consequences of community re-entry for women, male adolescents, and their families and communities. Am. J. Public Health 95, 1725–1736.

Hodgins, S., 2008. Violent behavior among people with schizophrenia: a framework for investigations of causes, and effective treatment, and prevention. Philos. Trans. R. Soc. Lond. B. Biol Sci. 363 (1503), 2505–2518.

Jackson, M., Hardy, G., 2011. ABI in the Victorian prison system. Department of Justice, Melbourne.

Livingston, J., Rossiter, K., Verdun-Jones, S., 2011. Forensic labelling: an empirical assessment of its effects on self-stigma for people with severe mental illness. Psychiatry Res. 188 (1), 115–122.

Maguire, T., Daffern, M., Bowe, S., et al., 2018. Risk assessment and subsequent nursing interventions in a forensic mental health inpatient setting: associations and impact on aggressive behaviour. J. Clin. Nurs. 27 (5–6).

Maguire, T., Young, R., Martin, T., 2012. Seclusion reduction in a forensic mental health setting. J. Psychiatr. Ment. Health Nurs. 19, 97–106.

Martin, T., Daffern, M., 2006. Clinician perceptions of personal safety and confidence to manage inpatient aggression in a forensic psychiatric setting. J. Psychiatr. Ment. Health Nurs. 13 (1), 90–99.

Martin, T., Maguire, T., Quinn, C., et al., 2013. Standards of practice for forensic mental health nurses: identifying contemporary practice. J. Forensic Nurs. 9 (3), 171–178.

Mason, T., Richman, J., Mercer, D., 2002. The influence of evil on forensic nursing practice. Int. J. Ment. Health Nurs. 11 (2), 80–93.

McKenna, B., Skipworth, J., Tapsell, R., et al., 2015. Prison mental health in-reach: the impact of innovation on transition planning, community mental health service engagement and re-offending. Crim. Behav. Ment. Health 25, 429–439.

McKenna, B., Thom, K., Simpson, A., 2007. Media coverage of homicide involving mentally disordered offenders: a matched comparison study. Int. J. Forensic Ment. Health 6 (1), 57–63.

Miles, H., Dutheil, L., Welsby, I., et al., 2007. 'Just say no': a preliminary evaluation of a three-stage model of integrated treatment for substance use problems in conditions of medium security. J. Forens. Psychiatry Psychol. 18 (2), 141–159.

Ogloff, J., Daffern, M., 2006. The dynamic appraisal of situational aggression: an instrument to assess risk for imminent aggression in psychiatric inpatients. Behav. Sci. Law 24, 799–813.

Prebble, K., Kidd, J., O'Brien, A., et al., 2011. Implementing and maintaining nurse-led healthy living programmes in forensic inpatient settings: an illustrative case study. J. Am. Psychiatr. Nurses Assoc. 17 (2), 127–138.

Simpson, A., Penney, S., 2011. The recovery paradigm in forensic mental health services. Crim. Behav. Ment. Health 21 (5), 299–306.

Timmons, D., 2010. Forensic psychiatric nursing: a description of the role of the psychiatric nurse in a high secure psychiatric facility in Ireland. J. Psychiatr. Ment. Health Nurs. 17, 636–646.

Wallace, C., Mullen, P., Burgess, P., 2004. Criminal offending in schizophrenia over a 25-year period marked by deinstitutionalisation and increasing prevalence of comorbid substance use disorders. Am. J. Psychiatr. 161 (4), 716–727.

Webster, C.D., Martin, M.L., Brink, J., et al., 2009. Short-Term Assessment of Risk and Treatability (START). St Joseph's Healthcare, Forensic Psychiatric Services Commission, Port Coquitlam, BC.

Young, A., 2006. Dual diagnosis and forensic care. Are the needs of service users being met? J. Psychiatr. Ment. Health Nurs. 13, 117–124.

CHAPTER 27

Mental health settings

Fiona Whitecross

KEY POINTS

- Mental health–related services are provided in a variety of settings. There are opportunities for mental health nurses to work across acute, community, subacute residential care, forensic settings, primary care and school settings, and with a range of consumer groups, across the lifespan.
- The aim of all service provision regardless of setting are the principles of mental health recovery, which are about self-direction, responsibility empowerment, peer support, a non-linear approach to recovery, respect, a strengths-based focus and hope (Keet et al. 2019).
- Mental health care in all settings should aim to be least restrictive, ensuring a person is able to maintain their autonomy, that their rights are respected and that their individual worth, dignity and privacy are maintained. Weighing up decisions regarding responsibilities and duty of care within this model can be challenging for professionals and families.
- At times, more restrictive care settings are needed to provide containment and assertive treatment in the context of acute deterioration in mental health and increased risk.
- In all settings the patient is supported as a person in interactions with others, rather than as someone suffering from a health problem or disability. Person-centred practice maximises and encourages participation and shared decision making.
- Stigma and discrimination remain a barrier for some accessing mental health care. Nurses have a role to play in addressing stigma and discrimination within the community and with the person themselves.

KEY TERMS

- Community care
- Inpatient care
- Least restrictive care
- Mental health recovery
- Recovery-oriented practice
- Supported decision making

LEARNING OUTCOMES

The material in this chapter will assist you to:

- define and describe the components of the Australian mental health care system
- describe the functions of the multidisciplinary team
- discuss the role of the nurse as recovery partner in care in various settings along with the principles of mental health recovery and supported decision making
- gain an understanding of the least restrictive care model and nursing care in a variety of settings.

Introduction

> $9.9 billion was spent on mental health expenditure in 2017–18
>
> (Australian Institute of Health and Welfare 2020)

As was noted in Chapter 1, according to the World Health Organization (2019), mental illness accounts for 10% of the total burden of disease in the developed world. In 2010, depressive disorders ranked second in the global burden of disability (and were also considered major contributors to the additional burden related to cardiovascular disease and suicide), and the World Health Organization has predicted they will be the leading cause of the global burden of disease by 2030 (Salleh 2018).

The Australian Government and all state and territory governments share responsibility for mental health policy and for providing support services for Australians living with a mental disorder. State and territory governments are responsible for funding and providing state and territory public specialised mental health services and associated psychosocial support services. The New Zealand Ministry for Health has overall responsibility for delivering mental health care in collaboration with District Health Boards.

These provisions are coordinated and monitored through a range of initiatives including nationally agreed strategies and plans. The Australian Government also subsidises mental health–related services through Primary Health Networks, headspace, the National Disability Insurance Scheme, the Medicare Benefits Schedule and prescribed medications through the Pharmaceutical Benefits Scheme and the Repatriation Schedule of Pharmaceutical Benefits. State and territory governments fund and deliver services and assist with broader needs such as accommodation support (Australian Institute of Health and Welfare 2018).

The concept of the multidisciplinary team arose out of the advent of improved treatments for mental illness and the recognition that professional discipline-specific assistance was needed to better transition people from the hospital setting into the community. A variety of health and social care professionals provide a range of mental health services to people in Australia and New Zealand. The professions that comprise the multidisciplinary team include mental health nurses (registered and enrolled nurses with specialist qualifications, skills and experience in mental health), psychiatrists, psychologists, social workers, occupational therapists and peer workers. The specialist skills and knowledge of mental health nurses extends their scope of practice within both acute and community settings. In addition, complementary therapists such as art or music therapists can be a valuable addition to the team.

In 2016 about one in 15 (6.8%) nurses (including both enrolled and registered nurses) employed in Australia indicated they were working primarily in mental health settings. At the same time, there were 85.1 FTE mental health nurses per 100,000 population working in Australia (Australian Institute of Health and Welfare 2018). In 2019 there were 58,206 enrolled nurses, registered nurses and nurse practitioners working across New Zealand. Currently more than 370 nurse practitioners are working in New Zealand (NZ Ministry of Health 2019).

This chapter provides an overview of the range of the key considerations regarding mental health nursing in community and inpatient settings. It will help you understand the different focuses of care in different mental health–specific settings, and how you as a nurse can partner with people experiencing mental illness in their recovery. Two clinical scenarios will enable you examine the role of the nurse across community and inpatient settings.

Mental health care settings

Acute care settings

- Acute care settings provide specialised short- to medium-term, 24-hour assessment and treatment for people experiencing acute episodes of mental illness who cannot be supported in a community setting.
- This setting admits both voluntary and involuntary patients. Involuntary patients are those who are admitted under the provisions of a mental health Act for further assessment or treatment.
- Inpatient specialist mental health care typically has the highest proportion of people being treated involuntarily compared with residential mental health care and community mental health care.
- During an admission the person's status can change between voluntary and involuntary depending on risk factors, treatment plans and person's response to treatment.
- The average length of stay in a specialist inpatient mental health setting is 16 days (Australian Institute of Health and Welfare 2018).
- Treatment is from a multidisciplinary team that usually comprises a consultant psychiatrist, registrar, nursing staff and allied health staff. Specialist positions such as consumer or carer peer workers, an Indigenous mental health worker or dual diagnosis workers may also contribute to the multidisciplinary team.
- Nurses in the acute care setting have a responsibility for working with large numbers of people with high acuity in ways that promote recovery and ensure safety for all.
- Nurses are well placed to understand how the environment of an inpatient unit influences behaviour.

Subacute residential care settings

- The focus of treatment in subacute residential care settings is more on the day-to-day functioning of

patients through assessing and developing the skills required to lead a meaningful life and less on illness management.
- Patients develop functional skills that enable activities of daily living such as being able to budget, plan meals and manage medication.
- Social competencies, such as being able to establish, maintain and utilise relationships with family and friends in recovery, are also addressed.
- The major goals of residential care are to assist people towards independent living and to help them successfully navigate their life in the community and to develop a sense of belonging.
- This focus is in keeping with recovery principles. These centre on individual wellbeing and quality of life, wellness and competence (rather than illness and disability), and on keeping the person out of hospital.

Community mental health settings

- In community mental health settings, the continuum of care extends into the community and the choice of service again depends on the patient's care needs at the time.
- Community services range from clinic-based services that patients attend, to assertive outreach services in patients' own environments (see the next section). These living environments are as diverse as the patients themselves.
- Services may be available during business hours only or they may have extended hours, with crisis-oriented services often being available 24 hours a day, seven days a week.
- Care coordination (initially referred to in the literature as 'case management') is now the predominant form of service delivery in the community.
- The coordination of care can be taken up by an individual clinician or by a team of clinicians.
- The original goals of case management were to reduce the person's length of time in hospital and to assist patients to navigate the community mental health system. The role has developed over the years (and with the adoption of a recovery orientation) to service delivery. The terms 'care coordinator', 'recovery partner' or 'key worker' are more likely to be used.

Forensic mental health settings

- People with a mental illness are over-represented in prisons (Singh & Castle 2007).
- Forensic services are addressed in more detail in Chapter 26, but it is important to recognise that within forensic services the mental health nurse can work in:
  - custody centres (for both youth and adults)
  - courts
  - custodial diversion services
  - prisons (both generalist health services and specialist mental health services)
  - specialised forensic mental health services for sentenced prisoners and those deemed unfit for trial due to mental illness.

Schools

- Nurses specifically educated in mental health are well placed to contribute to student and family counselling services within schools and to work closely with the team that provides for the wellbeing of students.
- They provide information and advice about healthy behaviours (mental health promotion) and link students and families to community-based health and wellbeing services.
- These roles also include assessment and early identification of mental health issues, as well as crisis intervention and linkage and referral to specialist mental health services.

Private practice and primary care

- Mental health nurses can work in primary care in collaboration with general practitioners and private psychiatrists.
- They may also choose to go into private practice, providing counselling and psychotherapy to individuals, families and/or groups, as well as clinical supervision and education to colleagues. Nurses choosing to take this career path need to consider:
  - their practice location
  - patient access to their services
  - business issues such as fees charged, the cost of running an independent practice, indemnity insurance and leave coverage.
- These mental health nurses often specialise in particular areas and hold postgraduate qualifications in therapies.
- The Australian College of Mental Health Nurses has a Primary Care Special Interest Group comprising members engaged in private practice and in primary care. The Nurse Practitioner Special Interest Group may also be a useful resource.

MENTAL HEALTH NURSE PRACTITIONERS

Mental health nurse practitioners have been in place in Australia since 1998. These positions can ameliorate some of the concerns about appropriateness, affordability and accessibility of quality mental health care. Nurses constitute 77% of the mental health workforce.

SCENARIO 27.1

Juan

Juan is a 19-year-old man from Columbia, having moved to Australia with his mother and sister a year ago. He is unemployed and supported by Centrelink and is living in share-house accommodation. He's had no previous contact with mental health services but says he experienced mental health issues in Columbia and had been in detox for marijuana use. He reports going to school up to the age of 15 and then studying business management. Most of his work in Australia has been manual labouring. He is currently unemployed and struggling on a Newstart Allowance.

In a recent incident, Juan saw a group of men walking by; one of them looked over and Juan thought they were talking about him. He threw a rock at them, and they proceeded to approach him. He took out the knife he was carrying and waved it at them. He was arrested and jailed for 3 days. The mental health nurse at the local magistrates court was concerned he was presenting with auditory hallucinations and persecutory ideation, putting himself at risk of harm to himself and others. The court placed Juan on a mental health Act assessment order and transported him to an emergency department.

On review in the emergency department Juan was pleasant and cooperative with the interview process. He reported experiencing auditory hallucinations and visual hallucinations from a young age and expressed paranoid ideation that his family was coming to harm. He was willing to come into hospital for assessment and treatment and was admitted to the psychiatric unit. He was commenced on quetiapine 25 mg in the emergency department and consented for his mother to be contacted.

Upon arrival to the ward the nurse notes Juan looks tired and on edge. He asked if he could go out for a cigarette and said he wanted to leave.

RED FLAGS

- Transition from the emergency department to the mental health unit can be a daunting experience, particularly for people presenting or being admitted for the first time.
- The risk of misinterpreting others is high when a person has active psychosis. Juan is yet to begin treatment and is experiencing distressing psychotic symptoms.
- Juan is suspicious of others and ambivalent about staying in hospital.
- During the initial treatment period Juan is reluctant to take medication.
- Juan's family are distressed and are seeking clarification about his prognosis and treatment.

PROTECTIVE FACTORS

Protective factors are characteristics that reduce the likelihood of poor mental health. They include characteristics within the individual or conditions in the family circumstances, peers, school and the broader community that help a person to successfully cope with life's challenges (see https://beyou.edu.au/).

Juan has supportive family, social supports and connections. He has consented for his mother to be involved in his care, indicating a positive relationship.

KNOWLEDGE

Avoiding conflict and restrictive interventions

- Safewards is a model that was developed in the United Kingdom by Professor Len Bowers and others. The model and associated interventions have been highly effective in reducing conflict and restrictive interventions (such as seclusion and restraint) and increasing a sense of safety and mutual support for staff and patients.
- Safewards specifically examines events known in the model as 'conflict' (events that threaten staff and patient safety such as self-harm, suicide, aggression and absconding) and 'containment' (things staff do to prevent or reduce harm to staff and patients, such as increased observation, use of extra medication and use of restrictive interventions) (Bowers 2014).
- The Safewards intervention known as 'mutual expectation' focuses on ensuring that people who come into an acute inpatient setting are given proper orientation, so they know what to expect during their stay. For example, on admission to the ward Juan expected there would be a place he would be allowed to smoke, so clear advice around the hospital's smoke-free policy and options for managing nicotine withdrawal are important nursing considerations.
- Safewards acknowledges that some of the difficult and challenging behaviours exhibited by patients are due in part to a lack of clarity about how they are expected

to behave or to a lack of consistency between the ward staff about what the expectations are.
- This ambiguity or lack of clarity is particularly problematic for people who may:
  - have difficulty thinking clearly
  - be distracted by psychotic thinking or preoccupations
  - find it hard to concentrate
  - have difficulty interpreting the verbal and non-verbal communications of others
  - be experiencing extreme emotional distress and changes to their mood, which may result in bias of their perception and interpretation of what is going on around them.
- These expectations work both ways. Just as the staff have expectations of patients, patients have expectations of staff (Bowers 2014).

Nursing observation

- Nursing observation is the purposeful gathering of information from people receiving care to inform clinical decision making (Department of Health Victoria 2013).
- Undertaking observation requires nurses to be person-centred and to engage therapeutically with those receiving care.
- Only through talking with people receiving care do nurses gain a comprehensive understanding of their most pressing issues.
- Underpinning all nursing observation should be the goal of supporting recovery. Implicit in this definition is promoting active engagement with people, rather than passively watching them from a distance.
- Observation is indelibly linked with nursing assessment.
- Nursing observation contributes information to the assessment of psychosocial functioning, physical health and safety, and decisions to undertake different forms of observation. In this way, various forms of assessment and observation are cyclical and should be a continuous feature of the care of people in psychiatric inpatient units.
- There are several core principles that underpin the practice of nursing observation. The principles hold that:
  - nursing observation is multifaceted
  - observation and assessment are interrelated
  - observation is grounded in therapeutic engagement with the person
  - nurses appreciate how inpatient environments influence behaviour
  - observations are communicated between colleagues
  - there is a clear process of documentation that is timely and descriptive.

ATTITUDES

- Nurses who ground their clinical practice within a recovery framework can form supportive and productive relationships with the people for whom they provide care.
- Mental health recovery can be defined as 'an overarching philosophy that encompasses notions of self-determination, self-management, personal growth, empowerment, choice and meaningful social engagement' (Department of Health Victoria 2011).
- To ensure care is provided using a recovery-oriented approach, nurses should make sure their practices are consistent with the principles promoted in the *Framework for recovery-oriented practice* (Department of Health Victoria 2011).
- The framework emphasises the following aspects of recovery-oriented care:
  - promoting a culture of hope
  - promoting autonomy and self-determination
  - collaborative partnerships and meaningful engagement
  - focusing on strengths
  - holistic and personalised care
  - family, carers, support people and significant others
  - community participation and citizenship
  - responsiveness to diversity
  - reflection and learning.
- More information about recovery can be found in Chapter 2.

NURSING ACTIONS AND INTERVENTIONS

Goals of care

- Provide a therapeutic milieu in which Juan feels emotionally safe, supported and understands how the ward operates.
- Practise therapeutic engagement that effects trust and supports safety and recovery.
- Engage Juan in understanding his treatment choices and support him in the shared decision-making process with the treating team. Empower him to participate and feel a genuine partner in care.

Biopsychosocial assessment

- All young people presenting with possible psychosis should have a comprehensive biopsychosocial assessment by an acute treating team. This should include:
  - developing an understanding of the personal context of illness
  - developing a case formulation
  - mental state examination
  - physical examination and investigations
  - cognitive assessment
  - assessment for comorbid disorders
  - risk assessment (Orygen 2016).
- Patients are also experts on their own values and what gives their life meaning, purpose and quality.

Transition and orientation

- Consider risks for those experiencing acute behavioural disturbance, particularly during transitions between care settings.
- Ensure Juan is oriented to the ward's routines and the environment including providing him information about his rights and responsibilities, meal times, visiting hours, how to escalate concerns, sexual safety and the smoke-free environment.

- Anticipate Juan's anxiety in an unfamiliar environment and provide reassurance.
- Be aware of the potential for patient distress when telling Juan that he is not able to smoke or to leave the hospital right away.

Observation in practice

- Nursing observation occurs through direct contact including:
  - sitting with the person
  - listening
  - understanding non-verbal and verbal indicators or cues
  - asking pertinent questions
  - developing an understanding of the most pressing issues in the person's everyday life
  - understanding how they might react to the stress of hospitalisation and all that is occurring in that environment.
- It's important for the nurse to be mindful of explaining the 'observation' process to Juan because he has not experienced this before.
- Talking to Juan about his safety and measures to support his safety form a crucial part of the observation process, along with the aims of building rapport and developing trust.

Empathy and the therapeutic relationship

- Developing the therapeutic relationship, discussing risk issues and, in collaboration with the patient, developing strategies that can be enacted when risk presents are key interventions.
- Engagement requires a series of actions that include:
  - establishing a relationship (a person-to-person connection)
  - conveying acceptance of different views
  - hearing, listening and understanding (Cutcliffe & Stevenson 2007).
- Engagement enables people to be active in the management of their health, which can lead to improved health outcomes.
- Nurses who can build rapport with people are in a stronger position to foster positive therapeutic outcomes.
- Nurses can build rapport with people through therapeutically engaging with them and practising in ways that appreciate the person's unique history, strengths and hopes for the future.

Shared decision making

- Shared decision making is a process in which clinicians and patients work together to make decisions and selects tests, treatments and care plans based on clinical evidence that balances risk and expected outcomes with the patient's preferences and values (Orygen 2016).
- A key role for the nurse here is to activate Juan to be capable of participating in the decision-making process. This involves monitoring Juan's engagement with the information provided and ensuring it is presented in an age-appropriate way.
- Juan's decisional capacity might fluctuate during his admission, highlighting the need to tailor the process.
- Using peer support workers, advocates or programs to facilitate shared decision making could also help.
- Clinicians should clearly communicate and document a discharge plan that is developed with the person and shared with their family, their general practitioner and any new service providers before discharge.

Assisting and involving family

- It is important to make an effort to fully understand how Juan and his family see the situation and try to convey to them the nature of what Juan is experiencing and to try to find some common ground with them about their difficulties, despite the psychosis.
- Assisting and supporting Juan to understand and make sense of his experience is an obvious and essential part of treatment. An equally important but often neglected element of treatment is to understand the needs of his family and to support them to understand their experience.
- When a son or daughter is first diagnosed with a psychotic illness, parents are likely to experience a range of emotions including guilt, anxiety, sadness or anger. Conveying a sense of understanding of this distress and providing Juan's family time to express their feelings is essential.
- It's also important to understand the meaning the family attaches to the illness and actively dispel common myths.
- There are many things you may need to consider when working with a person's family, including sharing with them that:
  - Most people recover from a first-episode psychosis.
  - Recovery is a gradual process and may take some time.
  - Psychosis is caused by an interaction between biological vulnerability and environmental stress – it is not their fault.
- Antipsychotic treatment is an important part of treatment but usually needs to be supplemented by psychosocial treatments.

TREATMENT MODALITIES

- For Juan, the psychosis has been detected and inpatient care provides immediate treatment.
- The initial focus of treatment is on controlling positive psychotic symptoms and secondary symptoms such as insomnia, agitation and poor self-care.
- Treatment will then gradually progress to helping the person make sense of the experience, preventing relapse and supporting recovery.
- It is important to discuss all treatment options with the patient and their family.

Least restrictive treatment

- To minimise as much as possible any iatrogenic trauma, mental health treatment should be provided in the least restrictive manner and in the least restrictive setting that will ensure the needs of the individual are met.
- Iatrogenic trauma occurs when a person is receiving treatment and an outcome of that treatment involves

more harm. For example, the process of receiving treatment in an inpatient unit could trigger a trauma response, particularly for patients with a history of trauma.
- Seclusion, physical and mechanical restraint, pharmacological restraint and locked wards are all restrictive care measures that could cause iatrogenic trauma. These are measures of last resort, and health services across Australia and New Zealand are working towards eliminating seclusion and restraint in mental health services.
- It is important to respond early to mental state deterioration and to escalate concerns to ensure behavioural disturbance is responded to in a timely and person-centred way. Enacting personal safety plans that identify early warning signs, patient preferences for calming and triggers for escalation are best practice (Australian Commission on Safety and Quality in Health Care 2017).
- See Chapter 3 for detailed information about trauma and the trauma-informed approach. See Chapter 26 for detailed information about applying least restrictive treatment options.

Medication

- Medication is a primary treatment for psychosis. This is the first time Juan has experienced psychosis. If untreated, his symptoms could develop into a full psychotic episode or may cause the illness to become more biologically entrenched and less responsive to treatment.
- The quality of the therapeutic relationship is key to improved medication adherence. A collaborative approach with the patient, taking note of their ideas and beliefs, is more likely to be successful than mere insistence. The nurse should explore the patient's fears or concerns and empower the patient to participate in decision making about their treatment. Shared and informed decision making is a key principle that respects patient autonomy.
- Someone who is experiencing a first psychotic episode is typically very sensitive to the pharmacological effects of antipsychotic medications and quite susceptible to possible side effects. The nurse should monitor carefully for any side effects including (but not limited to):
  - acute dystonic reactions – sudden, painful muscle spasms, commonly affecting muscles in the head and neck
  - pseudo-parkinsonism – muscle stiffness, tremor and hypokinesia (decreased bodily movement)
  - akathisia – a feeling of motor restlessness that makes the person feel they need to keep moving around.
- Potential side effects of antipsychotic medication (including metabolic side effects, weight gain, extrapyramidal motor symptoms and sexual side effects) should be noted and discussed with Juan using a shared decision-making approach before beginning pharmacotherapy, and then monitored, managed and addressed early, with a prevention model if possible (e.g. weight management strategies implemented before beginning treatment).
- Routine metabolic screening should guide intervention. Preventing physical ill health must be prioritised as part of routine early psychosis treatment (Orygen 2016).

Cognitive remediation

- Cognitive remediation programs and/or cognitive adaptation strategies should be offered to young people who have cognitive deficits that interfere with functional recovery.
- These are behavioural training-based interventions that aim to improve cognitive processes (attention, memory, social cognition and metacognition), with a goal of compensating for a cognitive deficit or restoring it.
- The training can be offered in sets of exercises or may be personalised to target specific deficits. When combined with psychosocial rehabilitation programs, outcomes are most significant (Orygen 2016).

See Chapter 12 for more detailed information about psychological treatments for people experiencing psychosis.

SCENARIO 27.2

Virginia

Virginia is 68-year-old woman who presented to the community aged psychiatry service with her youngest daughter, Jean. Jean describes her mother as having difficulty sleeping and being more irritable, noting Virginia's rapid speech and how difficult it is to interrupt her when she speaks. Virginia has a diagnosis of bipolar affective disorder and is being treated with lithium carbonate.

Virginia has been living in her own home, a two-storey terrace house, for almost 30 years. She has lived alone since her husband died two years ago following a cardiac arrest. Jean moved in with her mother a year ago after she lost her job. Virginia's eldest daughter, Catherine, lives interstate with her family.

Virginia is a retired schoolteacher and she and both daughters describe her as a very private woman who has never enjoyed having visitors in her home. Virginia took much encouragement to accept cleaning and shopping assistance once a week after her most recent admission for a manic relapse; however, she does not agree to an increase in service provision. Jean has an 'enduring power of attorney (EPOA) financial' – paperwork that indicates that Virginia appointed Jean as her financial guardian two years ago. She does not appear to have initiated an enduring power of guardianship (before September 2015) or an enduring power of attorney (medical treatment), so this means Jean's power of attorney is limited to managing Virginia's financial issues.

In discussion with Jean and Catherine, the nurse identifies that Jean and Virginia have always been very close and that there is a history of longstanding conflict between Catherine and Jean, which was exacerbated by the death of their father. Both daughters say they understand the impact of bipolar affective disorder on their mother's overall functioning, but they do not agree on what is the most appropriate treatment. Virginia says she will be fine once she gets home and is reluctant for her case manager to visit - demonstrating a lack of insight into her care needs. Repeated attempts to discuss options with all parties in the same room have not resulted in a decision that is agreeable to everyone. Virginia is adamant that she wants to return home to live with Jean, who she says can look after her despite having some significant health issues of her own.

RED FLAGS

- Virginia is at high risk of experiencing a manic relapse with the emergence of hypomanic symptoms.
- Virginia's lithium level might be subtherapeutic or toxic.
- Virginia's daughter is at risk of carer burnout; she also has her own physical health issues to deal with.
- There is a risk of relationship breakdown between Virginia and Catherine.

PROTECTIVE FACTORS

- Virginia is a woman who has had a professional career as a teacher and who has lived in her own home for 30 years.
- Despite the strained relationships between them, Virginia's daughters are concerned for the welfare of their mother.
- Jean has power of attorney over Virginia's finances and has arranged some social care support services.

KNOWLEDGE

- Bipolar disorder (formerly called 'manic depression') is a mental illness that involves the person having a least one manic episode or *nearly* manic episode (called 'hypomania', which is considered a less severe version of mania). The mood swings of this illness can last for weeks at a time.
- A person may feel euphoric and extremely energetic, only to drop into a period of paralysing depression, in a cycle of elation followed by sadness.
- The exact cause is unknown, and several factors may be involved, although a genetic predisposition has been clearly established (Bloch et al. 2017).
- It is estimated that around one in 50 Australians develops this illness, which affects men and women equally. Most of those affected are aged in their 20s when first diagnosed (Mitchell et al. 2010).

LITHIUM

- 'Lithium toxicity' is another term for lithium overdose.
- The right dose varies from person to person, but most people are prescribed between 900 mg and 1,200 mg per day.
- A safe blood level of lithium is 0.6 to 1.2 mL equivalents per litre (mEq/L).
- Lithium toxicity can occur at levels above 1.5 or higher. Toxicity can occur if the person becomes dehydrated and the concentration of the medication in the blood stream is increased or if there are interactions with other medications or problems with kidney function after dose increases or when too much lithium is taken (Corbett 2018).

NURSING ACTIONS AND INTERVENTIONS

Goals of care

- Ensure Virginia remains free from harm/injury and assist her to decrease her agitation and hyperactivity.
- Avoid lithium toxicity or subtherapeutic levels. Achieve adherence to the prescribed treatment.
- Explore carer respite options and support and develop an understanding of possible National Disability Insurance Scheme (NDIS) supports available to Virginia.

Assessment

- A comprehensive mental health assessment including a mental state examination, assessing for hypomanic or manic symptoms along with a review of any physical health concerns.
- A person experiencing mania may present with the following symptoms:
  - elevated mood
  - increased energy or overactivity
  - reduced need for sleep or food
  - irritability
  - rapid thinking and speech
  - grandiose plans and beliefs
  - lack of insight
  - distractibility.

Medication

- Ask questions about food and fluid intake and encourage fluids, particularly when it is hot or the person's exercise/activity is increased – dehydration can exacerbate lithium toxicity.
- Be aware to the symptoms of lithium toxicity such as:
  - vomiting
  - diarrhoea
  - tremors
  - drowsiness
  - stomach pains
  - muscle weakness
  - ataxia.
- Monitoring of the long-term side effects of lithium treatment is also an important responsibility for the multidisciplinary team. Long-term treatment can affect the kidneys and thyroid. Regular testing of lithium levels, thyroid and kidney function should form part of the community treatment plan.

Support to carers

- Providing direct support to carers is an important intervention for mental health nurses, who are well placed to provide information, navigate the family dynamics and foster links and support between all parties.
- A carer needs assessment is key. In Virginia's case, her daughters differ in their opinions about care. The case manager can bring families together to facilitate planning and decision making.
- Carer peer workers could also help Virginia's daughters to navigate their own understanding of the illness and to get the support and care they need.
- The healthcare system is complex to navigate. Nurses can help patients and families to access community-based supports that are relevant and that meet the person's needs. In this instance, the nurse might consider encouraging Virginia's family to apply for NDIS support to access in-home support. Currently Jean provides the main support, but she is experiencing carer burden and has her own health issues.

ATTITUDES

The following **values** underpin how mental health clinicians apply skills and knowledge when working with people, families, carers and communities:

- respect
- advocacy
- recovery
- working in partnership
- excellence in care.

Attitudes are also important and involve the interaction of beliefs, feelings and values, and a disposition to act in particular ways. The nurse's attitude defines how they see situations and individuals. Key attitudes include:

- respectful
- compassionate, caring and empathic
- ethical, professional and responsible
- self-aware
- culturally aware
- collaborative.

Relevant treatment modalities

- Careful assessment to rule out organic conditions is an important first step in managing hypomania/mania. Mood-stabilising agents, benzodiazepines or antipsychotics may be needed to treat psychotic symptoms, sleep disturbance and agitation. Monitoring serum drug levels for mood-stabilising agents is an important treatment function.
- Psychosocial strategies include education, support for the person and their family, stress management and support with medication decision making and adherence. Read more about psychological therapy of people with mood disorders in Chapter 10.

Peer support

A mental health peer worker is someone employed based on their lived experience of mental illness and recovery (consumer peer worker) or their experience of supporting family or friends with mental illness (carer peer worker). This lived experience is an essential qualification for their job, in addition to other skills and experience required for the particular role they undertake.

> Peer support is a system of giving and receiving help founded on key principles of respect, shared responsibility, and mutual agreement of what is helpful. Peer support is not based on psychiatric models and diagnostic criteria. It is about understanding another's situation empathically through the shared experience of emotional and psychological pain. When people find affiliation with others they feel are 'like' them, they feel a connection. This connection, or affiliation, is a deep, holistic understanding based on mutual experience where people are able to 'be' with each other without the constraints of traditional (expert/patient) relationships.
>
> (Mead 2001, p. 1)

Chapter summary

This chapter provided information about mental health treatment settings and mental health nursing across inpatient and community settings via two clinical scenarios. Several interventions and key knowledge and attitude requisites have been described to assist you to work with people who experience mental illness.

Regardless of the care setting the attitude the nurse brings is of fundamental importance. As a novice nurse, bringing a genuine compassion and willingness to understand will be enormously helpful. The skills, knowledge and attitudes you will acquire as your practice evolves will be enhanced by good clinical supervision and an attitude of life-long learning.

In the acute care setting nurses are regularly exposed to people who are at their most vulnerable; with this comes high levels of patient distress and behaviours of concern calling for regular and meaningful engagement via nursing observation and safety planning. The situation carries high emotion for the nurse, the patient and their family. The immense reward one feels working with people in this phase of illness gives a mental health nursing career meaning and purpose. This continues as nurses have the chance to work with people in the community setting in an ongoing way to partner in a person's recovery.

Useful websites

Bipolar disorder: https://www.sane.org/information-stories/facts-and-guides/bipolar-disorder
Early psychosis services: https://iepa.org.au/
National Disability Insurance Scheme (NDIS): https://www.ndis.gov.au/
Safewards interventions: https://www2.health.vic.gov.au/mental-health/practice-and-service-quality/safety/safewards
Stigma: https://www.sane.org/information-stories/facts-and-guides/reducing-stigma
Supported decision making: https://www2.health.vic.gov.au/mental-health/practice-and-service-quality/mental-health-act-2014-handbook/recovery-and-supported-decision-making

References

Australian Commission on Safety and Quality in Health Care, 2017. National Safety and Quality Health Service Standards, second ed. Australian Commission on Safety and Quality in Health Care, Darlinghurst.
Australian Institute of Health and Welfare, 2018. Patient-reported experience and outcome measures. In: Australia's Health 2018. AIHW, Canberra (Chapter 7.17).
Australian Institute of Health and Welfare, 2020. Mental health services in Australia. 30 January 2020 Revision. Available: https://www.aihw.gov.au/reports/mental-health-services/mental-health-services-in-australia/report-contents/summary-of-mental-health-services-in-australia.
Bloch, S., Green, S., Janca, A., et al., 2017. Foundations of Clinical Psychiatry. Melbourne University Press, Melbourne.
Bowers, L., 2014. Safewards: a new model of conflict and containment on psychiatric wards. J. Psychiatr. Ment. Health Nurs. 21, 499–508.
Corbett, B., 2018. Lithium toxicity. In: Nordstrom, K., Wilson, M. (Eds.), Quick Guide to Psychiatric Emergencies. Springer, Cham.
Cutcliffe, J.R., Stevenson, C., 2007. Care of the Suicidal Person. Churchill Livingstone, Edinburgh.
Department of Health Victoria, 2013. Nursing Observation Through Engagement in Psychiatric Inpatient Care Guideline. State Government of Victoria, Melbourne.
Department of Health Victoria, 2011. Framework for Recovery-Oriented Practice. State Government of Victoria, Melbourne.
Keet, R., de Vetten-Mc Mahon, M., Shields-Zeeman, L., et al., 2019. Recovery for all in the community; position paper on principles and key elements of community-based mental health care. BMC Psychiatry 19, 174.
Mead, S., 2001. Peer support: a theoretical perspective. Psychiatr. Rehabil. J. 25 (2), 134–141.
Mitchell, P.B., Loo, C.K., Gould, B.M., 2010. Diagnosis and monitoring of bipolar disorder in general practice. Med. J. Aust. 193 (4), S10.
NZ Ministry of Health, 2019. New Zealand's nursing workforce the largest its ever been [media release]. Available: https://www.health.govt.nz/news-media/media-releases/new-zealands-nursing-workforce-largest-its-ever-been.
Orygen, 2016. Clinical Practice in Youth Mental Health Shared Decision Making. The National Centre of Excellence in Youth Mental Health, Melbourne.
Salleh, M.R., 2018. The burden of mental illness: an emerging global disaster. J. Clin. Health Sci. 3 (1), 5–12.
Singh, B., Castle, D., 2007. Why are community psychiatry services in Australia doing it so hard? Med. J. Aust. 187 (7), 410–412.
World Health Organization (WHO), 2019. Mental health. who.int/news-room/facts-in-pictures/detail/mental-health.

Glossary

Acceptance and commitment therapy (ACT): develops acceptance of unwanted private experiences that are out of the person's control, and fosters commitment and action towards living a valued life.

Addiction: physical dependence on a drug to the extent that physical symptoms occur if the drug is withdrawn.

Adjustment disorder: a clinically significant emotional or behavioural response to a significant life change or stressor such as a relationship break-up, bereavement, divorce or illness.

Advance directive: a means by which clients can state their preferences for future healthcare.

Advanced practice: a level of nursing practice characterised by clinical expertise, application of research to practice, clinical leadership and postgraduate education.

Affect: the observable behaviours associated with changes in a person's *mood*, such as crying and looking dejected. Some terms for affect are 'blunted', 'flat', 'inappropriate', 'labile' and 'restricted'.

Ageism: the systematic stereotyping of and discrimination against people because of their age alone.

Aggression: actions or behaviours ranging from verbal abuse, insults and nonverbal gestures to violent physical acts such as kicks or punches.

Agitation: (also known as psychomotor agitation) excessive non-productive, repetitious motor activity associated with a feeling of inner tension (pacing, hand-wringing, fidgeting).

Agnosia: a failure to recognise objects.

Agoraphobia: anxiety about being in places or situations from which escape might be difficult (or embarrassing) or in which help might not be available.

Agranulocytosis: a blood disorder characterised by severe depletion of white blood cells, rendering the body almost defenceless against infection.

Akathisia: one of the side effects of antipsychotic medication; involves the person not being able to stay or remain still, being restless and suffering from leg aches.

Allostasis: the adaptation process of a person's physiological system to psychosocial, environmental or physical stressors.

Alzheimer's disease: a form of dementia that features memory impairment as well as one or more cognitive disturbances, including aphasia (impaired understanding of language in any form), apraxia (impaired motor activities), agnosia (failure to recognise objects) and disturbance in executive functioning.

Ambivalence: an individual's tendency to hold conflicting views and feelings about a person or situation, making decision making difficult.

Amnesia: an inability to remember events from a particular period. There are a number of different amnesias, including localised amnesia, selective amnesia, generalised amnesia and systematised amnesia.

Anhedonia: loss of the feelings of pleasure previously associated with favoured activities.

Anorexia nervosa: a mental illness characterised by an inability to maintain normal body weight for age and height; an intense fear of gaining weight; disturbed perception of body shape and size.

Anticholinergic: medication that blocks the action of acetylcholine thereby reducing the side effects of some psychotropic medication, including dry mouth, blurred vision, orthostatic hypotension, tachycardia, urinary retention and nasal congestion.

Antidepressant medication: medication that aims to elevate mood by enhancing the transmission of neurochemicals, particularly serotonin and noradrenaline, by blocking their reuptake at the synapse, inhibiting their metabolism and/or enhancing the activity of the receptors.

Antiparkinsonian medication: Medication used to treat Parkinson's disease or the extrapyramidal side effects of antipsychotic medication, including dystonia and akathisia.

Antipsychotic medication: also known as *neuroleptics*, these drugs were introduced in the 1950s for the treatment of mental illness. First-generation antipsychotics are dopamine antagonists that aim to reduce the 'positive' symptoms of schizophrenia. Second-generation antipsychotics also aim to reduce the 'positive' symptoms of schizophrenia and can also improve the 'negative' symptoms.

Antisocial: exhibiting disregard for the rights of others and engaging in reckless, aggressive, deceitful and impulsive behaviour.

Anxiety: a common human experience that is a normal emotion felt in varying degrees by everyone; also a state in which individuals experience feelings of uneasiness, apprehension and activation of the autonomic nervous system in response to a vague, nonspecific threat.

Anxiolytic medication: also known as anti-anxiety medication; used when anxiety symptoms becomes debilitating.

Apathy: indifference; lack of interest or feeling.

Aphasia: impairment in the understanding or transmission of ideas by language in any form (writing, reading, speaking) due to impairment of the brain centres involved in language.

Apraxia: impaired motor activities.

Assertive community treatment: a model of community care in which clinicians, often nurses, actively follow up clients with high needs in order to maintain community living and prevent hospitalisation.

Assertiveness: a communication skill that enhances one's interpersonal effectiveness and allows one the choice of how to respond to others. The assertive person protects the rights of each party and achieves their own goals without hurting others. This results in self-confidence and the ability to express oneself appropriately in emotional and social situations.

Asylum: a term for institutions developed in the 19th century intended to provide sanctuary and care for those with mental illness. Sometimes used to describe a place of withdrawal and refuge.

Ataxia: partial or complete loss of voluntary muscular movement and coordination.

Attachment: the strong bond or connection one feels for particular people in one's life; usually associated with the primary bond between infant and mother, which can influence one's self-concept, relationships and life experiences.

Autism: an individual's tendency to retreat into an inner world, resulting in social isolation or withdrawal and inflexible, repetitive patterns of thinking and behaviour.

Autism spectrum disorder: A range of disorders defined in DSM 5 which involve problems with attention, communication and social interaction.

Autonomy: the right of each person to make their own decisions, provided these decisions do not violate another person's autonomy. For people to be able to make autonomous decisions, they must be free of the control of others.

Avoidance behaviour: withdrawing or turning away from occupational and/or social activities because of fear of disapproval, rejection and ridicule.

Avoidant/Restrictive Food Intake Disorder: an eating disorder characterised by extreme dietary restriction, such that it causes weight loss or failure to grow or develop properly (in children and adolescents); unlike anorexia nervosa, the person does not experience distress around body image issues.

Behaviour therapy: therapy aimed at changing behaviour by changing the patterns of reinforcement that maintain behaviour. Behaviour therapy is usually highly structured with specific measureable goals, interventions to achieve goals and a timeline for goal achievement.

Beneficence: actions taken with the intention of benefitting others.

Bereavement: deprived by death of a friend or relative.

Binge eating disorder: a mental illness characterised by regular episodes of binge eating, which are accompanied by feelings of loss of control, guilt, shame and disgust. Unlike bulimia nervosa, the person does not use compensatory behaviours such as vomiting or excessive exercise after binge eating.

Biomedical model: a model based on the idea that normal behaviour occurs because of equilibrium within the body and that abnormal behaviour results from pathological bodily or brain function.

Biopsychosocial model of assessment: a comprehensive assessment of all aspects of information concerning the consumer—biological, psychological, sociological, developmental, spiritual and cultural.

Bipolar disorder: a diagnosis when a person has previously experienced at least one manic episode and a depressive episode.

Blunted affect: significant reduction in the intensity of emotional response.

Body image assessment: assessment of components of body image, including body image distortion, body image avoidance and body image dissatisfaction.

Body dysmorphia: a disturbance of cognition and affect that leads to a negative evaluation of physical appearance; frequently associated with depression, anxiety and feelings of shame.

Body mass index (BMI): a numerical measure, based on the height and weight of an individual, used to help determine the degree of starvation or obesity.

Bulimia nervosa: a mental illness characterised by binge-eating behaviour—eating much larger amounts of food than would normally be eaten in one sitting - and inappropriate, compensatory weight-loss behaviours such as self-induced vomiting or excessive exercise.

Bullying: unwanted and repeated aggressive verbal or physical behaviour towards a person often considered less powerful with the aim to control, harm and intimidate.

Burnout: a syndrome in which healthcare workers lose concern and feeling for consumers under their care, becoming detached and distancing themselves from the consumers; characterised by emotional exhaustion, depersonalisation and decreased personal accomplishment.

Carer: someone who provides assistance for family members or friends with care needs. Informal carers may be parents, children, partners, other relatives and friends. Formal carers are staff of support agencies who assist with a variety of personal care, healthcare, transport, household and other activities.

Case formulation: the process of developing, with the consumer, a summary of the various influences on the consumer's current problems, and how the consumer and clinician can work towards resolving those problems.

Case management: assessing, planning, linking, monitoring and evaluating services with the consumer, with caseloads shared among the multidisciplinary team.

Catatonia: a severe and debilitating condition with disorganisation of motor behaviour and inability to relate to external stimuli; can be a feature of mood disorder, psychotic disorder or schizophrenia.

Challenging behaviour: a term used to describe behaviour that disrupts relationships with others and complicates healthcare delivery—for example, aggression, manipulation and self-harm.

Circumstantiality: a disturbance in form of thought, in which speech is indirect and longwinded.

Clang association: a disturbance in form of thought, in which words are chosen for their sounds rather than their meanings; includes puns and rhymes.

Classification of mental disorders: systems of categorisation that enable mental disorders to be identified based on patterns of behaviour, thoughts and emotions. The most commonly used classification systems are the Diagnostic and Statistical Manual and the International Classification of Diseases.

Clinical formulation: the process of developing with the consumer a summary of the various influences on the consumer's current problems, and how the consumer and clinician can work towards resolving those problems.

Clinical supervision: a professional process that involves reflection on clinical interactions and interventions between a clinician (or group of clinicians) and a more experienced clinician for support, professional development, education and development of clinical practice skills.

Code of ethics: guidelines for members of professional groups as to the nature of proper ethical conduct and their obligations to consumers and to the public.

Coexisting/comorbid disorder: having more than one disorder at the same time, most commonly a mental health disorder and a substance use disorder. Similar terms are *comorbidity, co-occurring disorders,* and *dual diagnosis*. Also used to refer to coexisting mental disorder and intellectual disability.

Cognitions: knowing or perceiving something; related to intellect, logic and reason, not emotions and feelings.

Cognitive behavioural therapy (CBT): therapy that aims to help people to develop more efficient coping mechanisms by equipping them with strategies that promote logical ways of thinking about and responding to everyday situations.

Cognitive enhancers: drugs used in the treatment of cognitive impairment to improve memory, boost energy and alertness levels, and increase concentration.

Cognitive restructuring: an intervention that aims to monitor and reduce distressing negative cognitions (thoughts), especially in people who are depressed.

Collaborative prescribing: where members of the multidisciplinary health care team (including nurses, pharmacists and psychologists) prescribe medications for mental health consumers and work together to determine the pharmacotherapeutic needs of the consumer.

Community care: health services available from community mental health centres and emphasising the multidisciplinary team; includes services such as counselling, follow-up treatment, referrals and supported accommodation.

Community treatment orders: provisions within Mental Health Acts that enable the involuntary treatment of people with mental illness while they live in the community.

Comorbidity: see *coexisting/comorbid disorder* and *dual diagnosis.*

Compassion: sensitivity to suffering and a desire to alleviate distress.

Competence: Ability of a person to understand information and make decisions about their health care. Individuals are assumed to be competent unless there are strong reasons for thinking otherwise, confirmed by clinical assessment of competence.

Competencies: a specific framework that describes the expected clinical skill base of all practitioners within a specific discipline; set by regulatory bodies and professional nursing organisations.

Compulsions: repetitive behaviours (e.g. hand-washing, checking) or mental acts (e.g. praying, counting), the goal of which is to prevent or reduce anxiety or distress, not to provide pleasure or gratification.

Confabulation: filling in gaps in memory with imaginary experiences.

Confidentiality: maintaining privacy of consumers' personal information within the healthcare team.

Consultation-liaison: a role where a mental health nurse offers assessment services, advice and assistance to staff in non-mental health settings about the management of people with mental health problems.

Consumer: someone who has the lived experience of mental distress and who has received care from mental health professionals.

Containment: provision of a place of safety; the hospital can be seen as a refuge from self-destructiveness and an opportunity to reassure the consumer and others that illness will not overwhelm them.

Continuity of care: a continuous relationship between a consumer and an identified healthcare professional or agency who ensure that the consumer's health needs over time are met.

Coping: the way one deals with change, conflict and demands in life, which can be influenced by factors such as one's feelings, thoughts, beliefs and values.

Countertransference: the response of the therapist to the patient. Having strong feelings for the patient, either negative or positive, might be a cue that one is experiencing countertransference. See also *transference*.

Court liaison nurse: employed in courts to advise judges, lawyers and the police on issues regarding the mental health, addiction status and needs of people presenting to court.

Credentialling: a core component of clinical/professional governance or self-regulation where members of a profession set standards for practice and establish a minimum requirement for entry, continuing professional development, endorsement and recognition.

Crisis: an event that creates a sense of one's life being out of control, feeling that one is vulnerable and that events are unpredictable; can involve a significant loss for the person involved but also an opportunity for growth.

Crisis intervention: involves assessment, planning, intervention and resolution of a *crisis.*

Cultural assessment: a process of examining individuals, groups, and communities regarding their cultural beliefs, values, and practices as a means to determine needs and appropriate interventions.

Cultural competence: the ability to understand, communicate and interact with people from cultures different from one's own.

Cultural safety: care provided by a nurse who is aware of their own cultural identity and who acts to promote and protect the cultural identity of others.

Culture: a body of learned behaviours that is used to interpret individual experience and shape individual behaviour, emotion and social responses.

Cyclothymia: a condition characterised by mild depression alternating with mild manic symptoms.

Defence mechanisms: unconscious processes whereby anxiety experienced by the individual's ego is reduced by behaviours such as denial, repression, projection and displacement.

Deinstitutionalisation: closure of major psychiatric hospitals and expansion of community-based care for consumers, including relocation of inpatient psychiatric beds into general hospitals.

Delirium: a syndrome that constitutes a characteristic pattern of signs and symptoms that reduce clarity of awareness and impair the consumer's ability to focus, sustain or shift attention; tends to develop quickly and fluctuate during the course of the day.

Delirium tremens (DTs): a syndrome in which the client presents with agitation, disorientation, fever, paranoia, hallucinations, coarse tremors and seizures following withdrawal of a substance such as alcohol.

Delusion: a false belief, based on incorrect inference about external reality that is firmly sustained despite what almost everyone else from the person's cultural group believes. Types of delusion include bizarre, jealous, erotomanic, grandiose, control, reference, persecution, somatic, thought broadcasting and thought insertion.

Dementia: a progressive illness that involves cognitive, emotional and behavioural impairments; caused by a gradual failure of brain function.

Dependence (drugs or alcohol): can be both physical and psychological. Physical dependence is the body's adaptation to the presence of a substance and symptoms of *withdrawal* when the substance is discontinued. Psychological dependence is the craving for the substance when the person stops using it.

Depersonalisation: a form of *dissociation* in which there is a sense of personal reality being lost or altered, of being estranged from oneself, as if in a dream, or that one's actions are mechanical or otherwise detached from the body or mind.

Depot antipsychotic medication: long-acting, injectable form of antipsychotic medication, administered fortnightly or monthly. Used when the patient is unable or unwilling to take oral medication, or when the patient prefers the convenience of periodic injections over daily oral medication.

Depression: a disorder characterised by lowered mood, with feelings of hopelessness and helplessness, lack of pleasure or interest, appetite disturbance, sleep disturbance and fatigue.

Derailment: a disturbance in form of thought, in which thoughts do not progress logically and ideas are unconnected.

Derealisation: a form of dissociation in which the person feels disconnected to the outside world.

Detoxification: the process by which an alcohol- or drug-dependent person discontinues the use of a substance in a supervised environment so that withdrawal symptoms are minimised.

Developmental psychology: the scientific study of how and why human beings develop over the course of their life.

Developmental theories: theories that highlight the importance of the early months and years of one's life in laying a solid foundation for mental health and wellbeing in adulthood.

Diagnosis: a mental illness a consumer is considered to be experiencing; the act of identifying a mental illness through a process of assessment.

Dialectical behaviour therapy (DBT): similar to *cognitive behavioural therapy* but actively incorporates social skills training, dealing with *distress*, and validation and acceptance of the person.

Differential diagnosis: the process of distinguishing one illness from other illnesses presenting with similar signs and symptoms by listing, in order of likelihood, the most likely diagnoses.

Diminished capacity: a mitigating defence used to establish the absence of malice by a defendant who committed an illegal act. Not technically 'insanity', but a suspended mental state in which the defendant's thoughts and actions were dominated by passion and emotional stress, preventing them from acting rationally or being aware of the consequences of their actions. See also *competence*.

Disability: an individual's impairment in one or more areas of functioning.

Discontinuation syndrome: a withdrawal syndrome that can result from switching between or rapid withdrawal of one of the antidepressant or *antipsychotic medications*.

Discrimination: unfavourable treatment based on prejudice, especially regarding race, colour, age or gender.

Dissociation: being disconnected from one's own thoughts, feelings, emotions or identity, and unaware of the external environment. For example, daydreaming is considered a mild form of dissociation.

Distractibility: a disturbance in form of thought or attention, in which nearby various stimuli cause repeated changes in the topic of speech that interfere with ability to attend to activities or interactions.

Distress: an unpleasant subjective emotional state.

Distress tolerance: a consumer's capacity to recognise and manage their own experiences of distress.

Diversion: arrangements between mental health services and police so that consumers can be diverted from the criminal justice system to mental health services.

DSM-5: *Diagnostic and Statistical Manual of Mental Disorders*, 5th edition, published by the American Psychiatric Association. Sets out concise descriptions of each mental disorder organised by explicit diagnostic information about the diagnosis, risk factors and associated features of each disorder.

Dual diagnosis: having more than one disorder at the same time, most commonly a mental health disorder and a substance use disorder. See also *coexisting/comorbid disorder*.

Dual disability: having a comorbid intellectual or developmental disability.

Duty of care: the taking of reasonable care by a nurse to avoid acts or omissions that one can reasonably foresee would be likely to injure another.

Dysthymia: chronic mild *depression*.

Dystonic reaction: one of the side effects of some *antipsychotic medications*. May include painful muscle spasms in the head, back and torso that can last minutes or hours.

Early intervention: can be employed with people who are identified as at risk or already showing signs of emotional or behavioural problems; may also contribute to the prevention of some types of mental illness or disorder, or to reduced severity or duration of symptoms if a disorder does emerge.

Eating disorders: complex and serious disorders that involve disturbance of eating behaviours; examples include *anorexia nervosa*, *bulimia nervosa* and *binge eating disorder*.

Echolalia: a disturbance in form of thought, in which other people's words or phrases are echoed, often in a 'mocking' tone; not the same as repetition of the person's own words (*perseveration*).

Echopraxia: repetition by imitation of the movements of another person. The actions are involuntary and semi-automatic.

Egocentric: focusing on oneself to the degree that other people's needs are beyond one's awareness.

Ego-dystonic: when a patient's symptoms are experienced as distressing to the individual.

Elation: a feeling of exhilaration and intense pride and joy.

Electroconvulsive therapy (ECT): the application of electrodes to the head, through which an electric current is delivered. ECT is an effective intervention in the treatment of severe depression, although it remains controversial.

Emotional dysregulation: being easily overwhelmed by negative emotions and unable to regain a sense of emotional control. Often associated with maladaptive regulation strategies such as self-harm.

Empathy: observing, listening, understanding and attending; 'being' with the person physically, cognitively and emotionally, understanding their story, thoughts, feelings, beliefs and emotions.

Enabling environments: (also known as supportive environments) inherently helpful environments that in and of themselves enable people to move towards recovery.

Engagement: the process of establishing rapport with a consumer through interactions based on acknowledgement and a relationship based on trust.

Ethical conduct: health professional behaviour that is consistent with ethical principles of *autonomy*, *beneficence*, *non-maleficence* and *justice*.

Ethics: morals in human conduct; rules of conduct appropriate to a profession or area of life.

Ethnocentrism: the belief that one's own cultural values constitute the human norm and that difference is deviant and wrong.

Excessive exercise: a compensatory behavior commonly seen in people with eating disorders, where a person engages in exercise despite illness or injury, feels guilt or anxiety if not able to exercise and/or uses exercise to 'offset' caloric intake.

Externalising problems: personal problems that are expressed as problematic outward behaviour, including antisocial or undercontrolled behaviour, delinquency or aggression.

Extrapyramidal side effects: side effects of antipsychotic drugs on the extrapyramidal motor system; include dystonia, parkinsonism, *akathisia* and *tardive dyskinesia*.

Family-focused practice: an approach to care that takes a 'whole of family' perspective and identifies the relationships between mental health consumers and their key others. Involves systematically incorporating family members' health and wellbeing and the role of parenting into a family plan of care.

Family of origin: the family a person is born into, where the family includes parents and siblings of a child or adult with mental illness.

Family therapy: an approach to treatment based on the idea that when a family member has a problem, it usually involves the whole family. Family therapists aim to effect change in the entire family system.

Fear: a response to a known threat; manifests in the same way as *anxiety*.

Flight of ideas: a disturbance in form of thought, in which the person's ideas are too rapid for them to express and so their speech is fragmented and incoherent.

Forensic client: a person who has been charged with a crime while mentally ill and is remanded in custody in an approved mental health service, within a prison, remand centre or forensic psychiatric hospital.

Form of thought: the amount and rate of production of thought, continuity of ideas and language. Disturbances in form of thought include: *circumstantiality*, *clanging*, *derailment* (loosening of associations), *distractible speech*, *echolalia*, *flight of ideas*, *illogicality*, *incoherence*, *irrelevance*, *neologisms*, *perseveration*, *tangentiality*, *thought blocking*, *thought disorder* and *word approximations*.

Fugue: a dissociative state in which the person is unable to remember the past and may also be confused about their identity, or unable to remember their name or occupation.

Generalised anxiety disorder (GAD): excessive worry concerning events or activities occurring more days than not for a period of at least six months, and which the individual finds it difficult to control.

Geriatric Depression Scale (GDS): assessment tool designed to assist in making a diagnosis of *depression* in older persons and referral for treatment and to provide a baseline assessment with which to measure the outcome of treatment.

Gillick competence: the ability of young people to consent to medical treatment or seek medical consultation, as seen in their cognitive ability to make an informed judgement to give consent for treatment.

Glasgow Coma Scale (GCS): a standardised system for assessing the degree of impairment of consciousness and for predicting the duration and outcome of coma, primarily in clients with head injury.

Grandiosity: an inflated appraisal of one's worth, power, knowledge, importance or identity.

Grief: a natural process that can be experienced after loss; may be an emotional response of distress, pain and disorganisation.

Group cohesion: an important component in creating a climate of support and involvement in a group of people. Group cohesion is important in group therapy and in inpatient care settings.

Group therapy: engagement of two or more people in therapy at the same time. Interactions with others in a group situation, especially between people who experience similar difficulties.

Hallucination: a sensory perception that seems real but occurs without external stimulation. Types of hallucination include auditory, gustatory, olfactory, somatic, tactile and visual (see also *illusion*).

Harm reduction: the guiding principle used to identify a range of strategies that target the consequences of drug use rather than the drug itself.

Hazardous substance use: a repetitive pattern of use that poses a risk of harmful physical, psychological or social consequences.

Health of the Nation Outcome Scales (HoNOS): instrument used to gather information concerning key areas of mental health and social functioning for service monitoring and outcome measurement.

Histrionic: displaying theatrical, dramatic and exaggerated behaviour.

Holism: healing of the whole person by recognising the importance of the interrelationships between biological, psychological, social and spiritual aspects of a person.

Human rights: rights that are believed to belong to every individual. Human rights are protected by various domestic and international laws and conventions.

Hyperarousal: a state of heightened psychological alertness and physiological arousal associated with anxiety and with *post-traumatic stress disorder*.

Hypersomnia: excessive sleepiness; prolonged nocturnal sleep, difficulty in staying awake during the day and/or undesired daytime sleep episodes.

Hypertensive crisis: excessive and dangerous elevation in blood pressure.

Hypervigilance: a state of heightened awareness in which the person constantly scans the environment for evidence of threats.

Hypomania: a form of elevated mood less severe than mania.

ICD-11: *International Statistical Classification of Diseases and Related Health Problems*, 11th revision, published by the World Health Organization; provides a comprehensive listing of clinical diagnoses, each with its own numerical code.

Ideas of reference: belief that an insignificant or incidental object or event has special significance or meaning for that individual.

Identity: distinguishing characteristics of an individual, for example *culture*, gender, age, ability.

Illicit drugs: drugs that are classified as illegal.

Illusion: a misperception or misinterpretation of a real external stimulus, such as seeing a shadow on the wall as a person, or hearing rustling leaves as people speaking.

Impulsivity: a tendency to act in an unpremeditated fashion, suddenly and without reflection.

Incidence: the number of new cases of a condition, symptom, death or injury that develop during a specific time period, such as a year.

Incoherence: a disturbance in form of thought in which there is verbal rambling with no clear main idea.

Incongruent affect: a mismatch between a person's thoughts and their emotional expression.

Individual psychotherapy: one-on-one psychotherapy designed to effect change in the person's character; provides the client with opportunities to examine the historical experiences that have shaped who they are and influenced their life decisions.

Informed consent: consent to treatment that is (among other requirements) voluntary and specific and comes from a competent person.

Insane: a term usually used in a legal context to refer to severe mental disorder which is argued to justify a finding of not guilty.

Insight: the consumer's ability to understand the reason for and the meaning of their behaviour, feelings and life events.

Intellectual disability: a *disability* typified by major limitations in intellectual functioning and in conceptual, social and practical adaptive skills that originates before the age of 18.

Intergenerational mental illness: patterns of mental illness that occur across generations in a family.

Interpersonal therapy (IPT): therapy that targets relationships as a key factor in the contribution and maintenance of psychological or emotional disorders.

Internalising problems: the person's concerns are internalised, turned inwards or kept to themselves.

Intoxication: a reversible state that occurs when a person's intake of a drug exceeds their tolerance and produces behavioural and/or physical changes.

Involuntary admission and treatment: compulsory detention in a mental health facility for treatment that will alleviate the individual's symptoms of mental illness.

Justice (ethical principle): the equal or fair treatment of all individuals.

La belle indifference: 'beautiful indifference', where the client shows a marked indifference to or unconcern about their symptoms, even if the symptom is blindness or paralysis.

Labile: having rapidly shifting or unstable emotions.

Learned helplessness: both a behavioural state and a personality trait of a person who believes that their control over a situation has been lost. It can also relate to hopelessness and powerlessness—an inability to escape an intolerable situation, leading to the ultimate mode of adaptation: subjugation and acceptance.

Least restrictive alternative: the option of least restriction for the individual (e.g. in a community-based environment rather than hospital).

Limit setting: explaining to clients what behaviours are acceptable and what are unacceptable, and informing them of the consequences of breaking the rules; aims to offer the client a degree of control over their behaviour by setting firm, fair and consistent limits or rules.

Mad: Colloquial term for *mental illness* meaning to have lost reason and judgement.

Magical thinking: the erroneous belief that one's thoughts, words or actions will cause or prevent a specific outcome in some way that defies the laws of cause and effect.

Major depressive disorder: a condition involving seriously depressed mood and other symptoms defined by the DSM-5 that affect all aspects of a person's bodily system and interfere significantly with daily living activities.

Malingering: the intentional production of symptoms in order to avoid some specific duty or responsibility; the incentive to become sick is clearly identifiable.

Mania: a state of euphoria that results in extreme physical and mental overactivity.

Manipulation: managing a person or situation unfairly or unscrupulously to one's own advantage.

Medication adherence: formerly called compliance, this refers to maintaining a prescribed medication regimen.

Mental disorder: a diagnosable illness that significantly interferes with an individual's cognitive, emotional or social abilities; a condition in which an individual cannot cope and function as they did previously, causing considerable personal, social and financial distress.

Mental distress: an unpleasant, mental or emotional state which can impact on enjoyment of life, and on personal and social functioning.

Mental health: a state in which an individual has a positive sense of self, personal and social support with which to respond to life's challenges, meaningful relationships with others, access to employment and recreational activities, sufficient financial resources and suitable living arrangements.

Mental health assessment instruments: standardised measures for reliable, valid and consistent assessment of mental health and change that occurs with treatment.

Mental health legislation: legislation that establishes criteria for mental health detention and treatment without consent, and protects the rights of individuals.

Mental health policy: local, national and international policies governing the provision of mental health services and promoting mental health.

Mental health problem: diminished cognitive, emotional or social abilities but not to the extent that the criteria for a diagnosable *mental disorder* are met.

Mental health promotion: a population-health approach to mental health that attends to the mental health status and needs of the whole population, emphasising a continuum of care from universal prevention to long-term individual care with early intervention and treatment.

Mental illness: a condition of impairment resulting in significant changes in mental, emotional, psychological or social functioning. See also mental disorder.

Mental Status Assessment/Examination (MSA/MSE): an assessment of the person's current neurological and psychological status using several dimensions, such as perception, affect, thought content, form of thought and speech.

Mental wellbeing: state in which an individual realises their own abilities, can cope with normal stresses of life, can work productively and is able to make a contribution to their community.

Mentoring: process aimed at promoting growth and development in nurses by means of partnerships with other nurses in the workplace, involving problem solving, feedback, support and relationship building.

Metabolic syndrome: a group of risk factors that together predict cardiovascular disease and type 2 diabetes. Risk factors include hypertension, elevated triglycerides, elevated high-density lipoproteins and increased waist circumference. Metabolic syndrome is common in people with mental illness, and especially in those taking second-generation antipsychotic agents.

Milieu therapy: therapy that involves the environment in the treatment process, the participation of consumers and staff in decision making, the use of a multidisciplinary team, open communication and individualised goal-setting.

Mindfulness: deliberate awareness of the present; openly interested and receptive.

Mini-Mental State Examination (MMSE): a standardised assessment of mental state; based on observable behaviour in a client assessment interview; results in a score between 0 and 30.

Mood: a subjective emotion that colours the person's perception of the world (in contrast to *affect,* which is objective and observable, the visible expression of emotions).

Mood-stabilising medication: a medication primarily used for treating bipolar disorder. Treatment aims to stabilise a person's mood between depression and mania/hypomania.

Motivational interviewing (MI): a form of interviewing aimed at maximising a consumer's ability to change a problem behaviour; proceeds from the assumption that change is produced collaboratively and cannot be imposed from outside.

Mourning: an emotional response to the loss of a loved person or a valued part of someone's life. See also *grief.*

Multidisciplinary team (MDT): a team of clinicians from multiple disciplines, such as nurses, psychologists, psychiatrists, social workers and occupational therapists, working together to provide a holistic team approach to care.

Narcissistic: excessive love of self.

Nature versus nurture debate: discussion about the effects of biological phenomena and inheritance (nature) and the individual's environment and experiences in the world (nurture) and whether both are vital, inseparable, interdependent components of personality development that influence human behaviour.

Negative symptoms of schizophrenia: signs and symptoms such as blunting of *affect, avolition* and *anhedonia.*

Negligence: failure to take all reasonable action to provide an appropriate standard of care and to prevent harm.

Neologism: disturbance in form of thought, in which a person creates new words or expressions that have no recognised meaning.

Nutritional rehabilitation: nutritional recovery, the goals of which include achieving a healthy body weight and metabolic stability, reversal of any medical complications, improved eating behaviours and psychological functioning.

Neuroleptic malignant syndrome: a rare disorder caused by *antipsychotic medication* and characterised by fever, muscular rigidity, altered mental status and autonomic dysfunction; risk of death is high if it is not treated.

Neuropsychiatric disorders: disorders, such as Huntington's disease, in which the origin of the psychological disturbance lies in the neurological structure and function of the brain.

Neurosis: a historical term that was used in reference to madness caused by nervous system disease. Since Freud's time, 'neurosis' has been used to refer to non-psychotic disorder characterised mainly by anxiety.

Neurotransmitter: chemical messenger necessary for communication between neurons. Neurotransmitters involved in psychological functions include acetylcholine, noradrenaline, dopamine, serotonin (5HT) and gamma-aminobutyric acid (GABA).

Non-government organisations (NGOs): services that operate outside mainstream government authority and at a community level to support consumers and carers with a range of special needs, e.g. Association of Relatives and Friends of the Mentally Ill (ARAFMI).

Non-maleficence: an ethical principle that means above all to do no harm and implies both a duty of care to avoid actual harm and considering the risks of any potential harm.

Non-suicidal self-injury (NSSI): intentional, self-effected, bodily harm, commonly of low lethality and of a socially unacceptable nature, performed to reduce and/or communicate psychological distress.

Normalisation: a humanistic model of care in which people with an intellectual disability are given the same rights and opportunities as any other person and the support of appropriate services.

Novel psychoactive substance: an emerging class of substances of abuse, either in pure form or preparation (not controlled by 1961 *Single Convention on Narcotic Drugs* or the 1971 *Convention on Psychotropic Substances*), that may post a public health threat.

Nurse–client relationship: the nurse and the person work together towards the person's growth and independent problem solving. The relationship exists for the benefit of the client and at every interaction the nurse uses self therapeutically. This is achieved by maintaining the nurse's self-awareness to prevent unrecognised needs from influencing their perception of and behaviour towards the client.

Nurse practitioner: an advanced practitioner with a high degree of autonomy, who has extended education within a defined scope of practice and is licensed to practise within an extended role and to prescribe medication.

Observation: a continuous watchful presence in a non-threatening, non-intrusive manner to maintain safety and set reasonable limits on behaviour.

Obsessions: recurrent, persistent thoughts, impulses and images that are intrusive and inappropriate and cause marked anxiety or distress.

Obsessive-compulsive disorder: recurrent obsessions or compulsions that are severe enough to be time-consuming or cause marked distress or significant impairment.

Obstructive sleep apnoea: the most common form of sleep disordered breathing. Untreated, it is associated with high morbidity and mortality due to increased risks of cardio- and cerebrovascular disease, worsening of diabetes and hypertension.

Other Specified Feeding or Eating Disorder (OSFED): the person presents with many but not all of the symptoms of another eating disorder and as such, does not meet the full criteria for diagnosis; e.g. someone who meets all of the criteria for *anorexia nervosa* but who is not underweight.

Panic attack: a discrete period of intense fear or discomfort in the absence of real danger.

Panic disorder: the presence of recurrent, unexpected panic attacks followed by concern about having another panic attack or significant behavioural change related to the attacks.

Paranoia: unfounded suspicion and distrust of others and their actions.

Parkinsonism: one of the group of side effects of *antipsychotic medication*, with the person exhibiting a, mask-like facial expression, muscular rigidity, shuffling gait and drooling.

Passivity: a state of inactivity and submissiveness/ acceptance; can involve being influenced by the will of another.

Peer support: the provision of support to people with mental health challenges by people who have also experienced challenges with their mental health.

Perinatal depression: depression occurring in the antenatal (before birth) and postpartum (after birth) periods, characterised by depressed mood, excessive *anxiety*, insomnia and change in weight.

Perseveration: a disturbance in form of thought, in which the individual persistently repeats the same word or ideas; often associated with organic brain disease.

Personal agency: a *recovery* principle; discovering a more active sense of self.

Personality: characteristic patterns of expression of our feelings, thoughts and behaviour that begin in childhood and develop over time.

Personality disorder: a diagnosis made when manifestations of *personality* in an individual start to interfere negatively with the individual's life or with the lives of those close to them. Personality disorders include paranoid, schizoid, schizotypal, antisocial, borderline, histrionic, narcissistic, avoidant, dependent and obsessive-compulsive.

Personality traits: aspects of our *personality* that make us unique and differentiate us from each other.

Person-centred planning: a process of shared responsibility whereby a person is provided with the opportunity to take full control of setting lifestyle goals and negotiating with others how those goals will be achieved.

Pet therapy: use of pets and or companion animal robots to reduce agitation and improve quality of life.

Pharmacodynamics: the processes by which drugs and their metabolites influence biological functioning.

Pharmacokinetics: the study of the actions of drugs within the body, including the mechanisms of absorption, distribution, metabolism and excretion.

Phobia: an irrational fear of something, so that the person feels compelled to avoid it.

Polypharmacy: concurrent use of multiple *psychotropic medications*. Although polypharmacy might be useful in some instances, it is generally not advisable as it increases the chance of side effects and interactions. Polypharmacy can be extremely problematic in older people.

Positive symptoms of schizophrenia: signs and symptoms such as *delusions* and *hallucinations*.

Postpartum depression: a condition characterised by depressed mood, excessive *anxiety*, insomnia and change in weight occurring in the six months following giving birth.

Postpartum psychosis: a rare psychotic disorder in women who have recently given birth, characterised by *depression*, delusions and thoughts of harming herself or her infant.

Posttraumatic stress disorder (PTSD): a condition where the person experiences severe psychological distress as a result of a traumatic past experience or set of experiences.

Preceptoring: a relationship usually based in the clinical environment, occurring between a nurse who is new to an area and a preceptor (a more experienced nurse) who is allocated to support the nurse.

Pressure of speech: speech that is increased in amount, accelerated and difficult or impossible to interrupt.

Prevalence: the proportion of a population affected by a disease or who have a specific characteristic at a particular time.

Primary gain: results in relief from psychological pain, *anxiety* and conflict. For example, having physical symptoms gives legitimacy to feeling unwell.

Primary care: healthcare provided in community clinics as the first level of intervention by health professionals.

Primary mental healthcare: screening and assessment for mental illness and addiction. Includes early intervention, effective treatment and liaison with specialist mental health services.

prn (pro re nata) medication: medication that is given on an as-needed basis rather than at set times.

Prodrome/prodromal: an early or premonitory sign or symptom of a disorder.

Professional boundaries: limitations that need to be agreed upon in *therapeutic relationships* between the client and the nurse. These boundaries define acceptable and expected behaviour for both the nurse and the client that ensures a 'safe' environment based on ethical practice.

Progressive muscle relaxation (PMR): involves the progressive relaxation of the major muscles of the body while making a conscious effort to distinguish muscle tension from muscle relaxation.

Protective factors: a number of aspects that protect a person against mental health problems or *mental illness*; includes, for example, positive relationships, support from peers, and a sense of humour.

Psychotropic medication: medication that affects mental and emotional functioning.

Psychoactive drug: a drug that affects thinking, perception, emotion and/or behaviour. Includes stimulants, depressants and hallucinogens.

Psychoanalytic theory: developed by Freud, this theory places strong emphasis on the role of the unconscious in determining human behaviour. *Mental illness* is seen as a state of being fixated at a developmental stage or conflict that has not been resolved.

Psychodynamic theory: rooted in the belief that we develop a sense of self during childhood and that difficulties of living can be resolved by examining childhood development of the psyche that shaped the person's subsequent decisions.

Psychoeducation: information and education concerning a client's *mental illness* and treatment, aimed at promoting wellness and providing an opportunity for the person to gain *insight* into their condition.

Psychological first aid (PFA): designed to identify unobtrusively and quickly who is in need of immediate intervention. Rather than focusing on pathology, the emphasis is on reducing acute distress by encouraging adaptive coping.

Psychomotor retardation: marked slowing in mental and physical activity, often associated with *depression*.

Psychopathology: a term that refers to either the study of *mental illness* or mental distress or the manifestation of behaviours and experiences that may be indicative of mental illness or psychological impairment. It is also a synonym for mental illness.

Psychopharmacology: the use of medications to treat *mental disorders*. Psychopharmacology includes medication indications, interactions, side effects and precautions, consumer experience and education, and the issues of adherence and as-needed or prn administration.

Psychosis/psychotic disorder: a condition in which a person has impaired cognition, emotional, social and communicative responses and interpretation of reality.

Psychosocial rehabilitation: working with people who are mentally ill to assist them to regain personal and social skills, and reintegrate into the community.

Psychotherapy: a form of therapy that is concerned with the nature of the human experience; it has a number of interpersonal models with individual philosophy and set techniques, such as *cognitive behavioural therapy*, *motivational interviewing* and planned short-term *psychotherapy*.

Psychotropic/psychoactive medications: a collection of pharmacological agents in current psychiatric use: anti-anxiety sedatives, *antidepressants*, mood-stabilising, and antipsychotic drugs.

QT prolongation: a change in the part of the heart's electrical cycle known as the QT interval. This change is caused by many psychotropic medications.

Racism: an ideology of inferiority that labels some ethnic/racial groups as inferior to others. Characterised by avoidable and unfair actions that further disadvantage the disadvantaged and advantage the advantaged, expressed through beliefs, actions and prejudice.

Reality testing/confrontation: reflecting an individual's behaviour back to them; a form of giving information and sharing feelings in an acceptable way.

Recidivism: the repetition (relapse) of criminal behaviour.

Recovery: the process of healing and overcoming experiences of mental ill health and its associated challenges. This often includes people restoring a sense of relational connection with others, developing hope and a personally satisfying life in a community of choice, with or without the presence of mental health issues.

Refeeding syndrome: potentially fatal hormonal and metabolic changes that occur during refeeding a person who is malnourished.

Reflection: a process of critically reviewing experiences and using them to inform and change future practice in a positive way.

Reflective practice: processes that allow nurses to examine both their practice (actions) and the accompanying cognitions (thoughts) and affective meanings (feelings) in relation to their values, biases and knowledge, in the context of a particular situation.

Regulation: system whereby authorities set and monitor standards in the interests of the public and the professions, and maintain registers of individuals licensed to practise nursing.

Relapse prevention: programs that aim to teach consumers a set of cognitive and behavioural strategies to enhance their capacity to cope with high-risk situations that could otherwise precipitate relapse.

Relational recovery: an approach to recovery that considers family as important relationships in peoples' lives. Family relationships are understood to affect all aspects of a person's recovery from mental illness.

Resilience: a process of positive adaptation to significant stress or adversity that involves the interaction of personal characteristics (such as self-efficacy and optimism) and external resources (such as social support and financial resources).

Resocialisation: re-establishing social support networks and peer support through group therapy and individual goal setting.

Respite care: planned or emergency temporary care provided to carers that affords the carer an opportunity to attend to their personal everyday activities.

Risk assessment/management: assessment of a consumer with regard to various factors: risk of harm to self, risk of harm to others, risk of suicide, risk of absconding and vulnerability to exploitation or abuse. Identifying and estimating risk so that structured decisions can be made as to how best to manage a risk behaviour.

Rumination: repetitive and increasingly intrusive negative thoughts and ideas, which can eventually interfere with other thought processes.

Schizophrenia: a disorder characterised by major disturbances in thought, perception, thinking and psychosocial functioning; a severe mental illness.

Scope of practice: the range of roles, functions, responsibilities and activities that a registered nurse or enrolled nurse is educated, competent and has authority to perform.

Seclusion: a form of restraint in which a consumer is confined within a room from which they cannot freely exit. Initiated when other methods, such as talking, distraction, and medication have failed.

Secondary gain: the attention and support provided by others for a physical illness; can involve any benefit other than relief from anxiety.

Self-awareness: the process of becoming aware of and examining one's own personal beliefs, attitudes and motivations and recognising how these may affect others.

Self-disclosure: making knowledge about oneself known to others.

Self-efficacy: the person's expectation that they can cope with and master life events effectively, and that their efforts will achieve satisfactory outcomes.

Self-harm: harmful behaviour occurring along a continuum, from pulling one's own hair out to cutting, piercing and burning oneself, through to *suicide*. These behaviours may be a mode of emotional self-regulation for the client and can be comforting and confirming in a world that is out of control from their perspective.

Self-help: listening to one's own self-wisdom; can also involve seeking assistance and support from others who have had similar experiences to learn coping skills, tap into resources and find useful information.

Service user: an alternative term to 'patient', 'client' or 'consumer'.

Sexual abuse: unwanted sexual activity with the perpetrator using force, making threats or taking advantage of victims not able to give consent.

Sexual health: all aspects of sexual functioning and related healthcare, including relationships, screening for sexually transmitted diseases, sexual side effects of medications, and reproductive health.

Sexuality: involves people's gendered sex, their sexual feelings for others, their feelings about themselves as sexual beings, their sexual orientation and their sexual behaviour.

Sleep hygiene: the development of personal practices that assist in gaining adequate good-quality sleep.

Social determinants of health: the social and economic conditions in which people are born, grow, live, work and age.

Social ecological approach: refers to the dynamic interactions between a person and their environment or ecology that influence their health and wellbeing. This interaction involves a number of internal and external factors and processes.

Social inclusion: involves the provision of rights and opportunities to all individuals and groups in society, such as employment, adequate housing, healthcare, education and training.

Social skills training: helping people to learn the skills they need in order to engage with other people and the communities in which they live. Social skills training groups combine instruction, modelling, rehearsal and role-playing as well as coaching, feedback and reinforcement.

Sociological theories: theories that examine the influence of societal factors on the behaviour of individuals.

Socratic questioning: a common technique for encouraging self-understanding and motivation, which helps the client to come to an alternative belief of their own.

Solution-focused brief therapy (SFBT): encourages solutions rather than dwelling on problems; based on the strengths approach, SFBT works with the person's strengths and capacities and assumes that they are capable of knowing what is best for them and of achieving self-defined goals.

Somatisation: a psychological process whereby anxiety or psychological conflict is translated into physical complaints, although no mechanism has been found.

Spirituality: a person's sense of connection with a greater reality which may include a concept of God, sources of strength and hope, religious practices and meaning and purpose in the client's life.

Splitting: an attempt to divide a group by appealing to individual members, by sharing 'secrets' and suggesting that one person is the 'only one' who understands them or is approachable.

Stage theories: theories based on measuring and monitoring a person's individual development against a set of expected 'norms' as certain age milestones are achieved.

Standards of practice: professional standards that describe the expected performance of nurses providing mental healthcare; represent the commitment to accountability of mental health nurses. Mental health nursing standards of practice include a rationale and attributes for each standard.

Stepped care: mental healthcare that is staged to provide an appropriate level of intervention for the seriousness of an individual's mental illness or symptoms. Stepped care begins in *primary care* with stages from advice and guided self-help through to psychological intervention, medication and hospitalisation.

Stigma: devaluation of individuals by others on the basis of characteristic/s they possess, such as mental health issues.

Strengths: a person's knowledge, skills, talents, resources, and uniqueness; what a person can do and do well.

Strengths-based approach: proposes that all people have goals, talents and confidence, and that all environments contain resources, people and opportunities. Focusing on strengths and personal values promotes a person's resilience, aspirations, talents and uniqueness, what the person can do and how strengths can be mobilised to overcome current difficulties.

Stress: a psychological response to any demand or stressor; can be experienced as negative (distress) or positive. Individuals can respond differently to the same stressor.

Stress-diathesis model: a model used to understand how mental illness occurs; individuals are exposed to stressful events in the course of their lives and these events may precipitate symptoms in some people who have a predisposition to *mental illness*.

Stress management: managing the effects of the stress one is experiencing by changing the situation, increasing one's ability to deal with the situation, changing one's perception of the situation and/or changing one's behaviour.

Substance abuse: the use of drugs or alcohol in a way that disrupts prevailing social norms; these norms vary with culture, gender and generations.

Suicide: the intentional ending of one's life. In Australia, suicide is the leading cause of death due to injury. More people die each day by suicide than by motor vehicle accidents or murder.

Support worker: a non-professional mental health worker who works with people with *mental illness* to enable them to function well and achieve personal life goals.

Supportive environments: see *enabling environments*.

Tangentiality: a disturbance in form of thought in which the individual gives irrelevant or oblique replies to questions; the reply might refer to the topic but not be a complete answer.

Tardive dyskinesia: stereotypical involuntary movement of the tongue, lips and feet; results from prolonged use of first-generation antipsychotics antipsychotics.

Telephone counselling: method of crisis counselling that usually involves a single session and affords anonymity to the caller at a time when the person may be feeling vulnerable. The counsellor helps the person to cope with the crisis by working through feelings and problem solving.

Therapeutic alliance/relationship: the development of the trusting, beneficial and understanding partnership that needs to exist between the nurse and the client for a therapeutic relationship to develop.

Therapeutic community: an environment in which the emphasis is on normal functioning rather than on an illness or a disability. Decision making is shared and relationships between staff and residents are intended to be non-hierarchical.

Thought blocking: a disturbance in form of thought in which there are abrupt gaps in the individual's flow of thoughts; not caused by *anxiety*, poor concentration or being distracted.

Thought broadcasting: the belief that one's thoughts are being directed from one's head to the external world.

Thought disorder: disorganisation in either the form (structure, sequence, coherence) or content of thoughts.

Tic: an involuntary, sudden, rapid, recurrent, non-rhythmic, stereotyped motor movement or vocalisation.

Tolerance: with medication or substance use, needing more and more of the substance to get the effect you want. Results from the repeated effects of daily doses of drugs such as alcohol, methamphetamines, nicotine or opioids.

Toxicity: non-therapeutic, harmful effects of medication usually associated with high serum levels, sensitivity to the effects of the medication or impaired ability to metabolise or excrete the medication.

Transference: when a person transfers beliefs, feelings, thoughts or behaviours that occurred in a past situation to a situation happening in the present. The person with unconscious feelings or beliefs about someone in their past transfers these feelings or beliefs onto another, unfamiliar person. See also *countertransference*.

Trauma: a severe physical injury or a specific experience that triggers mental and emotional distress and results in suffering and disruption to the person's physical and/or emotional wellbeing.

Trauma informed care: core features of trauma-informed care are safety, trustworthiness, choice, collaboration and empowerment.

Treaty of Waitangi: a treaty first signed in New Zealand on 6 February 1840 by representatives of the British Crown and Māori chiefs. The purpose of the treaty was to enable the British settlers and Māori to live together under a common set of laws or agreements.

Tremor: involuntary and rhythmic muscle contractions and relaxation leading to twitching or shaking of one or more parts of the body.

Triage: a process for decision making that occurs when alternatives for acute care are being considered. A comprehensive assessment is undertaken, including the person's symptoms and current situation.

Victim: a person who has endured a form of physical and/or psychological or emotional harm at another's hand; for example, a person who has suffered sexual assault, domestic violence and/or rape.

Violence: physical or psychological attack where the intent is to cause harm to an individual or object.

Voluntary admission: admission of individuals, with their full *consent*, who require treatment in a mental health setting because of the severity or acuity of their *mental illness*.

Vulnerable: capable of being physically or emotionally harmed, wounded or hurt.

Withdrawal: the development of a substance-specific syndrome due to the cessation of (or reduction in) substance use that has been heavy and prolonged. Most individuals going through withdrawal have a craving to readminister the substance to reduce the symptoms.

z-track technique: a type of intramuscular injection technique used to prevent tracking (leakage) of medication into the subcutaneous tissue.

Index

b = box, f = figure, t = table

A

abnormal eating behaviour, 260
Abnormal Involuntary Movements Scale (AIMS), 374–375, 376b
ABS *see* Australian Bureau of Statistics
absolute neutrophil count (ANC), 378
abstraction, 337
acceptance and commitment therapy (ACT), 172, 319
'accidental crises,' 41t
ACE-R *see* Addenbrooke's Cognitive Examination-Revised
acetylcholinesterase inhibitor, 379
ACT *see* acceptance and commitment therapy
actuarial risk assessment methods, 64
acute agitation, medication for, 384, 386f
acute care services, 397
acute care settings, 455
acute dystonic reaction, as side effects of typical antipsychotics, 375t
acute intoxication, on alcohol/drugs, 202
acute stress disorder (ASD), 163t, 169
AD *see* adjustment disorder
Addenbrooke's Cognitive Examination-Revised (ACE-R), 116t
addiction, pharmacological aspects of, 196–197, 198t
adjustment disorder (AD), 163t, 169
adolescence
  childhood and
    behavioural issues, 300–301
    case study, 296–298, 301, 302–303
    critical thinking challenge, 291, 298, 299, 303, 306
    depression of, 302–303
    developmental issues on, 291
    eating disorder in, 251
    engaging with, 295–305
    exercise for class engagement, 308
    family work and, 305–306
    HEEADDSSS assessment for, 305b
    historical anecdote, 291, 292
    interventions in, 303–304
    psychosis and behaviour issues of, 299–300
    psychotropic medication use in, 386
    risk taking in, 304, 304b, 305b
    self-harm in, 303
    suicide in, 302–303
    vulnerability in, 295
  disorders of, 288–308
    assessment of, 292–293
    diagnosis of, 289
    nursing role in, 294–295
  engaging with, 299
  services for, 293–294, 294f
advance directive, 145b, 151–152
advanced practice, in expertise development, 100
affect, 183
  in mental state assessment, 124
age, of older adulthood, 426
ageing
  demography of, 312–313
  older age care and, 430
ageism, 312, 426, 431
aggression, safety in care during, 57–58
agitation, managing of, in emergency care, 411
agoraphobia, 163t, 165
agranulocytosis, 239
Ahpra *see* Australian Health Practitioner Regulation Authority
AIHW *see* Australian Institute of Health and Welfare
AIMS *see* Abnormal Involuntary Movements Scale
akathisia, 367t, 375t
alcohol, 182, 204t, 210t–211t
  consumption, 194
  withdrawal, 203–205, 205f, 206t
Alcohol, Smoking and Substance Involvement Screening Test (ASSIST), 214
Alcohol Use Disorder Inventory Test, 116t, 117
Alcohol Use Disorders Identification Test (AUDIT), 214, 215b
alkalosis, 414
allostasis, 76
alogia, 230
alternative, least restrictive, definition of, 145b
aminoindanes, 199t
amphetamines, 210t–211t
  withdrawal, 206–207
AN *see* anorexia nervosa
ANC *see* absolute neutrophil count
anhedonia, 230
anorexia nervosa (AN), 247–248, 260
  nurse's story, 263
anosognosia, 367t
antianxiety medications, 368–369
anticholinergic medications, 239–240
anticonvulsants, 368t, 373–374, 440
  for mood disorder, 186
antidepressant medications, 319, 369–372
antidepressants, 186
antiparkinsonian medications, 378, 379t
antipsychotic medications, 186, 239, 367t, 374–376, 375t, 376b
  atypical, 376–378, 378b
  in diabetes, 349
antisocial personality disorder, 276t–277t
anxiety
  ASD and, 338
  medications for, 368–369
  nature of, 414
anxiety disorder, 156–174, 159f, 161b, 162–167, 312
  aetiology of, 157–158, 157f, 158f
  agoraphobia, 163t, 165
  assessment of, 161–162, 161b
  awareness of, 161b
  case study, 166
  in children, 290t
  comorbidity in, 160
  consumer's story, 164, 170
  critical thinking challenge, 160, 167
  definition of, 157

anxiety disorder *(continued)*
diagnosis of, 161–162, 161b
epidemiology of, 159–160
generalised, 162–164, 163t
in Māori and Pacific peoples, 160
nursing interventions for, 169–173
obsessive-compulsive disorder, 163t, 164
in older adults, 316–317
panic disorder, 163t, 165, 165f
psychopharmacology of, 173
social, 163t, 166
specific phobia, 163t, 166–167
trauma- and stressor-related disorders of, 167–169
acute stress disorder, 163t, 169
adjustment disorder, 163t, 169
post-traumatic stress disorder, 163t, 167–169
treatment for, 169–173
acceptance and commitment therapy, 172
cognitive behaviour therapy, 171, 172t
cultural support, 173
digital mental health resources, 172–173
psychoeducation, 169–170
psychological formulations, 170
psychological interventions, 170–171
social support, 170
transdiagnostic approaches, 172
trauma-informed care, 170
appearance, in mental state assessment, 124
appetite, reduced, in depression, 181
APPs *see* Australian Privacy Principles
aripiprazole monohydrate, 385t
ASD *see* acute stress disorder
asociality, 230
assessment, 110–113
ageism in, 313
of body image, 257–258
class engagement exercise, 128–129
comprehensive process of, 118–122
critical thinking challenge, 110, 112, 116, 120, 121, 125
of eating disorder, 257–259
in mental health, 145b
for older age care, 428, 431
of stress, fear and anxiety, 161–162
ASSIST *see* Alcohol, Smoking and Substance Involvement Screening Test
ataxia, 367t
attention deficit/hyperactivity disorder, 379
atypical antipsychotics, 367t, 376–378, 378b
AUDIT *see* Alcohol Use Disorders Identification Test
auditory hallucinations, 229
Australasian triage scale, 126
Australian Bureau of Statistics (ABS), 7, 73, 400
Australian Health Practitioner Regulation Authority (Ahpra), 141
Australian Institute of Health and Welfare (AIHW), 294, 400
Australian National Survey of Mental Health, 7–8
Australian Privacy Principles (APPs), 142
autism, 331–343
autism spectrum disorder
in children, 290t
consumer's story, 339, 340–341
contributing factors in, 336
deinstitutionalisation in, 343
diagnostic criteria of, 334b
inclusion and exclusion in, 337
interventions of, 342–343
key points related to assessment of, 341–342
nurse's story, 335
physical health and, 340
prevalence of, 336
signs and symptoms of, 337–338
types of, 332–333
autonomy, 135
definition of, 134b
avoidance behaviours, 158, 167
avoidant personality disorder, 276t–277t
avolition, 230

B

'baby blues,' 178
'bath salts,' 197
BATOMI mnemonic, 123
BDI *see* Beck Depression Inventory
Beck Depression Inventory (BDI), 116t
bed-based services, 397
behaviour, in mental state assessment, 124
behavioural addictions, 193–195
ancient remedies for, 195
in Australia, 194
gambling disorders, 193–194, 193b
in New Zealand, 194–195
prevalence of, 194
behavioural flexibility, impaired, 337
beneficence, 135
definition of, 134b
benzhexol, 379t
benzodiazepines, 173, 204t, 368–369, 368t, 369b, 369t
withdrawal, 205, 207t
benztropine mesylate, 379t
bereavement, 39
binge eating disorders, 249
biopsychosocial assessment, 419f, 458
biopsychosocial domains, 417f
biperiden, 379t
bipolar disorder, 348–349, 357
in children, 290t
depressive phase in, 181
diagnoses relating to, 179
distinctive feature of, 181
DSM-5 diagnosis of, 181
main symptoms of a manic episode in, 181
manic phase of, 180
in pregnant women, 178
bisexual groups, women from, 435b
Bleuler, Eugen, 228
BMI *see* body mass index
body image, 257–258
body mass index (BMI), 257b, 377
borderline personality disorder (BPD), 134b, 276t–277t
BPD *see* borderline personality disorder
breastfeeding, medication during, 438
management of, 439
Bridger, Aldolphus, 195
brief intermittent psychosis, 231
Buddha *see* synthetic cannabinoids
buddying, in point-of-care learning, 95
bulimia nervosa, 247–248
buprenorphine taper, 206, 207t
burnout syndrome, 90–91

C

Cade, John, 186
CAM *see* Confusion Assessment Method
CAMHS *see* child and adolescent mental health services
cannabinoid withdrawal, 208
cannabinoids, synthetic, 197–200, 199t
cannabis, 195, 204t, 210t–211t
capacity, definition of, 145b
cardiac risks, related to psychotropic medications, 381
cardiometabolic health, 351, 352f

cardiovascular disease (CVD), 350–351, 352f
cardiovascular effects, of eating disorder, 255t, 256f
care/caring
  compassion and, 31–32
  emergency, 409–415
    approaches to mental health presentations in, 410
    attitudes in, 412, 414
    case scenario, 411, 413
    knowledge in, 411, 413–414
    protective factors in, 410–411, 413
    red flags in, 410, 413
    skills in, 412, 414
    treatment modalities and considerations in, 412–413, 414
care services
  acute, 397
  primary, 395–397
'carers,' 72
Cartwright, Samuel, 228
catatonic behaviour, 229–230
catecholamines, 414
CBT *see* cognitive behaviour therapy
central nervous system (CNS), 367
Centrelink or the Department of Housing, 187
CFT *see* compassion-focused therapy
child, behaviour checklist of, 290b
child and adolescent mental health services (CAMHS), 293
child and youth mental health services (CYMHS), 293
childhood
  and adolescence
    behavioural issues, 300–301
    case study, 296–298, 301, 302–303
    critical thinking challenge, 291, 298, 299, 303, 306
    depression of, 302–303
    developmental issues on, 291
    eating disorder in, 251
    engaging with, 295–305
    exercise for class engagement, 308
    family work and, 305–306
    HEEADDSSS assessment for, 305b
    historical anecdote, 291, 292
    interventions in, 303–304
    psychosis and behaviour issues of, 299–300
    psychotropic medication use in, 386
    risk taking in, 304, 304b, 305b
    self-harm in, 303
    suicide in, 302–303
    vulnerability in, 295
  behaviour checklist of, 290b
  engaging with, 296
  identifying vulnerability in, 295
  nurse's story, 307
childhood disorder, 288–308
  assessment of, 292–293, 293b
  critical thinking challenge, 291, 298, 299, 303, 306
  diagnosis of, 289
  historical anecdote, 291
  incidence of, 289–290
  mental illness in, 292
  overview of, 290t
children of parents with mental illness (COPMI), 74–75, 295
CHIME *see* connectedness, hope, identity, meaning and empowerment
Chisholm, Brock, 9
chronic obstructive pulmonary disorder (COPD), 355
chronic stress, 44, 157–158
civil commitment, 145b
Clark's cognitive model, 165
classification of personality disorder
  criteria for, 276t–277t
  suggestions for, 277t
clinical facilitation, 95
clinical formulation, 125, 126t
clinical management processes, 98
clinical supervision, 95–96, 96–97
  historical anecdote, 97
clinical support, in bed-based services, 397
clinical teaching, 95
clozapine, 136, 377, 378
CNS *see* central nervous system
coaching, definition of, 96
cocaine, 207
Code of Conduct for Nurses in Australia, 142
Code of Ethics for Nurses in Australia, 142
Codes of ethics, 133
coercion
  definition of, 145b
  working with, 147
cognition, in mental state assessment, 124
cognitive assessment tools
  for older adults, 316
  for older age, 316
cognitive behaviour therapy (CBT)
  in anxiety, trauma and stress, 171
  components of, 172t
  for eating disorders, 265–266
  in interactive therapy, 282
  in older adulthood, 317
  for substance use/misuse, 215
cognitive development, malnutrition and, 255t
cognitive effects, of eating disorder, 255t
cognitive enhancers, 379
cognitive remediation, 460
cognitive skills, forensic mental health nursing and, 447
cognitive therapy (CT), 319
cogwheeling rigidity, 367t
collaborative care planning, in primary and community care, 405
collaborative prescribing, in psychotropic medication use, 383
colleague-related stressors, 89
committal, 145b
committed, definition of, 145b
Commonwealth government, in primary care services, 395–397
communication, 431
  in cultural considerations, 12
community care, 399–406
  attitudes in, 402, 405
  case scenario, 401, 403–404
  knowledge in, 402, 404–405
  mental health skills in, 402–403, 405
  nursing actions and interventions in, 405
  presentations to, 400–401
  protective factors in, 401–402, 404
  red flags in, 401, 404
  treatment modalities and considerations in, 403, 405–406
community health, 397
community mental health settings, 456
community treatment orders (CTOs), 136, 145b, 149–150
compassion, caring and, 31–32
compassion fatigue, 89–90
compassion-focused therapy (CFT), 319
complex crises, 41t
comprehensive assessment process, 118–122
compulsory treatment, 145b, 146
conduct disorders, in children, 290t
confidentiality, 141, 306–307
Confusion Assessment Method (CAM), 116t, 320
connectedness, hope, identity, meaning and empowerment (CHIME), 77, 78b
consultation-liaison psychiatry, 419b, 421b, 423b

consumer-focused models, 53
Convention on the Rights of Persons with Disabilities, 133, 143, 145b, 150
co-occurring mental health disorders, 191–221
  case study of, 220
  consumer's story, 201–202
  critical thinking challenge, 220
  nurse's story, 208, 209, 220
co-occurring substance use disorders, 217–220
  clinical significance of, 218
  managing clients with, 218–219, 219b
coping strategies
  focus on strengths, 46–47
  mental illness, 43–44
  neurobiology and neuroplasticity, 44
  promote self-determination, 47
  protective and risk factors of, 43t
  work in partnership, 45–46
  working with people who experience mental health distress, 44–45
COPMI *see* children of parents with mental illness
Cornell Scale for Depression in Dementia (CSDD), 319
couples therapy, 438
criminal justice system, 445
crisis, mental health, 40–42
  common types of, 41t
crisis intervention, in personality disorder, 281
CSDD *see* Cornell Scale for Depression in Dementia
CT *see* cognitive therapy
CTOs *see* community treatment orders
cultural considerations, of mental health, 12
cultural determinants, of mental disorders, 21t
cultural diversity
  in assessment, 121
  in mental health problems, 12
cultural factors, safety in care and safety at work and, 52–53
cultural identity, 22
cultural safety, mental health care and, 12–13
cultural support, for anxiety, 173
CVD *see* cardiovascular disease
CYMHS *see* child and youth mental health services

D

dangerousness, definition of, 145b
DAO *see* duly authorised officer
DASA *see* Dynamic Appraisal of Situational Aggression
DBT *see* dialectical behaviour therapy
decision-making capacity, in legal issues, 151–152
deep acting, in emotional labour, 89
de-escalation techniques
  in safety care, 57–58, 59t–61t
  themes, principles and attributes of, 58
deinstitutionalisation, in ASD and intellectual disability, 343
delirium, 317t, 319–320
delta-9-tetrahydrocannabinol (THC), 197
delusional beliefs, 180
delusional disorder, 231
delusions, 229
dementia, 317t, 320–321
  clinical features of, 321
  nursing management for, 321
  prevalence of, 320
dental and oral effects, malnutrition and, 255t
deontology, 134
dependence, 192
dependent personality disorder, 276t–277t
depressants, 198t
depression, 178
  diagnoses relating to, 178
  in older age
    presentation of, 318
    screening and assessment for, 318–319, 319b
    treatment for, 319
  symptoms of, 180
depression insomnia, 181
'depression of the mind,' 178
depressive disorder, in children, 290t
detachment, burnout and, 90
detoxification, for substance use/misuse, 215–216
developmental crises, 41t
developmental history, in mental health assessment, 120
deviance, 40
diabetes, 348–349
diagnosis
  of childhood disorders, 289
  of stress, fear and anxiety, 161–162
Diagnostic and Statistical Manual of Mental Disorders, 5th edition (DSM-5), mood disorders, 178
Diagnostic and Statistical Manual of Mental Disorders (DSM), 125, 136
diagnostic criteria
  of autism spectrum disorder, 334b
  of intellectual disability, 335b
dialectical behaviour therapy (DBT), 282–283
diaries, 117
diazepam, 203–205
diet, in holistic self-care, 92
differential diagnosis, definition of, 128
digital/web-based interventions, for mood disorder, 187
direct causal relationship theory, 218
direct observation, 117
discontinuation syndrome, 136, 380–381, 381b
disorganised behaviour, 229–230
disorganised thinking, 229
dissociachotic phenomena, 232
dissociachotic theory, for psychosis and schizophrenia-related phenomena, 232
distress, 40
  managing of, in emergency care, 411
  mental
    epidemiology of, 6–10
    prevalence of, 6
  mental health, working with people who experience, 44–45
documentation, in mental state assessment, 123b
dopamine, 196
drapetomania, 228
Drug Use Disorders Identification Test (DUDIT), 214
DSM *see Diagnostic and Statistical Manual of Mental Disorders*
DSM-5 *see Diagnostic and Statistical Manual of Mental Disorders*, 5th edition
DUDIT *see* Drug Use Disorders Identification Test
duly authorised officer (DAO), 147, 148
Durie, Mason, 173
duty of care, 145b, 151–152
Dynamic Appraisal of Situational Aggression (DASA), 449b
dynamic risk factors, 449
dysfunction, 40
dyslexia, 166
dystonia, 367t

E

eating disorders, 246–269
  anorexia nervosa, 247–248
  assessment of, 257
  biological factors in, 251–252
  body image in, 257–258
  bulimia nervosa, 247–248, 248–249
  cardiovascular effects in, 255t
  in children and adolescence, 251

eating disorders *(continued)*
class engagement exercise, 269
cognitive changes in, 256t
consumer's story, 248–250, 261
contributing factors for, 251–254
critical thinking challenge, 251, 254
examples of, 259b
family relationships in, 253
gender and, 250–251
historical anecdote, 251
hospitalisation in, 260–261
incidence and prevalence of, 249–250
interventions for, 261–268
mental health in, 254–257
monitoring intake for, 264–265
nursing care in, 261
pharmacotherapy for, 268
physical health, 254
prevention and protection, 254
psychological factors in, 252
psychotherapeutic techniques in, 265
risk and protective factors, 251
self-help programs for, 267–268
signs and symptoms of, 254–257
sociocultural and environmental influences in, 252, 252b
specialist supportive clinical management for, 267
therapeutic relationships in, 262–263
treatment and recovery in, 259
ECG *see* electrocardiogram
echolalia, 229
ecological perspective, of mental health, 20
ECT *see* electroconvulsive therapy
EEG *see* electroencephalogram
electrocardiogram (ECG), 122
electroconvulsive therapy (ECT), 136–137
in ethical framework, 136–137
for mood disorder, 186
in older adulthood, 319
electroencephalogram (EEG), mental health assessment and, 122
electrolyte abnormality, malnutrition and, 255t
elimination disorders, in children, 290t
EMDR *see* eye movement desensitisation reprocessing
emergency care, 409–415
approaches to mental health presentations in, 410
attitudes in, 412, 414
case scenario, 411, 413
knowledge in, 411, 413–414
protective factors in, 410–411, 413
red flags in, 410, 413
skills in, 412, 414
treatment modalities and considerations in, 412–413, 414
emergency departments, 397
emotional distress, 39
emotional labour, 89
emotional support, in primary and community care, 403
empathy, 459
in nursing, 30, 88
in safe care, 57
employment, 118
endocrine disorder, 255t
engagement
in emergency care, 412
mood disorders and, 185
environment, stress and, 39
environmental factors, safety in care and safety at work and, 52
ethical dilemma, mental health nursing, 88
ethical framework, 133–141, 134b
class engagement exercise, 152–153
confidentiality in, 141
critical thinking challenge, 134, 140
electroconvulsive therapy in, 136–137
of interpersonal therapy, 140
involuntary treatment in, 139–140
in mental health practice, 135–141
principles of, 135
professional boundaries in, 140–141
of professional practice, 133–134
psychiatric treatment in, 136
psychopharmacology in, 136
seclusion and restraint in, 138–139
suicidal behaviour in, 139
exclusion, in ASD and intellectual disability, 337
exercise, in holistic self-care, 92
exhaustion, burnout and, 90
expertise development, 99–100
extrapyramidal side effects, 367t, 374–375
eye movement desensitisation reprocessing (EMDR), 169, 170

F

Fagerstrom nicotine dependence scale, 208, 208t
family assessment, 82b, 259
'family carers,' 72
family mental health, 71–84
assessment of, 120
challenges with, 73–75
childhood mental health, 74–75
class engagement exercise, 79
consumer's story, 78–79
defining, 72
eating disorder in, 259
family-focused practice, 79–83, 81t
gears, 76f
genogram of, 84f
range of, 80–82
recovery in, 77f, 78t
relational recovery, 77–79
resilience in, 76–77, 76b
stigma and, 75, 75b
strengths-based approach, 72–73
therapy, 82–83
young person, 75
family mental illness, case study, 83
'family of choice,' 72
'family of origin,' 72
'family of procreation,' 72
family-based treatment, for eating disorder, 266
family-focused practice, 79
FASD *see* fetal alcohol spectrum disorder
fear, aetiology of, 157–158, 157f, 158f
feeding and eating disorders, in children, 290t
fetal alcohol spectrum disorder (FASD), 196, 197t
fidelity
definition of, 134b
principle of, 140
fiduciary relationship, 140
fight/flight/freeze response, 157
FITT *see* frequency, intensity, time and type
flupenthixol decanoate, 385t
forced treatment, 145b
forensic consumers, legal status of, 446
forensic history, in mental health assessment, 121
forensic mental health
consumers, groups of, 446b
nursing, 444–452
actions and interventions, 448, 450–451
addressing stigma and, 451
attitudes for, 448
case scenarios, 445, 450
cognitive and social skills, 447
demographic characteristics, 447
discrimination and, 451
knowledge for, 446, 450
mental illness and risk to others, 447
pre-release planning and, 450–451
red flags on, 446, 450
relationship building and, 450–451

forensic mental health *(continued)*
risk assessment for, 448–449, 449b
social disadvantage and, 451
social skills and, 447
substance abuse, 447–448
treatment modalities for, 451
forensic mental health settings, 456
formalised risk assessments, in emergency care, 410
frequency, intensity, time and type (FITT), principle of, 355
Freud, Sigmund, 207
and psychoanalysis, 120

G

GABA *see* gamma-aminobutyric acid
GAD *see* generalised anxiety disorder
GAD-7, 162
gambling disorders, 193–194, 193b
gamma-aminobutyric acid (GABA), 368–369
gastrointestinal effects, malnutrition and, 255t
gay groups, women from, 435b
(GDS), 318, 319b
GDS *see* geriatric depression scale
gender identity, 22–23
general health, 121–122
General Health Questionnaire (GHQ-12), 116t
general practitioner (GP), 293
general screening questions, 161, 161b
generalised anxiety disorder (GAD), 162–164, 163t
generalist inpatient settings, 416–423
attitudes in, 422
case scenarios, 420, 421
ill-health experiences, 417, 417f, 418b
knowledge on, 420, 422
mental state, 417
alteration in, 418
assessing for deterioration in, 418–419, 419f, 423b
nursing actions and interventions in, 420–421, 422–423
protective factors in, 420, 421
red flags on, 420, 421
skills for, 420, 422
genetic difference, in ASD, 336
genetic factors, in eating disorder, 251–252
genogram, of family mental health, 84f
Geriatric Depression Scale, 428
Geriatric Depression Scale short form, 116t
GHB, 204t
GHQ-12 *see* General Health Questionnaire
Glasgow Coma Scale, 213, 213t
goals of care, for mental health care settings, 458, 461
GP *see* general practitioner
grandiose delusions, 229
grief, 40, 430
Guardianship and Administration Act 1986, 143
guardianship legislation, 142–143
gustatory hallucinations, 229

H

half-life, 367t
hallucinations, 229
hallucinogens, 198t, 210t–211t
haloperidol decanoate, 385t
harm minimisation, 217
harm reduction, 217
HCR-20 *see* Historical Clinical Risk Management Scale
HDL *see* high-density lipoprotein
HEADSS *see* Home, Education and Employment, Activities, Drugs, Sexuality, Suicide/Depression
healing, therapeutic use of self and, 29
health, mental, 38–42
crisis, 40–42, 41t
distress, working with people who experience, 44–45
nursing practice, 48
problems, 40
spectrum of, 37–48, 38f
stress, 39
Health and Disability Commissioner Act 1996, 142
health care
and holistic self-care, 94
mental, 10–12
cultural safety and, 12–13
'stepped care' model of, 10, 11b
money making and, 346
health history
mood disorders and, 182
in older age, 315–316
health networks, primary, in primary care services, 395–397
Health Practitioner Regulation National Law Act, 141
Health Practitioners Competence Assurance Act 2003, 141
Healthy Active Lives, 348, 349b
Herodotus, 184
high-density lipoprotein (HDL), 347–348, 349b
high-functioning autism, 333
Historical Clinical Risk Management Scale (HCR-20), 116t
histrionic personality disorder, 276t–277t
holistic approach, to mental health nursing, 28–29
holistic perspective, of mental health, 20
holistic self-care, 91–94
diet in, 92
exercise in, 92
general health care and, 94
mind-body practices in, 93, 93b
psychological strategies in, 92–93
resilience in, 93–94
rest in, 92
sleep in, 92
work-life balance in, 92
Home, Education and Employment, Activities, Drugs, Sexuality, Suicide/Depression (HEADSS), 115, 294
hope, 31
HPA *see* hypothalamic–pituitary–adrenal axis
human mind, 227
human rights, 66
in mental health legislation, 150
hygiene, sleep, 358b
hypothalamic–pituitary–adrenal axis (HPA), anxiety and, 157, 157f

I

iatrogenesis, 240
iatrogenic, definition of, 367t
IES-R *see* Impact of event scale-revised
ill-health experiences, 417, 417f, 418b
illicit substance use, 195
illness, mental, 42–47
coping, 43–44
epidemiology of, 6–10
prevalence of, 6–7
spectrum of, 37–48, 38f
Impact of Event Scale-Revised (IES-R), 162
inclusion, in ASD and intellectual disability, 337
indigenous Australians, substance use in, 195
indigenous people
of Australia and New Zealand, 12
stress, fear and anxiety of, 173
indigenous women, 435b
indirect causal relationship theory, 218
individualised care, 431
infant mental health, 434–442
assessing risk to baby, 437
attitudes for, 438, 441

infant mental health *(continued)*
barriers to screening of, 436
care planning for delivery and postnatal care, 441
case scenarios, 435–436, 439, 440–441
family approach for, 438
interprofessional collaboration and, 438
knowledge for, 436, 439, 440
nursing actions and interventions for, 441–442
protective factors for, 437
psychoeducation and, 438
red flags on, 436, 439
reflection on, 436
risk assessment for, 437
safety of, 437, 438
skills for, 438
support for, 438
therapeutic relationship on, 438
treatment modalities for, 437–438, 442
influence, manipulation *versus*, 63
information identification, in mental health assessment, 118
informed consent, 145b
psychotropic medications and, 383
inpatient mental health units, 397–398
inpatient order, 145b
inpatient settings, generalist, 416–423
attitudes in, 422
case scenarios, 420, 421
ill-health experiences, 417, 417f, 418b
knowledge on, 420, 422
mental state, 417
alteration in, 418
assessing for deterioration in, 418–419, 419f, 423b
nursing actions and interventions in, 420–421, 422–423
protective factors in, 420, 421
red flags on, 420, 421
skills for, 420, 422
insight, in mental state assessment, 125
insulin, 348–349
integument effects, malnutrition and, 255t
intellectual developmental disorder
consumer's story, 339, 340–341
contributing factors in, 336–337
deinstitutionalisation in, 343
diagnostic criteria of, 335b
inclusion and exclusion in, 337
interventions of, 342–343
key points related to assessment of, 341–342
nurse's story, 335
physical health and, 340
prevalence of, 336
signs and symptoms of, 339
types of, 333
intellectual disability
consumer's story, 339, 340–341
contributing factors in, 336–337
deinstitutionalisation in, 343
diagnostic criteria of, 335b
inclusion and exclusion in, 337
interventions of, 342–343
key points related to assessment of, 341–342
nurse's story, 335
physical health and, 340
prevalence of, 336
signs and symptoms of, 339
types of, 333
interactive therapy, 282–283
intergenerational mental illness, 79
International Classification of Diseases and Health Related Problems, 128
International Hearing Voices Network, for psychosis and schizophrenia-related phenomena, 233
International Organization of Physical Therapists in Mental Health (IOPTMH), 355
internet-based self-help treatments, 172
interpersonal relationships, 253
historical anecdote, 253
for mood disorders, 185
interpersonal therapy (IPT), 140, 266
intersex groups, women from, 435b
interventions, 62–63
in childhood and adolescence, 303–304
interviewing
in assessment, 112–113
concluding, 115
historical anecdote, 113
problems management of, 114–115
process management of, 114
safety in, 114
settings for, 113–114
summarisation of, 115
therapeutic communication and, 113, 113t
intimacy, older age care and, 431
intoxication, 192, 202, 202b, 203b
intramuscular injectable antipsychotics, 384, 385t
intravenous drug use, signs of, 213b
involuntary treatment, 139–140, 145b
IOPTMH *see* International Organization of Physical Therapists in Mental Health
IPT *see* interpersonal therapy

J

'Jekyll and Hyde' manifestation, in schizophrenia, 228
job–person fit, 98
judgement, in mental state assessment, 125
judicial review, 145b
justice, definition of, 134b, 135

K

K2 *see* synthetic cannabinoids
Kabat-Zinn, Jon, 93b
Keeping the Body in Mind (KBIM), program of, 356
ketamine, 204t
Kraepelin, Emil, 127–128
Kroc *see* synthetic cannabinoids

L

laboratory tests, 122
lactation, substance use in, 196, 197t
law issues, common, 66
legal context, 65–67
common law issues, 66
legislative frameworks, 66–67
reasonable force, 67
'legal highs,' 197
legal issues, 132–153
decision-making capacity in, 151–152
duty of care, 151–152
ethics and, 133–141, 134b
frameworks of, 133–134
in mental health practice, 135–141
principles of, 135
law and, 141–151
decision making in, 150–151
guardianship legislation in, 142–143
mental health legislation in, 143–150, 144t, 145b
privacy legislation in, 142
professional regulation in, 141–142
in mental disorders of childhood and adolescence, 307
professional practice for, 133–141
legislative frameworks, 66–67
lesbian groups, women from, 435b
life stressors, women experiencing, 435b
lifestyle, in primary and community care, 406

limit setting, in personality disorder, 281–282
lithium, 368t, 372–373, 373b
lithium carbonate, for mood disorder, 186
lithium toxicity, 461
Liverpool University Neuroleptic Side Effect Rating Scale (LUNSERS), 116t, 376b
longevity, 426
loss, 40, 430
LUNSERS *see* Liverpool University Neuroleptic Side Effect Rating Scale

M

Madrona, Lewis Mehl, 228
magnetic resonance imaging (MRI), mental health assessment and, 122
management processes, 98
managerial supervision, 98
manipulation, influence *versus*, 63
MANTRA, for eating disorder, 266
MAOIs *see* monoamine oxidase inhibitors
Māori and Pacific peoples, anxiety disorders in, 160
Maudsley family-based therapy (MFBT), 266
MBCT *see* mindfulness-based cognitive therapy
meaning making, as psychological strategy, 92
medical setting, general, 397
medication
  adherence to, 380–384, 380b
  on mental health care settings, 460, 462
  in primary and community care, 403
  sex and, 358
melancholia, 178
memory, in mental state assessment, 124
mental disorders, social and cultural determinants of, 21t
mental distress
  epidemiology of, 6–10
  prevalence of, 6
mental health, 5–16, 38–42
  assessment of, 257
  Australian national survey of, 7–8
  case study, 13
  class engagement exercise, 48
  consumer's story, 15, 41–42
  crisis, 40–42, 41t
  critical thinking challenge, 9, 12, 47
  cultural considerations of, 12
  cultural safety and, 12–13
  distress, working with people who experience, 44–45
  of eating disorder, 254–257
  epidemiology of mental distress and illness, 6–10
  forensic, nursing, 444–452
    actions and interventions, 448, 450–451
    addressing stigma and, 451
    attitudes for, 448
    case scenarios, 445, 450
    cognitive and social skills, 447
    demographic characteristics, 447
    discrimination and, 451
    knowledge for, 446, 450
    mental illness and risk to others, 447
    pre-release planning and, 450–451
    red flags on, 446, 450
    relationship building and, 450–451
    risk assessment for, 448–449, 449b
    social disadvantage and, 451
    social skills and, 447
    substance abuse, 447–448
    treatment modalities for, 451
  mental health care, 10–12
  nursing and, 14–15
  nursing practice, 48
  overview of, 6
  physical and, 9
  problems, 40
  scope of nursing practice and, 14
  self-harm and suicide, 10
  in setting, 393–398
    case scenario, 394
    integrating across service spectrum, 396, 396t
    nurses' roles and, 395–398
    red flags in, 394–395
    reflection points in, 394b
  spectrum of, 37–48, 38f
  stress, 39
  Te Rau Hinengaro: New Zealand mental health survey, 8–9
Mental Health Act, 142, 144t
mental health assessment, 109–129
  classification of, in psychiatry, 127–128
  clinical formulation for, 125, 126t
  comprehensive process of, 118–122
    cultural issues in, 121
    developmental history in, 120
    family history in, 120
    forensic history in, 121
    general health history in, 121–122
    historical anecdote, 122
    information identification in, 118
    laboratory investigations in, 122
    mental health history in, 119
    physical health assessment in, 122
    problem presentation in, 118–119
    social history in, 120
    spirituality in, 121
    substance use history in, 119–120
    trauma in, 120–121
  consumer's story, 127
  descriptive approach to, 112
  diagnosis on, 125
  mental state and, 123–125
    affect and mood in, 124
    behaviour and appearance in, 124
    cognition in, 124
    documentation in, 123b
    insight in, 125
    judgement in, 125
    memory in, 124
    orientation in, 124
    sensorium in, 124
    thought and speech in, 124
  methods of, 112–118
    diaries, 117
    direct observation, 117
    interviews, 112–113
    mnemonics, 115
    standardised tools, 115–117, 116t
    therapeutic communication, 113, 113t
    third-party information, 117–118
  narrative approach to, 112
  in primary and community care, 402
  professional standards and, 112
  of risk, 126–127
  of strengths, 127
  threads of, 111b, 111f
  triage in, 126, 126b
mental health care, 10–12
  cultural safety and, 12–13
  'stepped care' model of, 10, 11b
mental health care settings, 454–463
  assessment on, 461
  assisting and involving family on, 459
  attitudes in, 458, 462
  avoiding conflict and restrictive interventions on, 457–458
  avoiding conflict on, 457–458
  biopsychosocial assessment on, 458
  case scenarios, 457, 460–461
  cognitive remediation on, 460
  empathy on, 459
  goals of care for, 458, 461
  knowledge on, 457–458, 461
  least restrictive treatment and, 459–460
  lithium and, 461
  medication on, 460, 462

mental health care settings *(continued)*
nursing actions and interventions in, 458–459, 461
nursing observation on, 458, 459
observation in practice, 459
orientation and transition on, 458–459
peer support on, 462
primary care and, 456
private practice and, 456
protective factors in, 457, 461
red flags on, 457, 461
support to carers on, 462
therapeutic relationship on, 459
treatment modalities in, 459–460, 462
mental health disorders, in older age, 316
mental health history, 119
mental health legislation, 13–14, 143–150, 144t, 145b
assessment under, 146
in Australia, 148–149
civil commitment in, 144–146
coercion and compulsion in, 147
community treatment orders in, 149–150
compulsory treatment and, 146
concepts of, 145b
critical thinking challenge, 149, 150
duty of care in, 151–152
guidelines of, 144t
human rights and, 150
in New Zealand, 147–148
procedural justice in, 147
protective mechanisms in, 147
rationale for, 143–144
mental health nurse practitioners, 456–457
mental health nurses, 32
for mood disorder, 187
mental health nursing
assessment in, 110–111
childbirth in, 295
class engagement exercise, 102
consumer's story, 88
in context, 19–34
case study, 24
class engagement exercise, 33
compassion and caring, 31–32
consumer's story, 33–34
critical thinking challenge, 34
cultural, sexual and spiritual identities, 22–23
effective mental health nursing practice, 28–33
empathy and therapeutic use of self, 30
environment and identities, 22–23
hope and spirituality, 31
professional boundaries, 32–33
recovery-oriented care, 23–26
self-awareness, 30–31
self-disclosure, 33
social determinants of health, 20–21
social ecological approach to, 20–27
therapeutic alliance, 30
therapeutic relationship-consumer and nurse partnership, 29
therapeutic use of self, 29
trauma-informed care, 26–28
working within recovery-oriented and trauma-informed approaches of care, 23–26
critical thinking challenge, 102
ethical dilemma, 88
hope and spirituality, 121
interpersonal aspects of, 185
nurse's story, 90–91, 97, 101
perinatal, 295
professional boundaries in, 87
professional supportive relationships, 98
reflection in, 87–88
self-awareness in, 87
stress in, 88–91
therapeutic alliance in, 87–88
mental health nursing practice, effective, 28–33
mental health promotion, 428
mental health review tribunal, 145b
mental illness, 23, 42–47
ASD and, 338
class engagement exercise, 48
coping, 43–44
critical thinking challenge, 47
disorders and, 52
epidemiology of, 6–10
intellectual disability and, 339
nurse's story, 11, 46–47
prevalence of, 6–7
psychiatric symptoms in, 359
spectrum of, 37–48, 38f
women experiencing, 435b
working with families in, 73–75
mental state, 417
alteration in, 418
assessing for deterioration in, 418–419, 419f, 423b
mental state assessment, 123–125
affect and mood in, 124
behaviour and appearance in, 124
cognition in, 124
documentation in, 123b
insight in, 125
judgement in, 125
memory in, 124
orientation in, 124
sensorium in, 124
thought and speech in, 124
Mental State Examination (MSE), 438
for substance use/misuse, 214
mentoring, definition of, 96
metabolic health, screening for, 348, 349b
metabolic syndrome, 347–348, 348t, 349b, 377
primary and community care in, 404
methamphetamine, 207, 370
MFBT *see* Maudsley family-based therapy
migrant women, 435b
mind–body practices, in holistic self-care, 93, 93b
mindful handwashing, 93, 93b
mindfulness-based cognitive therapy (MBCT), 319
Mini-Mental State Examination (MMSE), 116t, 315
MMSE *see* Mini-Mental State Examination
mnemonics of assessment, 115
money making, health care and, 346
monoamine oxidase inhibitors (MAOIs), 371, 371b
mood, 183
in mental state assessment, 124
mood disorders, 177–189
assessment areas of, 181–182
cultural views, 184
health history, 182
physical health, 181, 182
psychological (cognitive and affective) state, 183
risk assessment, 184–185
social networks, 183
spiritual beliefs, 183
substance abuse, 182
consumer's story, 187–188
experience of, 180
factors contributing to, 180
interventions of, 185–187
digital/web-based, 187
interpersonal, 185
pharmacological, 186
nurse's story, 185–186
prevalence of, 179–180
role of nursing in, 187
signs and symptoms of, 180–181
types of, 178–179
mood-stabilising medications, 372–374, 440

Mosher, Loren, 179
motivational intervention, 266–267
motivational interviewing, for substance use/misuse, 214–215, 216b
MRI *see* magnetic resonance imaging
MSE *see* Mental State Examination
musculoskeletal effects, malnutrition and, 255t

N

narcissistic personality disorder, 276t–277t
narrative approach, to mental health assessment, 112
NCNZ *see* Nursing Council of New Zealand
negative symptoms, 230
neglect, physical health, 346–347, 347f
 class engagement exercise, 359
 critical thinking challenge, 350, 351, 354, 356, 357, 358
 nutrition in, 354
 oral health in, 356–357
 physical activity in, 354–355
 respiratory disease in, 355
 sexual health in, 357–359
 sleep in, 357, 358b
neologisms, 229
neurobiology, 44
neurodevelopmental disorders, in children, 290t
neurodiversity movement, 336
neuroleptic malignant syndrome (NMS), 374–375, 375t, 376b
neurological effects, of eating disorder, 255t
neuroplasticity, 44
neurotransmitters, 368–369
neurotypical thinkers, 338
New Entry to Specialty Practice (NESP) program, 111
New Zealand mental health survey, 8–9
NGOs *see* non-government organisations
nicotine/tobacco, 204t, 210t–211t
 withdrawal, 208, 208t, 209t
night eating syndrome, 249
NMBA *see* Nursing and Midwifery Board of Australia
NMS *see* neuroleptic malignant syndrome
non-benzodiazepine antianxiety medications, 369
non-government organisations (NGOs), 11
non-maleficence, definition of, 134b
non-malfeasance, 135
noradrenaline serotonin reuptake inhibitors (NSRIs), 368t, 372
novel psychoactive substances, 197, 199t
NSRIs *see* noradrenaline serotonin reuptake inhibitors
nurse–consumer relationship, 51
nurse roles
 in childhood and adolescent mental health, 294–295
 mental health in setting and, 395–398
 in physical health neglect, 357, 358
 in primary and community care, 400
 team approaches of, 284
nursing
 Australia and New Zealand, 14
 mental health, in context, 19–34
  case study, 24
  compassion and caring, 31–32
  effective mental health nursing practice, 28–33
  empathy and therapeutic use of self, 30
  environment and identities, 22–23
  hope and spirituality, 31
  professional boundaries, 32–33
  self-awareness, 30–31
  self-disclosure, 33
  social determinants of health, 20–21
  social ecological approach to, 20–27
  therapeutic alliance, 30
  therapeutic relationship, consumer and nurse partnership, 29
  therapeutic use of self, 29
  trauma-informed care, 26–28
  working within recovery-oriented and trauma-informed approaches of care, 23–26
 mental health and, 14–15
 role of, in mood disorders, 187
Nursing and Midwifery Board of Australia (NMBA), 112, 141
nursing care, in inpatient setting, 265
Nursing Council of New Zealand (NCNZ), 112
nursing observation, on mental health care settings, 458, 459
nursing practice
 and intervention, in eating disorder, 261
 scope of, mental health, 14
nutrition, 258, 354, 430
nutritional rehabilitation, 263–264

O

observation, older age care and, 428, 431–432
obsessive-compulsive disorder (OCD), 163t, 164
obsessive-compulsive personality disorder, 276t–277t
OCD *see* obsessive-compulsive disorder
ODT *see* open dialogue therapy
olanzapine, side effects of, 377
olanzapine pamoate, 385t
OLDCART mnemonic, 115
older adulthood, at risk of suicide, 427
older age
 anxiety disorders in, 316–317
 assessment of, 313, 315–316
 biopsychosocial factors and life-stage transition in, 313–314, 313f
 case study, 324
 chronic disease and mental health in, 314–315
 critical thinking challenge, 314, 316, 322, 326
 delirium in, 317t, 319–320
 dementia in, 317t, 320–321
 depression, 318–319
  critical thinking challenge, 314, 316, 322
 electroconvulsive therapy in, 319
 geriatric depression scale of, 318, 319b
 health history in, 315–316
 historical anecdote, 323
 mental health disorders of, 311–326
 nurse's story, 321, 324
 nursing management of, 324–325
 polypharmacy in, 325–326
  critical thinking challenge, 326
 schizophrenia in, 322
 screening for, 313
 substance misuse in, 322
 suicide in, 323–324
older age care, 425–432
 age-related considerations for, 427
 assessment for, 428, 431
 attitudes for, 427, 430–431
 care planning for, 431
 carer responsibilities for, 426
 case scenarios, 426, 429
 knowledge for, 427, 430
 monitoring and, 431–432
 nursing actions and interventions for, 431
 observation for, 428, 431–432
 protective factors in, 427
 red flags on, 426–427, 429–430
 sexuality and relationships, 430
 skills for, 428, 431

older age care *(continued)*
therapeutic relationship and, 428, 431
treatment modalities for, 428–429, 432
useful tools for, 428
older people, psychotropic medication use of, 386–387
olfactory hallucinations, 229
open dialogue therapy (ODT), for psychosis and schizophrenia-related phenomena, 232–233
opioid withdrawal, 205–206, 207t
opioids, 204t, 210t–211t
opium, 195
oral health, 356–357
organisational stressors, 88
orientation, in mental state assessment, 124
orphenadrine, 379t
OSFED *see* other specified feeding or eating disorder
other specified feeding or eating disorder (OSFED), 249
overwhelm, older age care and, 426

P

paliperidone palmitate, 385t
panic attacks, 165
panic disorder (PD), 163t, 165, 165f
panic symptoms, nature of, 414
paracetamol, 152–153
paranoid delusions, 229
paranoid personality disorder, 276t–277t
parens patriae power, 145b
parent–infant psychotherapy, 437
parenting
in ASD, 336
substance use in, 196, 197t
training programs, 437–438
parkinsonism, as side effects of typical antipsychotics, 375t
Parkinson's syndrome, 367t
participation, 337
partner violence, intimate, women experiencing, 435b
paternalism, 140
pathological gambling, 193
Patient Health Questionnaire (PHQ), 428
PD *see* panic disorder
PD-TS *see* personality disorder trait specified
peer relationships, 253–254
peer review, 96
peer support, on mental health care settings, 462
perception of danger, anxiety and, 159, 159f
performance review, 98
perinatal mental health, 434–442
assessing risk to baby, 437, 437b
attitudes for, 438, 441
barriers to screening of, 436
care planning for delivery and postnatal care, 441
case scenarios, 435–436, 439, 440–441
family approach for, 438
interprofessional collaboration and, 438
knowledge for, 436, 439, 440
nursing, 295
nursing actions and interventions for, 441–442
in partners, 437
problems, women at increased risk of, 435b
protective factors for, 437
psychoeducation and, 438
red flags on, 436, 439
reflection on, 436
risk assessment for, 437
safety of, 437, 438
skills for, 438
support for, 438
therapeutic relationship on, 438
treatment modalities for, 437–438, 442
perinatal period, 435
perseveration, 229
person-centred approach, in emergency care, 412
person-centred care, 432
person-centred manner, 52
personality, 274
personality disorder trait specified (PD-TS), 276t–277t
personality disorders, 273–285. *see also* personality
assessment of, 280–281
class engagement exercise, 284
classification of
criteria for, 276t–277t
suggestions for, 277t
consumer's story, 283
contributing factors of, 278
crisis intervention in, 281
experience of, 278
historical anecdote, 278, 280
interactive therapies of, 282–283
limit setting in, 281–282
nurse's story, 284
nursing approaches of, 284
pharmacological interventions for, 284–285
prevalence of, 275–278
principles of working with, 285b
self-harm and, 279
self-management in, 282
signs and symptoms of, 278–279
types of, 274–275
PGSI *see* Problem Gambling Severity Index
pharmacological interventions, for personality disorder, 284–285
pharmacological principles, 366–367
pharmacotherapy, 325, 432
for eating disorder, 268
phencyclidine-type substances, 199t
phenethylamines, 199t
phenothiazines, 374
PHQ *see* Patient Health Questionnaire
physical activity, 354–355
physical assessment, 257, 257b
physical health, 122, 253, 345–359, 427
mental health and, 9
mood disorders and, 181, 182
in primary and community care, 406
assessment of, 405
monitoring of, 405
promoting, forensic mental health nursing and, 451
protective and risk factors of, 43t
stress and, 39
substance use/misuse and, 209, 210t–211t
physical health neglect, 346–347, 347f
class engagement exercise, 359
critical thinking challenge, 350, 351, 354, 356, 357, 358
nutrition in, 354
oral health in, 356–357
physical activity in, 354–355
respiratory disease in, 355
sexual health in, 357–359
sleep in, 357, 358b
physical health promotion, for psychosis and schizophrenia-related phenomena, 240
physiological dependence, 192
physiological tolerance, 192
piperazines, 199t
point-of-care learning, 95
police power, 145b
polypharmacy, 367t
for older people, 325–326
postpartum/perinatal depression, 178
post-traumatic stress disorder (PTSD), in anxiety and trauma, 163t, 167–169
Power Threat Meaning Framework, for psychosis and schizophrenia-related phenomena, 232

preceptorship, in nursing, 95
preconception planning, 439
pregnancy, 384–386
  ethical considerations during, 440
  medication during, 438, 440
    management of, 439
  psychosocial screening during, 436
  substance use in, 196, 197t
pre-judgement, 339
prejudice, 339
presence, engagement and, 185
preterm births, 440
primary care, 399–406
  attitudes in, 402, 405
  case scenario, 401, 403–404
  knowledge in, 402, 404–405
  mental health skills in, 402–403, 405
  nursing actions and interventions in, 405
  presentations to, 400–401
  protective factors in, 401–402, 404
  red flags in, 401, 404
  treatment modalities and considerations in, 403, 405–406
primary care services, 395–397
primary health networks, in primary care services, 395–397
primum non nocere, 136
Privacy Act 1988, 142
Privacy Act 1993, 142
privacy legislation, 142
pro re nata (prn), 366, 367t, 379–379
problem gambling, 193
Problem Gambling Severity Index (PGSI), 193b
problem presentation, in mental health assessment, 118–119
procedural justice, 147
professional boundaries, 32, 87, 140–141
  preparedness for, 54, 55t
professional development, 95–97
  education and training for, 97
  point-of-care learning for, 95
  structured reflective practice relationships for, 95–97
professional practice, ethical framework of, 133–134
professional self-care, 86–102
  career maintenance for, 97–101
    clinical practice settings in, 99, 99t
    education in, 100
    expertise development in, 99–100
    management in, 100
    research in, 100–101
    transitions in, 97–98
    work environments in, 98
  challenges in, 88–91
  holistic, 91–94
    diet in, 92
    exercise in, 92
    general health care and, 94
    mind–body practices in, 93, 93b
    psychological strategies in, 92–93
    resilience in, 93–94
    rest in, 92
    sleep in, 92
    work-life balance in, 92
  lifelong learning as, 94–97
    early graduate programs for, 95
    growth mindset for, 94–95
    organisations for, 97
    professional development for, 95–97
    professional supports for, 97
  therapeutic use of, 87–88
professional supportive relationships, 98
Protection of Personal and Property Rights Act 1988, 143
protective factors, 449
protective mechanism, in legislation, 147
protest psychosis, 229
protocols, in emergency care, 411
pseudo-patients, 236
psychiatric diagnosis, 135–136
psychiatric symptoms, 359
psychiatric treatment, 136
psychiatry, consultation-liaison, 419b, 421b, 423b
psychoactive drugs, pharmacology of, 196–200
psychoeducation, 169–170, 267, 438
  in emergency care, 414
  in mental disorders of childhood and adolescence, 307
'psychological dependence,' 192
psychological factors
  in eating disorder, 252
  protective and risk factors of, 43t
psychological formulations, 170
psychological interventions, 170–171
psychological (cognitive and affective) state, mood disorders and, 183
psychology, stress and, 39
psychopharmacology, 365–387
  adherence and concordance in, 380–384, 380b
  for anxiety, 173
  case study, 381, 382, 383–384
  class engagement exercise, 387
  commonly used terms, 367t
  consumer's story, 371
  critical thinking challenge, 382–383
  discontinuation syndrome in, 380–381, 381b
  in ethical framework, 136
  nurse's story, 366, 373, 376
  principles of, 366–367
  for psychosis and schizophrenia-related phenomena, 239–240
  psychotropic medications, 367–378
    antianxiety or anxiolytic, 368–369
    antidepressant, 369–372
    antiparkinsonian, 378, 379t
    antipsychotic or neuroleptic, 374–376, 375t, 376b
    atypical antipsychotics, 376–378, 378b
    classification of, 368t
    mood-stabilising, 372–374
    pro re nata antipsychotic medications administration, 379–380
    special issues with, 378–379
psychosis, 226–243, 299–300
  alternative approaches to, 231–234
    dissociachotic theory, 232
    International Hearing Voices Network, 233
    open dialogue, 232–233
    Power Threat Meaning Framework, 232
  consumer's story, 233–234
  definition of, 227
  final word regarding stigma, 243
  nurse's story, 242
  nursing interventions of, 234–242
    assessment, 235
    physical health promotion, 240
    psychopharmacology, 239–240
    recovery-oriented care planning, 241–242
    relapse prevention, 241
    social advocacy, 240–241
    therapeutic communication, 236–239, 237t, 238t
  powerful role of language and labels in, 228–229
  prevalence and social determinants of, 227–228
  protest, 229
  signs and symptoms of, 229–230
  theories of causation/aetiology of, 234
  types of, 230–231
    brief intermittent psychosis, 231
    delusional disorder, 231
    schizoaffective disorder, 231
    schizophreniform disorder, 231
    substance-induced psychotic disorder, 230

psychosocial issues, 187
psychosocial risk factors, 437b
psychosocial screening, during pregnancy, 436
psychotherapy, 432
psychotropic medications, 367–378, 384–387
  in physical health, 356, 358
PTSD *see* post-traumatic stress disorder
purging disorder, 249, 263
Purple Haze *see* synthetic cannabinoids

Q

QTc interval, malnutrition and, 255t
quetiapine, side effects of, 377

R

rapid-cycling bipolar disorder, 181
reasonable force, 67
reciprocity, definition of, 134b
recovery
  of eating disorder, 259
  family mental health in, 78t
recovery-informed practice, traditional practice *versus*, 25t
recovery model, of care, 53
recovery-oriented approaches of care, working within, 23–26
recovery-oriented care, 23–26
refeeding syndrome, 262
reflection in nursing, 87–88
refrigerator mother, 336
relationships
  protective and risk factors of, 43t
  stress and, 39
renal dysfunction, 255t
research, in professional self-care, 100–101
'research chemicals,' 197
resilience
  family mental health of, 76–77
  holistic self-care and, 93–94
respiratory disease, 355
rest, in holistic self-care, 92
restraint, 138–139
  seclusion and, 57–58, 61b
review tribunal, 145b
revolving-door syndrome, 240
rights, definition of, 134b
risk assessment, 448–449, 449b
risperidone, 385t
role challenges, at workplace, 89
Rowland Universal Dementia Assessment Scale (RUDAS), 315
RUDAS *see* Rowland Universal Dementia Assessment Scale
Rush, Benjamin, 178

S

SAD *see* social anxiety disorder
SAD PERSONS mnemonic, 115
safe care, 50–68
  during aggression, 57–58
    and de-escalation techniques, 57–58, 59t–61t
    restraint and seclusion, 58, 61b
  case study, 54
  class engagement exercise, 67–68
  critical thinking challenge, 57, 58, 63
  deliberate self-harm and suicide, 58–63
    interventions, 62–63
    traumatic experiences, 58–62
  legal context, 65–67
    common law issues, 66
    human rights, 66
    legislative frameworks, 66–67
    reasonable force, 67
  manipulation of, 63
  models of care, 53–54
  nurse's story, 62
  preparedness for creating, 54–56
    emotional management, 55–56
    nurses' self-care, 54–55
    professional boundaries, 54, 55t
  principles for engaging consumers in, 56–57
    active listening, 56–57
    assertiveness, 57
    empathy, 57
    flexible, 56
    non-verbal interactions, 56
    verbal interactions, 56
  types of behaviour challenge in, 51
  understanding context of, 51–53
    consumer factors, 52
    cultural factors, 52–53
    environmental factors, 52
    social factors, 53
    staff factors, 51–52
  understanding safety risks in, 63–95
    assessment processes, 64
    community settings, safety and situational awareness, 64–65, 65t, 66b
    positive risk taking, 64
    summary of risk in mental health settings, 65
safe work, 50–68
  case study, 54
  class engagement exercise, 67–68
  critical thinking challenge, 57, 58, 63
  deliberate self-harm and suicide, 58–63
    interventions, 62–63
    traumatic experiences, 58–62
  human rights, 66
  legal context, 65–67
    common law issues, 66
    legislative frameworks, 66–67
    reasonable force, 67
  manipulation of, 63
  models of care, 53–54
  nurse's story, 62
  preparedness for creating, 54–56
    emotional management, 55–56
    nurses' self-care, 54–55
    professional boundaries, 54, 55t
  principles for engaging consumers in, 56–57
    active listening, 56–57
    assertiveness, 57
    empathy, 57
    flexible, 56
    non-verbal interactions, 56
    verbal interactions, 56
  types of behaviour challenge in, 51
  understanding context of, 51–53
    consumer factors, 52
    cultural factors, 52–53
    environmental factors, 52
    social factors, 53
    staff factors, 51–52
  understanding risks in, 63–65
    assessment processes, 64
    community settings-safety and situational awareness, 64–65, 65t, 66b
    positive risk taking, 64
    summary of risk in mental health settings, 65
safety, in emergency care, 412
schizoaffective disorder, 179, 231
schizoid personality disorder, 276t–277t
schizophrenia, 226–243, 346, 350, 357
  alternative approaches to, 231–234
    dissociachotic theory, 232
    International Hearing Voices Network, 233
    open dialogue, 232–233
    Power Threat Meaning Framework, 232
  in children, 290t
  consumer's story, 233–234
  final word regarding stigma, 243
  nurse's story, 242
  nursing interventions of, 234–242
    assessment, 235
    physical health promotion, 240
    psychopharmacology, 239–240
    recovery-oriented care planning, 241–242
    relapse prevention, 241

schizophrenia *(continued)*
social advocacy, 240–241
therapeutic communication, 236–239, 237t, 238t
in older adulthood, 322
powerful role of language and labels in, 228–229
prevalence and social determinants of, 227–228
protest, 229
signs and symptoms of, 229–230
theories of causation/aetiology of, 234
types of, 230–231
brief intermittent psychosis, 231
delusional disorder, 231
schizoaffective disorder, 231
schizophreniform disorder, 231
substance-induced psychotic disorder, 230
schizophrenia-related phenomena
alternative approaches to, 231–234
dissociachotic theory, 232
International Hearing Voices Network, 233
open dialogue, 232–233
Power Threat Meaning Framework, 232
types of, 230–231
brief intermittent psychosis, 231
delusional disorder, 231
schizoaffective disorder, 231
schizophreniform disorder, 231
substance-induced psychotic disorder, 230
schizophreniform disorder, 231
schizotypal personality disorder, 276t–277t
schools, for mental health, 456
screening
in emergency care, 414
in mental health assessment, 121
for metabolic health, 348
of sexual health, 358–359
of stress, fear and anxiety, 161b
seclusion, 138–139
seizures, as side effects of typical antipsychotics, 375t
selective noradrenaline reuptake inhibitor (SNRI), 166, 173
selective serotonin reuptake inhibitors (SSRIs), 166, 173, 268, 317, 368t, 371–372, 378–379
in cultural support, 173
for generalized anxiety disorder, 163
self-awareness, 87
in nursing, 30–31
self-compassion, 92
self-determination, promote, 47
self-disclosure, in mental health nursing, 33
self-harm, 10
deliberate, 58–63
in personality disorder, 279
of young people, 303
self-help
internet-based treatments, 172
programs, for eating disorder, 267–268
self-management, 282
self-rated instruments, 117
'self-stigma,' 75
sense of ineffectiveness, burnout and, 90
sensorium, in mental state assessment, 124
serotonin syndrome, 367t, 378–379
service spectrum, integrating mental health across, 396, 396t
setting, mental health in, 393–398
case scenario, 394
integrating across service spectrum, 396, 396t
nurses' roles and, 395–398
red flags in, 394–395
reflection points in, 394b
severe mental illness (SMI), 346, 347
sex, medication and, 358
sexual health, 357–359
screening, 358–359
shared decision making, 459
Short-Term Assessment of Risk and Treatability (START), 449b
situational crises, 41t
skin effects, malnutrition and, 255t
sleep, 357, 358b
disturbance, 357
in holistic self-care, 92
sleep disorders, nursing assessment and intervention of, 357
Smart, Positive, Active, Realistic, X-factor thoughts (SPARX), 173
SMI *see* severe mental illness
smoking
cessation, 351–353
during pregnancy, 196
SNRI *see* selective noradrenaline reuptake inhibitor
social advocacy, for psychosis and schizophrenia-related phenomena, 240–241
social anxiety disorder (SAD), 163t, 166
social communication, impaired, 337
social crises, 41t
social deprivation, in intellectual disability, 337
social determinants, of mental disorders, 21t
social disadvantage, 451
social ecological perspective, of mental health, 20, 21f
social environment, 43t
social factors, safety in care and safety at work and, 53
social history, in mental health assessment, 120
social isolation, 430
social mediation, 337
social networks, mood disorders and, 183
social support, 170
in bed-based services, 397
in primary and community care, 403
society, 337
Socratic questioning, 164
sodium valproate, for mood disorders, 186
solution-focused brief therapy
of care, 53
in emergency care, 412
somatic hallucinations, 229
SPARX *see* Smart, Positive, Active, Realistic, X-factor thoughts
specific phobia, 163t, 166–167
spectrum disorder, autism
consumer's story, 339, 340–341
contributing factors in, 336
deinstitutionalisation in, 343
diagnostic criteria of, 334b
inclusion and exclusion in, 337
interventions of, 342–343
key points related to assessment of, 341–342
nurse's story, 335
physical health and, 340
prevalence of, 336
signs and symptoms of, 337–338
types of, 332–333
speech, in mental state assessment, 124
Spice *see* synthetic cannabinoids
spiritual beliefs, mood disorders and, 183
spiritual care, 92–93
spiritual identity, 22
spirituality, 31, 121, 183
SSRI *see* selective serotonin reuptake inhibitors
staff factors, safety in care and safety at work and, 51–52
staffing, in emergency care, 411–412
standardisation, definition of, 117

standardised assessment, 126–127
  tools, 115–117, 116t
START *see* Short-Term Assessment of Risk and Treatability
static risk factors, 449
'stay low and go slow' approach, 239
stepped care, 173
  approach, 395, 396t
'stepped care' model of mental health care, 10, 11b
stimulants, 198t, 204t
strengths, focus on, 46–47
strengths assessment, 127
strengths-based approaches, 53
  of family mental health, 72
  working with families in, 72–73
stress, 23, 88–91
  aetiology of, 157–158, 157f, 158f
  and allostasis, 76
  chronic, 44
  fear and anxiety
    acceptance and commitment therapy in, 172
    acute stress disorder in, 163t, 169
    adjustment disorder in, 169
    agoraphobia, 163t, 165
    assessment and diagnosis of, 161–162
    assessment tools of, 162
    Clark's cognitive model in, 165, 165f
    class engagement exercise, 174
    cognitive behavioural intervention in, 171, 172t
    critical thinking challenge, 169
    cultural support in, 173
    eye movement desensitisation reprocessing in, 169
    nurse's story, 161, 171
    obsessive-compulsive personality disorder (OCD), 164
    panic disorder in, 163t, 165, 165f
    post-traumatic stress disorder, 163t, 167–169
    psychoeducation in, 169–170
    psychological intervention, 170–171
    psychopharmacology in, 173
    related disorders of, 163t, 167–169
    screening of, 161b
    self-help treatment in, 172
    social anxiety disorder in, 163t, 166
    social support in, 170
    specific phobia, 166–167
    stepped care in, 173
    trauma-informed care in, 170
    treatment and nursing in, 169–173
  mental health and, 39
  workplace, 88–91
    burnout and, 90–91
    compassion fatigue and, 89–90
    emotional labour and, 89
    trauma and, 901
'stress response,' 39
stress-vulnerability-protective factors model, 234
structured professional judgement, 64
subacute residential care settings, 455–456
substance abuse, 182, 447–448
substance-induced psychotic disorder, 230
substance use/misuse, 119–120, 191–221
  among specific populations, 195–196
    Indigenous Australians, 195
    New Zealand Māori, 195–196
    pregnancy, lactation and parenting, 196, 197t
  assessment areas of, 209–213
    history, 209–212
    key elements of, 212, 213t
    observations, 212–213, 213b, 213t
    presentation and setting, 209
    taking, 212
  case study, 220
  consumer's story, 201–202
  contributing factors of, 200, 200t
  critical thinking challenge, 220
  detoxification for, 215–216
  experience of, 200–201
  interventions for, 214–215
    cognitive behaviour therapy, 215
    early and brief, 214
    motivational interviewing, 214–215, 216b
  laboratory tests for, 214
  mental status examination for, 214
  nurse's story, 208, 209, 220
  in older adulthood, 322
  other healing approaches of, 216–217
  physical health and, 209, 210t–211t
  relapse prevention for, 216
  screening tests for, 214, 215b
  signs and symptoms of, 202–209
    intoxication, 202, 202b, 203b
    withdrawal, 202–209, 203b, 204t
  test for, 214
  types of, 192
    dependence, 192
    intoxication, 192
    tolerance, 192
    withdrawal, 192
suicidal behaviour, 139, 152–153
suicidal ideation, 426
suicidal thinking, 184
suicide, 10, 58–63, 184
  of childhood and adolescence, 302–303
  in older adulthood, 323–324, 427
supported decision making, 145b
surface acting, in emotional labour, 89
symptoms, older age care and, 427
synthetic cannabinoids, 197–200, 199t
synthetic cathinone, 199t

T

T2DM *see* type 2 diabetes mellitus
talking therapy, in primary and community care, 403, 405–406
tardive dyskinesia, 239, 367t, 375t
tardive syndrome, 367t
Te Rau Hinengaro, 8–9
Te Whare Tapa Wha model, 173
technology, young people and, 305
television, 355
Ten Basic Principles of Mental Health Care Law, 395
theory of mind, 337
therapeutic alliance, of mental health nursing, 30
therapeutic communication, 113, 113t
  for psychosis and schizophrenia-related phenomena, 236–239, 237t, 238t
therapeutic intervention
  interviewing in, 112
  laboratory tests in, 122
  mnemonics of, 115
  nurse's story, 111, 118
  professional standards in, 112
  standardised tools of, 115–117
therapeutic relationships
  consumer and nurse partnership, 29
  in eating disorder, 262–263
  empathy of, 30
  on mental health care settings, 459
  older age care and, 428, 431
  in primary and community care, 402–403, 405
  therapeutic alliance of, 87–88
  use of self in, 29, 87–88
third-party information, 117–118
thought, in mental state assessment, 124
thought broadcasting, 229
thought insertion, 229
thought withdrawal, 229
3-hour rule, 264
tidal model, of care, 53

tobacco consumption, 194–195
tobacco-related illness, 351–353
traditional practice, recovery-informed practice *versus*, 25t
tranquillisers, 136
transdiagnostic approaches, for anxiety, 172
transgender, 138–139
  groups, women from, 435b
Transtheoretical Model of Change, 214–215, 216b
trauma, 120–121
  in children, 290t
  disorders relating to, 167–169
    acute stress disorder, 163t, 169
    adjustment disorder, 163t, 169
    post-traumatic stress disorder, 163t, 167–169
  screening, anxiety and, 161
  workplace stress and, 901
trauma-genic neurodevelopmental model of psychosis, 234
trauma-informed care, 26–28, 53, 170
  essentials of, 27
  working within, 23–26
traumatic births, 440
traumatic experiences, 58–62
treatment
  of eating disorder, 259
  in stress, fear and anxiety, 169–173
Treaty of Waitangi, 148
triage, 126, 126b
tricyclic antidepressants, 370–371, 371b
trust
  definition of, 134b
  in primary and community care, 402–403
tryptamines, 199t
type 2 diabetes mellitus (T2DM), 348–349
typical antipsychotic medication, 367t

U

UCLA Loneliness Scale, 428
United Nations, Convention on Rights of Persons with Disabilities, 150
unstructured clinical judgement, 64
utilitarianism, 134

V

veracity, definition of, 134b
verbal de-escalation, in emergency care, 412
verbal interactions, 56
virtue ethics, 134
visual hallucinations, 229
voluntary treatment, 145b

W

walking, for mood disorder, 187
WBC *see* white blood cell
weight gain, 264
whakamaa, 12
white blood cell (WBC), 378
WHO *see* World Health Organization
Whytt, Robert, 178
withdrawal, 192, 202–209, 203b, 204t
  alcohol, 203–205, 205f, 206t
  amphetamine, 206–207
  benzodiazepine, 205, 207t
  cannabinoid, 208
  nicotine, 208, 208t, 209t
  opioid, 205–206, 207t
women
  psychotropic medication use of, 384–386
  in shared environment, 138–139
Woolf, Virginia, 179
work environments, 98
work-life balance, 92
workplace stress, 88–91
  burnout and, 90–91
  compassion fatigue and, 89–90
  emotional labour and, 89
  trauma and, 901
World Health Organization (WHO), 346, 395
  in legislation, 307
  in mental health, 6

Y

Yale-Brown Obsessive-Compulsive Scale (Y-BOCS), 162
Y-BOCS *see* Yale-Brown Obsessive-Compulsive Scale

Z

ziprasidone, side effects of, 377
zuclopenthixol decanoate, 385t